THE SOCIETY FOR HEALTHCARE EPIDEMIOLOGY OF AMERICA

A Practical Handbook for Hospital Epidemiologists

D1244318

THE SOCIETY FOR HEALTHCARE EPIDEMIOLOGY OF AMERICA

A Practical Handbook for Hospital Epidemiologists

Edited by Loreen A. Herwaldt, MD
Department of Internal Medicine
University of Iowa Hospitals and Clinics
College of Medicine
Iowa City, Iowa

Co-edited by Michael D. Decker, MD, MPH
Vanderbilt University
School of Medicine
Nashville, Tennessee

SLACK Incorporated, 6900 Grove Road, Thorofare, NJ 08086-9447

Publisher: John H. Bond
Editorial Director: Amy E. Drummond
Creative Director: Linda Baker

Cover design by Robyn Hepker, MS

A practical handbook for hospital epidemiologists/The Society for Healthcare Epidemiology of America; edited by Loreen A. Herwaldt; co-edited by Michael Decker.
    p. cm.
    Includes bibliographical references and index.
    ISBN 1-55642-302-0
    1. Nosocomial infections--Prevention. I. Herwaldt, Loreen, A. II. Decker, Michael, D. III. Society for Healthcare Epidemiology of America.
    [DNLM: 1. Cross Infection--prevention & control. 2. Epidemiologic Methods. 3. Risk Management. 4. Hospital Administration. WX 167 P895 1997]
    RA969.P73 1997
    614.4'5--dc21
    DNLM/DLC
    for Library of Congress   97-10168

Printed in the United States of America

Published by: SLACK Incorporated
                 6900 Grove Road
                 Thorofare, NJ 08086-9447 USA
                 Telephone: 609-848-1000
                 Fax: 609-853-5991
                 World Wide Web: http://www.slackinc.com

Contact SLACK Incorporated for more information about other books in this field or about the availability of our books from distributors outside the United States.

Last digit is print number: 10 9 8 7 6 5 4 3 2 1

Dedication

To my mentors who gave me the opportunities that I needed to learn and grow in my profession:

Archie A. MacKinney

Dennis G. Maki

Donald J. Krogstad

Richard P. Wenzel

Michael A. Pfaller

Contents

Support Functions

Special Topics

Contributors

Elias Abrutyn, MD

Brenda A. Barr, RN, MS, CIC

Consuelo Beck-Sague, MD

John M. Boyce, MD

Patrick J. Brennan, MD

John P. Burke, MD

Cheryl D. Carter, RN, BSN

David C. Classen, MD, MS

Donald E. Craven, MD

Michael D. Decker, MD, MPH

H. Gunner Deery II, MD

Louise M. Dembry, MD

Daniel J. Diekema, MD, MS

Bradley N. Doebbeling, MD, MS

Robert A. Duncan, MD, MPH

Michael Edmond, MD, MPH

Jonathan Freeman, MD, ScD

Richard A. Garibaldi, MD

Peter A. Gross, MD

Loreen A. Herwaldt, MD

Walter J. Hierholzer Jr., MD

William R. Jarvis, MD

Stephen B. Kritchevsky, PhD

Ludwig Lettau, MD, MPH

William J. Martone, MD

Joel Maslow, MD, PhD

R. Michael Massanari, MD, MS

John E. McGowan Jr., MD

Beverly G. Metchock, DrPH

Elyse D. Miller, MA

Maury Ellis Mulligan, MD

Mary D. Nettleman, MD, MS

Lindsay E. Nicolle, MD

Trish M. Perl, MD, MSc

Jean M. Pottinger, MA, RN, CIC

Gina Pugliese, RN, MS

David R. Reagan, MD, PhD

Marie-Claude Roy, MD, MS

William A. Rutala, PhD, MPH

Robert J. Sherertz, MD

Bryan P. Simmons, MD

Shannon D. Smith, MD

Kathleen A. Steger, RN, MPH

Sheri Swartzendruber, RN, BS

Michael L. Tapper, MD

August J. Valenti, MD

William M. Valenti, MD

Richard P. Wenzel, MD, MSc

R. Todd Wiblin, MD, MS

Kim Wilkerson, ART

Rebecca Wurtz, MD, MPH

Preface

I did not set out to edit a book on infection control and hospital epidemiology. I merely suggested to the SHEA board that we, as a society, needed a statement on ethics. Somehow that comment led to many other suggestions by the board members and I ended up editing this book.

This long arduous task has, like my mentors, given me an opportunity to learn and grow in my profession. Many people have not been blessed with mentors such as mine who were good examples and who taught and challenged me. My hope is that the Handbook will serve as a surrogate mentor to those who have not been as fortunate as I. I also hope that the Handbook will enable those who read it to learn and grow as well as to solve problems within their hospital epidemiology and infection control programs.

I am at most moments grateful to the board of SHEA who gave me this opportunity and challenge. I am truly grateful to the authors who took time out of their extraordinarily busy schedules to share their hard earned wisdom with you. To make matters worse, they had to endure the indignity of my editing. I am pleased that most of them are still speaking with me.

Lorene Bender, Lorraine Scoma, and Patsy McAtee spent countless hours typing revisions and corresponding with authors. Joan Benson and Elyse Miller helped me edit many of the chapters and Susan Cantrell and Michael Decker, my coeditor, refined the prose and style further. I am thankful to all of them for helping make this Handbook so readable. I am also grateful to Michael for his sage advice.

I want to thank the hospital epidemiology fellows at the University of Iowa who critiqued these chapters: Yasmina Berrouane, Daniel Diekema,

Patricia Meier, Edward Morales, Marie-Claude Roy, Shanon Smith, Constanze Wendt, Stefan Weber, and Todd Wiblin. Their comments helped improve this Handbook substantially. They have taught me more than I ever taught them. I am grateful that they continue to be my colleagues and my friends.

The nurse epidemiologists at the University of Iowa Hospitals and Clinics, Brenda Barr, Cheryl Carter, Jean Pottinger, and Marlene Schmid also made many contributions to this book. I am very grateful that they have allowed me to work with them and that they have taught me so much infection control.

Debra Christy and John Bond at SLACK Incorporated deserve special thanks for their flexibility and patience while working with this neophyte editor. I am thankful that they believed in this project.

Finally, I would like to thank my husband, Marc Abbott, who has loved and encouraged me throughout this long process. He helped me keep my head on straight and remember my priorities when I could not see past the next split infinitive or dangling modifier. He also kept me sane and working when it seemed like this project would never end. Just before the Handbook was completed, Marc gave me a plaque that now adorns my desk at work. I hope the Handbook will help hospital epidemiologists and infection control professionals avoid the fate described in the plaque's inscription:

Why do your disciples break the tradition of the elders?
They don't wash their hands before they eat!

Matthew 15:2

Loreen A. Herwaldt, MD

GETTING STARTED

CHAPTER 1

An Introduction to Practical Hospital Epidemiology

Loreen A. Herwaldt, MD

Hospital epidemiology and infection control have become increasingly complex fields. The complexity of these endeavors is illustrated by the size and weight of two recently published textbooks.[1,2] To help introduce newcomers to these professions, the Society for Healthcare Epidemiology of America (SHEA) has produced the *Practical Handbook for Hospital Epidemiologists.*

This new publication is aptly named. According to *Webster's Ninth New Collegiate Dictionary*[3] the word practical means:

- Actively engaged in some course of action or occupation.
- Of, relating to, or manifested in practice or action; not theoretical or ideal.
- Capable of being put to use or account (useful).
- Disposed to action as opposed to speculation or abstraction.
- Qualified by practice or practical training.
- Designed to supplement theoretical training by experience.

- Concerned with voluntary action and ethical decisions.[3]

Hospital epidemiologists and infection control professionals certainly are engaged actively in professions that require them to take actions or institute interventions that are not ideal. Persons in these professions are usually disposed to action not abstraction, and they also must make ethical decisions every day. Consequently, hospital epidemiologists and infection control professionals need practical or useful advice from persons who are qualified by practice and who have supplemented their theoretical training by experience. Or put in contemporary parlance, persons who have been there, done that.

A handbook is, as defined by *Webster's,* "capable of being conveniently carried as a ready reference," a "concise reference book covering a particular subject."[3] The SHEA Handbook certainly meets this definition. In addition, it is packed with pragmatic advice that will assist both neophyte and experienced epidemiologists and infection control professionals as they establish and operate successful hospital (or other healthcare) epidemiology programs.

I feel that this is an especially propitious time to launch this new venture because, as Faith Popcorn (futurologist and advisor to Fortune 500 corporations) stated, "these are bizarre times."[4] If the times are bizarre for Fortune 500 companies, the times are even more bizarre for healthcare providers who must respond to the demands of a myriad of discontented customers—patients, corporations, third-party payers, and the federal government—to name but a few.

As we can all attest, the golden era of unlimited budgets for healthcare is over. The economic and social forces that drive other businesses are no longer sparing hospitals. Because they must drastically reduce costs while increasing quality and accessibility, hospitals are being forced to shift the center of healthcare delivery from the inpatient to the outpatient setting and shift the focus of healthcare economics from generating revenue by fee for service to amassing capitated lives.

These cataclysmic shifts in healthcare delivery and economics will profoundly affect those practicing infection control. As hospital epidemiologists and infection control professionals, we can either resist these forces or we can anticipate trends and implement change. If we choose the former, we will be supplanted by those who respond quickly to the pressures but whose vision for health protection is blinkered. Whereas, if we choose the latter, we will help our hospitals survive and we will assure new and expanded roles for those trained in infection control. We would do well to heed Tom Peter's warning that businesses and individuals will survive in our ever more competitive economy only if they embrace and thrive on change.[5] Clearly, the future of hospital epidemiology and infection control depends not only on our epidemiologic skills but on how well we apply those skills within the changing environment.

The current healthcare climate discomfits and

challenges even experts in hospital epidemiology and infection control but daunts many who are just entering the field. Consequently, SHEA published *The Practical Handbook for Healthcare Epidemiology* to help hospital epidemiologists and infection control professionals improve their practice during this chaotic time.

The Society recognizes that several excellent academic textbooks of infection control and quality assessment[1,2,6,7] are available as references for hospital epidemiologists and infection control professionals. Therefore, the Handbook does not reproduce those scholarly works, but rather supplements them with pragmatic information from the literature and advice from individuals who have wrestled with relevant issues in their own practices. Although both fledgling and seasoned epidemiologists will benefit from the practical discussions, the Handbook emphasizes the basic information newcomers need to begin practicing hospital epidemiology.

To achieve this goal, we instructed the authors to write their chapters as if they were talking with a group of infectious diseases fellows who, on the eve of their graduation, realized that they soon will be running infection control programs and that they know nothing about this topic. The authors' task was to prepare these incipient hospital epidemiologists for their future careers by summarizing basic data from the literature and by providing essential references and resources. In addition, we asked the authors to share their own experiences of what works and what does not work in particular situations and to suggest where neophytes should focus their initial efforts.

To whet your appetite, I will briefly describe the subjects discussed in the Handbook. Because no one ever teaches hospital epidemiologists what overarching goals or ethical principles they should adopt to guide their practice, what they can do to educate themselves, or how they should negotiate with the administration and communicate with colleagues, we have included chapters on each of these topics. We have also included chapters on many nitty gritty aspects of hospital epidemiology including how to fulfill administrative responsibilities and how to choose surveillance and isolation systems.

To help hospital epidemiologists and infection control professionals expand their horizons beyond typical infection control issues, we have included chapters on using epidemiologic methods to assess quality of care and to study noninfectious adverse outcomes of medical care. For those like myself who are mathematically challenged and computer impaired, we have included chapters that simply and clearly explain the basic statistics and the computer hardware and software necessary to do hospital epidemiology, and a chapter on how to communicate with the computer wizards in your hospital's information department.

In the future, microbiologic and environmental issues will increasingly challenge the hospital epidemiologist's ingenuity and tenacity. To help them meet this challenge, we have included chapters which discuss the microbiologic and molecular epidemiologic services needed by a hospital epidemiology program, the basic principles of disinfection and sterilization, the essentials of a tuberculosis control plan, and infection control issues associated with construction and remodeling.

The hospital epidemiologist and the infection control professional of the future must expand their programs into new areas and guide their hospitals through inspections by outside agencies. Therefore, the Handbook tackles topics such as extending infection control programs into long-term care and outpatient facilities and surviving inspections by the Joint Commission on Accreditation of Healthcare Organizations (JCAHO) and the Occupational Safety and Health Administration (OSHA).

I hope that the Handbook will provide fledgling hospital epidemiologists with the information they need to successfully begin their practice. I also hope that the authors' opinions will provoke SHEA members to debate the purpose, content, and methods of hospital epidemiology. If the Handbook helps SHEA achieve those goals, we will all benefit because new colleagues and lively debate will energize our profession and our Society so that we can meet the challenges that lie ahead.

References

1. Mayhall CG, ed. *Infection Control and Hospital Epidemiology.* Baltimore, Md: Williams & Wilkins; 1996.
2. Wenzel RP, ed. *Prevention and Control of Nosocomial Infections.* 3rd ed. Baltimore, Md: Williams & Wilkins; 1997.
3. *Webster's Ninth New Collegiate Dictionary.* Springfield, Ill: Merriam-Webster Inc; 1986.
4. Popcorn F. *The Popcorn Report.* New York, NY: Doubleday Currency; 1991.
5. Peters T. Thriving on chaos. *Handbook for a Management Revolution.* New York, NY: Alfred A Knopf; 1988.
6. Bennett JV, Brachman PS, eds. *Hospital Infections.* Boston, Mass: Little, Brown and Company; 1992.
7. Wenzel RP, ed. Assessing quality health care. *Perspectives for Clinicians.* Baltimore, Md: Williams & Wilkins; 1992.

CHAPTER 2

The Hospital Epidemiologist: Practical Ideas

Richard P. Wenzel, MD, MSc

Abstract

The modern hospital epidemiologist has broad perspectives and influence across clinical departmental lines. The opportunities to improve patient care by expanding traditional areas of focus beyond infection control are great. Useful skills include epidemiology, communication, and respect for colleagues.

Introduction

With the increasing prominence of the hospital epidemiologist and the new opportunities emerging in the face of healthcare reform,[1] more is being written about this person's role in helping to provide high quality care.[2] Nevertheless, some specific and especially helpful views may have been omitted in deference to more scholarly perspectives. With the hope that ideas gleaned from experience may help the newcomer, it is my goal to provide a brief perspective of five issues with respect to hospital epidemiology: organization, surveillance, priorities, growth of the program, and the future.

Organization

The team leader should be supported adequately with infection control professionals, secretarial help, and computer hardware and programming capabilities. I think it is useful to develop an expert team consisting of the hospital epidemiologist and colleagues from the microbiology laboratory and the biostatistical group. I always have had a special microbiology laboratory for infection control, initially in my career overseen by me and more recently by the expertise of a skilled clinical microbiologist. In the same way, when one begins in the field, he or she can manage the basic data analysis. However, as the program grows, experts in data management and statistical issues should join the team. At some point, the position of hospital epidemiologist becomes increasingly demanding and the organization requires specialization.[3]

Although many persons in our field are content with a limited focus of hospital epidemiology or infection control, I have argued that it may be better to lead expanded programs. Our expertise in the field of epidemiology and experience working with

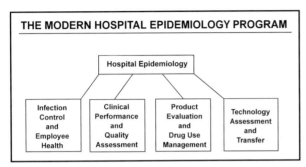

FIGURE 2-1. Four offices under the hospital epidemiology program.

both healthcare workers and the hospital's administrators have created special opportunities for us. Briefly stated, some institutions may wish to have at least four main offices under the program for hospital epidemiology:

1. Clinical performance and quality assessment.
2. Infection control and employee health.
3. Product evaluation and drug use management.
4. Technology assessment and transfer (Figure 2-1).

Our routine activities deal with all areas, and it makes some sense to coordinate those offices with the special skills of the hospital epidemiologist.

One also needs to forge good working relationships with clinicians, the director of the clinical microbiology laboratory, the pharmacist in charge of antibiotic oversight, and the director of the employee health program. Furthermore, from an administrative perspective, it is enormously important to have access to and the support of the senior members of the hospital's administrative staff.

Although much has been written already about the monthly infection control meeting,[4] I would emphasize its administrative and political importance. It would be folly to trivialize that meeting and consider it a bureaucratic waste of time. Nothing could be further from the truth. Instead, this is the moment to show your expertise and the time you have expended in the quest for quality healthcare. Most importantly, it is the time and

place to develop useful and important policies. As emphasized in earlier discussions, one should limit agenda items, be fully prepared, and be so well organized that a vote on one new policy or procedure takes place each month.[4]

Newcomers to the field frequently are tempted to bite off more than they can chew. Their motivation is admirable and energy quite high, but before long it becomes obvious that success has not been achieved in any single important goal. My recommendation is to have one long-term (annual) important goal and one or two short-term (3 to 6 months) goals. As examples, an important long-term goal would be the development of a comprehensive plan to manage tuberculosis exposure in the hospital and clinics. A short-term goal might be the development of an updated policy on the length of time central venous catheters are recommended to stay in place before removal. It takes hard work and some creativity to organize priorities, but one might begin by examining the problems identified by routine surveillance or by anticipating a problem emerging at other hospitals in the country. The main point is to have a limited number of short- and long-term priorities and then to follow through in a comprehensive manner with a policy that is adopted by the institution.

Surveillance

Surveillance is not the mere collection of data for purposes of calculating rates. Instead, it is part of a comprehensive program in infection control involving continuing visibility and consultation, feedback of data, Hawthorne effect, and networking with front-line healthcare workers.[5] That is why, although computer-assisted surveillance is attractive and useful,[6] I would be reluctant to take the infection control professional away from the patient care areas.

From my perspective, the value of surveillance seems obvious. One needs to know with some precision what the problems are first. The identification of endemic and epidemic rates and subsequent setting of priorities have their base in accurate and routine surveillance. Then one can build a database for long-term analyses and possibly for serious epidemiologic and intervention studies.

I also would suggest that it is of value is to prove that the data are accurate, to validate the surveillance system. The methods by which to do this have been described.[6] Although time consuming, the process of validation leads not only to an appreciation of the value of the infection control professionals, but also to credibility for the program and widespread acceptance of the data by the clinicians. This is extremely important because surveillance is the basis by which priorities are identified and policies are developed.

Even with limited resources, one should perform surveillance, perhaps only in critical care units or only for nosocomial bloodstream infections. These are important infections clinically, and a running tally of antibiotic resistance patterns, especially for bloodstream pathogens, is appreciated by the clinical staff (Figure 2-2). They are useful for the development of policy for prophylactic, empiric, and therapeutically directed antibiotic use.

Reports to the ward staff ideally should be brief, illustrated graphically, supported statistically, and accompanied by a summary message. The latter should focus on the basic change in rate or pattern and should include the practical recommendations of the hospital epidemiology team.

Before leaving the topic of surveillance, it would be useful to say that infection control professionals frequently are undervalued and unsung heroes and heroines. They need time away from surveillance to learn at conferences and to teach. Teaching provides an opportunity for them to use their knowledge and experience as well as their networking skills to promulgate policies developed by the infection control committee. Obviously, such a role provides a platform for infection control professionals and evidence of the confidence that the hospital epidemiologist has in them.

Priorities

In addition to the development of limited priorities for policy development, one may wish to consider limited priorities for organizational change, for new services, or for research. As with policy development, the message is the same: limit the number of goals, stay focused, and write a report.

One activity that is useful to help envision priorities and plan for the year is an annual retreat. At the retreat, which should be away from the usual areas of intrusion, one should organize group discussions on two or three main issues. One person should be assigned to lead each topic, and there should be 1 to 3 hours for discussion and development of a strategic plan. At the subsequent year's retreat, one can present the "report card" of success.

Evolution of the Effective Program

There are different skills involved in starting a good program versus maintaining it. I am frequently asked, "How do you keep it going...keep it interesting...keep it focused on important issues?" Growth requires the development of continuing education programs that are taught locally, visits by outside experts, invited critique, and attendance at scientific meetings yourself.

By teaching, one learns. In addition to conveying information to others, one maintains a high level of expertise and knowledge. Outside visitors who review the activities of an infection control program provide new perspectives that are quite stimulating, and invited critique is a healthy lens through which to view the activities of the program. Obviously, time away for national meetings is essential to fuel the fires of enthusiasm, as well as to gain new information and insight.

An important danger in an established program is that the next epidemic, the next policy need, or the next administrative problem will not be met with the same high level of enthusiasm as the first one. There may be a natural tendency to give less attention to an issue, and one needs to be aware of

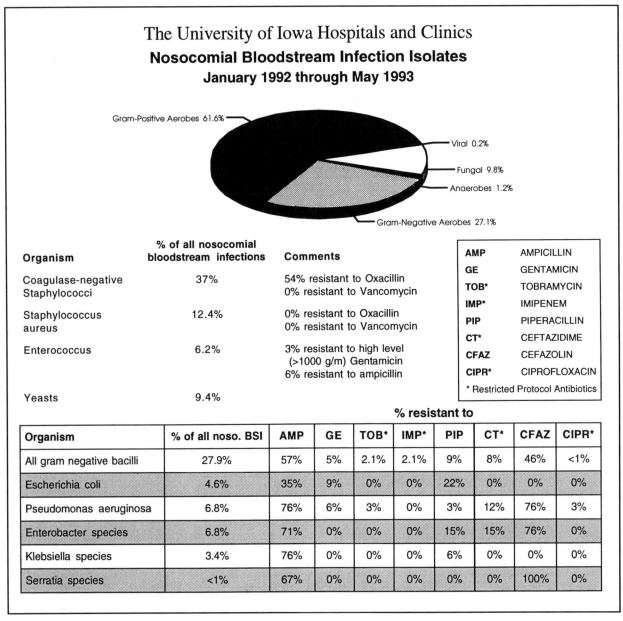

FIGURE 2-2. Graphic reports and tallies are helpful for presenting information to clinical staff.

this trap associated with experience. One also needs to continue to question the routines in administration. New problems need to be managed, not just dealt with in their urgency. Management implies planning and anticipation for purposes of control and for effective use of time. It has been my good fortune to be associated with a continued line of excellent fellows who continually breathe new life into our established program. I recommend

continual exposure of the team and its challenges to new and exciting young physicians and nurses.

The Future

The nature of the field of hospital epidemiology is change.[7] That is good news because change, although sometimes threatening, brings adventure and opportunity. To maintain a good program, one needs to adapt to the changing environment.

However, when I say adapt, I do not mean to imply waiting for change and finding a formula for fitting in. Instead, I am suggesting that the effective hospital epidemiologist be aware of the changing environment and anticipate the change. One should not wait and react, but instead one should anticipate and plan.

A second recommendation with respect to adapting is to try to understand the competing priorities of all stakeholders or partners. This skill may determine the success of the program as much as any others in our complex environment. In performing that task, my additional admonition is simply to do your best and to maintain your integrity.

References

1. Wenzel RP. Instituting health care reform and preserving quality: role of the hospital epidemiologist. *Clin Infect Dis.* 1993;17:831-834.

2. Wenzel RP. Quality assessment—an emerging component of hospital epidemiology. *Diagn Microbiol Infect Dis.* 1990;13:197-204.

3. Wenzel RP. Beyond total quality management. *Clinical Performance and Quality Health Care.* 1993;1:43-48.

4. Wenzel RP. Management principles and infection control. In: Wenzel RP, ed. *Prevention and Control of Nosocomial Infections.* 2nd ed. Baltimore, Md: Williams and Wilkins; 1993:207-213.

5. Wenzel RP, Streed SA. Surveillance and use of computers in hospital infection control. *J Hosp Infect.* 1989;13:217-229.

6. Broderick A, Mori M, Nettleman MD, Streed SA, Wenzel RP. Nosocomial infections: validation of surveillance and computer modeling to identify patients at risk. *Am J Epidemiol.* 1990;131:734-742.

7. Herwaldt LA. National issues and future concerns. In: Wenzel RP, ed. *Prevention and Control of Nosocomial Infections.* 2nd ed. Baltimore, Md: Williams & Wilkins; 1993:1001-1015.

CHAPTER 3

Educational Needs and Opportunities for the Hospital Epidemiologist

Louise M. Dembry, MD, Walter J. Hierholzer Jr., MD

Abstract

The role of the hospital epidemiologist has changed substantially over the last 30 years as medical care has become more complex. The hospital epidemiologist needs training in methods for surveillance, prevention, and control of nosocomial infections. The hospital epidemiologist also must know how to apply these methods to other areas, including the epidemiology of noninfectious adverse outcomes of medical care. Training in hospital epidemiology should be a defined part of every infectious disease fellowship training program. Ancillary and additional training is available from several sources.

Introduction

Over the past decade, hospital epidemiologists have expanded their roles by increasing their activities in the traditional realm of infection control—the surveillance, prevention, and control of nosocomial infections—and by applying epidemiologic techniques in new areas, such as the assessment of noninfectious adverse outcomes of care. Some hospital epidemiologists have moved beyond a narrow focus on infection control to evaluate a broad spectrum of healthcare outcomes. These persons have become institutional epidemiologists who can participate in or direct their institutions' comprehensive quality improvement programs.

Given recent changes in healthcare delivery, hospitals now admit more high-risk and immunosuppressed patients. In addition, hospitals are challenged to care for more patients with tuberculosis and bloodborne pathogens and, at the same time, to prevent transmission of resistant microorganisms and new environmental pathogens. With the shift in practice patterns, many patients who previously received care in the acute care setting now receive care in outpatient, long-term care, and rehabilitation facilities. Thus, individuals practicing infection control must develop new approaches to prevent the spread of infections within the healthcare setting.

Furthermore, to survive the dramatic changes in healthcare delivery and financing, hospitals have been forced to optimize the process of care and to balance cost and outcomes. Moreover, to decrease costs, numerous hospitals have compelled outcome measuring groups—quality improvement, risk

TABLE 3-1
BASIC KNOWLEDGE AND SKILLS REQUIRED FOR HOSPITAL EPIDEMIOLOGISTS

- Principles of epidemiologic investigations
- Techniques of data acquisition, management, and analysis
- Methods for controlling nosocomial infections
- Biostatistics
- Computer skills
    Word processing
    Information analysis
    Graphics
- Communication and management skills
- Laboratory skills
    Evaluation of antibiotic resistance
    Molecular typing techniques
    Environmental sampling

management, and infection control—to cooperate. Thus, individuals who can apply the basic techniques of epidemiology, biostatistics, surveillance, and informatics to a broad range of problems— both infectious and noninfectious—could help their hospitals meet these challenges and, at the same time, ensure their job security.

The skills described above are essential to individuals practicing infection control. Hospital epidemiologists who wish to succeed in the future should obtain training in these essential areas (Table 3-1). In addition, the hospital epidemiologist must learn to apply these skills in new settings, such as clinics, and to new problems, such as the epidemiology of noninfectious adverse outcomes of care.

Persons interested in hospital epidemiology may choose one of several options for training. Persons interested in clinical practice, clinical research, or infection control could select infectious disease fellowship programs that offer training in hospital epidemiology and infection control during the fellow's clinical and research years. A limited number of infectious diseases fellowship programs offer this training. Individuals could choose to do specific fellowships in hospital epi-

demiology and infection control. Such fellowships could be done either as part of an infectious disease training program or as additional training in clinical epidemiology or in epidemiology and public health. Others might choose to augment training in infectious diseases or general medicine by taking one of the several summer epidemiology programs offered through schools of public health.

Individuals who have completed their training or who have limited time should consider taking a short course offered by the Society for Healthcare Epidemiology of America (SHEA), in conjunction with the Centers for Disease Control and Prevention (CDC) and The American Hospital Association (AHA); the Association for Professionals in Infection Control and Epidemiology (APIC); or various university medical centers. In addition, SHEA and APIC each offer continuing medical education during their annual national meetings. We would recommend that persons who do not complete a formal fellowship in hospital epidemiology should avail themselves of several training opportunities, including short courses, summer programs, and national meetings.

In addition, persons interested in hospital epidemiology can educate themselves by reading appropriate literature. Several major textbooks of infection control and hospital epidemiology are available, and three journals, which are cited and abstracted by the National Library of Medicine, provide extensive peer-reviewed literature, as do several infectious disease and microbiology publications.

In the following sections, a number of training opportunities are described briefly. Interested individuals may obtain detailed information regarding each program from the sponsoring institutions. The institutions' addresses are listed at the end of this chapter.

Fellowships

The University of Texas Medical Branch in Galveston offers a 2-year fellowship in hospital epidemiology, which can accommodate one fellow during each 2-year cycle. Applicants must be board eligible in internal medicine and infectious diseases. Fellows receive training in basic infection control theory and practice, including the principles of surveillance, isolation techniques, infection control policies, and problem solving. They participate in outbreak investigations, conduct research, and learn to apply computer technology to hospital epidemiology. Fellows are encouraged strongly to take courses in biostatistics. The program plans to offer training in quality management principles.

The Department of Internal Medicine at the University of Iowa College of Medicine offers training in clinical epidemiology. The training program is offered for physicians who wish to have postgraduate training in hospital epidemiology. The fellowship program varies in length from 1 to 3 years and includes training in both academic and practical aspects of hospital epidemiology. Fellows participate in a variety of conferences, in specific research projects with faculty members, and in the day-to-day practice of hospital epidemiology, including outbreak investigations. Fellows may choose from a broad range of research projects, including clinical trials, epidemiological studies of nosocomial pathogens, cost-benefit analysis, statistical modeling, and molecular epidemiology. Many fellows obtain a Master of Science in Epidemiology through the Department of Preventive Medicine and Environmental Health.

Some infectious disease fellowship programs allow second- or third-year fellows to work with the hospital epidemiologist. The hospital epidemiologist, usually a member of the infectious diseases section, serves as a mentor and supervises the fellow's research. The level to which such fellows may participate in the infection control program varies. Programs that allow fellows to do research and to participate actively in the day-to-day activities of the infection control program, including the administrative aspects, offer the most well-rounded

experiences outside of the formal fellowships in hospital epidemiology.

Training Courses

APIC has designed short courses for new infection control professionals who have minimal experience in the field. APIC offers the Basic Training Course three times each year in various locations in the United States. The course, which lasts 4 to 7 days, addresses surveillance methodology, basic microbiology and immunology, definitions of nosocomial infections, infection control precautions, methods for calculating nosocomial infection rates, and methods for investigating outbreaks. New hospital epidemiologists could benefit from APIC's course, because it discusses the fundamental information and skills that infection control personnel need to build their programs. APIC also offers an Advanced Practice Course for those persons who have experience in infection control.

SHEA, in conjunction with the CDC and the AHA, offers short training courses for new hospital epidemiologists, infectious disease fellows, and infection control professionals. This course, which lasts 3 to 4 days, is offered twice each year in different locations in the United States. The course covers core infection control topics including the epidemiology of nosocomial infections, isolation systems, disinfection and sterilization, employee health, the role of the hospital epidemiologist, and compliance with standards set by regulatory agencies. The course also introduces methods for surveillance and for epidemic investigations. The course includes problem-solving sessions that teach trainees to detect, investigate, and control various nosocomial problems.

The Department of Continuing Education at the Harvard Medical School, Boston, Massachusetts, offers the course "Nosocomial Infectious Diseases and Healthcare Epidemiology." The Children's Hospital Epidemiology Program presents this 3-day course every 2 years in the fall. The course is geared toward persons with some experience or interest in infection control and provides indepth discussions of contemporary issues in hospital epidemiology. The format includes lectures, mini-symposia on critical issues in hospital epidemiology, and one-half day workshops.

The Program of Hospital Epidemiology at The University of Iowa Hospitals and Clinics, Iowa City, Iowa, in cooperation with The University of Iowa Colleges of Nursing and Medicine, offers a 5-day course that is designed primarily for professionals in infection control. However, physicians could benefit from the course, especially from the surveillance tutorial. The course also teaches individuals to apply epidemiologic principles to the study of noninfectious adverse outcomes of care, and it uses unique computer simulations to teach students to investigate outbreaks. Other topics include the principles of epidemiology, criteria development, the epidemiology of important nosocomial pathogens, disinfection and sterilization, infection control in anesthesia and in the outpatient setting, and the infection control committee.

The *American Journal of Infection Control* (*AJIC*), published bimonthly, has a section entitled "Educational Calendar" that is a good resource for individuals desiring more training in infection control and hospital epidemiology. The section lists programs that range from basic infection control courses to updates on infection control issues and practices.

Summer Courses

Several schools of public health offer graduate summer programs in epidemiology. These courses, which vary in length from 1 to 4 weeks, are an alternative way for novice hospital epidemiologists to learn the principles of epidemiology. The courses also help more experienced individuals augment their knowledge and practical skills.

Generally, the summer epidemiology programs offer graduate level, basic, and secondary courses in epidemiology, biostatistics, and study design and analysis. The programs usually also address specific topics including the epidemiology of acute and chronic diseases, occupational and environmental health, health policy, clinical epidemiology, and others. Some programs offer courses in hospital epidemiology, the epidemiology of infectious diseases, and methods in quality assessment. Several programs also offer courses on how to use microcomputers in epidemiology. Some programs provide graduate-level credit through their respective universities.

The Graduate Summer Session in Epidemiology is an independent course taught by faculty members from numerous institutions. The Session currently is held at the University of Michigan School of Public Health in Ann Arbor. This program offers several courses lasting from 1 to 3 weeks, including courses in the fundamentals of epidemiology and biostatistics, a course in microcomputer applications for epidemiology (3 weeks), the epidemiology of infectious diseases (1 week), infection control (1 week), and methods in medical quality assessment (1 week).

The New England Epidemiology Institute, Newton Lower Falls, Massachusetts, sponsors the annual New England Epidemiology Summer Program held at Tufts University. The program covers the theory and practice of epidemiology, several levels of biostatistics, methods for epidemiologic and clinical research, and epidemiology in public health practice.

The McGill University Department of Epidemiology and Biostatistics in Montreal, Quebec, Canada, offers a summer program intended for clinicians and other health professionals. The courses all last 4 weeks and include training in epidemiology, biostatistics, principles of epidemiologic research, risk assessment and management, and the epidemiology of infectious and parasitic diseases.

The Graduate Summer Program in Epidemiology at The Johns Hopkins University School of

Hygiene and Public Health, Baltimore, provides courses in the principles and methods of epidemiology and biostatistics. Other courses address methods for case-control studies, the epidemiologic basis for tuberculosis control, the epidemiology of infectious diseases, and the use of microcomputers in epidemiology.

Continuing Education

Both APIC and SHEA hold annual meetings that provide continuing education opportunities to attendees. APIC's meeting, held in late spring or early summer, provides scientific and practical information relevant to the practice of infection control. The SHEA meeting, held in early spring, includes workshops, symposia, and sessions for poster and oral presentations of original scientific work. The broad areas covered include nosocomial infections, occupational risks of healthcare workers, and quality assessment. Both meetings enable infection control personnel to learn about new developments and discoveries regarding the causes, modes of transmission, diagnosis, prevention, and control of nosocomial infections. In addition, division "L" of the American Society for Microbiology (ASM), comprised of individuals who are interested in hospital epidemiology, sponsors sessions at the ASM national meetings that are relevant to hospital epidemiologists. Finally, the Infectious Diseases Society of America devotes significant portions of its national meetings to important infection control topics.

Book and Journals

Several textbooks, including *Hospital Infections*,[1] *Prevention and Control of Nosocomial Infections*,[2] and *Hospital Epidemiology and Infection Control*,[3] discuss the principles and practice of infection control and provide good reference lists. The textbooks are particularly useful for persons who previously have learned basic epidemiologic concepts.

APIC publishes the bimonthly journal *AJIC*. *AJIC* includes original articles that focus on the basic infection control practices, a commentary section, and APIC Guidelines for Infection Control Practice. *AJIC* also publishes information on upcoming meetings and courses in infection control.

The official journals of SHEA are *Infection Control and Hospital Epidemiology*, which is published monthly, and *Clinical Performance and Quality Health Care* (*CPQHC*), which is published quarterly. *Infection Control and Hospital Epidemiology* includes editorials on topical issues in hospital epidemiology, original articles, review articles, consensus papers, and special topics such as practical hospital epidemiology and molecular epidemiology, as well as information regarding the SHEA Annual Meeting and the SHEA/CDC/AHA Training Course. *CPQHC* publishes articles that address appropriateness of care, quality of care, outcome assessment, the application of practice guidelines, and the economic aspects of quality improvement and assessment.

The Hospital Infection Society (HIS), based in the United Kingdom, publishes the *Journal of Hospital Infection*. The journal publishes original articles, as well as a series of practical articles entitled "How to Do It." HIS also supports educational programs as a part of its national and international meetings.

Other Needs

Molecular typing techniques, which are used to determine genetic relatedness of organisms, have become important tools for investigating endemic and epidemic nosocomial infections. Organized training in this field is limited, although laboratories performing these techniques often are willing to train interested persons on an individual basis. The American Tissue Type Collection, Rockville, Maryland, offers workshops such as "Basic Techniques in Molecular Mycobacteriology," and the CDC occasionally offers similar workshops in molecular epidemiologic techniques. Expertise in molecular epidemiology is most important for persons who direct a laboratory that uses these techniques. However, hospital epidemiologists must know when molecular typing would be helpful, understand the strengths and weaknesses of each technique, and must know the principles of interpreting the results. We recommend that hospital epidemiologists who do not have experience with molecular typing read one of several good reviews on the topic.[4,5]

Other skills such as preparing grant proposals and manuscripts are helpful, particularly for hospital epidemiologists practicing in an academic setting. Persons still in fellowship training should participate in these activities under the supervision of a mentor. Medical schools often conduct seminars and workshops on these topics. Interested persons should inquire about resources available in their geographic area.

Addresses

Administrative Coordinator
Graduate Summer Session in Epidemiology
The University of Michigan School of Public Health
109 S Observatory St
Ann Arbor, MI 48109-2029
Telephone: 313-764-5454

American Journal of Infection Control
11830 Westline Industrial Dr
St Louis, MO 63146-3318
Telephone: 314-453-4351

American Society of Microbiology
1325 Massachusetts Ave, NW
Washington, DC 20005-4171
Telephone: 202-737-3600

American Type Culture Collection
12301 Parklawn Dr
Rockville, MD 20852
Telephone: 301-231-5566

Association for Professionals in Infection Control and Epidemiology
1016 Sixteenth St, NW, 6th Floor
Washington, DC 20036
Telephone: 202-296-2742

Extension Training Program for Infection Control Professionals
The University of Iowa Hospitals and Clinics
200 Hawkins Dr, Room C-41 GH
Iowa City, IA 52242-1009
Telephone: 319-356-1606

Loreen A. Herwaldt, MD
Associate Professor
Hospital Epidemiologist
Division of General Medicine, C-41 GH
The University of Iowa Hospitals and Clinics
Iowa City, IA 52242-1081

Infection Control and Hospital Epidemiology
6900 Grove Rd
Thorofare, NJ 08086
Telephone: 609-848-1000

Infectious Diseases Society of America
1200 19th St, NW, Suite 300
Washington, DC 20036-2401
Telephone: 703-299-0200

The Journal of Hospital Infection
WB Saunders
24-28 Oval Rd
London, NW1 7DX, United Kingdom

C. Glen Mayhall, MD
Division of Infectious Disease, Rte 1092
Former Shriner's Burns Building, Room 2-64B
University of Texas Medical Branch
Galveston, TX 77555-1092

New England Epidemiology Institute
Department PA-5
One Newton Executive Park
Newton Lower Falls, MA 02162-1450
Telephone: 617-244-1200

Nosocomial Infectious Diseases and Healthcare
Epidemiology Course, Harvard MED-CME
PO Box 825
Boston, MA 02117-0825
Telephone: 617-432-1525

Program Coordinator
Graduate Summer Program in Epidemiology
Johns Hopkins University School of Hygiene and Public
Health
615 North Wolfe St
Baltimore, MD 21205
Telephone: 410-955-7158

The Society for Healthcare Epidemiology of America
19 Mantua Rd
Mt Royal, NJ 08061
Telephone: 609-423-0087

Summer Program Coordinator
Department of Epidemiology and Biostatistics
McGill University
1020 Pine Ave, W, Room 38BJ
Montreal, Quebec, H3A1A2, Canada
Telephone: 514-398-3973

References

1. Bennett JV, Brachman PS, eds. *Hospital Infections.* 3rd ed. Boston, Mass: Little, Brown and Co; 1992.

2. Wenzel RP, ed. *Prevention and Control of Nosocomial Infections.* 2nd ed. Baltimore, Md: Williams & Wilkins; 1993.

3. Mayhall CG, ed. *Hospital Epidemiology and Infection Control.* Baltimore, Md: Williams & Wilkins, 1995.

4. Sader HS, Hollis RJ, Pfaller MA. The use of molecular techniques in the epidemiology and control of infectious diseases. *Contemporary Issues in Clinical Microbiology.* 1995;15:407-431.

5. Arbeit RD. Laboratory procedures for the epidemiologic analysis of microorganisms. In: Murray PR, Baron EJ, Pfaller MA, Tenover FC, Yolken RH, eds. *Manual of Clinical Microbiology.* Washington, DC: ASM Press; 1995:190-208.

CHAPTER 4

Negotiating With the Administration— or How to Get Paid for Doing Hospital Epidemiology

H. Gunner Deery II, MD

Abstract

Many hospital administrators acknowledge the value of a hospital epidemiologist. However, many hospital epidemiologists are not being paid for their work. To eliminate this inequity, hospital epidemiologists must negotiate contractual relationships successfully with their hospitals or healthcare systems. This chapter reviews an approach to rectifying this problem that is based on practical experience.

Introduction

My credentials for writing this chapter include the following:

- I have worked as a hospital epidemiologist for free.
- I have been paid.
- I have been fired.
- I have been rehired.
- I have been reorganized.

As this litany implies, the relationship between physicians and hospitals or healthcare systems can be tumultuous and complex. The relationship also can be highly productive and enjoyable, if both parties feel they are being treated fairly and the roles and responsibilities are delineated clearly in a contractual relationship.

Working for Free

If you currently are working as a hospital epidemiologist or if you chair an infection control committee and you are not being paid, please resign today! What do you have to lose? If the hospital values your work, they will open negotiations with you. If they prefer not to pay you, you know how much they value you and your work. You also will eliminate at least one meeting per month and will give yourself the gift of more time.

But what about your "citizenship" obligation to your hospital? No problem. You can offer to be on the education committee, red code committee, or any other committee that does not represent the bread and butter of your specialty. Do your surgical colleagues operate au gratis for the hospital? Do the cardiologists donate a catheterization per day to the hospital? Those who do hospital epidemiology for free undermine the value of our profession as a whole. Remember, hospitals pay for the services they value.

Hospitals or healthcare facilities that have never paid physicians for administrative services may be exceptions to the rule of getting paid for your work. For example, small rural hospitals may not have paid physicians to do administrative work and may not know the value that a hospital epidemiologist adds to their programs. In such hospitals, you may need to work for a defined period of time (1 to 2 years) to demonstrate your value. We all would hope that this probationary period could be avoided if we educated the hospital administrators adequately and explained to them how a hospital epidemiologist could help to reduce costs and liability by decreasing nosocomial infection rates. However, if you must donate your services to prove your assertions, I would recommend that you do so only for 1 to 2 years. If you are not able to negotiate payment for your work by the end of this period, then you should resign from the hospital epidemiology duties and enjoy your free time. After several months without your direction and leadership, the hospital may realize your value and capitulate. Also, the medical staff may rally around you and insist that the hospital pay you for your services. An outbreak could accelerate this process.

I work in a rural-based group practice in a multispecialty clinic that admits patients to a 299-bed, nonteaching, community, regional-referral hospital. When I began working for this group in 1982, neither the clinic nor the hospital understood what an infectious disease specialist and hospital epidemiologist could contribute. I did not know how to negotiate, and I felt that I could not persuade the hospital administration of my value. Consequently, for the first 18 to 24 months, I worked as a hospital epidemiologist for free. However, after this period (of sin), I began negotiations to establish hospital epidemiology as a paid position. I subsequently became the first physician in our hospital, excluding the pathologists, who was paid to perform hospital administrative services.

The Society for Healthcare Epidemiology of America (SHEA) recently completed a membership survey,[1] and the preliminary results reveal that an astounding 268 of the 532 respondents (50.4%) were *not* paid for their infection control activities. If you are one of these individuals, please resign today, if not for yourself then for your profession.

How to Get Paid

I believe that hospital administrators who understand the value of hospital epidemiologists will pay for this expertise. What and where is our value? The hospital epidemiologist's marketable skills are myriad (Table 4-1). However, hospital epidemiologists no longer just can tell administrators or other physicians that infection control has value. Neither can hospital epidemiologists just demonstrate their value by doing good work for the hospital. Instead, we must use these components to build a powerful and effective negotiating position.

If you and your hospital or healthcare system are new at this, you may need to consider working for free, as mentioned earlier, for a limited period of time. During this period, you absolutely must demonstrate your value. To reach this goal, you should identify a few projects that are achievable and that reduce costs. Once you have completed the projects, you should summarize your efforts and present the data to the infection control committee, the directors of major clinical departments, the medical executive committee, and the hospital board. During this process, you can build support among the medical staff as well.

Although you would never wish for an outbreak, you can use them to your advantage if they do occur. A properly conducted outbreak investigation will terminate the outbreak and prevent similar problems in the future. You can thereby prevent nosocomial infections and avoid the associated morbidity and mortality, reducing costs. Outbreaks usually represent extra-systemic (special cause) defects that occur rarely. Outbreaks, therefore, do not account for most of the costs associated with nosocomial infections. However, outbreaks may allow

---

TABLE 4-1
A HOSPITAL EPIDEMIOLOGIST'S MARKETABLE SKILLS

- Supervises and collaborates with the infection control professionals
- Chairs infection control committee
- Supervises collection of surveillance data
- Analyzes surveillance data and implements control strategies
- Validates the surveillance system
- Supervises projects to decrease endemic "common-cause" nosocomial infections
- Investigates outbreaks
- Analyzes antibiotic resistance patterns and interprets their significance relative to antibiotic utilization
- Evaluates new products (eg, intravenous catheters, etc.)
- Evaluates the scientific validity of policies and procedures
- Interprets and implements, in a cost-effective manner, standards from regulatory agencies that are applicable to infection control, employee health, etc
- Consults with medical staff, hospital staff, and administration on epidemiologic matters
- Analyzes trends in employee illness
- Supervises vaccination programs for medical staff and hospital employees
- Supervises preemployment screening of new hospital employees
- Supervises the follow-up process for hospital employees who are exposed to infectious diseases (eg, bloodborne pathogens, tuberculosis, varicella, herpes zoster, meningococcus, etc.)
- Directs and supervises AIDS-related issues (eg, hospital employee education, case reporting, etc)
- Consults with staff in the microbiology laboratory regarding the appropriate use of laboratory tests, antibiotic susceptibility reports, analysis of new rapid lab tests, etc

- Consults with architects, engineers, and contractors regarding infection risks associated with construction projects
- Consults with staff in risk management regarding actual or potential malpractice claims related to nosocomial infections
- Consults with the hospital's public relations personnel regarding release of information about outbreaks, endemic nosocomial infections, quality of care, and epidemiologically based report cards, etc
- Serves as a liaison between hospital and medical staff in quality improvement initiatives
- Consults with other staff regarding epidemiologic evaluations of noninfectious disease problems (eg, falls, decubitus ulcers, etc)
- Supervises or consults with the hospital's pharmacokinetic dosing service
- Supervises the epidemiologic initiatives in the hospital's long-term care facility
- Directs the infection control and employee health initiatives in an expanded healthcare setting that includes the hospital or healthcare system, a home nursing program, and a home infusion therapy program
- Helps to develop an epidemiologically based quality management approach to noninfectious adverse outcomes of care
- Assists in outcome management initiatives
- Assists other staff as they develop clinical practice guidelines
- Serves as a liaison with staff from the local public health department

---

you to identify (common-cause) defects within the system that increase endemic infection rates. If you can correct the systemic defects, you will decrease the rate of endemic infections and substantially decrease the overall cost of nosocomial infections.

From a hospital's perspective, the 1990s mantra "Provide high-quality care at low cost" represents our fundamental opportunity. Thus, the primary benefit that hospital epidemiologists can offer beleaguered administrators in any market is reduced nosocomial infections and the associated

reduced costs. In addition, the hospital epidemiologist must communicate openly with the appropriate administrator. Frequently, this is like mixing oil and water. However, if you develop a nonadversarial relationship or, even better, a congenial social relationship, you can help the administrators understand your value and increase the likelihood that you can negotiate a contractual relationship. I would term this process a "Slamaization," in honor of the master of this technique, Dr. Thomas Slama, of Indianapolis, Indiana.

Negotiating a Contract

In business, you don't get what you deserve, you get what you negotiate. Unfortunately, negotiation may not come naturally to you. Remember, negotiation really is joint problem solving. The two major models of negotiation are the confrontational approach (win-lose) and the collaborative model (win-win). The win-lose model appeals to many people, because it enables them to win a few battles quickly. However, the win-lose approach usually produces angry losers who will resist vigorously any projects that you attempt in the future. The win-win approach is slower, but it is more likely to help you build relationships and long-term trust. Thus, over the years, you will be able to accomplish more with the win-win model of negotiation.

Despite demonstrating their worth and using a collaborative style of negotiating, hospital epidemiologists may still be faced, as I was, with intransigent administrators, at which point, you will be forced, as I was, to use a confrontational approach and hope that subsequently you can collaborate again. My first experience with being fired illustrates this process. After approximately 10 years of relative stability, the administration of our hospital changed. The new administration canceled all administrative contracts with physicians. After attempting to reason with the new administrator, I stopped providing hospital epidemiology services. I resigned as Chairperson of the Infection Control Committee and the Pharmacy and Therapeutics Committee. I also refused to participate in any of our ongoing projects. Unfortunately, this left our infection control professional in a compromised position. She understood, in principle, what I was doing, but questioned whether my response was ethical. In addition, the burden of work fell on her shoulders. The medical staff, however, supported my position. Despite considerable effort, the new administrator was unable find physicians who would lead the Infection Control Committee and the Pharmacy and Therapeutics Committee.

Our outstanding infection control professional maintained essential infection control and employee health activities, but she had no guidance from physicians. During this period, the infection control professional identified an apparent cluster of pneumonias caused by *Serratia marcescens* in our intensive care unit. The administration asked me to assist in the investigation. My response remained hard-line. I would assist, but only if paid $1,000 per hour as a consultant. After 6 months of this contentious relationship, the administration reopened negotiations for a new contract. I used this opportunity to increase my compensation by over 50%.

If you are trying to obtain a contract, it may be worthwhile to ask an expert in negotiations to advise you or to negotiate for you. Your practice administrator may be able to help you. If you feel powerless or intimidated by a large healthcare system or hospital, you should get some help. However, if you have someone negotiate for your contract, you cannot be passive. You must be well prepared, and you must specify what you want in your contract. Furthermore, before beginning to negotiate, you must gather essential background information. When you negotiate with the administrators for a contract and for your salary, you should know what other hospital epidemiologists do and what they are paid. Data from your state and region will be more compelling than data from distant locations. The likelihood that you can negotiate a satisfactory contract will be increased if other epidemiologists in your city, region, or state are paid for their services. Your state SHEA liaison may be able to help you obtain this information.

A contract is simply a written set of promises: "I promise to do something for you and, in return, you promise to do something for me." The core components of a contract should define the hospital epidemiologist's roles and responsibilities, the expected time commitment, the lines of authority, and the compensation package. The contract also might specify the hospital epidemiologist's access to data, computers, computer software, space, laboratory support, and secretarial support. The contract also could allocate money for books, journals, and continuing medical education.

How to determine appropriate compensation is an extremely important and difficult issue. Hospital epidemiologists could be paid by the hour for the services they provide, or they could receive a fixed salary based on hospital size (a per-bed rate). Many hospitals prefer to pay hospital epidemiologists for each hour of service, because contracts with other employees specify an hourly wage and because they may be able to defend this cost structure more easily to auditors from Medicare. I personally dislike this approach, because I do not really "punch in and out" with a time-clock mentality. I integrate my epidemiologic activities into my daily work, and I find it difficult to put on and take off the "hat" of hospital epidemiology. As a professional, I prefer to receive a salary commensurate with my job description. When I first was paid for my services as a hospital epidemiologist, I received a set salary. However, when the relationship between the clinic and the hospital was restructured, the hospital insisted on finding a more "objective" method for compensation. I reluctantly agreed to receive an hourly wage for my epidemiologic services.

What is the appropriate hourly rate for hospital epidemiologists? The practice administrator and the president of our multispecialty group negotiate hourly wage rates for me and all clinic physicians who provide administrative services for the hospital. The basic formula multiplies the Medical Group Management Association (MGMA) gross median production per specialty (excluding academic faculty, ancillary services, technical components, and physician extenders) by our actual overall clinic collection rate, to get the net production. The net production then is divided by 2,080 hours (40 hours per week × 52 weeks) to obtain the net rate per hour. The net rate per hour then is multiplied by the hours an individual is expected to work

for the hospital. A 1-month time-study is required to validate the time commitment. The number of hours in the physician's time-study is multiplied by 12 to obtain the total time spent per year. The logic behind this formula is that we could generate revenue in our clinical practices during the time we give to the hospital. The MGMA gross median production serves as an external standard and helps to support the calculation. The 1994 MGMA gross median production for infectious disease specialists in multispecialty clinics was $253,068.[2] Our clinic collection rate for 1994 was 66%. Using this formula, the 1994 net rate per hour for infectious disease at our clinic was $80.30 per hour.

This approach poses some significant problems. The current number of infectious diseases specialists in multispecialty clinics on which MGMA calculated the gross mean production was very small (n=31). Also, in my opinion, revenue generated by performing clinical consultations in infectious disease is not related directly to the value of hospital epidemiology services. Moreover, the amount of money generated by clinical infectious disease specialists varies tremendously by the setting in which they practice (eg, hospital practice, office practice, infusion program, teaching hospital, clinical research, geographic location, etc). I also think that the income generated by infectious diseases consultants is an inappropriate and inadequate basis on which to determine remuneration for hospital epidemiologists. On the other hand, the MGMA assessment is a place to start negotiating (your "line in the sand"). Be aware that the hospital administrators may argue that this calculation does not include the overhead from your practice or your benefits. They will argue that they should not have to cover overhead and benefits, and they will try to decrease the rate per hour. The hospital administrators also may argue that you do not actually give up practice time, but you simply add the hospital epidemiology time commitment to your day or week. After negotiating some of these points, my 1994 net rate per hour was $152.17, nearly twice the base rate calculated from the MGMA formula.

Alternatively, the hourly rate for hospital epidemiology services could be based on the fees paid in your state or region to experts who review medical records for litigation. These fees range from $200 to over $500 per hour. I like this approach, because it is simple, and it considers the intangibles of your experience and expertise. Another approach is to base the hospital epidemiologist's salary on the number of hospital beds. In the 1990s, this method is antiquated, because the number of hospital beds is decreasing but the number of services may not decrease equally, and the proportion of critically ill patients in hospitals is increasing. Furthermore, more procedures are performed in outpatient clinics, which broadens the scope and complexity of the hospital epidemiologist's responsibilities. Information regarding the level and manner of compensation of other hospital epidemiologists in your state and region may help you determine your remuneration and help you negotiate with your administrators. The SHEA state liaisons might be able to collate data from their area. The SHEA membership survey conducted in 1995 might provide some benchmarks.

In addition to the compensation issues, the contract must define explicitly the hospital epidemiologist's lines of authority and communication. Much of the turmoil I have experienced over the years was due, in part, to the fact that I did not know where I was located in the hospital administrative structure. I'm not sure it matters where you are located, as long as it makes sense for your particular situation. The 447 hospital epidemiologists who responded to the SHEA membership survey[1] reported to various individuals or departments: 196 (44%), medical director; 68 (18%), quality management; 44 (10%), nursing; 20 (4%), risk management; and 118 (26%), other. In the past, I reported to the vice president of operations; I now report to the hospital's medical director (vice pres-

ident of medical affairs), which is a very positive change. My ability to communicate with the hospital administration has improved since I have begun reporting to another physician.

The contract can delineate roles and responsibilities generically or very specifically. The hospital epidemiologist could participate in many specific activities, some of which are outlined in Table 4-1. A few caveats pertain: You should never agree to do things that cannot be accomplished or in which you have responsibility but no authority. You should not spread yourself so thin that you cannot do anything well; you will be better off doing a few things well. Once you have won the confidence and respect of your colleagues and the administration, you can work to expand your responsibilities and the associated compensation.

Keeping Your Job

The healthcare environment is changing rapidly. It is now replete with cost constraints, managed care programs, quality improvement initiatives, ways to assess outcomes, and groups that develop clinical pathways. All of these efforts could benefit from the expertise offered by hospital epidemiologists. Thus, the changing healthcare environment could provide many opportunities for us. However, these opportunities are accompanied by a new level of accountability. No longer can we simply say that we are good and that our services are necessary. Rather, we must demonstrate that we can help clinicians improve the quality of medical care while they decrease costs. Moreover, hospital epidemiologists can perform an invaluable service for patients, clinicians, and administrators, if they can demonstrate that medical care that is done correctly (quality) produces fewer adverse outcomes and thus saves money. Hospital epidemiologists then could argue that quality, not cost, should be the primary driving force.

I have a few practical suggestions for new hospital epidemiologists who are trying to survive in this competitive and chaotic environment. You should pick one or two major projects and perhaps two minor projects each year. Once you have chosen your projects, you should develop a strategic plan for implementing them, and then you should get busy and do them. When you have finished your projects, you may want to use cost-benefit analysis to demonstrate the success of your efforts. Do not be afraid to share your victories with the hospital administrators, your medical colleagues, and important committees. They need to know that your efforts help the entire health center reach its goal of providing excellent care at a reasonable cost. In addition, to keep your job, you must deal proactively with potential problems and communicate openly with physicians, nurses, directors of other departments, and your supervisor.

Conclusion

Your skills as a hospital epidemiologist are extremely valuable and, when used properly, improve patient care. If you believe in your value, you will demand appropriate recognition and reimbursement. It's the right thing to do! After all, as George Bernard Shaw once said "A day's work is a day's work, neither more nor less, and the man who does it needs a day's sustenance, a night's repose, and due leisure, whether he be painter or plough-man."[3]

References

1. Membership survey. *SHEA Newsletter.* 1996;6:5.

2. Medical Group Management Association. *Physician Compensation and Production Survey: 1995 Report Based on 1994 Data.* Englewood, Colo: MGMA; 1995.

3. *Webster's Book of Quotations.* New York, NY: PMC Publishing Co Inc; 1994:239.

Recommended Reading

Gross PA. The future of the hospital epidemiologist in the 1990s: presidential address, SHEA annual meeting. April 1994. *Infect Control Hosp Epidemiol.* 1995;16:179-182.

Karrass CL. *The Negotiating Game.* Rev. ed. New York, NY: HarperCollins Publishers, Inc; 1992.

Simmons BP, Parry MF, Williams M, Weinstein RA. The new era of hospital epidemiology: what you need to succeed. *Clin Infect Dis.* 1996;22:550-553.

Wenzel RP. Instituting health care reform and preserving quality: role of the hospital epidemiologist. *Clin Infect Dis.* 1993;17:831-836.

CHAPTER 5

The Infection Control Committee

R. Todd Wiblin, MD, MS, Richard P. Wenzel, MD, MSc

Abstract

Hospital epidemiologists translate their expertise into institutional policy and gain the support of administrators through the infection control committee. Committee members have the important task of helping disseminate information to all important hospital constituencies. The infection control team can facilitate its goals by properly preparing committee members for the meeting. A well-educated committee will approve policies efficiently. The committee should periodically reassess its accomplishments and goals. This chapter will explore the workings of the infection control committee and suggest strategies that the hospital epidemiologist can use to make the committee an asset rather than a hindrance.

Introduction

Healthcare has become such a big business that an administrative bureaucracy has evolved to manage its resources and actions. The infection control committee is the arm of hospital administration that regulates most infection control activities throughout the organization. While the Joint Commission on Accreditation of Healthcare Organizations (JCAHO) no longer requires hospitals to have an infection control committee, the committee retains importance at many institutions. A well-run committee facilitates the work of the hospital epidemiologist; a poorly run committee will, at best, waste the time of infection control personnel (and other busy people), and at worst, hinder the implementation of needed infection control actions.

Purpose of the Infection Control Committee

You must first recognize what the committee can and cannot do. The committee's purpose is to ratify the ideas of the infection control team and to disseminate infection control information. The committee provides the political support that empowers the infection control team to implement infection control policies. Committee members who understand the policies will take critical information to their work areas where they can relay it to peers. However, the committee itself does not do the actual work of infection control and rarely generates independent ideas. For example, many committee members may be unaware that the incidence of vancomycin-resistant enterococci (VRE) is rising nationwide. Likewise, most members will not have time to research extensively risk factors for VRE or to develop a detailed infection control policy regarding antibiotic-resistant organisms. They can, however, learn about VRE and your newly proposed policy at the committee meeting. Subsequently, they can explain to their peers why infection control personnel have recommended that staff wash their hands with chlorhexidine and obtain surveillance stool cultures from patients.

Committee Membership

The hospital epidemiologist should recruit people who can help the committee meet its goals. The committee should include a core group that does the real day-to-day work of infection control. This infection control "team" includes the hospital epidemiologist, the infection control professionals, the clinical microbiologist, and the employee health director—the people who perform surveillance, analyze trends, and develop policies. The other members should represent the important constituencies of the healthcare organization: administration, nursing, family practice, internal medicine, surgery, pediatrics, pharmacy, and central services. Depending on the structure of the individual institution, the committee may benefit from representatives from other areas, such as respiratory therapy or laundry services. All members should ideally be very interested in infection control, wield authority in their areas, and communicate, if not charismatically, at least tactfully. The total size of the committee is unimportant. The core group, however, should not grow beyond six or seven, because larger groups hinder day-to-day consensus building.

Committee Chair

The chair of the infection control committee is usually the hospital epidemiologist. He or she is often an infectious disease specialist or medical microbiologist with training in infection control. A clinician may be better able to command the respect of staff physicians than someone from a non-clinical department. Regardless, continuity in leadership over time is necessary to preserve the infection control program's goals.

Logistics

The committee should meet at a set time and place monthly or quarterly, on the same week of the month and day of the week. This routine will help committee members remember the meeting. The setting should be comfortable. Committee members may be more likely to attend if a meal or refreshments are provided. The committee members should receive the agenda several days in advance to remind them of the meeting and to allow them to prepare for it.

Getting Things Done

To keep things running smoothly in today's bureaucratic environment, the hospital epidemiologist must prepare extensively before each meeting. You must know who is in the local power structure and gain their support ahead of time. In particular, you must know which administrator has the authority to make decisions. If you meet with these administrators one-to-one in a non-threatening venue, you will often be able to implement policies more readily. Infection control personnel must remember to convey their messages in the language of the administrators, and to explain clearly the benefits for important organizational constituencies. For example, when developing an infection control policy for varicella, you should delineate for the administrators the financial and legal hazards of an exposure, including estimates of how much work time employees lose and the resources expended to contain an outbreak. Administrators will be particularly interested in cost/benefit analyses that compare the costs of furloughing employees with the costs of vaccinating seronegative healthcare workers. Once you have gained the administration's approval, you should have the authority to implement the policy as needed.

In addition to discussing issues with the administration, the hospital epidemiologist should consult with persons who have expertise in the area addressed by the proposed policy. You would be wise to have the experts present relevant background data at the infection control meeting. By including them in the policy formation process, you will not only learn useful information, but you will also assure the experts that you will not invade their turf. Thus, they will be more likely to support your position. For instance, having the local mycobacteriologist as an ally is very important when you propose a new tuberculosis (TB) isolation policy. Similarly, when developing a plan to stop the spread of VRE on the bone marrow transplant unit, you should involve the medical director of the unit.

Finally, you should identify people who are likely to oppose your goal. If you talk with opponents individually in a non-confrontational manner before the meeting, you may disarm them and win them to your viewpoint. If this strategy is unsuccessful, you should enlist allies who are not members of the infection control team, but who can provide counter arguments at the meeting. If you take this approach, infection control committee members are less likely to think you are forcing them to approve unpopular policies.

Minutes

The minutes of the infection control committee are a legal document. They record the topics that the committee discussed and the policies or procedures that the committee approved. An appointed secretary should compose them with care. Copies should be sent to committee members for review. The committee should approve the minutes at the next scheduled meeting.

Meeting Agenda

You should structure the agenda so that the meeting will finish within its allotted time. "Old business" should be limited to updates on items of ongoing interest, for example, outbreaks, TB, or antibiotic-resistant organisms. "New business" at each meeting should include a brief summary of surveillance data. Overly detailed reports of infection rates usually do not interest the full committee. One way to retain members' attention is to highlight a specific topic during each meeting. For example, infection control personnel can discuss changes in antibiotic susceptibility patterns of important nosocomial pathogens, or review rates of particular infections, such as *Clostridium difficile* colitis. If available, reports from the state or local area health department may provide additional insight into trends seen within an institution.

Finally, you should discuss new policies or procedures and substantial revisions to current protocols. You should try to approve one new policy or procedure per meeting. However, do not schedule a policy for discussion until your team has thoroughly reviewed the literature and sought the advice of clinical experts. When your team has synthesized all pertinent information, you should present the options to the committee. Concise handouts with excellent illustrations will often clarify your recommendations. Once the committee has heard and discussed all of the data, the members should immediately vote on the policy. We recommend that you deal with items requiring the committee's approval in a single meeting, because meetings easily bog down if debate drags out from month to month. The infection control team can prevent many of these impasses by working to gain the support of committee members before the meeting.

Reassessment

The infection control committee should periodically reassess its performance. Infection control team members should list and evaluate their accomplishments and state their priorities. You should not be afraid to ask hard questions. Has the TB isolation policy reduced exposures? Have the rates of VRE bacteremia increased? Does your surveillance system identify surgical site infections in patients undergoing operative procedures as outpatients? Has the committee passed 12 new or revised policies over the past 12 months? During this process, you should also eliminate policies and procedures that are inefficient or no longer necessary. If the infection control team critically assesses its priorities and performance, it can adapt to changes in the healthcare environment. Revitalized, it will be able to greet the new challenges with insight and energy.

Recommended Reading

Ayliffe GA. Infection control in the United Kingdom. *Chemotherapy.* 1988;34:536-540.

Brachman PS, Haley RW. Nosocomial infection control: role of the hospital administrator. *Rev Infect Dis.* 1981;3: 783-784.

Haley RW. The "hospital epidemiologist" in US hospitals, 1976-1977: a description of the head of the infection surveillance and control program. *Infect Control.* 1980;1: 21-32.

Shands JW, Jr, Wenzel RP, Wolff SM, Eickhoff TC, Fields BN, Jackson GG. Hospital epidemiology and infection control: the changing role of the specialist in infectious diseases. *J Infect Dis.* 1982;144:609-613.

Wenzel RP. Management principles and the infection-control committee. In: Wenzel RP, ed. *Prevention and Control of Nosocomial Infections.* 2nd ed. Baltimore, Md: Williams & Wilkins; 1993:207-213.

CHAPTER 6

Developing Policies and Guidelines

Patrick J. Brennan, MD, Elias Abrutyn, MD

Abstract

Practice guidelines are proliferating in the era of managed care. Hospital epidemiologists frequently are asked to author guidelines for infection control. The greatest challenge in the process is not writing the guidelines but implementing them. This chapter offers practical advice on which topic to select and on how to develop and implement guidelines.

Introduction

Practice guidelines, critical pathways, and policies are overlapping terms used to denote documents that describe the parameters within which clinical practice should occur in a healthcare organization. The hospital epidemiologist long has held the responsibility to create infection control guidelines at the institutional level, and this role is more important than ever in the era of managed care and cost containment.

The Institute of Medicine has defined practice guidelines as "systematically developed statements to assist practitioner and patient decisions about appropriate healthcare for specific clinical circumstances."[1] The preferred term, "practice guideline," implies a nonbinding document that allows the practitioner to exercise clinical judgment; thus, we will use this term throughout this discussion. In contrast, "policy" suggests a binding rule that eliminates clinical judgment and thus carries undesirable overtones.

Although guidelines are not new, they have proliferated in recent years. The American Medical Association has published a directory of approximately 1,500 practice guidelines.[2] Hospitals, federal agencies, insurers, and physician organizations have developed guidelines to satisfy a variety of agendas.[3-5] A physician's age and practice type affect the physician's knowledge of the guidelines and trust in their content. Also, physicians generally judge guidelines disseminated by professional organizations as more credible than those disseminated by insurers.[6] The greatest challenge for the guideline writer, then, is not identifying a topic or writing the document, but developing one that is credible and widely implemented after the writing is finished.

Rationale

In general, the object of guidelines is to reduce variations in practice to achieve an organization's desired outcomes.[4] The benefits of practice guidelines include medical education, establishment of a better standard of care, better clinician compliance with recommended practices, and improved clinical results.[7] By creating practice guidelines, the hospital epidemiologist will help the institution establish performance standards, comply with regulatory requirements, meet accreditation requirements, and improve the quality of care while decreasing costs.

Creation of Institutional Performance Standards

Most industries establish standards for workers to minimize variations in performance that may lower quality and increase cost. Such standards also permit industry to measure productivity and outcomes. Examples of such standards in the healthcare industry are the hospital infection control manual and departmental infection control guidelines. The person in the organization with infection control oversight, the hospital epidemiologist or infection control professional, should write and revise the manual. Each department should write and implement department-specific guidelines, frequently with input from the hospital epidemiologist.

Compliance with Regulatory Requirements

Laws, local ordinances, regulations, and standards of municipal, county, state, and federal authorities influence activities in healthcare institutions. As a result, the hospital epidemiologist may need to develop guidelines to help clinicians comply with extramural regulations. The hospital epidemiologist may need to write institutional guidelines on the reporting of communicable diseases, consent requirements for HIV antibody testing, constraints on the professional activities of healthcare workers with bloodborne diseases, reporting of communicable diseases to emergency services personnel under the Ryan White Act, and procurement of cadaveric organs for transplantation.

Meeting Accreditation Requirements

The Joint Commission on the Accreditation of Healthcare Organizations (JCAHO) currently requires that hospitals have written infection control policies and documentation of procedures needed to conduct the organization's mission effectively.[8] The infection control officer should ensure that each of these documents exists. Examples of the required documentation include a definition of the program for nosocomial infection surveillance, prevention, and control; departmental infection control guidelines; and the institutional statement of the infection control officer's authority.

Achieving Quality Improvement and Cost Containment

As purchasers of healthcare services capitate care, healthcare organizations find it increasingly important to channel patients through prescribed regimens to achieve desired clinical and financial outcomes. Practice guidelines and critical pathways have become important tools to reduce lengths of stay and costs. Physicians have not viewed as credible the guidelines established by insurers for this purpose.[6]

Developing Practice Guidelines

Woolf has described methods that the hospital epidemiologist can use to develop practice guidelines (Table 6-1).[4] Each approach has inherent strengths and weaknesses. The consensus approach favors speed but may lack validity. Evidence-based development introduces scientific rigor, but its role may be limited in areas where evidence to support a guideline is lacking. Explicit guideline development combines elements of several approaches to specify the benefits and costs of interventions. The analyses may exceed institutional capabilities. Figure 6-1

TABLE 6-1

METHODS FOR PRACTICE GUIDELINE DEVELOPMENT[4]

- Informal consensus: the opinion of experts
- Formal consensus development: National Institutes of Health Consensus Statement Model
- Evidence-based: grounded in scientific evidence
- Explicit guideline development: uses scientific evidence and analytic methods to assess the benefits, harms, costs, and probability of various outcomes

shows a schematic of the process that one institution used to develop practice guidelines. An evidence-based approach predominates, but the process also includes elements of consensus development.

Selecting a Topic for Guideline Development

To ensure a successful outcome, the hospital epidemiologist must choose the right topic. Clinicians may suggest topics and advise the hospital epidemiologist on specialty and subspecialty concerns. Clinicians who recently have joined the staff can provide fresh insights into long-entrenched practices. However, in some matters, the hospital epidemiologist will have no choice of topic. A law, federal mandate, or a Type I citation from JCAHO may force the issue. In discretionary areas, the hospital epidemiologist should choose topics carefully. Although cost containment may be the impetus for a guideline, above all else, the hospital epidemiologist must focus on improving the quality of care. If the epidemiologist determines that a standard clinical procedure is an unnecessary intervention, then a new practice guideline could improve quality and reduce costs.

The hospital epidemiologist should use infection control data to identify areas of need. Infection rates that exceed benchmarks are good targets for improvement through guideline development. If the hospital's infection rates exceed published rates or rates from similar hospitals, the epidemiologist has a powerful tool to convince staff of the need for a change. For example, our rates of bloodstream

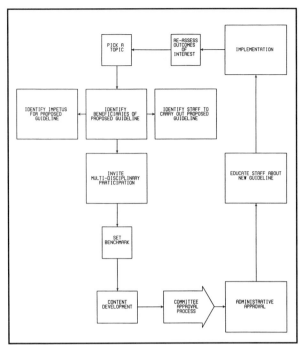

FIGURE 6-1. Schematic of the process used by one institution to develop practice guidelines.

infections were higher than those published by the National Nosocomial Infection Surveillance System at the Centers for Disease Control and Prevention. When we began examining the cause of our high rates, a new staff member expressed concern that the methods for inserting and maintaining central venous catheters were inadequate. After we observed the practices in our intensive care unit and compared these practices with those at peer institutions, we formed a multidisciplinary committee that developed a new practice guideline. The guideline standardized insertion and care of central venous catheters, significantly reducing bloodstream infection rates.

Tackling Larger Issues

Ensuring compliance with infection control practices and developing guidelines for insertion and care of central venous and urinary catheters may seem daunting, but the results of improved practices in important areas are likely to have a greater impact on quality of care than smaller, more easily achieved

TABLE 6-2
SUGGESTED TOPICS FOR PRACTICE GUIDELINE
DEVELOPMENT

Device Use

- Management of bladder catheters
- Management of ventilatory support equipment
- Sterilization of critical devices
- Maintenance of sterilizers

Patient Care

- Discontinuation of isolation precautions
- Triage of patients suspected of having tuberculosis
- Isolation of patients suspected of having tuberculosis
- Postoperative wound care
- Administration of nutritional supplements

Cost-Effectiveness

- Appropriate use of specific microbiology tests
- Appropriate blood culture techniques

Antimicrobial Therapy

- Indications for vancomycin use
- Perioperative antimicrobial prophylaxis

Procedures

- Central venous catheter insertion practices
- Operating room traffic control
- Performance of cough-inducing procedures

Quality Improvement

- Sterile production of pharmaceuticals

Regulatory Requirements

- Respirator training program
- Notification of emergency medical personnel following exposure to transmissible diseases

objectives. Your organization will measure your credibility by your choice of appropriate targets for practice guideline development. Don't squander your credibility on small matters. We list possible topics for practice guidelines in Table 6-2.

Answering the Important Questions and Choosing the Participants

Guideline writers can avoid problems by answering several questions before sitting down at the word processor. First, what is the impetus for the guideline? Second, who is likely to benefit from the guideline? Third, who will execute the new

guideline? If the impetus is a need that is widely perceived and improvement will benefit patients and staff, there may be a groundswell of support. If the impetus for action is unclear or the benefits uncertain, you may have chosen the wrong topic and should reconsider. At the very least, you may have difficulty finding support for such an undertaking. The answers to these questions could help the hospital epidemiologist to identify individuals who should participate in the process.

Any change in practice is likely to encounter opposition, but some changes are more difficult to promote than others. Mandates of regulatory agencies, such as the Bloodborne Pathogens Standard of the Occupational Safety and Health Administration, are among the most difficult policies to translate into hospital practice. People at any level of an organization may oppose mandates. Healthcare workers may find mandates onerous to execute; administrators find them costly to implement; and patients may feel isolated by them. Infection control officers may have little personal enthusiasm for such mandates, yet must bring the hospital into compliance with the new rule. Although professional organizations can pressure agencies over mandates that lack credible scientific underpinnings, in the end, the hospital epidemiologist must protect the interests of the institution. Hospital epidemiologists defy such mandates at their own peril. The hospital epidemiologist may have to convince administrators to implement expensive yet unproven measures so that the hospital can avoid substantial fines. Both staff and administrators must recognize that failing to comply may lead to such fines.

Hospital epidemiologists can learn from the federal mandate process and prevent institutional resistance to practice guidelines by bearing in mind our third question, "Who executes the policy change?" Although federal mandates allow for a period of public comment and debate, the scale of a national rule-making process leaves the clinicians who are responsible for implementing the mandate feeling isolated and disempowered. Clinicians then view the final rule as an arbitrary pronouncement that is distant from the reality of clinical practice. At the institutional level, we have learned by hard experience that guideline pronouncements grounded in sound principles of infection control flounder unless key individuals in the departments buy into the process. The hospital epidemiologist can achieve "buy in" by actively including opinion leaders in the development process. The resulting committee process may be time-consuming, but the benefits far outweigh the burdens. Staff in key departments will accept, understand, and cooperate with a guideline that their departmental leaders or deputies helped to develop. Table 6-3 lists key individuals who helped to develop our infection control guideline for central venous catheter insertion. Participants in the process become resources who bring information to the table, as well as educators who take the final product back to their constituents.

After selecting key representatives to initiate guideline development, the hospital epidemiologist must establish a timetable. Open-ended processes punctuated by monthly meetings may drag on indefinitely without ever gaining momentum. Meetings held at shorter intervals (every 2 weeks) allow participants sufficient time to complete the necessary intermeeting homework and to build momentum and enthusiasm for the objective. The hospital epidemiologist should ask various individuals to obtain needed data and to present these data at subsequent meetings.

The Content

Choosing Benchmarks

A guideline should describe in clear, straightforward language *one* of an organization's processes. Overreaching content tends to tread on other policies and practices, creating confusion. The approach to developing the content of the guideline

TABLE 6-3

KEY PARTICIPANTS IN DEVELOPMENT OF INFECTION CONTROL CENTRAL VENOUS CATHETER PRACTICE GUIDELINE

- Hospital epidemiologist
- Physician directors
    Cardiac care unit
    Medical intensive care unit
    Surgical intensive care unit
    Neonatal intensive care unit
- Chief residents
- Trauma surgeon
- Nurse administrator
- Infection control professional
- Nurse managers
- Staff nurses
- Medical intensivist
- Nurse clinical specialists

(see Table 6-1) will vary by institution, by the topic chosen, and by the availability of scientific evidence and local experts. If you present a document without a supporting bibliography, clinicians may respond: "Show me the data." Guidelines should cite pertinent literature; institutional experience, if appropriate; and the consensus of local or national expert panels. This information will educate the users of the document and may mollify some of those resistant to change. The necessary elements are described below.

Introduction. This section provides the rationale and background for the document and sets out the objectives for creating the guideline and the factors leading to its development. The introduction may contain a glossary of key terms used in subsequent sections.

Scope. This section defines the circumstances and individuals to whom the guideline may apply.

Responsibility. This section identifies the individuals who will ensure compliance and enforce the policy.

Implementation. This section should contain an unambiguous, step-by-step description of the process and a list of equipment essential to the process. Accompanying diagrams may clarify procedures.

Appendices. Some guidelines may overlap areas in which separate or complementary guidelines already exist. Take care not to contradict these preexisting documents (eg, nursing practice manuals). If you cross-reference these documents or include them as appendices to the guideline, you may avoid confusion.

Conclusion. At the end of the guideline, you should list the address and the telephone number of people who can answer questions or clarify the document. When the appropriate hospital authority, usually the hospital epidemiologist, signs and dates the guideline, the document is complete. Remember to review guidelines periodically to ensure that they still are current. For example, the JCAHO requires that policies and procedures be reviewed periodically. Document the review process and enter the documentation in the infection control committee minutes.

Implementation

Memos, Movies, and More Work

Once the guideline has been written, the real work has just begun. Nothing is more frustrating than to have spent months developing a sound piece of work and then to have it lie dormant and unnoticed in a policy manual. The first step in implementing the written document is the administrative approval process. Stepwise approval, starting with the hospital infection control committee and moving upward to medical staff committees and ultimately hospital administration, is necessary before implementation can occur. You very well may have to appear at one or more committees to answer questions and ensure smooth passage.

If the guideline is to have a life after it is approved, the institution must intensively educate its personnel. Memos announcing the new guide-

line are of little value, as staff seldom read and never remember them. Inservice educational programs are essential for all staff members who fall within the scope and responsibility of the guideline but traditional lecture techniques often fall short on content, given the time limitations of such workday presentations. Demonstrating new procedures, either in person or by videocassette, may be more effective. Strategically placed posters and repeated presentations for house staff as they move from one intensive care unit to another may reinforce the changes. Nursing staff development educators are ideal persons with whom to conduct inservice programs for nurses. Educating physicians is more difficult because, traditionally, they have practiced autonomously. Perhaps more important than any of these tools is the support of hospital and departmental leaders. If an intensive care unit director makes the reduction of infection rates a high priority, it is likely to translate into practice.

Measuring the Outcome

The coin of the realm in healthcare is improving performance. Therefore, successful implementation of the new practice guideline is not the final step in the process. To bring the process full circle, institutions continuously must measure the outcome of interest and determine any impact of the guideline. The outcome of interest may be bloodstream infection rates, as in the example of a central venous catheter insertion guideline. To determine whether the practice guideline or the "Hawthorne Effect" improves rates, the hospital epidemiologist will need to measure compliance. For example, the epidemiologist could directly observe practice. If the guideline introduced a new product, the epidemiologist could assess how often healthcare workers use the product.

Conclusion

Practice guidelines will increase in importance as managed care strengthens its hold on the healthcare marketplace. Currently, many physicians remain unfamiliar with the content of guidelines, although aware of their existence.[6] Healthcare epidemiologists will be challenged to write clear, credible guidelines that are grounded in science and to bring them into practice through persistent and creative peer education.

References

1. Institute of Medicine. In: Field MJ, Lohr KN, eds. *Clinical Practice Guidelines: Directions for a New Program*. Washington, DC: National Academy Press; 1990.

2. American Medical Association. *Directory of Practice Parameters: Titles, Sources, Updates*. Chicago, Ill: Annual Meeting; 1992.

3. Woolf SH. Practice guidelines: a new reality in medicine, 1: recent developments. *Arch Intern Med*. 1990;150:1811-1818.

4. Woolf SH. Practice guidelines: a new reality in medicine, 2: methods of developing guidelines. *Arch Intern Med*. 1992; 152:946-952.

5. Audet AM, Greenfield S, Field M. Medical practice guidelines: current activities and future directions. *Ann Intern Med*. 1990;113:709-714.

6. Tunis SR, Hayward RS, Wilson MC, et al. Internists' attitudes about clinical practice guidelines. *Ann Intern Med*. 1994;120:956-963.

7. Woolf SH. Practice guidelines: a new reality in medicine, 3: impact on patient care. *Arch Intern Med*. 1993;153:2646-2655.

8. Joint Commission on Accreditation of Healthcare Organizations. Surveillance, prevention, and control of infections. *Comprehensive Accreditation Manual for Hospitals. The Official Handbook*. Oakbrook Terrace, Ill: JCAHO; 1996:IC1-IC-25.

CHAPTER 7

Intramural and Extramural Communication

Ludwig Lettau, MD, MPH

Abstract

Effective communication with hospital administrators, with medical staff, with the media, and with peers in healthcare epidemiology is a vital skill for hospital epidemiologists. This chapter will describe a number of practical ways to improve such communication based on the author's experience, on interviews with senior members of the Society for Healthcare Epidemiology of America, and on relevant articles from the literature.

Introduction and Methods

Hospital epidemiologists must communicate regularly with hospital administrators, medical and nursing staff, and staff in other hospital departments. In addition, many hospital epidemiologists also must communicate with peers at scientific meetings and with collaborators from outside institutions, such as other hospitals, medical schools, local and state health departments, and federal agencies such as the Centers for Disease Control and Prevention. Finally, hospital epidemiologists also might need to speak with members of the press or the public. Thus, effective communication is a vital skill for a hospital epidemiologist.

Basic principles of effective communication can be found in textbooks or may be taught in school, but there is little in the literature that specifically addresses the needs of a hospital epidemiologist. Articles, books, and courses may help hospital epidemiologists improve their communication skills. However, one usually learns to communicate more effectively through hard experience. Therefore, to provide a broader background for this chapter, I interviewed eight senior members of the Society for Healthcare Epidemiology of America (SHEA). These experts provided practical advice about improving intramural communication and dealing with the media. They also suggested ways to approach problems in presenting and publishing epidemiologic data. I collated their responses, my own experience, and relevant articles from the literature to form the basis of this chapter.

Intramural Communication

Hospital Administration

One of the hospital epidemiologist's vital functions is to communicate with administrators. The hospital epidemiologist must communicate regularly and effectively with administrators not only to solve ongoing problems such as outbreaks, but also to maintain resources for the infection control program—perhaps even the salaries of the infection control professional and the hospital epidemiologist.

The hospital epidemiologist needs a clearly defined chain of reporting and access to the chief administrator. This chain usually includes an administrative representative who is a member of the infection control committee and who communicates routine committee business to upper level administrators. However, for more important or urgent issues, the hospital epidemiologist needs more direct access to the chief administrator. Ideally, the hospital epidemiologist would be able to speak directly to the chief administrator but, if necessary, could gain access through the medical director or through a senior hospital administrator.

New hospital epidemiologists should meet with key hospital administrators at the beginning of their tenure to lay the foundation for their relationship and to discuss mutual expectations. The hospital epidemiologist should "market" himself or herself actively during regular meetings with the chief administrator. In this manner, the hospital epidemiologist will maintain visibility, and such meetings also serve to reinforce the utility of the infection control program. The frequency of these meetings will vary depending on the needs of the individual administrator and of the infection control program. The hospital epidemiologist also must be aware that administrators do not like surprises. Thus, when the hospital epidemiologist identifies an important problem, he or she should talk with the administrators at the outset and as often as necessary to inform them of pertinent developments.

Medical Staff

Successful interaction with the medical staff often requires both delicate and complex communication. The hospital epidemiologist should have some credibility with the medical staff because of his or her dual role as a clinician. However, some skeptical and defensive physicians may construe the hospital epidemiologist to be an unfriendly policeman, who enforces unpopular policies and procedures. Others might consider the hospital epidemiologist to be a spy who uses surveillance activities or special investigations to collect data that potentially are biased and damaging. Such perceptions by physicians may be discomforting, particularly for hospital epidemiologists who also are infectious disease specialists and whose clinical livelihoods depend on consultations from the medical staff.

Before a controversial change in policies or the enforcement of unpopular existing policies, the hospital epidemiologist first should acquire or reaffirm the approval of all appropriate committees, including the infection control committee, the quality committee, and the pharmacy and therapeutics committee. Thereafter, the persons who enforce the changes or policies should emphasize that the infection control committee or other appropriate committees developed and approved the policies, which should serve to take some of the onus away from the hospital epidemiologist. In addition, the hospital epidemiologist might be able to avoid the role of enforcement agent by emphasizing the process of continuous quality improvement (CQI). This approach will be most useful in hospitals that currently have successful CQI programs. However, physicians remain paranoid about being deselected during this era of managed care and competition, and the paradigm shift to CQI may take many years to accomplish in hospitals that have not implemented this methodology. The hospital epidemiologist who uses the CQI approach in such a hospital could engender even a more violent response than he or she would have done simply by enforcing the policy.

The infection control committee minutes, which may be accompanied by summary reports of surveillance data, are the usual means by which the infection control staff communicate to the medical staff and to other hospital departments. The hospital epidemiologist or the infection control committee chairperson should review the report carefully and edit the minutes before they are distributed to ensure that the information is stated clearly and the data are accurate.

The hospital epidemiologist should help to determine the quantity of epidemiologic information that the infection control program communicates to various departments, as well as the method of data communication. For example, results of surveillance for surgical site infections could be presented on paper to the department of surgery, by an infection control professional or by the hospital epidemiologist. When choosing the appropriate vehicle, the hospital epidemiologist should consider whether the data or the associated recommendations might be misunderstood or will engender controversy. In addition, the hospital epidemiologist should consider whether the recipient of the data would respond better to a physician than to the infection control professional and whether the latter can respond effectively to strong criticism.

In general, the hospital epidemiologist should not confront medical staff directly about undesirable results, such as high infection rates, because the staff are likely to respond defensively. A gentler, more positive approach of alignment with the medical staff with the intent of helping and protecting them often is more productive. To help solve contentious problems, the hospital epidemiologist should arrange informal meetings (ie, without official minutes) in which he or she presents the data to the service chiefs or individual practitioners and then asks them to identify possible interventions. Hospital epidemiologists who act as facilitators not only reassure the clinicians that their input is necessary and valuable but also allow the persons most

familiar with the process to identify the interventions that are likely to work.

Attempts to correct an undesirable behavior, such as lack of compliance with handwashing, could stir up conflict with the medical staff. The infection control professional might be able to address and resolve such issues, but ultimately the hospital epidemiologist is responsible to deal with the situation if the infection control professional is not successful. If such problems arise, the hospital epidemiologist first should attempt to communicate his or her concerns privately to the offending medical staff. The hospital epidemiologist should state the rationale and recommendations sensitively and explicitly. If this approach is unsuccessful, the physician medical director for clinical affairs may need to mediate the discussion. If the medical director cannot resolve the conflict, the infection control committee, quality assurance committee, or medical care committee may need to address the problem. The hospital epidemiologist must be very careful not to send mixed, nonverbal messages by exhibiting less than scrupulous adherence to the practices that he or she (or the infection control professional) advocates. The hospital epidemiologist must be aware that the medical and nursing staff do observe the handwashing practices of infection control personnel.

Other Departments

The hospital epidemiologist and the infection control professionals regularly interact with a number of other hospital departments, including quality assurance (QA) or risk management. In fact, some hospital epidemiologists actively participate in or direct QA programs. The hospital epidemiologist should communicate immediately with the risk management department if he or she detects adverse nosocomial events that could lead to litigation. The hospital epidemiologist might wish to review infection-related lawsuits that are filed against the hospital. He or she should document such "freebies" and remind the administration of this valuable service to the hospital during the annual performance review. Hospital epidemiologists who help their hospitals save litigation costs may have an easier time justifying or increasing their salaries.

Extramural Communication

Interaction with the Mass Media

The general public has an insatiable appetite for news about healthcare. Newspapers and television stations frequently contact hospitals and ask for information about new developments and current issues in medical practice. The hospital should designate a spokesperson in advance who can handle routine media inquiries. However, the appropriate person to respond to a specific media request will vary depending on who is available and who has the needed expertise. The hospital epidemiologist often will be the spokesperson, especially for infectious disease issues, but public relations staff, the chief of the medical staff, the chief administrator, or a physician director for clinical affairs also could respond to inquiries. A wise hospital epidemiologist will be available to respond to routine media requests, so that he or she can establish some goodwill and rapport with the press. This relationship may be helpful at a later date in the event of an outbreak or other adverse nosocomial event. Routine requests from the media also allow the hospital epidemiologist an opportunity to educate the public and the media about epidemiology and infectious diseases.

The degree of media interest in nosocomial infections intensifies in direct proportion to the severity and communicability of the infection. In addition, some types of infection (such as "flesh-eating" group-A streptococcus) and involvement of well-known persons are hot topics. Large nosocomial outbreaks that cause deaths predictably will spark a media frenzy. Conflict, controversy, and criticism increase their audience, so that members of the media eagerly seek aspects of stories that provide these elements.

As a rule, the public relations department either should handle or assist in the response to all media inquiries involving the hospital. In particular, the hospital epidemiologist initially should refer all media requests for information about an outbreak or other adverse hospital-related event to the public relations department. The public relations department, the hospital epidemiologist, a hospital administrator, and other appropriate persons together then should formulate the hospital's response to such a query. The hospital may wish to proactively carefully craft a statement that is released to the media when it appears inevitable that they will publish or broadcast news of a major hospital-related adverse event or circumstance. The media often still will ask to interview the principals involved to obtain information not covered in the press release. If numerous groups request interviews, the hospital should coordinate a single press conference, so that the spokespersons can communicate the information efficiently and consistently. During major events, such as the hospitalization of a well-known person or an ongoing severe outbreak, key hospital personnel should meet as often as necessary to review events and coordinate their responses to minimize controversy and conflict. The patient's and the family's confidentiality always takes precedence over the public's right to know.

Particularly during crises, the hospital epidemiologist should not refuse a direct request for an interview, because the media then may seek answers from other sources who may not have the appropriate background or facts to be able to respond accurately. The press even may publish inaccurate information just to goad the hospital epidemiologist to respond. Hospital epidemiologists who must respond under such circumstances must remain honest and forthright, and should emphasize the positive aspects of the institution's response.

Physicians, as a rule, have not been trained to interact with the media. The hospital epidemiologist can do several things to prepare for meeting the press. First, he or she should know with whom he or she is dealing. Media representatives vary tremendously in their strengths and weaknesses, in their standards, and in their knowledge about the subject of the interview. The public relations department should be able to help the hospital epidemiologist learn more about the reporter. The hospital epidemiologist can prepare for the interview better if he or she knows what prompted the media interest (eg, a wire service story) and the slant or angle the reporter wants for the story. In addition, the hospital epidemiologist could inquire in advance about specific questions to be asked in the interviews.

Television stations usually use videotaped interviews rather than live interviews. They typically broadcast only short excerpts from a lengthy question-and-answer session. Therefore, the hospital epidemiologist must formulate in advance key points that he or she wishes to make. The bridging technique allows the hospital epidemiologist to use his or her response to a question as a way to introduce more important information. For example, he or she could say "Yes, I agree that patients can acquire infections in the hospital, but I think the most important lesson to be learned is..." The hospital epidemiologist should use simple language, and give short answers, preferably not more than 40 to 60 seconds long. Preparation and rehearsal will help, but practical experience will make the fourth interview go much better than the first one.

The press can use any statement out of context. Therefore, the hospital epidemiologist should not make off-hand comments that put the hospital in a bad light and should avoid inflammatory words such as "terrifying," "scary," or "deadly." The press certainly will broadcast colorful, pithy statements referred to as "sound bites" (eg, "The crowded emergency room was a tuberculosis time bomb"). Consequently, the hospital epidemiologist must stick to the facts and avoid humor, satire, and sarcasm. The hospital epidemiologist also should avoid medical jargon, but, if it is necessary to use medical terms such as "colonization" the term should be explained. Whenever possible, the hospital epidemiologist should use simple analogies that humanize the response. Hospital epidemiologists who express concern and compassion for patients will make a positive impression on the public.

During provocation, the hospital epidemiologist must remain calm and collected and should try to respond to negative questions with a positive answer. Reporters often use hypothetical questions to trap the interviewee. The hospital epidemiologist should answer such questions warily or not at all. If the reporter's information or interpretation is incorrect, the hospital epidemiologist should challenge that individual or correct the misinformation, but should not argue. The viewing public will remember appearance, tone of voice, and demeanor much longer than content. Unfortunately, style often outweighs substance on television.

The same principles apply when the hospital epidemiologist interacts with reporters for the print media, but these interviews usually proceed at a more leisurely pace. The hospital epidemiologist should try to avoid telephone interviews with local reporters. A face-to-face meeting allows both the interviewer and interviewee to discern emphasis and nuance better. Newspaper reporters generally are not permitted to let the interviewee review the story before it goes to press. If the hospital epidemiologist wants to review the article before it is published, he or she should discuss this before the interview, while he or she still can bargain. It is reasonable for the hospital epidemiologist to request to review an advance fax copy of direct quotes or at least to have the reporter read them to him or her over the telephone before the article is published. The hospital epidemiologist might consider recording interviews about particularly contentious issues or if there is a track record of prior misquotes.

Problems in Communication of Data

The hospital epidemiologist may encounter two types of conflicts when trying to communicate epidemiologic data to peers at a scientific meeting. First, collaborating investigators or institutions might dispute the right to present or publish the data. Second, hospital administrators, public relations personnel, or risk managers may want to suppress extramural communication or publication of hospital data, because they fear lawsuits, adverse publicity, or loss of managed care contracts.

When the hospital epidemiologist plans a collaborative study, he or she should specify various needs (eg, typing of bacterial isolates) and expectations to the collaborating investigator or institution. After the initial contact, he or she may want to write a letter that specifies his or her understanding of the collaborative effort, including publication plans. Despite careful planning and good intentions, collaborators still may dispute the relative degree of contribution to the study and about publication rights. As Robert Weinstein commented, "The sum of contributions claimed always exceeds 300%" (Oral communication, May 4, 1992)." In such a case, the hospital epidemiologist should settle up, based on what was done and whose work was most important. If the individuals who cared for the study patients did not contribute substantially to the investigation, they should not be listed as co-authors, but still can be included as part of the investigative group. This concession may allow the hospital epidemiologist to maintain a relationship with the clinicians while satisfying the current stringent guidelines for authorship.

Hospital administrators, risk managers, or public relations staff may oppose a hospital epidemiologist who wants to publish unflattering data, such as an outbreak or high infection rates. However, if the study legitimately contributes to the literature, helps other healthcare workers improve the quality of patient care, and decreases nosocomial infection rates, the hospital epidemiologist should publish the data. Hospital epidemiologists in teaching hospitals can plead academic freedom.

Risk managers and hospital attorneys are concerned that publication of sensitive data will precipitate lawsuits. If given the opportunity, hospital attorneys often want to edit manuscripts extensively to reduce the possibility of litigation. However, nosocomial infections are not a common cause of lawsuits, and I am unaware of any successful lawsuits prompted solely by the publication of an article in the field of hospital epidemiology.

If the administration is likely to oppose publication, the hospital epidemiologist could publish the manuscript without informing the hospital administration, knowing that it is easier to get forgiveness than permission. Because studies often are published months or years after the problem occurred, the local press and the administrators may miss it, unless the journal happens to be the *Journal of the American Medical Association* or the *New England Journal of Medicine*. However, if the hospital epidemiologist chooses this approach, he or she might win the battle but lose the war. The hospital epidemiologist also might consider disguising the institution's identity by excluding all references to the institution's name, bed size, city, etc. The journal editor may be able to help the hospital epidemiologist in this regard.

Conclusion

Effective communication is vital to the successful practice of hospital epidemiology. The hospital epidemiologist must balance the need to communicate clearly and simply with the need to give sufficient information accurately. This balancing act takes considerable effort, but the hospital epidemiologist will improve with practice, and the effort expended is always worthwhile.

Peter Sandman[1] has suggested some general communication guidelines for epidemiologists, including the following:

- Tell the people who are most affected by what you have found, and tell them first.
- Make sure the people understand what you are telling them, and what you think its implications are.
- Show respect for public concerns even when they are not "scientific."
- Involve people in the design, implementation, and interpretation of the study.
- Decide that communication is part of your job, and learn the rudiments—it is easier than epidemiology.[1]

Acknowledgments

The author interviewed eight SHEA members by telephone, all of whom contributed practical suggestions and advice to this chapter: Robert Weinstein, MD; Glen Mayhall, MD; Bryan P. Simmons, MD; Michael D. Decker, MD, MPH; John Weems, MD; William Scheckler, MD; Joel Ehrenkranz, MD; and John E. McGowan Jr., MD.

References

1. Sandman PM. Emerging communication responsibilities of epidemiologists. *J Clin Epidemiol*. 1991;44(1 suppl):41S-50S.

Recommended Reading

Bander MS. The scientist and the news media. *N Engl J Med*. 1983;308:1170-1173.

DeVries WC. The physician, the media, and the 'spectacular' case. *JAMA*. 1988;259:886-890.

Glanz K, Yang H. Communicating about risk of infectious diseases. *JAMA*. 1996;275:253-256.

Kleiman MB. The media and illness in a public figure: enough is never enough. *Pediatr Infect Dis J*. 1992;11:513-515.

Smith MS, Shesser RF. The emergency care of the VIP patient. *N Engl J Med*. 1988;319:1421-1423.

CHAPTER 8

Ethical Aspects of Infection Control

Loreen A. Herwaldt, MD

Abstract

This chapter describes ethical dilemmas faced routinely by infection control personnel and outlines the basic principles of ethics as applied to the practice of infection control and hospital epidemiology.

Introduction

Hospital epidemiologists and infection control professionals make countless decisions every day. In general, we do not make life and death decisions such as whether to withdraw life support or whether to withhold possibly life sustaining therapies. Few of our decisions require court injunctions or provide the fodder for eager journalists. We simply decide whether to isolate patients, whether to let healthcare workers continue to work, or whether to investigate clusters of infections—all very routine decisions in the life of anyone who practices infection control. These decisions are so ordinary that they could not possibly have any ethical implications. Or could they?

In fact, of the many decisions we make everyday in our practices as hospital epidemiologists and infection control professionals, most are merely

decisions of the sort training programs equipped us to make. But more than a few are also ethical decisions—which is to say, they compel us to choose between competing values. Such choices are rarely easy, and their intrinsic difficulty is not eased by the fact that few of us have received more than cursory training in ethics. Moreover, if we attempt to train ourselves, we find that essentially nothing has been written about the ethics of our specialty, infection control.

Common Infection Control Decisions That Have Ethical Aspects

We may easily overlook the ethical component of our everyday decisions; thus, we may misconstrue the decision confronting us, thinking that it is without ethical consequences when, in fact, ethical principles are at stake. Take, for example, the practice of isolating a patient colonized with a resistant organism. Isolating a patient constrains the patient's freedom of movement but protects the rights of other patients to be treated in an environment without unnecessary risk. Similarly, restricting healthcare workers with contagious diseases from patient care follows from epidemiologic data but also from the ethical concept of utility—which means that one should strive to maximize good outcomes and minimize harm. In such cases, we restrict the freedom of healthcare workers to obtain the greater benefit of protecting patients and fellow workers. Or, when stocking the hospital formulary, we consider the efficacy and cost of drugs, but we also balance the benefit of lower cost to the patient and the hospital against the risk of selecting resistant microorganisms and against physicians' freedom to prescribe any available drug.

Infection control personnel confront additional ethical dilemmas in many of their daily activities. For example, when managing an outbreak, infection control personnel must identify the source and mode of transmission of the offending pathogen and then intervene appropriately. This is simple enough, if the reservoir is a contaminated drain that is easy to replace or a nursing assistant with no political clout in the hospital. But what if the reservoir is a powerful physician with a huge ego, a hot temper, a large practice, and tremendous influence with the administration. Or what if the administration might think your recommendations are too expensive and excessive? Would you bow to the pressures and recommend interventions that in your mind are less than optimal, or would you risk the wrath of the physician or the administration and state your best advice regardless of the consequences?

Infection control personnel frequently must inform patients or healthcare workers that they have been exposed to an infectious disease. When the agent is varicella-zoster virus the problem is relatively simple. Yet infection control personnel must still consider ethical issues. Do you permit some susceptible employees to continue working if they wear masks, but restrict others? Or do you restrict all susceptible healthcare workers regardless of their position or their economic status? If you are very busy at work or have plans for the evening, do

you delay your response or ignore the exposure altogether? Other exposures, such as those to the hepatitis B virus, the human immunodeficiency virus, or to the Creutzfeldt-Jakob agent, provoke volatile emotions and raise challenging ethical questions. For example, what do you tell employees in the pathology laboratory who were not informed that the patient might have Creutzfeldt-Jakob Disease (CJD) and, therefore, did not use special precautions when they processed the brain tissue? Do you recall and resterilize instruments used for the implicated brain biopsy? Do you notify patients who subsequently had surgery and might have been exposed to instruments that were not sterilized in the manner recommended to kill the agent?

Other routine infection control decisions, such as whether to label the medical records or laboratory specimens of patients who have bloodborne diseases, have substantial ethical implications. Do you choose to not mark the records and specimens because the label would violate the patients' privacy and because employees should use standard precautions? Or do you choose to label these items, reasoning that employees can protect themselves more effectively if they know?

When your institution transfers a patient who is colonized with a resistant organism or who is infected with a bloodborne pathogen, do you provide this information to the receiving institution? If so, how do you maintain the patient's confidentiality? If not, do you think you have any responsibility to healthcare workers and patients at that institution?

If a colleague at another healthcare facility asks you for rates of nosocomial infections or for your policies regarding particular procedures, do you share the information to help another program provide good care? Or do you decline to provide the requested information in order to protect your own hospital from legal entanglements?

Infection control personnel are frequently asked to mediate disputes among different departments, between administrators and clinicians, or between unions and the hospital. Sometimes the party that approaches you hides the central dispute and simply requests information on the best way to manage "X." Unless you ask questions, you are unlikely to learn that more than one party is interested in your answer and that the background information given to you does not tell the entire story. To avoid falling into such a trap, you should, before responding, ask many questions, identify the controversy, review pertinent literature, and consider the ethical implications.

Infection control personnel must frequently make choices in the face of inadequate or conflicting data. Consequently, you may have difficulty choosing the most efficacious and ethically sound alternative. In such cases, you would be wise to document both the current state of knowledge and the controversial issues, and then choose the alternative that appears to maximize good outcomes. After choosing a course, you must monitor the results and be ready to alter your plan if you do not get the desired results.

As funds for healthcare are reduced, infection control personnel will have a more active role in evaluating products, assessing changes in practice, considering reuse of single-use items, and advising architects and engineers regarding construction projects. For example, infection control personnel must decide whether to recommend expensive products purported to lower rates of nosocomial infections, such as specialized intravenous and urinary tract catheters. Infection control personnel will also be asked with increasing frequency to answer questions such as, "Do we really need dedicated equipment for an isolation room?" "Can we let intravenous fluids hang longer?" "Can we store cardioplegia solutions for longer periods?" "Can we reprocess and reuse single-use electrophysiology catheters?" "Can we use plaster board instead of an expensive, impervious material for the walls in the cardiac catheterization laboratory?" "Can we

install fewer sinks?" "Do we really need to build all these negative pressure rooms?" To answer these questions, infection control personnel will need to consider not only the current literature, their hospital's needs, the costs of the various alternatives, and the legal requirements, but also the ethical implications of each possible solution. Furthermore, as the number of externally mandated policies and procedures multiply, infection control personnel may sense subtle pressure to apply policies inequitably—to save money or to limit inconvenience for prominent individuals.

As the number of patients and healthcare workers infected with the human immunodeficiency virus increases, infection control personnel are likely to receive information on the HIV-status of coworkers, neighbors, friends, or family members. One must use this information only for legally mandated infection control purposes. To do otherwise would be illegal and a serious ethical breach.

I hope this brief review has enabled you to see that ethical considerations abound within the practice of infection control. Clearly, ethics is not the esoteric discipline many of us misunderstand it to be. Not only is ethics relevant to our daily practice, but we cannot entrust our ethical decisions to others no matter whether they are professional ethicists, hospital managers, accountants, or lawyers.

The following is but a glancing introduction to the intricate intersection of ethics and infection control.

Ethical Principles in Hospital Epidemiology

Most discussions of medical ethics ignore the epidemiologist-population relationship to concentrate on the clinician–patient relationship.[1,2] Infection control personnel are frequently clinicians; however, we must differentiate their clinical and epidemiologic roles because their fiduciary duties do not always coincide. Medical ethics are "person-oriented," while epidemiologic ethics are "population-oriented" (Table 8-1).[3,4] Even so, the

TABLE 8-1
EPIDEMIOLOGIC VERSUS MEDICAL ETHICS—GENERAL
SIMILARITIES AND DIFFERENCES

Epidemiologic	Medical
Population-oriented	Person-oriented
Non-maleficence	Non-maleficence
Confidentiality	Confidentiality
Investigation and reporting	Privacy
Justice	Autonomy

TABLE 8-2
EPIDEMIOLOGIC VERSUS MEDICAL ETHICS—AS APPLIED
TO A PATIENT WITH A TRANSMISSIBLE DISEASE

Epidemiologic	Medical
Treat colonization or infection	Treat infection
Place signs on door	Maintain confidentially
Place labels on chart	Maintain patient's privacy
Confine patient in room	Maintain patient's freedom
Require patient to wear gowns and masks	Maintain patient's dignity
Require healthcare workers to wear gloves, gowns, and masks	Maintain human contact

fundamental principles of medical ethics apply to hospital epidemiology. Those principles are:

- Autonomy (respecting patient rights).
- Beneficence (doing good).
- Non-maleficence (doing no harm).
- Justice (equitable allocation of resources).[5,6]

However, the principles are applied according to the public health model,[6] which requires commitment to improving the health of populations, rather than to the patient care model.[7] Although both medical and epidemiologic ethics stress non-maleficence and confidentiality, medical ethics emphasizes privacy and epidemiologic ethics emphasizes investigation and reporting to protect the population. Furthermore, medical ethics stresses autonomy, whereas epidemiologic ethics seeks justice. Put more practically, medical ethics demands that the clinician treat an infected patient while maintaining the patient's confidentiality, privacy, dignity, freedom, and contact with other human beings (Table 8-2). In contrast, epidemiologic ethics might stress treating both infected and colonized patients to protect patients and healthcare workers. In particular cases, epidemiologic ethics might require healthcare workers to post labels on medical records and on the doors to the patients' rooms; patients to stay in their rooms except when going to essential tests, in which case they must wear gowns, gloves, and masks; and healthcare workers to wear gowns, gloves and masks to avoid direct contact with patients.

Consider, for example, the case of a dialysis nurse who is sexually active and a hepatitis B car-

rier. Writing from the perspective of clinicians, Perkins and Jonsen conclude that "fiduciary duties to this patient are very strong, and duties to her contacts appear to be much weaker...Therefore, there is little to argue for severe restrictions on this patient's professional and personal life."[8] They add, "the physician's obligations to protect others are weightier only when the harm is very certain, very severe, and to specific others."[8] However, after reviewing the same case, infection control personnel—responsible for protecting patients and healthcare workers against hospital-acquired adverse outcomes—might well conclude otherwise.

Given the complexity of such an ethical decision, the carefully detailed, stepwise approach to resolving these problems suggested by Soskolne might be useful:

1. Collect all relevant background data.
2. Identify the ethical dilemma.
3. Specify alternative courses of action.
4. Choose the alternative that best balances the competing values.
5. Act on that choice and evaluate the outcome.[9]

In the above case, the interested parties include the dialysis nurse, the patients treated in the dialysis center, other healthcare workers in the center, and the center's administrators. Clinical and epidemiologic data about hepatitis B, including the availability of an effective vaccine (not available when Perkins and Jonsen published the case), are pertinent. The critical ethical task balances the right of the nurse to work and to maintain privacy against the right of the patient to be treated under conditions that minimize transmission of disease. The alternative courses of action include: doing nothing, removing the nurse from patient care; transferring the nurse to a clinical unit where fewer invasive procedures are done; requiring the nurse to wear gloves for patient contact; and vaccinating all dialysis patients and healthcare workers.

Because the risk of transmission from a nurse to a patient during dialysis is minimal, removal of the nurse from the dialysis unit or from clinical work is unwarranted. However, requiring the nurse to wear gloves when inserting needles would be prudent. Vaccination of dialysis patients and healthcare workers would also be prudent (if only because of the general risk for hepatitis B in dialysis units). Additionally, although infection control personnel cannot control the private lives of healthcare workers, one could advise the nurse to use protection during sexual intercourse and could encourage the nurse to inform all sexual contacts that they have been exposed to hepatitis B.

Differences in the ethical obligations of clinicians and infection control personnel are especially pronounced, emotionally charged, and politically and legally complex when applied to individuals with HIV infections. Clinicians are responsible to treat the HIV-infected person while maintaining confidentiality. Infection control personnel are also obliged to protect confidentiality, but they must also protect the health of patients and healthcare workers. The latter responsibility might require one to collect and analyze data, report cases, notify contacts, place blood-precaution labels on charts and specimens, or furlough healthcare workers, all of which infringe on privacy rights and might harm those persons constrained from working.

Given the excessive demands on our time and our lack of explicit training in ethics, we might be tempted to leave ethical decisions to professional ethicists, yet that course is hardly practical because we make such decisions daily. Fortunately, not all decisions require the complex constructs proposed by Soskolne and others.

As an aid to understanding and resolving the ethical questions that face infection control personnel, we must develop case studies specifically for our profession. Programs in medical ethics have used such studies effectively, and hospital epidemiology programs would benefit from using case studies that present specific infection control problems. As we develop and struggle with case studies, we hone our ability to make ethical decisions and, perhaps as important, to recognize the ethical implications of everyday decisions. For example, the case discussed above could be modified to present other ethical dilemmas. The healthcare worker could be a gynecologist, who routinely does procedures in which a needle is guided by finger contact, increasing the risk of exposing patients to the healthcare worker's blood. To make the case yet more challenging, the healthcare worker could be an HIV-infected person who does not perform invasive procedures; or an HIV-infected healthcare worker who does invasive procedures with high risk for contamination by the healthcare worker's blood.

Ethical Codes

Ethical codes emphasize a profession's core values and may help guide decisions and behavior. To my knowledge, neither the Society for Healthcare Epidemiology of America nor the Association for Professionals in Infection Control and Epidemiology, the two societies concerned with infection control, have developed codes of ethics. Currently, at least three epidemiologic organizations are developing written ethical guidelines.[7] These efforts could help infection control personnel formulate an ethical code appropriate for their profession. To the guidelines

TABLE 8-3
ETHICAL OBLIGATIONS OF INFECTION CONTROL
PERSONNEL

I. Obligations to the Subjects of Research

To protect their welfare

To obtain their informed consent

To protect their privacy

To maintain confidential information

II. Obligations to Society

To avoid conflicts of interest

To avoid partiality

To widen the scope of epidemiology

To pursue responsibilities with due diligence

To maintain public confidence

III. Obligations to Funders and Employers

To specify obligations

To protect privileged information

IV. Obligations to Colleagues

To report methods and results

To confront unacceptable behavior and conditions

To communicate ethical requirements

Reprinted from Beauchamp TL, Cook RR, Fayerweather WE, et al. Appendix: ethical guidelines for epidemiologists. Journal of Clinical Epidemiology. *1991;44:1515-1695, with kind permission from Elsevier Science Ltd, The Boulevard, Langford Lane, Kidlington 0X5 1GB, United Kingdom.*

recommended by Beauchamp and colleagues for epidemiologists in general[7] (Table 8-3), I would add the following suggestions for hospital epidemiologists and infection control professionals:

V. Obligations to patients (inpatients and outpatients): to protect them from adverse outcomes of medical care, to investigate clusters of adverse outcomes, to maintain confidentiality, to identify and implement effective interventions, and to monitor the efficacy of the interventions.

VI. Obligations to the hospital: to investigate clusters of adverse outcomes, to identify and implement cost-effective interventions, to monitor the efficacy of the interventions, to avoid conflicts of interest when recommending products and equipment, to protect the health of employees, and to report and interpret results honestly.

A well-developed and clearly stated ethical code is an essential guide, yet it is also insufficient. A code of ethics cannot identify all of the ethical dilemmas that individuals will face in the course of their practice. Nor, despite the fond hopes of professional school administrators, does the graduation recitation of such a code inoculate us against temptation. Alone, an ethical code cannot ensure ethical behavior. It must be taught, learned, affirmed, and lived if it is to affect our practice. As William Diehl writes in *The Monday Connection: A Spirituality of Competence, Affirmation, and Support in the Workplace*:

Formal codes of ethics are hot items these days. [But one] thing is certain: any organization that requires all its employees to review and sign its ethics code each year, and then does nothing else to encourage high moral behavior, is wasting its time on the code.[10] Any institution that acts not as it preaches, wastes time, and also, at least implicitly encourages unethical behavior. Institutions reward the conduct they prize. It should be a warning to us that, at present, we are more likely to hear of inconsiderate behavior excused on the grounds of a colleague's brilliance than to hear an individual praised for making a difficult but ethically sound decision. No wonder—we were taught that intelligence and success within the system are the highest values, whereas perhaps none of our textbooks quoted Ralph Waldo Emerson's startling and humbling words: "character is higher than intellect."

As our financial and staff resources are stressed without limit and as the pressures under which we work intensify, temptation amplifies. Barbara Ley Toffler of Resources for Responsible Management states:

For many employees, being ethical is getting to be too risky—something they can't afford any more...The problem grows out of what I call the "move it" syndrome...That's when the boss tells a subordinate to "move it"—just get it done, meet the deadline, don't ask for more money, time, or people, just do it—and so it goes on down the line.

For American companies, this peril from within is as serious as outside threats from competitors. As more employers are forced to "move it," companies are increasingly vulnerable—legally, financially, and morally—to the unethical actions of decent people trying to [move it just to keep their jobs].[11]

To move it, we may find ourselves declining to issue appropriate sanctions in an outbreak because we are loath to alienate an important doctor or lose referrals from a powerful practice group. Or, fearing management anger over bad publicity and loss of revenue, we may decide against closing a ward affected by an outbreak. Under pressure to reduce budgets, we may approve questionable practices or eliminate effective infection control programs. During this time of uncertainty, we may be tempted to treat preferentially influential administrators or practice groups because they control our budgets or could recommend our programs' demise. We may be tempted to recommend a particular product because we have received grants from the company or we have purchased their stock. Or perhaps we condone the alteration of hospital records to keep accreditation. Finally, we may withhold information regarding resistant organisms so that we can transfer patients to other institutions and shorten their length of stay in our hospital.

Practical Advice

What can you as an individual hospital epidemiologist or infection control professional do? I would recommend that you think about your job and identify the most common questions that you answer. Once you have identified the questions, you can try to identify the ethical dilemmas presented by those decisions. You can then develop a plan for dealing with the issues before you face them again, as one can usually think more clearly

and dispassionately when not in the middle of a crisis. When designing such plans, you should obtain help, if necessary or prudent, from experts in medicine, law, ethics, or other appropriate disciplines.

I have described but a few of the manifold temptations confronting us. Against their appeals to our ambition or their playing on our fears, we have only our values and continual self-examination to rely on. Are we here to serve ourselves? Or to protect the health of patients and healthcare workers? Are we seeking beneficial knowledge? Or merely to keep our jobs during this tumultuous time?

As difficult as these questions may be, we must ask them or risk a gradual slide into unethical conduct. In the quiet of our consciences, we must grade our answers strictly, guarding against our formidable capacity for rationalization. We cannot afford to ignore the ethical aspects of infection control, because in neglecting ethics we risk the soul of our profession.

Acknowledgments

The author thanks Brenda A. Barr, Cheryl D. Carter, Jean M. Pottinger, and Marlene Schmid for sharing their invaluable ideas, and Patti Meier, Yasmina Berrouane, Constanze Wendt, R. Todd Wiblin, and Stefan Weber for critiquing the manuscript.

Note

Sections of this chapter are reprinted with permission from Herwaldt LA. National issues and future concerns. In: Wenzel RP, ed. *Prevention and Control of Nosocomial Infections.* 2nd ed. Baltimore, Md: Williams & Wilkins; 1993.

References

1. Jonsen AR. Do no harm. *Ann Intern Med.* 1978;88:827-832.
2. Last JM. Ethical issues in public health. In: *Public Health and Human Ecology.* East Norwalk, Conn: Appleton & Lange; 1987:351-370.

3. IEA workshop on ethics: health policy and epidemiology. IEA guidelines on ethics for epidemiologists. [American Public Health Association 1991 Section Newsletter] *Epidemiol.* 1990;Winter.

4. Beauchamp TL, Childress JF. *Principles of Biomedical Ethics.* 2nd ed. New York, NY: Oxford University Press; 1983.

5. Soskolne CL. Epidemiology: questions of science, ethics, morality, and law. *Am J Epidemiol.* 1989;129:1-18.

6. Herman AA, Soskolne CL, Malcoe L, Lilienfeld DE. Guidelines on ethics for epidemiologists. *Int J Epidemiol.* 1991;20:571-572. Letter.

7. Beauchamp TL, Cook RR, Fayerweather WE, et al. Appendix: ethical guidelines for epidemiologists. *J Clin Epidemiol.* 1991;44(1 suppl):151S-169S.

8. Perkins HS, Jonsen AR. Conflicting duties to patients: the case of a sexually active hepatitis B carrier. *Ann Intern Med.* 1981;94:523-530.

9. Soskolne CL. Ethical decision-making in epidemiology: the case study approach. *J Clin Epidemiol.* 1991:44 (1 suppl);125S-130S.

10. Diehl WE. *The Monday Connection: A Spirituality of Competence, Affirmation, and Support in the Workplace.* New York, NY: Harper Collins Publishers; 1991:85-135.

11. Toffler BL. When the signal is 'move it or lose it.' *The New York Times.* 1991; Nov.17:Sect F:13.

Recommended Reading

Chavigny KH, Helm A. Ethical dilemmas and the practice of infection control. *Law Med Health Care.* 1982;10:168-171,174.

Childress JF. Hospital-acquired infections: some ethical issues. In: Wenzel RP, ed. *Prevention and Control of Nosocomial Infections.* Baltimore, Md: Williams & Wilkins; 1987:49-55.

Cook RR. Code of ethics for epidemiologists. *J Clin Epidemiol.* 1991;44(1 suppl):135S-139S.

Feinleib M. The epidemiologist's responsibilities to study participants. *J Clin Epidemiol.* 1991;44(1 suppl):73S-79S.

Feinstein AR. Scientific paradigms and ethical problems in epidemiologic research. *J Clin Epidemiol.* 1991;44(1 suppl):119S-123S.

Gordis L. Ethical and professional issues in the changing practice of epidemiology. *J Clin Epidemiol.* 1991;44(1 suppl):9S-13S.

Hogue CJ. Ethical issues in sharing epidemiologic data. *J Clin Epidemiol.* 1991;44(1 suppl):103S-107S.

Last JM. Obligations and responsibilities of epidemiologists to research subjects. *J Clin Epidemiol.* 1991;44(1 suppl):95S-101S.

MacMahon B. A code of ethical conduct for epidemiologists? *J Clin Epidemiol.* 1991;44(1 suppl):147S-149S.

Sandman PM. Emerging communication responsibilities of epidemiologists. *J Clin Epidemiol.* 1991;44(1 suppl):41S-50S.

Schulte PA. Ethical issues in the communication of results. *J Clin Epidemiol.* 1991;44(1 suppl):57S-61S.

Stolley PD. Ethical issues involving conflicts of interest for epidemiologic investigators. A report of the Committee on Ethical Guidelines of the Society for Epidemiologic Research. *J Clin Epidemiol.* 1991;44(1 suppl):23S-24S.

Tancredi L, ed. *Ethical Issues in Epidemiologic Research.* Vol. 7 New Brunswick, NJ: Rutgers University Press; 1986.

Waters WE. Ethics and epidemiological research. *Int J Epidemiol.* 1985;14:48-51.

Weed DL. The merger of bioethics and epidemiology. *J Clin Epidemiol.* 1991;44(1 suppl):15S-22S.

SURVEILLANCE AND ANALYSIS

CHAPTER 9

Basics of Surveillance—An Overview

Jean M. Pottinger, MA, RN, CIC, Loreen A. Herwaldt, MD,
Trish M. Perl, MD, MSc

Abstract

Surveillance of nosocomial infections is the foundation of an infection control program. This chapter describes components of a surveillance system, methods for surveillance, methods for case-finding, and data sources. The epidemiology team is encouraged to use this background information as they design surveillance systems that meet the goals of their individual institution's infection control program.

Introduction

Surveillance is a dynamic process for gathering, managing, analyzing, and reporting data on events that occur in a specific population. As the foundation of hospital epidemiology programs, surveillance provides data that enable the epidemiology staff to determine baseline rates of nosocomial infections or other adverse events, detect changes in the rates or the distribution of these events, investigate significantly increased rates, institute control measures, and determine whether the interventions were effective. The epidemiology staff also can use surveillance data to monitor compliance with established hospital practices, detect areas where breaks in technique occur, evaluate changes in practice, and identify topics for further study.

Historically, the Centers for Disease Control and Prevention (CDC), accrediting agencies, and hospital administrators accepted surveillance for nosocomial infections as an important element of an infection control program. In 1974, the CDC initiated the Study on the Efficacy of Nosocomial Infection Control (SENIC) to examine whether infection control programs reduced rates of surgical site infection (SSI), pneumonia, urinary tract infection (UTI), and bacteremia. The SENIC investigators found that different combinations of infection control practices helped reduce infections at each site. However, surveillance was the only component essential for reducing infections at all four sites.[1]

Components of Surveillance

The building blocks of surveillance comprise collecting relevant data systematically for a specified purpose and during a defined period of time, managing and organizing the data, analyzing and interpreting the data, and communicating the results to those empowered to make beneficial changes. Surveillance should enable the epidemiology staff to identify new problems quickly and to intervene immediately after they determine the probable causes. In this chapter, we primarily will discuss surveillance for nosocomial infections. However, an epidemiology team could apply the same principles to surveillance for noninfectious adverse outcomes of care.

Definitions

Epidemiology staff first must identify the event and the population they will study. Next, the staff should develop written definitions that are exact, concise, and nonambiguous. Once they begin collecting data, infection control personnel must apply the definitions consistently. Ehrenkranz recently described the severe consequences that may occur if the staff collects data but does not use objective, written definitions.[2] Over a 3-year period, an infection control team recorded SSI rates of 3% to 11% for a particular surgeon. The infection control committee considered these rates excessive and repeatedly investigated this surgeon. After the surgeon decided to stop operating, the hospital administrator consulted with infection control experts. During their investigation, the consultants found that infection control staff did not use a specific definition of SSI. The consultants concluded that a surveillance error, not poor operative technique, accounted for the surgeon's high infection rates.

When writing definitions for their hospital, infection control personnel should review the definitions developed by the CDC.[3,4] Some hospitals can use the CDC's definitions exactly as they are written; other hospitals may be able to use some, but not all of the CDC's definitions; and other hospitals will need to modify the CDC's definitions or develop their own definitions. Regardless, the definitions should be the same or similar to those

developed by the CDC or those used by other investigators if the hospital wants to compare their results with those of other healthcare institutions.

An infection is classified as nosocomial if it was not present or incubating at the time the patient was admitted to the hospital. Thus, an infection is not considered nosocomial if it represents a complication or extension of an infectious process present on admission. In general, infections that occur more than 48 to 72 hours after admission and within 10 days after hospital discharge are defined as hospital-acquired. The time frame is modified for infections that have incubation periods less than 48 to 72 hours (eg, gastroenteritis caused by Norwalk virus) or longer than 10 days (eg, hepatitis A). SSIs are considered nosocomial if the infection occurs within 30 days after the operative procedure or within 1 year if a device or foreign material is implanted. Infections should be considered nosocomial if they are related to procedures, treatments, or other events that occur immediately after the patient is admitted to the hospital. For example, bloodstream infections associated with central venous catheters, pneumonia associated with mechanical ventilation, or UTIs associated with urethral catheterization should be considered nosocomial, even if the onset of infection occurs within the first 72 hours of hospitalization.

Collecting Data

Surveillance can be performed either concurrently or retrospectively. In concurrent surveillance, epidemiology staff collect data at the time the event occurs or shortly thereafter. This surveillance method allows infection control staff to review the medical record, assess the patient, and discuss the event with caregivers. Because the data are collected close to the time the event occurs, additional information may be available, such as ward log books and nursing reports, that is not a part of the medical record. In retrospective surveillance, the epidemiology team collects data after the patient is discharged. The two methods have similar sensitivities, but retrospective surveillance depends on the completeness, accuracy, and quality of the medical records.[5] Because data are collected after the event, retrospective surveillance does not identify problems as promptly as concurrent surveillance.

The epidemiology staff usually choose highly sensitive methods for case-finding, so that they will not miss important cases. However, they also should refine surveillance to increase specificity and thus reduce time wasted collecting irrelevant data. Because the surveillance system's purpose is to identify trends and potential problems, epidemiology staff should collect only the information they need to adequately analyze and interpret the data. If these data suggest a potential problem, the epidemiology team can design a more comprehensive study.

When an infection control program begins a new surveillance project, the staff periodically should look for flaws in the data, the collection tool, the data sources, and the surveillance process. In this manner, epidemiology personnel can identify problems or errors and correct them before reaching the end of the study. Infection control staff can determine the project's sensitivity and specificity by examining a random subset of medical records for a defined time period and comparing the number of events identified by this review with those identified by the usual surveillance system. In addition, epidemiology staff should validate the surveillance system when they add a new item, modify definitions, or change the personnel who collect the data.

Managing Data

Epidemiology personnel will be able to identify patterns and trends only if the data are organized in a meaningful fashion. Thus, epidemiology staff should record surveillance data systematically on a flow sheet or line-listing. Pads of columnar accounting paper may suffice as a database in small hospitals, but relational databases on computers are better solutions for larger hospitals. Once the data are in a database, infection control personnel easily can plot the numbers or rates over time to identify possible trends.

Analyzing Data

If the epidemiology team does not analyze their data, they have wasted the time, money, and effort they spent collecting and recording the data. Epidemiology staff should analyze the data promptly, because the purpose of surveillance is not merely to count and record infections but to identify problems quickly and make changes that reduce the risk of infection. Infection control staff should decide how frequently to analyze the data, based on the nature of the nosocomial event and the purpose of surveillance. They must strike a balance between analyzing the data frequently enough to detect clusters promptly and collecting data for a long enough period of time to ensure that variations in rates are real.

Epidemiology personnel commonly report only the number of events that occur in a specified time period (numerator). However, to compare data over time, one must calculate the incidence of the event being studied, which requires both a numerator and a denominator—the population at risk during the same time period. The following example illustrates why the epidemiology team must select the appropriate denominator. Suppose 10 patients in a hospital developed pressure sores during 1 month. If the hospital discharged 1,000 patients that month, the incidence rate of new pressure sores acquired in the hospital would have been 1%. However, if all 10 patients were on the medical service, which discharged 600 patients, the incidence rate of patients with pressure sores on the medical service would have been 1.7%. If 8 of the 10 patients developed pressure sores while in the medical intensive care unit (MICU), which discharged 90 patients, the incidence rate in the MICU would have been 9%. Thus, infection control staff can assess the true incidence of an event in a defined population only if they use a denominator that accurately represents the patients who are at risk of experiencing the event.

Similarly, if infection control personnel evaluate only summary reports of microbiology data, they may not recognize important trends in specific units. For example, the summary reports may obscure the fact that 90% of the *Pseudomonas aeruginosa* isolated from patients in the MICU are resistant to gentamicin, piperacillin, and cefotaxime. Stratton demonstrated that yearly summaries showed little variation in antimicrobial susceptibility patterns within the whole hospital. Focused microbiologic surveillance on specific units, in contrast, showed that the predominant pathogens and their antimicrobial susceptibility patterns differed among specialty units and the entire hospital.[6]

The infection control team can discern the endemic (baseline) rate after they have collected data for a period of time. Subsequently, the epidemiology staff could determine whether the current rates were substantially different from the baseline rate. In addition to calculating overall rates, the epidemiology staff can analyze the data further by calculating attack rates for specific nursing units, services, or procedures. The latter rates enable the staff to identify significant changes and important trends within subgroups of patients that might be missed if only the entire population were analyzed, as in the example of the pressure sores. When comparing data, either within an institution or with data from another institution, the epidemiologist must use comparable surveillance methods, definitions, and time frames. The epidemiology staff can use statistical tests of differences to determine whether the rates have changed significantly over time.

Finally, the epidemiology team must interpret the data. If the rate of a particular event increases substantially, the epidemiology staff should analyze the data thoroughly to determine if a problem exists. The analysis should include assessing whether the increase is statistically significant. However, even if the increase is not statistically significant, it may be clinically significant and warrant control measures. Furthermore, the team should assess whether the incidence of an event is acceptable. For example, even if the rate of SSI is stable, the incidence may be higher than that reported by comparable institutions or may be higher than it would be if the process of care was improved. A study by Classen et al demonstrated that examining the process of care can decrease the rate of SSI significantly.[7] In their study, the SSI rate for patients who received prophylactic antibiotics within the 2-hour period before surgery was significantly lower than for the patients who received their antibiotics either early (ie, 2 to 24 hours before surgery) or postoperatively (ie, more than 3 hours after the incision but less than 24 hours after surgery). Therefore, an infection control team that wants to decrease SSI rates in their hospital might want to review the time at which the prophylactic antimicrobial agents are given.

Communicating Results

Finally, the infection control staff must communicate the data to the persons who need the information and who have the power to authorize changes. The epidemiologist most likely will report on a regular basis to the infection control committee or to the quality or performance improvement committee. Epidemiology staff also should communicate with key persons on individual nursing units, in each clinical service, in the nursing administration, and in the hospital administration. In addition, infection control personnel may need to report their data to the education service, the intensive care unit committee, or the safety committee. When reporting data in any setting, epidemiology personnel must maintain confidentiality for patients and employees.

Simple reports that the target audience can understand in a few seconds (the amount of time usually given to a report at a busy committee meeting) are most effective. Epidemiology staff should consider using graphs and charts to display the data, because these formats present the important trends in pictures that can be grasped more quickly than text. Moreover, individuals who are unfamiliar with infection control issues may not understand the importance of a problem if they are presented only with the data. This is true particularly if the number of cases is small or the etiologic agent has not been discussed in the popular press. Thus, epidemiology staff should include their assessment and conclusions in the report, so that they can persuade clinicians or hospital administrators that corrective action is necessary to reduce the number of cases.

Surveillance for Nosocomial Infections

Data Sources

Many different sources provide information about patients with infections (Table 9-1). In addition, infection control personnel can obtain data from databases maintained by other departments such as medical records, pharmacy, respiratory therapy, admissions, risk control, and financial management. However, these databases were not designed for collecting data on infections. Therefore, the infection control team must determine whether those databases provide the actual data needed for surveillance and whether the data are complete and accurate. For instance, in one hospital, the infection control professional (ICP) who conducted surveillance used the daily surgery schedule to obtain the number and classification of operative procedures instead of using the list of completed operative procedures. The ICP was unaware that surgeons added, canceled, and changed operative procedures during the day. Thus, the denominator for calculating surgical site infection rates was inaccurate.

TABLE 9-1
DATA SOURCES FOR SURVEILLANCE SYSTEMS*

Patient Based
    Patient examination
    Clinical rounds
    Communication with staff
    Patient medical record
    Kardex review
        Treatments
        Wound-dressing changes
        Intravenous fluids
        Urinary catheter
        Surgery
        Isolation precautions
        Antibiotics
    Medication records
    Temperature records
    Radiology reports
Laboratory Based
    Bacteriology reports
    Mycology reports
    Parasitology reports
    Serology reports
    Virology reports
    Pathology reports
    Antimicrobial susceptibility patterns
Other Departments, Services, or Agencies
    Admissions department
    Operating suite
    Emergency department
    Outpatient clinics
    Risk control (for incident reports and other data)
    Employee health
    Home-care agencies
    Multicenter surveillance systems
    Local and state health departments

Adapted from Perl TM.[26]

Surveillance Methods

Each infection control team must determine which of many surveillance methods is best for their hospital. To help infection control personnel choose an appropriate approach, we have described five basic surveillance methods, and we have summarized their advantages and disadvantages (Table 9-2).

TABLE 9-2
ADVANTAGES AND DISADVANTAGES OF VARIOUS SURVEILLANCE METHODS FOR NOSOCOMIAL INFECTIONS*

Method	Advantages	Disadvantages
Hospital wide	Collects comprehensive data on all infections in the facility Establishes baseline infection rates Identifies patterns of infections Recognizes outbreaks early Increases visibility of ICP	Expensive, labor intensive, and time-consuming Yields excessive data Leaves little time to analyze data and initiate changes Detects infections that cannot be prevented Overall infection rate not valid for interhospital comparison
Periodic	Increases efficiency of surveillance Liberates ICP to perform other activities	Provides data only during periods in which surveillance is conducted May miss clusters or outbreaks during nonsurveyed periods
Prevalence	Documents nosocomial infection trends Identifies risk factors Relatively quick and inexpensive Identifies areas that need additional surveillance	Data collection may be tedious Must collect data in short time period Data are restricted to a specific time period Cannot compare prevalence rates with incidence rates Few studies on prevalence rates published May miss clusters or outbreaks
Targeted	Concentrates limited resources on high-risk areas Focuses on infections with known control measures to reduce infection risk Can determine valid denominator Flexible, can be mixed with other strategies Increases efficiency of surveillance Liberates ICP to perform other activities	Collects data only for targeted patients or risks May miss clusters or outbreaks in nonsurveyed areas or populations
Outbreak thresholds	Automatic, ongoing monitor Thresholds are institution-specific Investigation is prompted by objective threshold	Does not provide data on endemic rates Difficult to compare rates with those of outside institutions

ICP = infection control professional.
Adapted from Perl TM.[26]

Hospital Wide Traditional Surveillance

Hospital-wide surveillance, the most comprehensive method, first was described by the CDC in 1972.[8] In this method, the ICP prospectively and continuously surveys all care areas to identify patients who have acquired infections during hospitalization. The ICP gathers information from daily microbiology reports and from the medical records of patients who have fever or positive cultures and of patients who are receiving antibiotics or are on isolation precautions. The ICP also garners important information by frequently (daily if possible) talking with nursing staff and by occasionally seeing patients. In addition, the ICP periodically reviews all autopsy reports and employee health records.[8] Each month, the infection control team calculates the overall hospital infection rates and infection rates by site, nursing unit, physician service, pathogen, or operative procedure.

Traditional hospital-wide surveillance is comprehensive. However, these systems are very costly, and they identify many infections that cannot be prevented. Consequently, many infection control programs have developed other surveillance methods that require fewer resources.

Periodic Surveillance

There are several ways to conduct periodic surveillance. In one method, the infection control program conducts hospital-wide surveillance only during specified time intervals, such as 1 month each quarter. Infection control programs that use this method frequently conduct targeted surveillance (see under "Targeted Surveillance") during the alternate periods. In another method, the infection control program conducts surveillance on one or a few units for a specified time period and then shifts to another unit or units. By rotating surveillance from unit to unit, the infection control team is able to survey the entire hospital during the year.

Prevalence Survey

In a prevalence survey, the ICP counts the number of active infections during a specified time period.[9] Active infections are defined as all infections that are present during the time of the survey, including those that are newly diagnosed and those that are being treated when the survey begins. The total number of active infections is divided by the number of patients present during the survey. Because new and existing infections are counted, the rates obtained from prevalence surveys are usually higher than incidence rates. Prevalence surveys can focus on particular populations such as patients

with central venous catheters or patients receiving antimicrobials. Prevalence studies also are useful for monitoring the number of patients colonized or infected with important organisms such as vancomycin-resistant enterococci (VRE) or methicillin-resistant *Staphylococcus aureus* (MRSA).

Infection control programs also can use prevalence studies to assess risk factors for infection in a particular population. To determine why patients in this population are developing infections, the epidemiology staff could collect additional data about potential risk factors from all patients surveyed. Because prevalence studies assess all patients in the target population regardless of whether they have infections, infection control personnel can compare the rate of infection in patients who have the risk factor with the rate in those who do not have the risk factor.

Targeted Surveillance

There are several approaches to targeted surveillance. Many infection control programs focus their efforts on selected geographic areas such as critical-care units or selected services such as cardiothoracic surgery. Other programs focus surveillance on specific populations such as patients at high risk of acquiring infections (eg, transplant patients), patients undergoing specific medical interventions (eg, hemodialysis patients), or patients with infections at specific sites (eg, bloodstream or surgical site). Some infection control staff target surveillance to infections associated with specific devices such as ventilator-associated pneumonia (VAP). By limiting the scope of surveillance, infection control personnel can collect data on entire patient populations. Thus, the staff can assess accurately the incidence of infections in the surveyed populations.

Some infection control programs use data from the microbiology laboratory to limit their surveillance. For example, the epidemiology team may focus either on specific microorganisms such as

Legionella species or on organisms with particular antimicrobial susceptibility patterns such as VRE or MRSA.

Outbreak Thresholds

Some investigators have conducted surveillance to assess their baseline infection rates. On the basis of their data, they developed outbreak thresholds. Subsequently, they stopped conducting routine surveillance and only evaluated problems when the number of isolates of a particular species or the number of positive cultures exceeded outbreak thresholds.[10,11] For example, McGuckin used a threshold of an 80th percentile above the baseline for each bacterial species from a particular nursing ward for a specified time period.[10] Similarly, Schifman established a threshold of double the baseline positive culture rate.[11]

Case-Finding Methods

Before we discuss methods for identifying patients who have nosocomial infections, we offer the following caveat. Infection control personnel should collect data only on infections that were acquired in their own facility or as a consequence of procedures or treatments done in their hospital or clinics. For example, a patient may become infected with *Clostridium difficile* while in Hospital A and then transfer to Hospital B while still infected. Infection control personnel in Hospital B should not include this infection in their rates, even though it was acquired in a hospital. Infection control personnel who include these infections in their rates will overestimate the extent of their problem and will underestimate the efficacy of their own program. It seems intuitively obvious that one would not want to include these infections in their nosocomial rates. However, the authors are aware of hospitals that do so. Although not included in the nosocomial infection rates, infection control personnel may want to identify all patients who on admission carry or are infected with particular organisms such as *C diffi-*

cile, VRE, MRSA, and respiratory syncytial virus. Such data allow infection control personnel to estimate the entire population of patients affected by these organisms. By determining the proportion of patients that acquires the organism in the hospital, infection control personnel can evaluate the efficacy of their infection control efforts.

Investigators have described various methods used to identify patients with nosocomial infections. We will review some of these methods in the following paragraphs and in Table 9-3.

Total Chart Review

When using the total chart review method, the ICP reviews nurses' and physicians' notes, medication and treatment records, and radiology and laboratory reports for each patient one to two times per week.[1,12] In addition, many ICPs review notes from respiratory therapy, physical and occupational therapy, dietetics, or any other specialty caring for the patient. Because the ICP requires between 10 and 30 minutes to review each medical record, this method is time-consuming and costly.

Laboratory Reports

Clinical laboratory reports often are the primary source for identifying infections, particularly if the ICP reviews virology and serology reports in addition to bacteriology results.[12-14] The ICP may find some nosocomial infections directly from reports of positive cultures. For example, the ICP could conclude that a patient had a nosocomial infection if a blood culture, which was obtained 10 days after admission, was positive for *S aureus*. In other instances, a laboratory report might prompt the ICP to review the patient's medical record. While reviewing the medical record, the ICP might identify a nosocomial infection for which a culture was not obtained. For example, a patient might have a blood culture from which *Klebsiella pneumoniae* was isolated. In the medical record, the ICP might learn that the chest radiographs

TABLE 9-3
CASE-FINDING METHODS*

Method	The Data Source Reviewed	Sensitivity[†]	Estimated Time (Hours)/ 500 Beds[‡]	Reference
Total chart review	Review all patient medical records	0.74-0.94	35.7-53.6	5,12
Selective medical record review based on§:	Only those medical records selected by screening:			
Laboratory reports	Microbiology reports to identify patients with positive cultures	0.77-0.91	23.2	12,13
Kardex screening	Patient kardex to determine patients at high risk for infection	0.75-0.94	14.3-22.3	12
Fever	Temperature record to identify patients with temperature > 37.8°C	0.09-0.56	8	12,13
Antibiotic use	Medication record to identify patients receiving antibiotics	0.57	14.3	12
Fever and antibiotic use	Temperature record to identify patients with fever >37.8°C, and medication record to identify patients receiving anti-biotics	0.70	13.4	12
Readmission	Admission record for patients readmitted with infection	0.08	Not specified	13
Autopsy reports	Autopsy reports to identify patients with infections	0.08	0.53	27
Ward liaison surveillance	Patients reported by nursing staff to have an infection	0.62	17.6	14
Laboratory-based ward liaison surveillance	Microbiology reports to identify patients with a positive culture and patients reported by nursing staff to have an infection	0.76-0.89	31.8	14
Risk factor based surveillance	Nursing reports and medication records to identify patients with risk factors for infection	0.50-0.89	32.4	14
Infection control sentinel sheet system	"Sentinel sheet" to identify patients reported by nursing staff to have symptoms of infection	0.73	‖	15

Adapted from Stratton et al.[6]

[†]*Sensitivity of the case-finding method is reported for the number of nosocomial infections identified by the method but not for the number of patients with nosocomial infections identified by the method.*

[‡]*Number of hours per week required for an infection control professional to perform surveillance in a 500-bed hospital.*

§*If these data are in a computer database, infection control staff can review this information on the computer or can review computer printouts.*

‖ *Case-finding method suitable for intensive care and specialty units; requires 1 minute per chart per day.*

revealed a new pulmonary infiltrate and the Gram stain of the sputum revealed many white blood cells and Gram-negative rods. This information might lead the ICP to conclude that the patient had pneumonia and a secondary bacteremia caused by *K pneumoniae*. Alternatively, a positive urine culture might prompt the ICP to review a patient's medical record. While reviewing the record, the

ICP might discover a nosocomial pneumonia caused by another organism.

Most laboratories maintain log books or notebooks that ICPs can scan quickly to obtain preliminary results. In addition, the laboratory staff often are willing to notify infection control personnel of positive tests. This is especially true if the epidemiology personnel visit the laboratory frequently and develop rapport with the laboratory staff. Nonetheless, laboratory reports have some substantial limitations, and the infection control program should not use them as the only source of data for identifying patients with nosocomial infections. For example, clinicians may not obtain cultures from patients with clinical evidence of SSI or UTI, but instead may treat these patients empirically. In addition, cultures from some sites of infection may be negative. This is particularly true if the patient is on antimicrobial therapy or if the organism is fastidious or does not grow on routine culture media. Consequently, the sensitivity of laboratory records is directly affected by the number of infections from which cultures are obtained and the culture methods used by the laboratory.

Kardex Screening

The ICP surveys the nursing kardex one to two times each week to determine whether patients are receiving antibiotics, intravenous fluids, or parenteral nutrition and whether the patient has an indwelling urinary catheter, special orders for wound-dressing changes, or orders for isolation precautions.[12] If the ICP identifies one of these "clues" or other information that suggests the patient is at risk of nosocomial infection, the ICP reviews the patient's record. If the kardex is complete and current, the method is highly sensitive and enables the ICP to spend less time reviewing charts.

Clinical Ward Rounds

Infection control professionals who regularly visit clinical wards can gain excellent information about patients, infections, and other adverse events, because much important information is not included in the patients' records.[14,15] This method allows the ICP to be highly visible in patient-care areas, to observe infection control practices directly, and to talk with the healthcare workers caring for patients. In this manner, the ICP not only can collect data on patients with nosocomial infections but also assess compliance with isolation precautions, answer questions on infection control issues, and conduct informal educational sessions.

Postdischarge Surveillance

As patients are discharged from hospitals earlier, the infection control team will have increasing difficulty detecting hospital-acquired infections unless the team conducts postdischarge surveillance. Infection control teams that do not conduct postdischarge surveillance will identify spuriously low nosocomial infection rates because traditional hospital-based surveillance methods identify only events that occur while the patient is in the hospital. In fact, studies have documented that postdischarge surveillance identifies 13% to 70% more SSIs than do methods that survey only inpatients.[16]

Most investigators who have studied methods for postdischarge surveillance have not evaluated all discharged patients, but have focused on specific populations such as postoperative patients, postpartum women, or neonates. Investigators have assessed various methods for identifying infections after these patients are discharged, including directly assessing the patients, reviewing records from visits to clinics or emergency rooms, and contacting physicians or patients by mail or telephone. Although all of the methods identify patients who developed infections after discharge, the methods are time-consuming and can be insensitive. None of these methods have been accepted widely.

Which Case-Finding Method Is Best?

Each case-finding method has some merit, but

each also has limitations. There is no agreement on which case-finding method is best. Some infection control personnel consider total chart review to be the gold standard for identifying nosocomial infections. However, in two studies that compared total chart review with combinations of two or more case-finding methods, the former method identified only 74% to 94% of the infections identified by the combined methods.[5,12] Investigators were unable to identify all infections by reviewing only the medical record, because:

- The records did not document all data required to determine whether the patients met criteria for specific infections.
- Laboratory or radiology reports were missing.
- Records were not available.
- The reviewer could not examine the patient.

Consequently, total chart review is no more sensitive than other case-finding methods or combination of methods.

Nettleman and Nelson conducted surveillance to identify adverse occurrences among patients hospitalized on general medical wards.[17] They used numerous data sources and found that no single source identified all adverse occurrences. In fact, the number of adverse occurrences the investigators identified in each category was dependent on which data source the investigators used. Certain data sources efficiently identified specific adverse occurrences. For example, the authors identified 77% of medication-related errors by reviewing the medication administration record, but detected only 10% of these events by reviewing the physicians' progress notes. Conversely, the authors identified 100% of procedure-related adverse occurrences by reviewing the physicians' progress notes, but did not detect any of these events by reviewing the medication administration record.

Therefore, the infection control team must select case-finding methods that best will identify the nosocomial infections they choose to study. For example, the ICP could identify most bloodstream infections by reviewing microbiology reports, but would find very few bloodstream infections by observing the patient directly. On the other hand, the ICP might identify most SSIs by observing surgical wounds directly, but not by reviewing microbiology reports. In addition, particular practices in individual hospitals can decrease the efficacy of particular case-finding methods. For example, if physicians routinely diagnose uncomplicated UTIs based on urinalysis and symptoms, but do not obtain cultures, infection control teams that use reports of urine cultures to identify these infections would underestimate the incidence of UTIs substantially. On the other hand, some practices that are unique to individual hospitals can help the infection control team identify patients who have infections at specific sites. If dicloxacillin and hot packs are used routinely to treat intravenous catheter-site infections, the ICP could review nursing care plans and medication records to identify patients receiving that treatment regimen rather than examining each intravenous catheter site.

National Nosocomial Infections Surveillance System

In 1970, the CDC enrolled a sample of hospitals, which voluntarily agreed to collect data on nosocomial infections, into the National Nosocomial Infections Surveillance (NNIS) system. Currently, 202 hospitals participate in the program, and NNIS is the only source of national data on nosocomial infections in the United States.[18] The hospitals participating range in size from 80 to 1,200 beds and include state, federal, profit, and nonprofit institutions. The NNIS program has several goals:

- To estimate the incidence of nosocomial infections.
- To identify changes in the pathogens causing nosocomial infections, the frequency of nosocomial infections at specific sites, the predominant risk factors, and the antimicro-

bial susceptibility patterns.

- To provide data on nosocomial infections with which hospitals can compare their data, including the distribution of nosocomial infections by major sites, device-associated infection rates by type of intensive care unit, and SSI rates by operative procedure.
- To develop strategies that infection control personnel can use for surveillance and assessment of nosocomial infections.

Initially, all hospitals participating in NNIS conducted prospective, traditional, hospital-wide surveillance. The CDC investigators subsequently identified methodological problems that made comparisons of data among hospitals unreliable. Thus, in 1986, the NNIS program created three surveillance components in addition to hospital-wide surveillance: the adult intensive care unit or the pediatric intensive care unit, the high-risk nursery, and all surgical patients or patients undergoing specific procedures. The revised NNIS system has some advantages. First, the new components require infection control personnel to collect data on exposure to devices or to specific operative procedures. Thus, the CDC can adjust infection rates in the surveyed units for exposure to these devices and procedures. Hospitals that participate in NNIS regularly receive reports that compare their adjusted data with the aggregate adjusted data. Infection control personnel in hospitals that do not participate in NNIS can compare their adjusted rates with the adjusted rates published by the CDC. Second, each hospital can choose the surveillance component in which it will participate. Thus, each infection control program can both design a surveillance program that meets the needs of their institution and participate in NNIS.

Nosocomial Infection Rates

Overall Hospital Infection Rates

Infection control programs that conduct hospital-wide surveillance sometimes track their overall infection rate. This rate is calculated by dividing the number of nosocomial infections identified in a given month by the number of patients admitted or discharged during the same month. However, the overall hospital infection rate has several inherent disadvantages.

- The overall rate treats all infections as though they are of equal importance, furthermore, changes in uncommon but important infections (eg, bacteremia) might be hidden in the larger volume of common but less important infections (eg, urinary tract infections).
- The overall rate does not distinguish between patients who had one infection and those who had numerous infections.
- The overall infection rate may not be accurate and may underestimate the true rate, because the ICP often cannot identify all nosocomial infections.
- The overall rate does not account for patients who are at increased risk for becoming infected because of their underlying diseases or exposure to procedures and medical devices, therefore, the overall infection rate tends to obscure important trends in intensive care units or among high-risk patients.
- The rate does not adjust for length of stay.
- The rate is not risk adjusted, therefore, it cannot be compared with rates from other hospitals.

In short, the accuracy and usefulness of the overall infection rate is limited. Therefore, we recommend that infection control personnel stop calculating their overall infection rate and begin calculating adjusted infection rates.

Adjusting Rates

Infection control personnel calculate infection rates so that they can identify problems and assess the effectiveness of their interventions. In addition, infection control staff follow their rates over time to identify significant increases above their baseline rates and to assess the efficacy of their program. In addition, to determine whether they actually have a problem, infection control personnel often compare their rates with those of other institutions. However, comparisons within a single hospital over time may not be valid, because the patients or patient care may have changed substantially. Further, comparisons among hospitals may not be valid, because healthcare facilities are not standardized.[19] Patients in different hospitals have different underlying diseases and different severities of illness. In addition, patients who have the same disease and the same severity of illness but who are in different hospitals could undergo different diagnostic and therapeutic interventions and stay in the hospital for different periods of time. Each hospital also has its own unique environment, patient-care practices, and healthcare providers. Infection control programs also vary substantially in the intensity of surveillance, the methods used for surveillance, the definitions of infections, and the methods used for calculating infection rates.

Consequently, infection control personnel must use adjusted rates if they want to assess their rates over time or to compare their rates with those in other hospitals. In the following paragraphs, we will discuss several methods for adjusting rates.

Adjusting Rates for Length of Stay

Infection rates more accurately reflect the risk of infection when they are adjusted for length of stay. Infection control staff have attempted to control for the length of stay by calculating the number of nosocomial infections per patient day. This method uses the total number of nosocomial infections in a month as the numerator and the total number of patient days (ie, the sum of the number of days that each patient was on the unit) in that month as the denominator. For example, an obstetrics ward admits many patients who stay in the hospital for a very brief time and whose risk of infection is low, but a rehabilitation ward admits a few patients who stay for long periods of time and

whose risk of infection is high. If the number of patients admitted to these units were used as the denominators, the rate for obstetrics probably would underestimate the risk of infection, whereas the rate on the rehabilitation ward most likely would overestimate the risk of infection. By using the number of patient-days as the denominator, infection control staff control for the effect of length of stay on the infection rate. However, this method does not control for the effect of other risk factors such as devices or for the severity of the patient's underlying illness.

Adjusting Rates for Exposure to Devices

Device-associated infection rates control for the duration of exposure to a device, which is one of the major risk factors for these infections. Therefore, device-associated rates can be compared more reliably over time and among institutions than can overall infection rates. To obtain this rate, the infection control team first chooses the device (eg, ventilators) and specifies the population (eg, patients in the MICU) to be studied. Next, the team identifies the device-associated infections (eg, VAP) that occur in the selected population during a specified time period. The number of infections is the numerator. To obtain the denominator, the team sums the number of patients exposed to the device during each day of the specified period. For example, if the team surveyed the MICU for 7 days and the number of patients on ventilators each day was four, three, five, five, four, six, and four, respectively, the number of ventilator days would have been 31. If the team identified three cases of VAP during the week, the VAP rate would have been 0.097 cases per ventilator-day or 97 per 1,000 ventilator days.

Adjusting Rates for Severity of Illness

One would expect that a 28-year-old man who does not have underlying medical illnesses and who is undergoing an elective herniorrhaphy would have a lower risk of acquiring an SSI than would a

65-year-old man who has chronic lung disease treated with steroids, diabetes mellitus, and heart disease and who is undergoing an emergency exploratory laparotomy. Several investigators have developed scores to determine a patient's severity of illness. These scores range from simple, subjective scales based on clinical judgment to commercially available, computerized programs that use objective clinical data to assess the severity of a patient's underlying illnesses. Unfortunately, the currently available severity of illness scores cannot identify patients who are at high risk of developing a nosocomial infection. Thus, most infection control programs do not use these scores to risk-adjust nosocomial infection rates.

The risk index with which infection control personnel are most familiar is the surgical-wound classification that separates procedures into four categories: clean, clean-contaminated, contaminated, or dirty.[20] The incidence of infection increases as the wound classification changes from clean to dirty. However, this system does not account for each patient's intrinsic susceptibility to infection. Consequently, its ability to predict which patients are at highest risk of SSI is limited. Investigators in the SENIC and NNIS projects have developed risk indices that include variables assessing the patients' intrinsic risk of infection.[21,22] Culver et al[22] used the NNIS risk index to stratify the risk of SSI and to standardize SSI rates. However, other investigators tested the validity of the NNIS risk index and found that it did not predict which patients were at highest risk of developing an SSI after cardiothoracic surgery.[23] Hence, before risk indices can be used to identify high-risk patients or to adjust rates, they must be validated, and the population for which they are most predictive must be defined.

Planning a Surveillance System

Many infection control programs established surveillance systems because the CDC recommended doing it, regulatory agencies required them, or other hospitals in the community had established programs. Such hospitals may not have established their own goals and priorities. Consequently, data collection became an end unto itself. The ICPs routinely collected data on all nosocomial and community-acquired infections, dutifully recorded the data, calculated the overall hospital infection rates, and presented the information at infection control committee meetings. Unfortunately, the surveillance data had little influence on the infection rates.

To be successful, a surveillance system needs goals that are clear and specific. When an infection control team is developing a new surveillance system or revising an existing system, the staff first must define the priorities of the infection control program, so they can determine what type of surveillance they should conduct and what types of data they should collect. After the epidemiology staff have analyzed preliminary data from their own institution (ie, data obtained either through the previous surveillance system or through a hospital wide prevalence survey), they can custom design a surveillance system specific for their own facility.

When developing a surveillance program, infection control personnel should consider characteristics of the institution, including the size, the hospital type (eg, private, university, federal, teaching, nonteaching), the patient populations served, the procedures and treatments offered, and the proportion of care that is done in the hospital compared with that given in the outpatient setting. Epidemiology staff also should consider the resources available to the infection control program, including the budget, the number of personnel and their level of training and experience, and the computer hardware and software that can be used by the staff. Infection control staff should design a surveillance system that requires fewer resources than are available, so the staff can accomplish their other responsibilities (eg, analysis, reporting, developing interventions, monitoring efficacy, etc).

TABLE 9-4
INFORMATION TO COLLECT ON INFECTIONS

General Information for all Definitions

Patient name

Patient identification

Age

Gender

Nursing unit

Service

Admission date

Date of onset

Site of infection

Organism

Antimicrobial susceptibility pattern

Primary diagnosis[*]

Medications (antibiotics, steroids, chemotherapeutic agents)[*]

Exposure or risk factor (immunosuppression, instrumentation, procedures)[*]

Date of exposure or risk factor[*]

Comments

Information for Surveillance on Resistant Organisms

Underlying disease

History of antibiotic use

Current or prior roommates

Previous rooms during this admission

Previous hospitalizations in this hospital

Previous hospitalizations in another hospital

Previous stay in a long-term care facility

Information for Selected Sites

Surgical site infection

Surgical procedure

Surgery date

Surgeons

ASA score

Wound classification

Perioperative antibiotic(s)

Time antibiotics administered[*]

Time procedure began[*]

Time procedure finished[*]

Other members of the surgical team[*]

Operating room[*]

Bloodstream infection

Intravascular catheters present (yes/no)

Location of intravascular catheter insertion site

Number of days catheter in place

Type of catheter[*]

Persons who inserted catheter[*]

Pneumonia

Endotracheal intubation (yes/no)

Number of ventilator days

Date patient intubated

Urinary tract infection

Urethral catheter present (yes/no)

External catheter present (yes/no)

Number of days catheter in place

Persons who inserted catheter[*]

Other urinary tract instrumentation[*]

ASA = American Society of Anesthesiologists.

*Information to be collected under particular circumstances such as an outbreak.

Infection control personnel must consider which events they will study and the data sources that are available in their hospital when they choose data sources and case-finding methods. The staff should consider the advantages and disadvantages of surveillance methods (see Table 9-1) and the sensitivity of case-finding methods (see Table 9-2) as they design their surveillance system. The ICP should collect basic information on all patients with nosocomial infections (Table 9-4). The ICP

also may need to collect additional data for some infections (eg, VAP or central venous catheter-associated bacteremia) or during certain time periods (eg, when conducting a study to evaluate the prevalence of certain infections and to identify risk factors for those infections [Table 9-4]). Thus, the infection control team could change which data elements they collect for different studies, different sites of infection, or different pathogens.

Infection control programs that have bountiful

TABLE 9-5
EXAMPLES OF PRACTICES THAT AFFECT OBSERVED INFECTION RATES

Change in Practice	Apparent Effect on Infection Rate
Shift locus of treatment from the hospital to the outpatient setting	Decrease overall infection rate, because surveillance rarely is performed in the outpatient setting
Length of hospital stay decreases as patients are discharged earlier	Decrease overall infection rate
Length of stay in hospital after operative procedures	Decrease surgical site infection rate, because surveillance rarely is performed in the outpatient setting
Low-risk operative procedures performed in separate ambulatory surgical facility	Increase surgical site infection rates, because patients who have a higher risk of infection have operative procedures performed in the hospital
Patients residing on a boarding unit are not counted as hospital admissions: thus, these patients are not included in the denominator	Increased infection rate if surveillance is conducted on these units, especially if outbreaks of infections (eg, gastroenteritis, *Clostridium difficile*) are detected
Patients counted as an admission each time they are transferred to a different unit	Decreased overall infection rate, because denominator is inflated artificially
The accounting office changes from charging one general cost for a central-line insertion to charging for each catheter opened	Decreased infection rate associated with central lines, because the denominator (ie, the number of central lines inserted) appears to increase
Business office assigns surgical procedure to admitting physician, regardless of that physician's specialty, rather than to the surgeon doing the procedure	Inaccurate surgeon-specific infection rates, because some surgical site infections will be assigned to the wrong physician
Physicians treat patients empirically for possible infections without obtaining cultures	Decreased infection rates if case-finding method relies solely on microbiology report
Microbiology laboratory changes screening criteria for processing specimens	Decreased infection rates if case-finding method relies solely on microbiology reports
Definitions used inconsistently or absence of written definitions	Inaccurate infection rates
ICD 9 codes used to identify patients with nosocomial infections	Inaccurate infection rates

ICD = International Classification of Diseases.

resources may want to continue doing hospital-wide surveillance so that they can detect nosocomial infections in all patient populations. However, programs that find themselves in this enviable position should develop innovative methods for conducting hospital-wide surveillance and not just use the traditional labor-intensive method—total chart review. Most infection control programs have severely limited budgets, and the staff therefore must decide how to use these precious resources. We believe that most infection control programs

should not conduct hospital-wide surveillance. Instead, they should limit their surveillance to specific infections, pathogens, or patient populations.

We recommend that infection control staff focus on infections that can be prevented, occur frequently, cause serious morbidity, increase mortality, are costly to treat, or are caused by multiresistant organisms. Instead of collecting data on all patients who have urinary tract infections, infection control personnel could evaluate only those infections associated with indwelling catheters or those caused by resistant organisms. Medical devices increase the risk of infections, and device-related infections may be preventable. Therefore, infection control personnel may want to limit surveillance to device-related infections in intensive care units. Nosocomial infections caused by *Legionella* sp or *Aspergillus* sp occur infrequently. However, these infections cause substantial mortality, and environmental controls can prevent most cases. Therefore, the infection control staff may want to use microbiology laboratory data (and other sources of data if necessary) to identify all of these cases. Vancomycin-resistant enterococci and other multiresistant bacteria can spread rapidly within hospitals. Infections caused by these organisms can be very costly to treat, or they may not be treatable. Therefore, infection control personnel may want to use microbiology data to do surveillance for patients who are infected with or who carry these organisms. Infection control personnel may choose to study infections that are relatively minor but occur frequently, because these infections will increase the total cost to the healthcare system substantially. For example, saphenous vein harvest site infections are less severe than sternal wound infections after coronary artery bypass graft (CABG) procedures. However, at least two thirds of the SSIs after CABG are harvest site infections, which have an attributable cost of nearly $7,000 per infection.[24,25] Because harvest site infections occur much more frequently than do serious sternal infections, the total cost to a healthcare system for the former approximates that of the latter. Furthermore, harvest site infections may be caused by technique problems and thus could be prevented if the surgical technique was improved. Therefore, infection control personnel might want to develop a surveillance system that is able to detect harvest site infections.

As medical care moves from the hospital to the outpatient setting, the infection control team should consider how they can identify infections acquired by patients treated in the ambulatory-care setting.

Unless infection control teams expand their boundaries, they will underestimate the frequency of infections associated with medical care. At present, many infection control programs monitor patients who develop SSI after ambulatory operative procedures. In addition, infection control staff might consider using surveillance to identify patients who acquire infections associated with outpatient treatments such as dialysis, chemotherapy, and intravenous therapy (eg, antimicrobials, antiviral agents, and parenteral nutrition) or in programs such as hospital-based home care.

Assessing a Surveillance System

At least annually, the epidemiology team should evaluate the surveillance system to determine if it provided meaningful data. The staff should ask themselves a series of questions.

- Did the surveillance system detect clusters or outbreaks?
- Which patient-care practices were changed based on surveillance data?
- Were the data used to develop methods to decrease the endemic rate of infection?
- Were the data used to assess the efficacy of interventions?
- Were the data used to ensure that infection rates did not increase when procedures were changed?
- Are administrative and clinical staff aware of surveillance findings?

If no one, including the infection control staff, uses the data to alter practice, the epidemiology team must conclude that their current system is not working. Infection control personnel would achieve more if they stopped collecting data, analyzed the data they had collected previously, and then devised a new strategic plan for the program. The strategic plan should include goals and priorities for the surveillance system and specific plans for how the data will be used. If appropriate, the epidemiology team could develop interventions on the basis of the data that are currently available. The staff could plan how they subsequently will use the revised surveillance system to monitor the efficacy of the interventions.

The epidemiology staff periodically must verify that the surveillance system is actually getting the data the staff thinks they are getting. Infection control personnel should be aware that hospital departments, which provide data for the program, may change their procedures. If the departments notify infection control staff, they can modify surveillance appropriately. However, departments often change important procedures without informing staff in other departments. Some changes could affect the infection rates substantially; other changes do not affect the infection rates directly, but alter the surveillance system's ability to obtain necessary data. Table 9-5 identifies several changes in practice that may affect infection rates. Because changes instituted by other departments can affect infection rates substantially, infection control personnel would be wise to investigate dramatic changes in the rates or other important results.

The ICP in one hospital calculated the proportion of S aureus isolates identified each month that were resistant to methicillin. When the proportion dropped precipitously from 34% to 0%, members of the Infection Control Committee were elated. The ICP, however, was suspicious that the decrease was not real. Because many of the MRSA isolates previously had been isolated from surgical wounds, the ICP checked to see if the surgeons had changed the way they managed possibly infected wounds. The ICP discovered that the surgeons now were treating SSI empirically without first obtaining wound cultures. Upon further investigation, the ICP discovered that the laboratory had changed the criteria for performing wound cultures. Laboratory personnel no longer plated specimens from wound cultures if the Gram stain did not show any white blood cells. The two unrelated changes reduced the proportion of S aureus isolates that were resistant to methi-

cillin. Unfortunately, the reduction was factitious.

The overall infection rate in another hospital suddenly decreased. The infection control team discovered that the fiscal department had changed the bed-count procedure so that a patient was counted as an admission each time the patient transferred to another unit. Thus, the denominator was inflated and the infection rate appeared low.

Conclusion

We believe that the surveillance systems of the 1990s must be extremely flexible so that they can be adapted to meet the needs of rapidly changing healthcare systems. We also think that effective infection control teams will not use a one-size-fits-all approach to surveillance, but will mix and match different case-finding methods and surveillance methods to create a surveillance system that meets the needs not only of their entire healthcare system but also of the individual components (eg, intensive care units and ambulatory-surgery center). In addition, we think infection control personnel must learn to use computers and must develop surveillance systems that use the computerized databases already present in their hospital (eg, databases from the laboratory, surgical services, and financial management). Furthermore, the infection control team should collaborate with personnel from the information systems department to develop algorithms that a computer uses to identify patients with possible nosocomial infections and thresholds that the computer uses to identify likely outbreaks. As hospitals develop electronic patient records, computer-based surveillance should become easier. However, we would encourage infection control personnel not to wait until their hospital has electronic patient records, but to use whatever resources are available currently to streamline surveillance. Finally, computerized models that predict which patients are at highest risk of infection would allow infection control personnel to improve the efficiency of surveillance and stratify infection rates more appropriately. However, these models are not currently available. We would encourage the infection control community to make development of such models a priority for the future.

Acknowledgments

The authors thank H. Jay Rothenberg for his careful and humorous critique of this work.

References

1. Haley RW, Culver DH, White JW, et al. The efficacy of infection surveillance and control programs in preventing nosocomial infection in US hospitals. *Am J Epidemiol.* 1985;121:182-205.

2. Ehrenkranz NJ, Richter EI, Phillips PM, Shultz JM. An apparent excess of operative site infections: analyses to evaluate false-positive diagnoses. *Infect Control Hosp Epidemiol.* 1995;16:712-716.

3. Garner JS, Jarvis WR, Emori TG, Horan TC, Hughes JM. CDC definitions for nosocomial infections. *Am J Infect Control.* 1988;16:128-140.

4. Horan TC, Gaynes RP, Martone WJ, Jarvis WR, Emori TG. CDC definitions of nosocomial surgical site infections: a modification of CDC definitions of surgical wound infections. *Am J Infect Control.* 1992;20:271-274.

5. Haley RW, Schaberg DR, McClish DK, et al. The accuracy of retrospective chart review in measuring nosocomial infection rates. *Am J Epidemiol.* 1980;111:516-533.

6. Stratton CW, Ratner H, Johnston PE, Schaffner W. Focused microbiologic surveillance by specific hospital unit: practical application and clinical utility. *Clin Ther.* 1993;15(suppl A):12S-20S.

7. Classen DC, Evans RS, Pestotnik SL, Horn SD, Menlove RL, Burke JP. The timing of prophylactic administration of antibiotics and the risk of surgical-wound infection. *N Engl J Med.* 1992;326:281-286.

8. US Department of Health, Education, and Welfare. *Outline for Surveillance and Control of Nosocomial Infections.* Atlanta, Ga: Centers for Disease Control; 1972.

9. US Department of Health and Human Services. *Prevalence Survey for Nosocomial Infections.* Atlanta, Ga: Centers for Disease Control; 1980.

10. McGuckin MB, Abrutyn E. A surveillance method for early detection of nosocomial outbreaks. *APIC J.* 1979;7:18-21.

11. Schifman RB, Palmer RA. Surveillance of nosocomial infections by computer analysis of positive culture rates. *J Clin Microbiol.* 1985;21:493-495.

12. Wenzel RP, Osterman CA, Hunting KJ, Gwaltney JM. Hospital-acquired infections I: surveillance in a university hospital. *Am J Epidemiol.* 1976;103:251-260.

13. Gross PA, Beaugard A, Van Antwerpen C. Surveillance for nosocomial infections: can the sources of data be reduced? *Infect Control.* 1980;1:233-236.

14. Glenister H, Taylor L, Bartlett C, Cooke M, Sedgwick J, Leigh D. An assessment of selective surveillance methods for detecting hospital-acquired infection. *Am J Med.* 1991;91(suppl 3B):121S-124S.

15. Ford-Jones EL, Mindorff CM, Pollock E, et al. Evaluation of a new method of detection of nosocomial infection in the pediatric intensive care unit: the infection control sentinel sheet system. *Infect Control Hosp Epidemiol.* 1989;10:515-520.

16. Holtz TH, Wenzel RP. Postdischarge surveillance for nosocomial wound infection: a brief review and commentary. *Am J Infect Control.* 1992;20:206-213.

17. Nettleman MD, Nelson AP. Adverse occurrences during hospitalization on a general medicine service. *Clinical Performance and Quality Health Care.* 1994;2:67-72.

18. Emori TG, Culver DH, Horan TC, et al. National nosocomial infections surveillance system (NNIS): description of surveillance methods. *Am J Infect Control.* 1991;19:19-35.

19. Nosocomial infection rates for interhospital comparison: limitations and possible solutions. *Infect Control Hosp Epidemiol.* 1991;12:609-621.

20. Garner JS. Guideline for prevention of surgical wound infections. *Am J Infect Control.* 1986;14:71-80.

21. Haley RW, Culver DH, Morgan WM, White JW, Emori TG, Hooten TM. Identifying patients at high risk of surgical wound infection. *Am J Epidemiol.* 1985;121:206-215.

22. Culver DH, Horan TC, Gaynes RP, et al. Surgical wound infection rates by wound class, operative procedure, and patient risk index. *Am J Med.* 1991;91(suppl 3B):152S-157S.

23. Roy MC, Herwaldt LA, Embrey R, Kuhns K, Wenzel RP, Perl TM. Does the NNIS risk index (NRI) predict which patients develop wound infection (SWI) after cardiothoracic (CT) surgery? In: Program and Abstracts of the 34th Interscience Conference on Antimicrobial Agents and Chemotherapy. Orlando, Fla: 1994:196. Abstract.

24. Roy MC, Herwaldt LA, Embrey R, Kuhns K, Perl TM. A 3-year wound surveillance study in cardiothoracic (CT)

surgery. In: Program and Abstracts of the 34th Interscience Conference on Antimicrobial Agents and Chemotherapy. Orlando, Fl: 1994. Abstract.

25. Morales E, Herwaldt L, Embrey R, et al. The epidemiology of saphenous vein harvest site wound infections (SVHSI) after cardiothoracic surgery. In: Program and Abstracts of the 33rd Interscience Conference on Antimicrobial Agents and Chemotherapy. New Orleans, La: 1993:131. Abstract.

26. Perl TM. Surveillance, reporting, and use of computers. In: Wenzel RP, ed. *Prevention and Control of Nosocomial Infections.* 2nd ed. Baltimore, Md: Williams & Wilkins; 1993.

27. Crossley K, Johnson J, Mudge R, Crossley L. An evaluation of autopsy review as a technique for infection control: a procedure of questionable value. *Infect Control.* 1983;4:29-30.

CHAPTER 10

Hospital-Acquired Pneumonia: Perspectives for the Healthcare Epidemiologist

Donald E. Craven, MD, Kathleen A. Steger, RN, MPH

Abstract

Nosocomial pneumonia is defined as an infection of lung parenchyma that was neither present nor incubating at the time of the patient's admission to the hospital. In the United States, hospital-acquired pneumonia is the second most common nosocomial infection and accounts for the most deaths. We describe how infection control personnel can use targeted surveillance to identify clusters of cases and to prevent pneumonia. We also discuss common pathogens that cause nosocomial pneumonia; ventilator-associated pneumonia; and strategies for prevention of hospital-acquired pneumonia.

Introduction

Osler's observations on medicine are nearly a century old, but they still apply to the diagnosis, pathogenesis, and prevention of hospital-acquired pneumonia. Pneumonia is the second most common nosocomial infection. Moreover, in the United States, nosocomial pneumonia is associated with more deaths than any other nosocomial infection.[1-5] The mortality directly attributable to nosocomial pneumonia has been difficult to determine, but is estimated to be approximately 30%. Despite the frequency and severity of nosocomial pneumonia, clinicians and researchers still are trying to determine which diagnostic criteria are most sensitive and specific, and which diagnostic method provides the best outcome.

In this chapter, we provide background information on nosocomial pneumonia, and discuss methods for surveillance, diagnosis, and prevention of this infection. We emphasize bacterial nosocomial pneumonia in mechanically ventilated patients, but we also discuss hospital-acquired pneumonia caused by respiratory viruses and fungi. Selected references that are relevant for infection control personnel are cited.

TABLE 10-1

LIMITATIONS AND ADVANTAGES OF CURRENT METHODS USED FOR THE DIAGNOSIS OF NOSOCOMIAL PNEUMONIA

Method of Diagnosis	Advantages	Limitations
Clinical[6,7]	• Based on widely available clinical data: fever, leukocytosis, purulent sputum, Gram stain, cultures, new and persistent pulmonary infiltrate on chest radiograph • Noninvasive • Relatively inexpensive • Gram stain and culture easy to perform • Serial Gram stains in intubated patients, when correlated with clinical condition, may provide a clue to guide the initial choice of antimicrobial agents and the interpretation of sputum culture results	• Poor specificity, especially in patients on ventilators or with diffuse infiltrates on chest radiograph (eg, ARDS or CHF) • Poor sensitivity for immunocompromised patients or unusual organisms • Poor specificity of nonquantitative sputum cultures • Quality of specimen varies • Processing and interpretation of Gram stain varies • Culture results not available for 24 to 48 h • Presence of potential pathogen suggestive, *not* diagnostic • *Legionella* cultures often not available (urine antigen may be helpful)
CPIS[9,10]	• CPIS correlates with diagnosis by bronchoscopy and PSB in ventilated patients • Uses quantitative bacteriology to increase specificity	• Quantitative endotracheal cultures are not widely available • Results may be altered by prior treatment with antimicrobial agents
Bronchoscopy With PSB or BAL[6,7]	• Better specificity in some mechanically ventilated and/or immunocompromised patients • PSB sensitivity (for >10^3/mL) 80% to 90% and specificity 95% when done by experienced staff • BAL sensitivity (for >10^4/mL) 86% to 100% and specificity 95% to 100% when done by experienced staff • Decreases unnecessary antibiotic use and development of antibiotic-resistant organisms • Useful for a patient who does not respond to initial antimicrobial therapy	• Relies on quantitative bacteriology • Prior treatment with antimicrobial agents may decrease sensitivity • May miss early cases of VAP • Bronchoscopy is relatively costly, invasive, and is not always available • Culture results not available for 24 to 48 h • BAL may have greater complication rate than PSB • Specimens must be processed promptly and meticulously • Efficacy, risk, cost of PSB or BAL versus clinical diagnosis for various populations are not well-defined

Background Information

Diagnosis

Infection control personnel must have an accurate definition of nosocomial pneumonia before they can perform surveillance or investigate outbreaks.[6-10] The diagnosis of nosocomial pneumonia often is made clinically, particularly in nonventilated patients, and usually is based on findings such as fever, leukocytosis, purulent tracheo-bronchial secretions, a suggestive Gram stain, and a new, persistent pulmonary infiltrate on chest radiograph (Table 10-1). These clinical criteria appear to have reasonable sensitivity, but limited specificity, especially in mechanically ventilated patients. Clinicians should be cognizant that pneumonia may be mimicked by adult respiratory distress syndrome, congestive heart failure, atelectasis, pulmonary edema, tumors, or pulmonary emboli.

TABLE 10-1 (continued)
LIMITATIONS AND ADVANTAGES OF CURRENT METHODS USED FOR THE DIAGNOSIS OF NOSOCOMIAL PNEUMONIA

Method of Diagnosis	Advantages	Limitations
Nonbronchoscopic BAL[6,10]	• Simpler, less expensive than bronchoscopy with PSB or BAL; appears to have comparable diagnostic yield • Useful for following response to treatment with antimicrobial agents	• Quantitative cultures are more costly than routine cultures • Procedure requires skilled technicians • Data on risk, benefit, and cost compared with clinical diagnosis and bronchoscopy are limited
QEA[6,8]	• Simpler, less expensive than bronchoscopy or nonbronchoscopic BAL • 65% correlation between QEA and bronchoscopy with PSB and BAL, but less specific • Good negative predictive value (~70%)	• Threshold for diagnosis of VAP varies among studies • Requires quantitative bacteriology
Transthoracic aspirates	• Good sensitivity and specificity	• Complications (eg, pneumothorax, hemorrhage) are relatively frequent; procedure is not used in most hospitals • False-negative results
Autopsy	• May increase diagnosis of unsuspected pathogens, such as *Legionella* sp, *Aspergillus* sp, *Candida* sp, CMV, and PCP	• No clinical value for patient • Infrequently performed in many hospitals

ARDS = adult respiratory distress syndrome; CHF = congestive heart failure; CPIS = clinical pulmonary infection score; PSB = protected specimen brush; BAL = bronchoalveolar lavage; VAP = ventilator-associated pneumonia; QEA = quantitative endotracheal aspirates; CMV = cytomegalovirus; PCP = Pneumocystis carinii pneumonia.

The definition of nosocomial pneumonia used by the infection control program will depend on which diagnostic techniques are available, the hospital's resources, and the question being addressed. Thus, we feel that infection control personnel should understand the strengths and weakness of the tests used to diagnose pneumonia. Because we do not have a gold standard diagnostic test, clinicians and epidemiologists still debate which tests are the most accurate, safe, and most cost-effective for diagnosing ventilator-associated pneumonia (VAP).[6-10] If a potential pathogen is isolated from cultures of the pleural fluid or blood, the clinician may establish a diagnosis of pneumonia more readily. However, these findings often are absent, or, if cultures are obtained, the results are not available for 24 to 48 hours. In addition, lower respiratory tract coloniza-

tion may be difficult to distinguish from tracheobronchitis and pneumonia. Moreover, upper respiratory secretions may leak around the endotracheal tube. Thus, bacterial pathogens that grow in cultures of endotracheal aspirates may be colonizing the lower respiratory tract rather than causing infections.

Some investigators have suggested that the standard diagnostic methods for VAP are bronchoscopy with protected specimen brush (PSB) or bronchoalveolar lavage (BAL) coupled with quantitative bacteriology.[7] However, these methods are not used widely. For bacterial nosocomial pneumonia, PSB ($\geq 10^3$ organisms/mL) has a sensitivity of 80% to 90% and a specificity of 95%, and BAL ($\geq 10^4$ organisms/mL) has a sensitivity of 86% to 100% and a specificity of 95% to 100%. Because these techniques are based on quantitative bacteriology, they may miss early cases of pneumonia, and prior antibiotic treatment may decrease the sensitivity and accuracy of these methods.[6]

Because bronchoscopy is an invasive technique that is costly and not readily available, some investigators have suggested that nonbronchoscopic, or "blind," BAL is an effective alternative diagnostic method.[8-10] Quantitative endotracheal aspirates are simpler, less expensive, and appear to provide results that are similar to those obtained by bronchoscopy. Serial quantitative cultures, when correlated with clinical infection scores,[9,10] appear to diagnose pneumonia more accurately than do clinical criteria.

Clinicians must decide which diagnostic approach is optimal for specific patients in their clinical setting. This decision should be based on outcome data, demonstrating decreased morbidity, mortality, antibiotic use, and cost of the various diagnostic approaches.

Rates of Nosocomial Pneumonia

Healthcare epidemiologists should consider several factors when they review published rates of nosocomial pneumonia.[11-13] First, rates of nosocomial pneumonia will be affected by the methods used for diagnosis. In addition, many studies have been conducted in populations of high-risk patients who were hospitalized in university teaching hospitals rather than in community hospitals or long-term care facilities. Moreover, many of the studies were conducted in the United States. Thus, the rates reported in these studies may not be consistent with those found in other hospitals or in other countries.

Currently, nosocomial pneumonia accounts for 13% to 18% of all hospital-acquired infections in the United States. The rate of nosocomial pneumonia is 4 episodes per 1,000 hospitalizations in nonteaching hospitals and 7 episodes per 1,000 hospitalizations in university hospitals.[1-5] Several studies have indicated that approximately 10% to 25% of patients in intensive care units (ICUs) develop

pneumonia.[11,13] In fact, rates of nosocomial pneumonia in these patients are 10- to 20-fold higher than rates for patients on general medical and surgical floors. For example, lower respiratory tract infections are diagnosed in 0.8% to 0.9% of medical and surgical patients, in 17.5% of postoperative patients, and in 7% of patients in neonatal intensive care units.

Rates of pneumonia are increased 4- to 21-fold for intubated patients. Crude rates of VAP are 1% to 3% per day of intubation and mechanical ventilation. The incidence of VAP in different study populations has ranged from 6 to 30 cases per 100 ventilated patients. However, rates that are calculated with the number of patients as the denominator do not adjust for duration of mechanical ventilation. Thus, rates calculated per 1,000 ventilator days more accurately assess the risk of VAP. Moreover, this method allows infection control personnel to identify trends in rates more readily and to compare rates among several ICUs in the same hospital or in different hospitals. Data from the National Nosocomial Infection Surveillance System indicate that rates of pneumonia have ranged from 5 per 1,000 ventilator days in pediatric ICUs to 34 per 1,000 ventilator days in patients with thermal injury. Rates of VAP are approximately 15 per 1,000 ventilator-days for patients in medical and surgical ICUs, but often are higher for patients in medical ICUs.

Etiologic Agents

Bacterial nosocomial pneumonia usually is polymicrobial, and the etiologic agents reflect the technique used for diagnosis.[11-13] The frequency of different etiologic agents causing pneumonia also varies by type of hospital, patient population at risk, diagnostic methods, time of onset, and the microbial flora in the ICU (Table 10-2).[14-20] In general, Gram-negative bacilli, such as *Pseudomonas aeruginosa, Klebsiella pneumoniae,* and *Acinetobacter* sp have been implicated in 40% to 60% of cases, and

Staphylococcus aureus has been implicated in 20% to 40% of cases.[11-14] Anaerobic bacteria are isolated from 0% to 35% of cases. However, anaerobes rarely are isolated from intubated patients, perhaps because high levels of oxygen and changes in the airways and lungs due to mechanical ventilation impede the growth of these organisms. The rates of pneumonia caused by some pathogens, such as *Legionella pneumophila,* influenza, and respiratory syncytial virus (RSV), vary by season and hospital type. In addition, the etiologic agents vary with the time of onset. Early-onset bacterial nosocomial pneumonia occurs during the first 4 days of the acute hospital stay and usually is caused by *Streptococcus pneumoniae* (pneumococcus), *Moraxella catarrhalis,* or *Haemophilus influenzae.*[11,13] Late-onset pneumonia occurs after 4 days and most commonly is caused by *P aeruginosa, K pneumoniae, Acinetobacter* sp, or *S aureus.* Patients with late-onset pneumonia are more likely than those with early-onset pneumonia to have a serious underlying disease, previous hospitalization, or prior antibiotic therapy.

Other factors that may influence the organism-specific pneumonia rates include the availability of data from autopsies and the availability of appropriate diagnostic cultures for viruses and for bacterial pathogens that require special culture media and methods (Figure 10-1).

Legionella pneumophila

L pneumophila causes 0% to 10% of all nosocomial pneumonia cases and also has been responsible for numerous nosocomial outbreaks.[11,21-25] However, the incidence of legionnaires' disease probably is underestimated, because the tests required to identify *Legionella* sp are not performed routinely. Because the incubation period of legionnaires' disease generally is 2 to 10 days, cases that occur more than 10 days after admission are considered to be nosocomial, and those that develop between 4 and 10 days after admission are

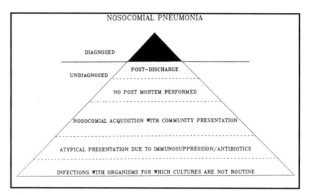

FIGURE 10-1. The "iceberg" of nosocomial pneumonia demonstrates that many cases were underdiagnosed or misclassified. Cases that were not diagnosed may have been misclassified as community-acquired, only identified at post mortem, diagnosed in the outpatient setting, or after discharge from the hospital. In addition, nosocomial pneumonia caused by *Streptococcus pneumoniae, Haemophilus influenzae,* or *Pneumocystis carinii* may be misclassified as community-acquired. Moreover, pneumonia caused by some pathogens such as *Legionella* sp may not be diagnosed because appropriate cultures were not obtained. Reprinted with permission from Craven DE, Steger KA. Epidemiology of nosocomial pneumonia: new perspectives on an old disease. *Chest.* 1995;108:1S-16S.

considered to be possibly nosocomial. Patients who are immunocompromised, critically ill, or receiving steroids are at highest risk of infection. Mortality rates from nosocomial pneumonia caused by *L pneumophila* are approximately 40%, which is nearly twofold higher than in cases of *Legionella* pneumonia that are acquired in the community.

Influenza Virus

Respiratory viruses cause nosocomial pneumonia uncommonly, but are probably underdiagnosed[11,26-29] (see Table 10-2). Most nosocomial viral infections, such as influenza, are seasonal and follow or parallel outbreaks in the community. Influenza pneumonia occurs most commonly during the winter months in patients who are elderly, immunosuppressed, or have chronic underlying diseases. The clinical disease caused by the influenza virus may be difficult to differentiate from that caused by other respiratory viruses. Therefore,

TABLE 10-2

SELECTED COMMON PATHOGENS CURRENTLY ASSOCIATED WITH NOSOCOMIAL PNEUMONIA

Pathogen	Frequency or Range (%)*	Comments
Early-Onset Bacterial Pneumonia		
Streptococcus pneumoniae (pneumococcus)	5-15	• Person-to-person spread has been documented • MDR strains are problematic • Subtyping and antibiograms are helpful to document transmission
Haemophilus influenzae (type b and nontypeable)	< 5	• Nosocomial outbreaks have been reported in pediatric and elderly patients
Anaerobic bacteria	0-35	• Rare cause of VAP
Late-Onset Bacterial Pneumonia		
Aerobic Gram-negative bacilli *Pseudomonas aeruginosa, Enterobacter* sp, *Acinetobacter* sp, *Klebsiella pneumoniae, Serratia marcescens, Escherichia coli*	40-60	• Endogenous colonization and nosocomial transmission • Gram-negative bacilli in food, water, and enteral feedings; on hands of hospital personnel; and on equipment and devices • MDR strains are a concern • Molecular typing is helpful in understanding epidemiology
Staphylococcus aureus	20-40	• Sources include other patients, hospital personnel, and fomites • MRSA is an important nosocomial pathogen • Molecular typing is useful
Mycobacterium tuberculosis	< 1	• MDR strains are an emerging nosocomial pathogen • Transmission is increased in AIDS patients • Molecular typing is important

either cultures of respiratory secretions or serologic tests must be done to confirm the diagnosis.

Respiratory Syncytial Virus

Respiratory syncytial virus infections are most common during infancy and early childhood. Disease often is mild, but may be particularly severe in children who are immunocompromised or have chronic cardiac or pulmonary disease. The clinical syndrome caused by RSV may be difficult to distinguish from that caused by other respiratory tract viruses. Culture remains the gold standard for diagnosis, but RSV antigen detection systems are rapid and have acceptable sensitivity and specificity. Once the laboratory has confirmed RSV from one hospitalized patient, subsequent patients who have a compatible clinical syndrome may be diagnosed presumptively and included in the surveillance data.

Aspergillus Species

Aspergillus pneumonia is uncommon, but associated mortality rates are high. Nosocomial respiratory infection caused by *Aspergillus* sp usually occurs in immunocompromised patients, particularly in patients undergoing chemotherapy or organ

TABLE 10-2 (continued)
Selected Common Pathogens Currently Associated With Nosocomial Pneumonia

Pathogen	Frequency or Range (%)*	Comments
Late-Onset Bacterial Pneumonia		
Legionella pneumophila	0-10	• Hospital water supply is the most common source • Molecular typing is helpful
Viruses		
Influenza A and B	Variable	• Person-to-person transmission • Associated with outbreaks in community
Respiratory syncytial virus	Variable	• Common on pediatric wards
Fungi/Protozoa		
Aspergillus	< 1	• Airborne spread to immunosuppressed patients • Associated with construction
Candida albicans	< 1	• Seen in critically ill or immunosuppressed patients treated with steroids or numerous antibiotics
Pneumocystis carinii	< 1	• Circumstantial evidence for nosocomial transmission

MDR = multidrug-resistant; VAP = ventilator-associated pneumonia; MRSA = methicillin-resistant Staphylococcus aureus; *AIDS = acquired immunodeficiency syndrome.*

*Crude rates of pneumonia taken in part from the Centers for Disease Control and Prevention's data and may vary by hospital, patient population, and method of diagnosis. Tablan et al.[11]

Reprinted with permission from Craven DE, Steger KS. Nosocomial pneumonia in mechanically ventilated adult patients: epidemiology and prevention. Semin Respir Infect. *1996;11:32-53.*

transplantation, but also in patients with acquired immunodeficiency syndrome (AIDS). Nosocomial outbreaks usually occur in bone marrow transplant patients who are granulocytopenic and receiving corticosteroids. Risk factors for invasive aspergillosis include granulocytopenia, high-dose corticosteroids or other cytotoxic drugs, and exposure to airborne spores.[11,30] Nasopharyngeal colonization may precede respiratory tract infection.

It often is difficult to diagnose *Aspergillus* pneumonia. Invasive tests, such as bronchoscopy with BAL or biopsy, usually are needed to discriminate between airway colonization and tissue invasion. Other diagnostic tests are less than optimal. For example, systemic antibody tests are unreliable, blood cultures are insensitive, and antigen assays are not available for routine clinical use.

High-risk patients who have a positive sputum culture and pulmonary signs or symptoms should be evaluated carefully.

Candida albicans

Candida albicans commonly is isolated from sputum cultures, but is an uncommon cause of nosocomial pneumonia. Patients who are immunosuppressed, receiving cytotoxic agents, steroids, or broad-spectrum antibiotics are at highest risk. We suspect that the incidence of nosocomial *C albicans* pneumonia will increase. Therefore, clinicians should consider the diagnosis in immunocompromised or critically ill patients who are treated for long periods with broad-spectrum antibiotics. Further research is needed to define the frequency of *Candida* pneumonia and to identify risk factors

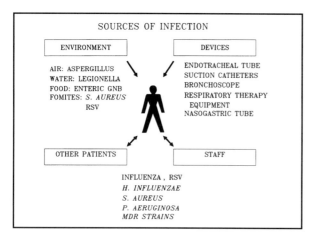

FIGURE 10-2. Summary of the modes by which various nosocomial respiratory tract pathogens are transmitted. Microorganisms may originate from the environment, contaminated devices, other patients, or hospital staff. Abbreviations: GNB = Gram-negative bacilli; RSV = respiratory syncytial virus; MDR = multidrug-resistant (in this case, it refers to multidrug resistant strains of various nosocomial pathogens including *Staphylococcus aureus* and *Mycobacterium tuberculosis*). Reprinted with permission from Craven DE, Steger KA. Epidemiology of nosocomial pneumonia: new perspectives on an old disease. *Chest.* 1995;108:1S-16S.

for this infection.

Epidemiology of Selected Pathogens

Nosocomial pathogens may be transmitted through the air, by contaminated water or colonized devices (Figure 10-2), by patients, or by healthcare workers. Gram-negative bacilli and *S aureus* may colonize healthcare workers' hands transiently, but colonization may persist in some persons, particularly those with dermatitis.[18,19] Proper handwashing, before and after patient contact, usually removes transient bacteria. Gloves and gowns also may help prevent healthcare workers from acquiring organisms while caring for patients. Gloves and gowns can become contaminated when the healthcare worker touches a patient or an environmental surface. Therefore, healthcare workers must remove gloves and gowns and wash their hands before they leave the patient's room.

Healthcare workers and infection control personnel sometimes fail to appreciate that common community-acquired bacterial respiratory pathogens, such as pneumococcus and *H influenzae,* can be transmitted within hospitals. Investigators in Spain and South Africa have documented that prior hospitalization and antibiotic use are risk factors for acquisition of multidrug-resistant pneumococci. Goetz et al recently documented transmission of nontypeable *H influenzae* among patients in a nursing home (as shown in Figures 10-3a and 10-3b).[17]

Nosocomial pneumonia caused by *L pneumophila* usually occurs in immunosuppressed patients.[21-25] The risk of infection is increased substantially if the hospital's water supply contains the organism. Inhalation of aerosols from showers, faucets, and respiratory therapy equipment or aspiration of contaminated potable water have been proposed as methods of transmission. Molecular typing techniques have helped investigators identify the reservoir for nosocomial outbreaks. For example, while investigating a common source outbreak of VAP, Venezia et al identified *L pneumophila,* Serotype 6, in specimens from the patients and in high concentrations in the hospital's potable water supply (>10^4 colony-forming units/mL [Figures 10-4a and 10-4b]).[23] Pulsed field gel electrophoresis revealed that the strain isolated from the potable water was identical to that isolated from patients with VAP. The investigators discovered that nurses used potable water to administer medications through nasogastric tubes and to dilute solutions for enteral tube feedings. The outbreak subsided after the temperature of the hot water at the faucet was increased to 131°F, and nurses began using sterile water to administer medications and to dilute solutions for enteral feedings.

Nosocomial transmission of multidrug-resistant *tuberculosis* is uncommon, but it has occurred in the United States. Recently, several outbreaks of multidrug-resistant tuberculosis have occurred in hospitals and outpatient clinics caring for patients with AIDS.[15] These outbreaks underscore the impor-

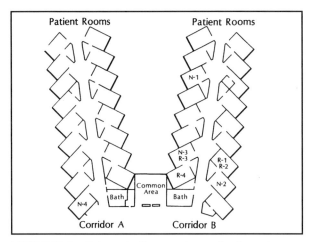

FIGURE 10-3a. Schematic diagram of a nursing home in which a strain of nontypeable *Haemophilus influenzae* caused an outbreak of pneumonia and respiratory tract colonization. Patients who developed pneumonia are designated N1 to N4, and asymptomatic roommates with oropharyngeal carriage are designated R1 to R4. Reprinted by permission of the publisher from Goetz MB, O'Brien H, Musser JM, Ward JI. Nosocomial transmission of disease caused by nontypeable strains of *Haemophilus influenzae. Am J Med.* 1994;96:342-347. Copyright 1994 by Excerpta Medica Inc.

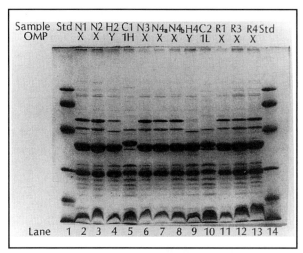

FIGURE 10-3b. Lanes 2 and 3, 6 through 8, and 11 through 13 contain outer membrane proteins (OMP) of *Haemophilus influenzae* isolates from patients in the nursing home. N4a and N4b denote two morphologically distinct isolates obtained from the same patient. All isolates from the nursing home had the same OMP profile that was named X. Lanes 5 and 10 contain OMPs from two well-characterized isolates of *H influenzae* type b (profiles C1 and C2). Lanes 4 and 9 contain OMPs from two *H influenzae* isolates obtained at a local hospital (profile Y). Lanes 1 and 14 contain the molecular weight standards which are 94 kd, 43 kd, 30 kd, 20 kd, and 14.4 kd. Reprinted by permission of the publisher from Goetz MB, O'Brien H, Musser JM, Ward JI. Nosocomial transmission of disease caused by nontypeable strains of *Haemophilus influenzae. Am J Med.* 1994;96:342-347. Copyright 1994 by Excerpta Medica Inc.

tance of instituting proper isolation precautions for all patients who have respiratory tract infections and who are at high risk of having tuberculosis until the diagnosis is established and proper treatment is instituted.[31]

Influenza virus, which probably is spread from person to person by large droplet nuclei, is transmitted in hospitals rarely. By comparison, nosocomial RSV is transmitted commonly on pediatric services, particularly during the winter months. RSV is present in high concentrations in respiratory secretions. The virus can be transmitted from person to person by large respiratory droplets that are inhaled. Alternatively, persons can acquire RSV by contact with infectious secretions or by touching contaminated fomites and then touching their conjunctiva or nasal mucosa.

Aspergillus sp commonly are found in soil, water, and decaying vegetation. *Aspergillus fumigatus* and *Aspergillus flavus* are the species most frequently isolated from patients. *A fumigatus* has

been obtained from unfiltered air in hospitals and from ventilation systems. The number of *Aspergillus* spores in the air may increase substantially during hospital construction and renovation. Even one case of nosocomial *Aspergillus* pneumonia should lead infection control personnel to look for previous cases that may have been missed and to investigate possible reservoirs within the hospital.[11,30] Patients who are neutropenic or immunocompromised may be at high risk of developing *A fumigatus* infections during periods of construction around the facility.[30] In contrast to *Aspergillus* species, *C albicans* frequently is isolated from endotracheal cultures, but has been an uncommon cause of nosocomial pneumonia. Although most patients become infected with endogenous

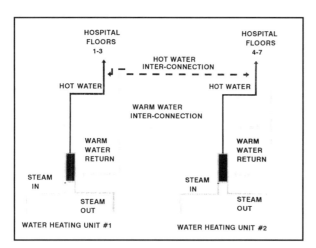

FIGURE 10-4a. Schematic diagram of the water supply system in a hospital that experienced an outbreak of pneumonia caused by *Legionella pneumophila* Serogroup 6.

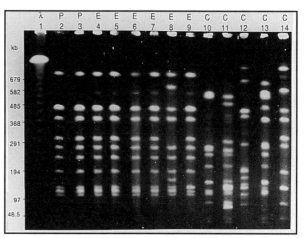

FIGURE 10-4b. Pulsed-field gel electrophoresis patterns of chromosomal DNA from *Legionella pneumophila* isolates. Lanes 2 and 3 contain chromosomal DNA obtained from patients' isolates; lanes 4 through 9 contain chromosomal DNA from isolates found in the hospital water (E), lanes 10 through 14 (C) contain chromosomal DNA from unrelated control strains. Lane 1 contains the molecular weight standard (labeled λ). Reprinted with permission Venezia RA, Agresta MD, Ahnley EM, Urquhart D, Schoonmaker MS. Nosocomial legionellosis associated with aspiration of nasogastric feedings diluted in tap water. *Infect Control Hosp Epidemiol.* 1994;15:529-534.

Candida strains, nosocomial transmission of *Candida* sp has been reported.

Pneumocystis carinii pneumonia (PCP) usually is not considered to be a nosocomial pathogen.[15] However, several clusters of cases among immunocompromised patients, including patients with acute leukemia, neutropenia, transplants, or AIDS, suggest that this organism may be transmitted within hospitals.[15] Although it has been difficult to prove that PCP was transmitted nosocomially, we believe that the circumstantial evidence is compelling.

Surveillance Methods

Previous studies have indicated that hospitals with effective surveillance and infection control programs have rates of pneumonia that are 20% lower than rates in hospitals without such programs.[11] Despite these data, advisory agencies, regulatory agencies, and medical societies have not made specific recommendations regarding surveillance for nosocomial pneumonia.

Surveillance for nosocomial pneumonia is time-consuming and thus, in our opinion, never should be considered routine, particularly in this era of limited resources. We recommend that infection control personnel perform surveillance to address questions germane to their hospital. Once the studies are com-

pleted, epidemiology personnel should share the results with hospital staff, so that together they can develop appropriate preventive strategies. Therefore, surveillance activities will differ by the size and type of hospital, the priorities of the infection control unit, and the available resources. We suspect that the spectrum of problems related to nosocomial pneumonia will be greater in large university hospitals than in small community teaching hospitals.

We recommend that infection control programs that wish to survey for nosocomial pneumonia design a system to meet the specific needs of their hospital and that they primarily should survey patients who are immunocompromised or who are hospitalized in ICUs. Infection control personnel should use a standardized definition for pneumonia and tracheobronchitis that ideally includes definitions for definite, probable, and possible nosocomial pneumonia. As discussed above, there are many techniques that can be used to diagnose nosocomial pneumonia, each of which has a different sensitivity and specificity, and there is no gold standard for diagnosis. We suggest that infection control programs tailor their definition of nosocomial pneumonia to fit the diagnostic tests that are available in their hospitals. Accurate culture or serologic data may help clinicians make a more accurate diagnosis and may help infection control personnel categorize patients correctly.

Microbiologic surveillance may help infection control personnel identify clusters of cases or outbreaks that are caused by specific pathogens, unusual organisms, or multidrug-resistant pathogens and that require the epidemiology staff to increase targeted surveillance or to conduct a thorough epidemiological investigation. The focus of the investigation will depend on the epidemiology of the organism responsible. If possible, the laboratory should save isolates obtained from patients and from possible reservoirs for serotyping or molecular typing to confirm the epidemiologic data. In some outbreaks, infection control personnel may need to include patients who have nasopharyngeal colonization, as well as patients who have infection, in their analysis, so that they have greater power to identify the source. Outbreaks caused by some pathogens, such as *S aureus,* might be associated with hospital staff who carry the epidemic strain. Thus, during outbreaks, infection control personnel may need to culture the nares or skin of staff, particularly those with dermatitis or skin lesions. When investigating some outbreaks of pneumonia, epidemiology staff may need to survey high-risk populations in the outpatient setting or in chronic-care facilities. Infection control personnel should use the epidemiologic data to design specific prevention strategies and appropriate feedback for hospital staff.

In summary, we believe that infection control staff should not collect rates of nosocomial pneumonia routinely, especially if the epidemiology staff and staff in units caring for high-risk patients do not analyze the data carefully. Infection control teams that follow trends in VAP should calculate the rates per 1,000 patient-ventilator days to adjust for length of stay and duration of mechanical ventilation. Infection control, epidemiology, and pathology staff, together with the hospital's infection control committee, should review carefully all cases of nosocomial pneumonia caused by special pathogens such as *L pneumophila, A fumigatus,* or *M tuberculosis.* Infection control personnel also should investigate clusters of cases caused by the same organism, by unusual pathogens, or by multidrug-resistant pathogens.

Pathogenesis

Although the pathogenesis of nosocomial pneumonia can be complex, hospital epidemiologists should focus on aspiration of bacteria from the oropharynx as the primary and most frequent route by which bacteria enter the lower respiratory tract (Figure 10-5).[11-13] In ventilated patients, bacteria may leak around the cuff of the endotracheal tube and colonize the patient's lower respiratory tract, increasing the risk of purulent tracheobronchitis and pneumonia. The patient's risk of pneumonia most likely is related to the quantity and virulence of the bacteria that reach the lower respiratory tract, the ability of the pulmonary defenses to protect the host, and the inflammatory response to infection.

Researchers have used both univariate and multivariate analysis to identify several risk factors for pneumonia.[11-15] Some of the putative risk factors include host factors, the types of bacteria colonizing the pharynx, and prior use of antibiotics. Mechanically ventilated patients often have devices such as nasogastric tubes and nasotracheal tubes that increase the risk of nosocomial sinusitis and VAP. Ventilated patients often have an increased risk of gastric, oropharyngeal, and tracheal colonization with hospital-acquired pathogens.[11-13] Other risk factors for gastric, oropharyngeal, and tracheal colonization with nosocomial pathogens include advanced age, achlorhydria, tube feeding,

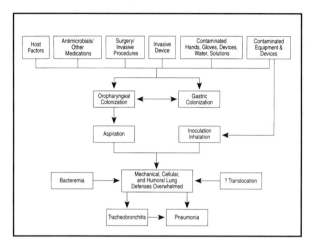

FIGURE 10-5. Summary of risk factors contributing to colonization and infection of the lower respiratory tract. Other factors include the number of organisms inoculated, the virulence of the infecting agents, and the host's defenses in the lung. Abbreviation: CASS = continuous aspiration of subglottic secretions.

gastrointestinal disease, malnutrition, and probably the use of antacids or histamine type 2 (H_2) blockers to prevent stress bleeding.

Prevention of Nosocomial Pneumonia

Healthcare epidemiologists should make prevention of pneumonia one of their priorities. However, experts do not agree about the efficacy of all preventive strategies, and particular strategies may not apply to all hospitals. Despite the limitations of the data, we believe that healthcare epidemiologists should try to institute practices and procedures that are cost-effective in their institutions and that decrease the risk of nosocomial pneumonia. Detailed information and recommendations are available in the 1994 "Guideline for Prevention of Nosocomial Pneumonia," issued by the Centers for Disease Control's Hospital Infection Control Practice Advisory Committee (CDC/HICPAC).[11] These data and recommendations are an important resource for healthcare epidemiologists and other infection control personnel. We have reviewed selected risk factors for nosocomial pneumonia, appropriate control measures, and the recommenda-

tions of CDC/HICPAC in Table 10-3. In addition, we strongly support using appropriate isolation precautions for patients admitted with undiagnosed respiratory tract infection to prevent nosocomial spread of respiratory pathogens. Once the diagnosis is established and proper therapy is initiated, the infection control team can reassess whether the patient needs to be in isolation. Furthermore, we think that infection control personnel should work with staff in the ICUs to develop appropriate strategies for reducing the risk of nosocomial pneumonia, including developing and instituting strict infection control policies, controlling the use of antibiotics, and developing mechanisms that limit the spread of multidrug-resistant organisms. In the following paragraphs, we discuss some specific recommendations that have been reviewed in detail by other authors.[11-13,18-20]

Host Factors

Host factors such as advanced age, lifestyle factors (eg, smoking and other substance abuse), and underlying diseases significantly increase the risk of colonization of the upper airway and of subsequent pneumonia. However, once the patient is hospitalized, these factors generally cannot be altered, and therefore these factors are inappropriate targets for the prevention of nosocomial pneumonia. In contrast, the risk of postoperative pneumonia may be decreased if patients ambulate soon after surgery, use incentive spirometry, and practice deep coughing.

Prescribed Drugs

Overuse of antibiotics may increase the risk of colonization with antibiotic-resistant nosocomial pathogens. Thus, we recommend controlling the use of antibiotics, especially in ICUs. We also recommend that physicians use sedatives prudently, because somnolent patients can aspirate their oropharyngeal contents and subsequently develop pneumonia. Stress bleeding prophylaxis with antacids, H_2 blockers, and sucralfate for mechanically ventilated patients has not been approved by the Food and Drug Administration, but is used widely and probably overprescribed. Several controversial studies have found lower rates of VAP in patients given prophylaxis with sucralfate compared with patients given antacids or H_2 blockers.[11,13] This may be related to the effects of H_2 blockers and antacids on gastric acid secretion, colonization, or host defenses.

Endotracheal Tubes

Aspiration and gastric reflux are common in mechanically ventilated patients. The risk of aspiration may be reduced by elevating the patient's head to 30° and by administering enteral feedings through oral or nasogastric tubes carefully. The HICPAC has recommended these practices.

Endotracheal tubes circumvent the defenses in the upper respiratory tract, impair mechanical clearance from the lower airway, and allow oropharyngeal secretions to leak around the cuff into the lower airway (Figure 10-6). Continuous aspiration of subglottic secretions, a relatively simple, safe, and inexpensive technique that removes contaminated secretions, reduces the risk of early onset VAP. Nasotracheal tubes increase the risk of maxillary sinusitis and VAP. Therefore, oral tracheal tubes should be used, if possible. Moreover, all invasive devices should be used only if essential for the patient's care.

Endotracheal Suction Catheters

Tracheal suction catheters, which are used on ventilated patients, may carry bacteria directly into the lung, increasing the risk of tracheal colonization. Healthcare workers should use the aseptic technique when suctioning endotracheal secretions and should use only sterile solutions to rinse these catheters. Closed, multiuse suction systems may be more convenient and safer for hospital personnel than single-use catheters and may cause less hypoxia for the patient than do the single-catheter systems.

Gastric Tube and Enteral Feeding

Nearly all patients receiving mechanical ventilation have a gastric tube inserted to manage gastric secretions, to prevent gastric distention, or to provide nutritional support. The risk of nosocomial sinusitis and VAP caused by the nasogastric tube can be decreased by the use of an oral gastric tube. When initiated early, enteral feeding through a gastric tube helps maintain the gastrointestinal epithelium and reduces the need for stress bleeding prophylaxis. We would encourage clinicians to assess accurately each patient's nutritional status and to avoid unnecessary parenteral nutrition, because these precautions may reduce the risk of nosocomial pneumonia. On the basis of data from Venezia et al[23] and Marrie et al,[25] we advocate using sterile water when diluting tube feedings and when flushing gastric tubes, to reduce colonization and the risk of pneumonia. However, the CDC/HICPAC has not made a recommendation on this practice. Likewise, this group has not made recommendations regarding the following important issues:
- Whether metoclopramide should be used to increase gastric emptying.
- Whether tube feedings should be administered continuously or in boluses.
- Whether the stomach contents should be monitored to determine if feeding solutions are present and, if a residual volume is found, whether it should be removed.

Finally, experts do not agree on which size feeding tube is best, which location in the gastrointestinal tract is optimal, and whether acidified enteral feedings are useful.

Respiratory Therapy Equipment

Ventilator breathing circuits that have humidifying cascades should be changed no more frequently than every 48 hours and may remain in place longer. In fact, these circuits may be changed as clinically indicated (Figure 10-7). Because condensate in ventilator circuits often contains mil-

TABLE 10-3
RISK FACTORS AND APPROPRIATE CONTROL MEASURES FOR NOSOCOMIAL PNEUMONIA

Risk Factors	Control Measures	CDC/HICPAC Category
Host		
Age	Primary prevention	NS
Multiple trauma or head trauma	Kinetic beds/continuous lateral rotational therapy	NR
Underlying disease, acute or chronic	Treat underlying condition (eg, COPD), use incentive spirometry and vaccines as indicated	II
Immunosuppression	Consider tapering steroids, cytotoxic, and immuno-suppressant agents; consider using granulocyte colony stimulating factor for neutropenic patients	IA
Malnutrition/obesity	Nutritional support or weight control as indicated	NS
Smoking	Nicotine patches, counseling, and support	NS
Alcohol abuse	Addiction counseling	NS
Parenteral drug use	Counseling, access to drug treatment	NS
Depressed level of consciousness	Judicious use of sedation to prevent decreased consciousness	NS
Coma	Reduce risk of aspiration by placing the patient in a semiupright position and administering enteral feedings properly	IB
Aspiration	CASS	NR*
	Semiupright position	IB
	Judicious use of enteral feedings	IB
Surgery		
(Head/neck, chest/abdominal)	Use proper antibiotic prophylaxis	IA
	Properly position patients	IA
	Rapidly ambulate the patients	IB
	Control pain	IB
	Use incentive spirometry	II
	Encourage postoperative patients to cough and breath deeply	IB
Medications		
Antimicrobial agents	Use antimicrobial agents judiciously for prophylaxis	IA
	Avoid routine SDD	NR*
Antacids/H2 blockers	Use sucralfate rather than antacids +/-H_2 blockers, stress bleeding prophylaxis is indicated	II
Neuromuscular blockers	Limit to specific clinical indications	NS
Environmental		
Seasonal	Increase awareness of seasonal pathogens through education	NS
Water	Conduct surveillance for *Legionella pneumophila* infections	IA
	Use sterile water for tube feedings and to prepare medications for high-risk patients	NS
Air	Use proper filters for *Aspergillus* sp in areas housing high-risk patients	IB
	Monitor airflow in hospital	NS
Cross-infection		
Patient to patient	Educate and train personnel in proper techniques for asepsis and isolation	IA
Staff to patient	Proper isolation for patients with possible respiratory infections	NS
	Encourage proper handwashing	IA
	Use gowns and gloves when appropriate	IA
	Feedback nosocomial data from infection surveillance	IA

TABLE 10-3 (continued)
RISK FACTORS AND APPROPRIATE CONTROL MEASURES FOR NOSOCOMIAL PNEUMONIA

Risk Factors	Control Measures	CDC/HICPAC Category
Devices/Equipment		
Invasive devices/equipment	Remove devices expeditiously	IB
	Clean and disinfect or sterilize equipment properly	IA
Endotracheal tube/intubation	Use oral tracheal tubes and avoid nasotracheal tubes; maintain cuff pressure >20 cm H_2O	NS
	Keep cuff inflated; aspirate subglottic secretions before deflating cuff	IB
	Use CASS	NR*
	Prevent patients from removing their endotracheal tubes	IA
	Keep patients in a semiupright position	IB
Nasogastric tube	Use orogastric tube when possible	NS
	Remove tube as soon as possible	IB
	Use sterile water rather than tap water to flush tube or to dilute enteral feeding solutions	NS†
Ventilator circuits	Change humidified ventilator circuits no more than every 48 hrs	IA
	May change these circuits as clinically indicated (over 48 hrs)	NR
Tubing condensate	Drain condensate in ventilator tubing away from patient and then discard	IB
	Use hygroscopic condenser/humidifiers or heat/moisture exchangers	NR
In-line nebulizers	Disinfect between treatments	IB
	Replace between patients	IB
	Sterilize between patients	IA
Spirometers, 0_2 sensors, and hand-powered resuscitation bags	Clean and disinfect between patients; use filter to prevent contamination	IA
Tracheal suction catheters	Use aseptic technique	IA
	Use closed circuit tracheal suction catheters	NR
	Use sterile catheter for open system	II
Tracheostomy care	Use aseptic technique when changing tubes	IB
Enteral feeding	Use oral gastric tube rather than nasogastric tube	NS†
	Remove tube as soon as possible	IB
	Elevate head of bed to 30°-45° if not contraindicated	IB
	Routinely assess patient's intestinal motility and adjust rate	IB
	Use small- or large-bore gastric tubes	NR
	Acidify gastric feedings	NR
	Check placement of tube	IB
	Use intermittent versus continuous enteral feedings	NR

CDC = Centers for Disease Control and Prevention; HICPAC = Hospital Infection Control Practices Advisory Committee; COPD = chronic obstructive pulmonary disease; CASS = continuous aspiration of subglottic secretions; SDD = selective decontamination of digestive tract; H2 = histamine type 2.
CDC/HICPAC categories: IA = strongly recommended for all hospitals and strongly supported by well-designed experimental or epidemiologic studies. IB = strongly recommended for all hospitals; viewed as effective by experts in the field and a consensus of HICPAC members, based on strong rationale and suggestive evidence, even though definitive scientific studies may not have been done. II = suggested for implementation in many hospitals; recommendations may be supported by suggestive clinical or epidemiologic studies, a strong theoretical rationale, or definitive studies that are applicable to some, but not all, hospitals. NR = no recommendation; unresolved issue is defined as "practices for which there are either insufficient data or no consensus regarding efficacy."[2] NS = not specified in CDC/HICPAC guideline.
*SDD not recommended for routine use; CASS system not yet available in United States.
†The authors recommend use of oral gastric tube and advocate the use of sterile water to administer medications and to dilute tube feedings.

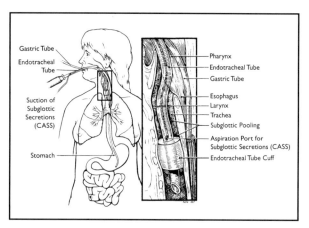

FIGURE 10-6. Schematic drawing of a patient with an oral endotracheal tube and an orogastric tube rather than a nasogastric tube to reduce the risk of nosocomial sinusitis. Note also the use of continuous aspiration of subglottic secretions. Reprinted with permission from Craven DE, Steger KS. Nosocomial pneumonia in mechanically ventilated adult patients: epidemiology and prevention. *Semin Respir Infect.* 1996;11:32-53.

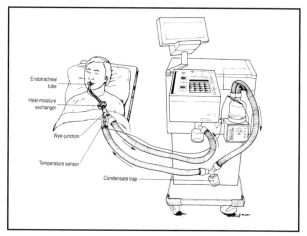

FIGURE 10-7. Diagram of a patient receiving mechanical ventilation. The compressed air from the ventilator is bubbled through the humidifying cascade, the inspiratory phase tubing, and the endotracheal tube to the patient. The expired gases travel through the expiratory tubing through a trap. The medication nebulizer is shown in the inspiratory phase circuit. A heat-moisture exchanger inserted in the Wye junction can be used instead of a bubbling humidifier.

lions of bacteria, healthcare workers must handle the tubing in a manner that prevents reflux into the patient's trachea. Heat and moisture exchangers, which recycle exhaled moisture and eliminate condensate, are tolerated well by most ventilated patients and are useful particularly in postoperative or lower-risk patients. Resuscitation bags, spirometers, and oxygen analyzers are potential sources of cross-contamination and must be cleaned and disinfected properly before they can be used for other patients.

Cross-Infection

Gram-negative bacilli and *S aureus* can be spread easily from patient to patient on the hands of healthcare workers. Handwashing removes transient bacteria effectively. Because healthcare workers frequently do not wash their hands, some experts have advocated the use of gloves and gowns for contact with all ventilated patients. In fact, investigators have shown that the use of gloves and gowns can decrease rates of nosocomial pneumonia and overall rates of nosocomial infections significantly. However, healthcare workers always

must change their gloves and wash their hands between patients.

Selective Decontamination of the Digestive Tract

The purpose of selective decontamination of the digestive tract (SDD) is to reduce oropharyngeal and gastric colonization by aerobic Gram-negative bacilli, thereby reducing the rate of VAP. SDD regimens usually include both systemic cefotaxime, trimethoprim, or a quinolone, and several nonabsorbable oral local antibiotics, such as an aminoglycoside, polymyxin B, and amphotericin B, which are applied in a paste to the oropharynx and are ingested by mouth or through the nasogastric tube.[11,13] Several investigators have studied the efficacy of SDD and have demonstrated dramatically reduced rates of respiratory tract colonization and infection. Some SDD regimens that included a broad-spectrum systemic antibiotic reduced mortality rates as well. However, the studies had very different designs, evaluated different populations, and used inconsistent definitions of respiratory tract infection, sometimes including tracheobronchitis.

The CDC/HICPAC guideline[11] did not make a recommendation regarding SDD. However, we cannot recommend routine use of SDD, because these regimens may select multidrug-resistant nosocomial pathogens and increase the frequency of infections caused by Gram-positive pathogens.[13]

Strategies for Preventing Pneumonia Caused by Specific Pathogens

The 1994 CDC/HICPAC "Guideline for Prevention of Nosocomial Pneumonia" summarizes strategies for the prevention of Legionnaires' disease.[11] The guideline presents two general approaches. First, Yu and coworkers[22] have recommended that hospitals routinely culture their potable water for *L pneumophila*. The advantage of this strategy is that clinicians and infection control personnel are aware that *L pneumophila* is present in the hospital's water supply and therefore will consider this pathogen in the differential diagnosis for patients with nosocomial pneumonia. However, *Legionella* sp contaminate the water systems in many hospitals that do not have cases of Legionnaires' disease. Thus, the CDC recommended that clinicians maintain a high index of suspicion for Legionnaires' disease and that infection control personnel obtain cultures of the hospital's water supply only when they identify a laboratory-confirmed case or two possible cases of nosocomial *Legionella* pneumonia. Neither Yu nor the CDC recommend treating water supplies in the absence of clinical cases.

Influenza may be prevented by vaccination if the implicated strain is in the vaccine and the host responds to the vaccine. Prophylactic amantadine or rimantadine may be useful to control nosocomial outbreaks of influenza A, but these drugs, especially amantadine, have notable side effects. Other preventive measures include placing infected patients on droplet isolation precautions in a private room or cohorting infected patients and limiting elective admissions and the number of visitors.[31]

Respiratory syncytial virus can spread easily in the hospital. Once the first case of RSV has been identified, the infection control program should institute contact isolation precautions with gowns and gloves for all children admitted to the hospital who have symptoms of respiratory infection or who develop such symptoms while hospitalized. Healthcare workers must change their gloves and wash their hands between patients, and they should avoid touching their eyes or noses. The use of gowns appears to prevent transmission after contact with the environment. Special efforts, such as private rooms or cohorting staff and infected patients, may be needed to protect high-risk patients.

Control of *Aspergillus* pneumonia is based on decreasing the exposure of high-risk patients to spores. The 1994 CDC/HICPAC guideline recommends methods for evaluating air handling systems and discusses, in detail, the current recommendations for the use of air filters and for the number of air exchanges.[11] Hospitals that are planning construction or renovation projects should follow these guidelines carefully.

Conclusion

Our understanding of the epidemiology and prevention of nosocomial pneumonia has increased substantially over the past decade. Well-designed studies are needed to improve and standardize diagnostic methods and to determine whether preventive strategies are beneficial and cost-effective. In addition, we must refine our understanding of the host's responses to colonization and infection and to immune stimulators that might prevent nosocomial pneumonia or might enhance the efficacy of antimicrobial therapy.

Nosocomial pneumonia is an important problem for healthcare epidemiologists and infection control staff, because these infections are common, and they are associated with substantial morbidity, mortality, and cost. Infection control personnel should choose their surveillance methods after defining their objectives and the needs of the specific healthcare facility. We recommend that infection control personnel cease to collect pneumonia rates routinely and, instead, institute targeted surveillance and methods for quickly identifying clusters and "red-flag" organisms such as *L pneumophila, M tuberculosis,* RSV, *A fumigatus,* or multidrug-resistant strains of bacteria. We believe that infection control personnel should aim to do the following:

- Promptly institute respiratory isolation for appropriate patients.
- Identify patients at high risk of nosocomial pneumonia.
- Educate healthcare workers regarding risk factors for nosocomial pneumonia.
- Work closely with appropriate healthcare workers to design methods that prevent colonization and cross-transmission of nosocomial pathogens.
- Develop policies that define appropriate use of invasive devices and antimicrobial agents.
- Identify environmental sources of nosocomial pneumonia, as necessary.

Despite limitations in our knowledge, healthcare epidemiologists and infection control staff must lead their hospital's efforts to prevent nosocomial pneumonia. However, they cannot accomplish this Herculean task on their own. To prevent nosocomial pneumonia successfully, infection control personnel must collaborate closely with physicians, nurses, respiratory therapists, nutritionists, microbiologists, healthcare administrators, and other hospital staff. The healthcare epidemiologist's challenge is to identify the primary remedial risk factors in the patient population and then to coordinate a vigorous multidisciplinary response.

Acknowledgments

The authors thank Maria Tetzaguic for helping us prepare the manuscript, and Drs. Robert Duncan and Michael Niederman for giving us helpful comments and suggestions.

References

1. Pennington JE, ed. *Respiratory Infections: Diagnosis and Management.* 3rd ed. New York, NY: Raven Press; 1994.

2. Niederman MS, Sarosi GA, Glassroth J, eds. *Respiratory Infections: A Scientific Basis for Management.* Philadelphia, Pa: WB Saunders; 1994.

3. Craven DE, Steger KA, Duncan RA. Prevention and control of nosocomial pneumonia. In: Wenzel R, ed. *Prevention and Control of Nosocomial Infections.* 2nd ed. Baltimore, Md: Williams & Wilkins; 1993.

4. Mayhall CG, ed. *Hospital Epidemiology and Infection Control.* Baltimore, Md: Williams & Wilkins; 1995.

5. Craven DE, Steger KA, LaForce FM. Nosocomial pneumonia. In: Bennett JV, Brachman PS, eds. *Hospital Infections.* 4th ed. Philadelphia, Pa: Lippincott-Raven Press; 1997.

6. Niederman MS, Torres A, Summer W. Invasive diagnostic testing is not needed routinely to manage patients suspected of having ventilator acquired pneumonia. *Am J Respir Crit Care Med.* 1994;150:565-569.

7. Chastre J, Fagon JY. Invasive diagnostic testing should be routinely used to manage suspected pneumonia in mechanically ventilated patients. *Am J Respir Crit Care Med.* 1994;150:570-574.

8. El-Ebiary M, Torres A, Gonzalez J, et al. Quantitative cultures of endotracheal aspirates for the diagnosis of ventilator-associated pneumonia. *Am Rev Respir Dis.* 1993;148:1552-1557.

9. A'Court CHD, Garrard CS, Crook D, et al. Microbiological lung surveillance in mechanically ventilated patients, using non-directed lavage and quantitative culture. *QJM.* 1993;86:635-648.

10. Pugin J, Auckenthaler R, Mili N, Janssens JP, Lew PD, Suter PM. Diagnosis of ventilator-associated pneumonia by bacteriologic analysis of bronchoscopic and nonbronchoscopic blind bronchoalveolar lavage fluid. *Am Rev Respir Dis.* 1988;138:117-120.

11. Tablan OC, Anderson LJ, Arden NH, et al. Guidelines for prevention of nosocomial pneumonia—1994. *Infect Control Hosp Epidemiol.* 1994;15:587-627.

12. Craven DE, Steger KA, Barber TW. Preventing nosocomial pneumonia: state of the art and perspectives for the 1990s. In: Martone WJ, Garner JS, eds. Proceedings of the Third Decennial International Conference on Nosocomial Infections. *Am J Med.* 1991;91(suppl 3B):44S-53S.

13. Craven DE, Steger KS. Nosocomial pneumonia in mechanically ventilated adult patients: epidemiology and preven-

tion. *Semin Respir Infect.* 1996;11:32-53.

14. Johanson WG Jr, Pierce AK, Sanford JP, Thomas GD. Nosocomial respiratory infections with gram-negative bacilli: the significance of colonization of the respiratory tract. *Ann Intern Med.* 1972;77:701-706.

15. Craven DE, Steger KA, Hirschhorn LR. Nosocomial colonization and infection in persons infected with human immunodeficiency virus. *Infect Control Hosp Epidemiol.* 1996;17:304-318.

16. Leu HS, Kaiser DL, Mori M, Woolson RF, Wenzel RP. Hospital-acquired pneumonia: attributable mortality and morbidity. *Am J Epidemiol.* 1989;129:1258-1267.

17. Goetz MB, O'Brien H, Musser JM, Ward JI. Nosocomial transmission of disease caused by nontypeable strains of *Haemophilus influenzae. Am J Med.* 1994;96:342-347.

18. Maki DG. Control of colonization and transmission of pathogenic bacteria in the hospital. *Ann Intern Med.* 1978;89:777-780.

19. Weinstein RA. Epidemiology and control of nosocomial infections in adult intensive care units. In: Martone WJ, Garner JS, eds. Proceedings of the Third Decennial International Conference on Nosocomial Infections. *Am J Med.* 1991;3B(suppl):179S-184S.

20. Torres A, Serra-Battles J, Ros E, et al. Pulmonary aspiration of gastric contents in patients receiving mechanical ventilation: the effect of body position. *Ann Intern Med.* 1992;116:540-543.

21. Kirby BD, Synder KM, Meyer RD, et al. Legionnaires' disease: report of sixty-five nosocomially acquired cases and review of the literature. *Medicine.* 1980;59:188-205.

22. Yu VL, Kroboth FJ, Shonnard J, et al. Legionnaire's disease: new clinical perspective from a prospective pneumonia study. *Am J Med.* 1982;73:357-361.

23. Venezia RA, Agresta MD, Ahnley EM, Urquhart D, Schoonmaker MS. Nosocomial legionellosis associated with aspiration of nasogastric feedings diluted in tap water. *Infect Control Hosp Epidemiol.* 1994;15:529-534.

24. Blatt SP, Parkinson MD, Pace E, et al. Nosocomial Legionnaires' disease: aspiration as a primary mode of disease acquisition. *Am J Med.* 1993:95:16-22.

25. Marrie TJ, Haldane D, MacDonald S, et al. Control of endemic nosocomial Legionnaires' disease by using sterile potable water for high risk patients. *Epidemiol Infect.* 1991;107:591-605.

26. Hoffman PC, Dixon RE. Control of influenza in the hospital. *Ann Intern Med.* 1977;87:725-728.

27. Valenti WM, Hall CB, Douglas RG, et al. Nosocomial viral infections: epidemiology and significance. *Infect Control.* 1979;1:33-37.

28. Hall CB. Nosocomial viral respiratory infections: perennial weeds on pediatric wards. *Am J Med.* 1981;70:670-676.

29. Leclair JM, Freeman J, Sullivan BF, Crowley CM, Goldmann DA. Prevention of nosocomial respiratory syncytial virus infections through compliance with glove and gown isolation precautions. *N Engl J Med.* 1987;317:329-334.

30. Arnow PM, Anderson RL, Mainous PD, et al. Pulmonary *Aspergillosis* during hospital renovation. *Am Rev Respir Dis.* 1978;118:49-53.

31. Garner JS, the Hospital Infection Control Practices Advisory Committee, Centers for Disease Control and Prevention. Guideline for isolation precautions in hospitals. *Infect Control Hosp Epidemiol.* 1996;17:53-80.

CHAPTER 11

Basics of Surgical Site Infection Surveillance

Marie-Claude Roy, MD, MS, Trish M. Perl, MD, MSc

Abstract

Surgical site infections, the third most common class of nosocomial infections, cause substantial morbidity and mortality and increase hospital costs. Surveillance programs can lead to reductions in surgical site infection rates of 35% to 50%. In this chapter, we will discuss the practical aspects of implementing a hospital-based surveillance program for surgical site infections. We will review surveillance methods, patient populations that should be screened, and interventions that could reduce infection rates.

Introduction

Our understanding of the pathogenesis and risk factors for surgical site infections (SSIs) has changed substantially over time. During the early years of modern surgery, many patients died from wound sepsis. Despite our increased knowledge, SSIs, as they are called today, continue to cause substantial morbidity, and they burden healthcare systems with immense costs. Currently in the United States, SSIs are the third most common nosocomial infection, accounting for 15% of all nosocomial infections reported to the National Nosocomial Infections Surveillance (NNIS) System in 1991.[2] In one study, SSIs accounted for 14% of all adverse events in hospitalized patients.[3] The average SSI prolongs the hospital stay by 7.3 days.[2] These infections also contribute 42% of the extra charges attributed to nosocomial infections,[4] which was estimated to be $3,152 per SSI in 1992.[2] On average, patients with an SSI incur 4.6 extra ambulatory-care visits than do patients who do not acquire these infections.[5] In NNIS hospitals, 0.62% to 1.9% of patients with SSIs died from these infections.[2] These numbers highlight the tremendous human and financial costs that SSIs add to the healthcare system and therefore the importance of controlling them.

The Centers for Disease Control and Prevention (CDC), motivated to document the cost-effectiveness of infection control activities, conducted the Study of the Efficacy of Nosocomial Infection Control (SENIC).[6] The investigators concluded that an infection surveillance program that reported SSI rates to surgeons could decrease overall SSI rates by approximately 32%.[6] Furthermore, Olson and Lee[7] and Cruse and

Foord[8] have demonstrated that active surveillance with feedback of SSI rates to individual surgeons decreased SSI rates by 50%; thus, research has documented that surveillance can reduce the incidence of SSIs significantly. However, several important questions about surveillance for SSIs remain unanswered.

- Which surveillance methods should we use?
- Which surgical patients should we survey?
- Should we conduct postdischarge surveillance, and, if so, how?

The purpose of this chapter is to answer some of the unanswered questions and to summarize the basic steps required to implement an in-hospital surveillance program for SSIs.

How to Do Surveillance

Objectives

When developing a surveillance system, an infection control program first must establish its objectives. The first objective is to reduce SSI rates, thereby reducing morbidity and improving care. To achieve this goal, infection control personnel must determine endemic or baseline rates of SSIs. As they follow these rates over time, epidemiology staff will be able to identify both clusters of infections and specific problems that increase SSI rates over the endemic rates. However, doing surveillance is more than collecting data, going to the microbiology laboratory, and spending many hours tabulating monthly infection rates. Surveillance programs should help infection control personnel to identify and implement preventive strategies and control measures, to assess the effect of these measures, and, ultimately, to decrease morbidity and hospital costs. Furthermore, epidemiology staff also may use the SSI surveillance program to review protocols for antimicrobial prophylaxis or the efficacy of aseptic precautions used in the operating theater. Infection control personnel also should feed back surveillance data to surgeons and

other members of the surgical team to educate them and to review their progress in preventing SSIs.

Definition

Before implementing an SSI surveillance system, infection control personnel must write a precise definition for SSIs. Ideally, in each hospital, the definition should remain unchanged, so that epidemiology and surgical staff can compare data over time and can evaluate interventions implemented to reduce these rates. The definition also should be simple to use and should be accepted by nurses and surgeons. Infection control personnel also must apply the definition consistently.

Ehrenkranz et al powerfully demonstrated why we must use objective criteria to identify SSIs, and why we must apply such definitions consistently.[9] The infection control professional (ICP) at a 200-bed general community hospital reported that a neurosurgeon's SSI rates ranged from 3% to 11%. The infection control committee considered these rates to be excessive and repeatedly investigated the surgeon's practice. When the surgeon proposed to terminate his practice, the hospital administrator asked consultants from the Florida Consortium for Infection Control to perform an independent investigation. Ehrenkranz and colleagues determined that the ICP used a definition of SSI that lacked objective criteria (ie, "recovery of potentially pathogenic bacterial species from the operative site or a physician's notation of a nosocomial infection").[9] Consequently, the ICP had falsely categorized noninfected patients as infected. The consultants recommended that the infection control committee establish clear standards for confirmed SSIs, which would be used routinely. Over the next 2 years, none of the surgeon's patients were reported to have had SSI.

The Joint Commission on Accreditation of Healthcare Organizations soon may require all hospitals in the United States to use a standard definition of SSI, so that rates can be compared among hospitals and surgeons. In 1992, a consensus group from the Association for Professionals in Infection Control and Epidemiology, the Society for Healthcare Epidemiology of America, and the Surgical Infection Society modified the definition of surgical wound infections and changed the name to surgical site infections.[10] According to this new definition, SSIs are categorized as incisional and organ-space SSIs. Incisional SSIs are classified further as involving only the skin and subcutaneous tissue (superficial-incisional SSI) or involving deep soft tissues of the incision (deep-incisional SSI) (Figure 11-1). The definition of superficial-incisional SSI requires that at least one of the following occur within 30 days of the operative procedure:

- Purulent drainage from the superficial incision.
- Organisms isolated from an aseptically obtained culture of fluid or tissue from the superficial incision.
- At least one of the following signs or symptoms of infection: pain or tenderness, localized swelling, redness, or heat, and the surgeon deliberately opened the superficial incision, unless incision is culture negative.
- The surgeon or attending physician diagnosed a superficial incisional SSI.

In addition, infections that occur within 1 year of a procedure in which an implant is placed also are considered to be nosocomial SSI. Deep-incisional and organ-space SSI are defined similarly.[10]

Surveillance Methods

Hospitals use many different surveillance methods to identify nosocomial infections. The sensitivity and specificity of several surveillance methods have been assessed for nosocomial infections in general,[11,12] but not specifically for SSIs. Nevertheless, we will review several common surveillance methods and discuss whether each method can be used effectively to survey for SSIs. Table 11-1 summarizes the sensitivity of several

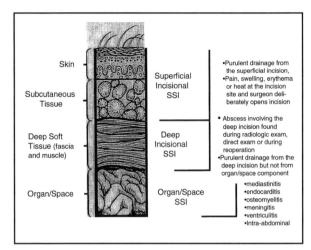

FIGURE 11-1. Schematic of surgical site infection (SSI) anatomy and appropriate classification. This figure depicts the cross-sectional anatomy of a surgical incision upon which is superimposed the most recent classification for SSI and the definition of an infection at each site.[10]

methods and specifies which have been studied for SSI surveillance.

Daily Wound Examination and Chart Review

After conducting prospective SSI surveillance for 10 years, Olson and Lee concluded that daily hospital chart review and examination of postoperative wounds probably are the most sensitive and rigorous ways to perform SSI surveillance.[7] Although these methods are tedious and time-consuming, some experts still consider them to be the gold standard and recommend that surveillance for SSI includes daily examination of operative wounds. To facilitate this method, infection control personnel or surgeons could train staff nurses who see the wounds during routine care to recognize signs of infection and report all clinically suspicious wounds to the ICP. The ICP then could examine all such wounds and determine which meet the criteria for infection.[13]

Cardo et al compared surveillance performed by an ICP who reviewed the patients' medical records and discussed each patient's progress with nurses and physicians with surveillance performed by a hospital epidemiologist who reviewed the

TABLE 11-1
SURVEILLANCE METHODS*

Surveillance Methods	Type of Nosocomial Infections Surveyed	Sensitivity	Reference
Physician self-report forms	All	0.14-0.34	41
Retrospective chart review	SSI	0.73-0.80	15
	All	0.90	11
Microbiology reports	All	0.33-0.71	11,42
Antibiotic use	All	0.81	18†
	All	0.48	11
Selective chart review using Kardex clues	All	0.85	11

SSI = surgical site infection.
Adapted from Perl TM[12] and Yokoe DS, Platt R.[43]
†Evaluated all nosocomial infections in patients who had cesarean sections.

patients' medical records and examined their wounds. The ICP identified 84% of SSIs noted by the hospital epidemiologist. The authors concluded that accurate data on SSIs could be collected by persons who do not examine the operative wounds directly.[14] Haley et al have corroborated this finding.[15] However, the quality of the information gleaned from medical records depends on their completeness and on the reviewer's experience. Furthermore, if the infection control team has limited resources for surveillance, they will not be able to review the medical records of all surgical patients. Such programs either must focus on specific surgical subpopulations or must use other less time-consuming surveillance methods.

Selective Chart Review With Kardex Review

Wenzel et al studied the sensitivity of reviewing selected medical records compared with reviewing all medical records.[11] With selective chart review, the ICP searched the kardex for clues such as fever or antibiotic use. If one or more clues were noted, the ICP evaluated the patient's medical record more thoroughly. In Wenzel's study, the ICP, using kardex review, correctly identified 82% to 94% of nosocomial infections identified when all medical records were reviewed. The kardex method saved 15 to 19 hours of the ICP's time.[11] The kardex may be a good source of information about patients at high risk of certain infections, but it probably would not be a good source of information on patients with SSIs. Indeed, fever and antibiotic use are not necessarily good indicators of SSI. Unfortunately, more useful indicators, such as the frequency with which wound dressings are changed and descriptions of discharge from the wound, are not readily available from the kardex. Moreover, the accuracy of this method is limited by the completeness and accuracy of the data in the kardex.

Microbiology Reports

Surveillance for all nosocomial infections that relies only on microbiology data has a sensitivity of only 33% to 65%.[11,12] Furthermore, only two thirds of inpatients' wounds and even fewer outpatients' wounds are cultured, despite clinical evidence for SSI.[16] Therefore, surveillance for SSI that uses only microbiology data will be even less sensitive than that for total nosocomial infections. Frequently, surgeons do not obtain cultures because they prefer to treat SSI with operative drainage, and thus feel that they do not need to know the etiologic agent or its antibiotic susceptibility. On the other hand, a positive wound culture does not prove that the patient has an SSI. Instead, the organisms may be colonizing the wound. The opposite also is true: a negative culture does not eliminate the diagnosis of SSI. For example, wound cellulitis often yields negative cultures. In addition, organisms such as *Mycobacterium tuberculosis,* other *Mycobacterium* sp, and *Legionella* sp are not detected by routine culture methods.

Furthermore, other factors, such as culture techniques or the time required to transport specimens to the laboratory, may affect the results. Although many programs have used microbiology data to detect SSIs, we feel that these data are severely limited and should not be used as the sole source of case-finding.

Pharmacy Files

Nosocomial infection surveillance that relies on data in the pharmacy's files has low sensitivity.[11,12] Some investigators suggest that antimicrobial use is an indicator of nosocomial infections. However, most studies that evaluated pharmacy data did not evaluate SSIs specifically. For example, Broderick et al found that the number of days the patient received antibiotics independently predicted which patients developed nosocomial infections (relative risk [RR], 5.61 for 1 to 5 days of antimicrobial treatment; RR, 31.30 for more than 5 days of antimicrobial treatment).[17] Likewise, Hirschhorn et al suggested that parenteral antibiotic treatment for at least 2 days after the first postoperative day was a marker for nosocomial infections among patients undergoing cesarean section.[18] They were able to discriminate between antimicrobials received for prophylaxis and those received as treatment.[18]

We think there are several reasons why infection control programs should not use pharmacy data alone when conducting surveillance for SSIs. Some patients may continue to receive prophylactic antibiotics postoperatively, and some patients receive antimicrobial agents for infections that were present preoperatively (eg, peritonitis caused by a ruptured appendix). On the other hand, a patient whose infected wound is drained but who does not receive antimicrobials would not be identified by this surveillance method. Furthermore, this method would not identify SSIs that manifest postdischarge.

Other Methods

Other traditional methods for identifying patients with SSI include talking with nurses and physicians on surgical wards and screening admission records to identify patients who are readmitted for SSIs. Some infection control programs are trying to identify new methods by which they can identify patients with SSIs, particularly those whose signs and symptoms occur after discharge. For example, Sands et al evaluated whether the individual components of an automated screening system could identify SSIs.[5] They determined that:

- Coded diagnoses, tests, and treatments in the ambulatory medical record had a sensitivity of 84% and a predictive value positive of 17%.

- Pharmacy records indicating that the patient received an antibiotic commonly used to treat soft-tissue infections had a sensitivity of 50% and a predictive value positive of 19%.

- Any hospital readmission, any emergency room visit, or emergency room visits with ICD-9 codes suggestive of SSI, records of blood and wound cultures, patient questionnaires, and surgeon questionnaires all had sensitivities of less than 40% and positive predictive values of less than 45%.[5]

Unfortunately, many programs will not be able to use alternative data sources at present, because their hospitals do not have integrated computer systems that enable infection control personnel to access the data.

Infection control personnel could consider combining two or more surveillance methods to increase their sensitivity. For example, infection control staff could review both the medical records and the pharmacy files of selected patients. However, investigators have not determined whether combined methods are efficacious when used for SSI surveillance.

Summary of Surveillance Methods

When selecting surveillance methods, infection control personnel must consider their objectives. We feel in-hospital surveillance for SSIs should include either concurrent chart review, kardex review, or direct examination of the wounds. We would not recommend review of the pharmacy records or microbiology reports as the sole method of identifying patients who have SSIs. Furthermore, infection control personnel should consider the various sources from which the necessary data may be obtained. Indeed, infection control personnel may identify some components of the CDC's definition by reviewing the patients' records and others by examining wounds or talking with physicians. For example, diagnostic procedures, such as computerized tomography or magnetic resonance imaging, may help physicians identify deep or organ-space infections; the operating room logbook may allow epidemiology staff to identify patients who return to the operating room for drainage and debridement. Computers and computerized databases can help infection control professionals perform surveillance efficiently. The availability of these resources will determine, in part, which surveillance methods are most useful in individual healthcare facilities. Finally, when choosing a surveillance method, infection control personnel must consider not only the sensitivity of the surveillance method and the sources for data but also the human and financial resources allotted for SSI surveillance.

Collecting Data

Data collected during surveillance can be classified into three categories (Figure 11-2): host factors, surgical and environmental factors, and microbial factors. Host factors are conditions that reflect the patient's intrinsic susceptibility to infection. These conditions usually are present when the patient is admitted to the hospital. Some of these factors increase the risk of SSI after many different operative procedures (eg, remote infection, age, preoperative length of stay),[19,20] while others increase the risk only after specific opera-

tive procedures (eg, obesity and cigarette smoking are associated with infections after cardiac surgery).[21] Surgical and environmental factors reflect the probability of bacterial contamination at the time of the surgical procedure. Variables specific to the surgical procedure or to the surgeon may increase the risk of SSI; for example, a contaminated wound, a long procedure, or poor surgical technique are risk factors for SSI.[19] Microbial factors, such as the virulence of the organism or the ability of the organism to adhere to sutures, may alter the risk of SSI, but few studies have addressed these issues systematically. Furthermore, to conduct routine surveillance for SSI, infection control personnel rarely need to know whether the patient carries specific organisms. However, during outbreaks, or when trying to answer specific research questions, infection control personnel may need to obtain preoperative surveillance cultures from specific body sites.

The amount of data that infection control personnel should collect depends largely on the purpose of the surveillance program. In general, the basic data that should be collected include the following: patient's identification, date of admission, date of surgery, type of procedure, wound category (ie, clean, clean-contaminated, contaminated, dirty), surgeon's identification code, the date that the SSI was diagnosed, and the type of infection (ie, superficial, deep, or organ space). Other useful data are the American Society of Anesthesiologists' (ASA) score, the procedure's duration and urgency, the organism identified, and type and timing of perioperative antibiotics.

Because surgical patients are readily identifiable, the denominator is easier to obtain than for other nosocomial infections such as pneumonia, urinary tract infection, or bacteremia, for which the number of ventilator days, Foley-catheter days, or intravenous-catheter days must be determined retrospectively. All surgical patients can be included in a registry at the end of the operative proce-

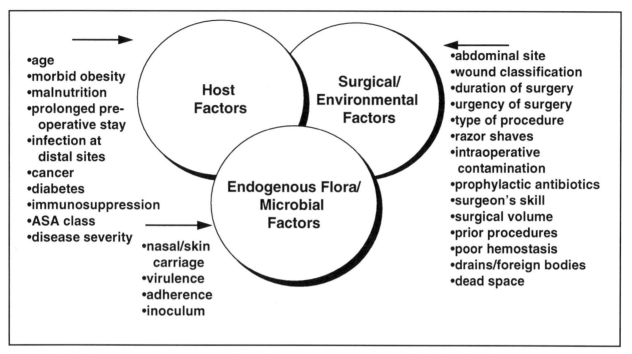

FIGURE 11-2. Risk factors for surgical site infections. This figure indicates that the patient's risk of developing a surgical site infection (SSI) varies with numerous host factors, surgical and environmental factors, and microbial factors. A complex interaction of these factors determines whether the patient will acquire an SSI. Abbreviation: ASA = American Society of Anesthesiologists.

dure. Indeed, many hospitals maintain operating room logbooks or have computer databases for financial management or for the surgical services that allow infection control staff to identify the appropriate denominators. Hospitals that have a separate database for the surgical services already may collect demographic data and some patient, operative, and environmental risk factors that are useful to the infection control program. In hospitals that do not collect these data, infection control personnel should consider seriously what information they need before they spend many hours collecting data. Indeed, numerous infection control programs have stopped collecting many variables, because the data were never used. Furthermore, several investigators have found that they collected data on variables that ultimately did not help them determine which patients were at highest risk of developing an infection.[22]

Which Patients Should Be Screened?

General Principles
Some infection control programs cling to the idea that they should survey all surgical patients, even healthy, young patients undergoing minor procedures. However, full-house surveillance consumes so much time that many programs must do some form of targeted surveillance.

In general hospitals, approximately 70% of operative procedures are categorized as clean operations (Table 11-2). Some hospitals survey only clean operative procedures, assuming that SSIs in the other categories are rarely preventable. However, the SENIC project demonstrated that surveillance for SSIs after contaminated or dirty procedures reduced SSI rates as effectively as did surveillance for SSIs after clean or clean-contaminated cases.[23] Therefore, we advocate SSI surveillance that includes all categories of operative procedures.

TABLE 11-2
RISK INDICES FOR SSI SURVEILLANCE: TRADITIONAL
WOUND CLASSIFICATION[24]

Class	Definition	Risk of Infection (%)
Clean	Uninfected, uninflamed operative wound where the respiratory, alimentary, genital, or uninfected urinary tracts are not entered	1-5
Clean-contaminated	Uninfected operative wound where the respiratory, alimentary, genital, or urinary tract is entered under controlled circumstances without unusual contamination	5-10
Contaminated	Acute, nonpurulent, inflamed operative wound or open, fresh, accidental wound or an operative procedure with major breaks in sterile technique or gross spillage from the GI tract	10-15
Dirty	Clinically infected operative wound or perforated viscera or old, traumatic wounds with retained devitalized tissue	>25

GI = gastrointestinal.

Targeted surveillance may be more effective when focused on specific operative procedures. For example, SSIs after craniotomies or coronary artery bypass procedures cause higher morbidity and mortality than do SSIs after hernia repairs. Therefore, infection control personnel might want to focus surveillance on the former procedures, so that they can intervene immediately if the SSI rates on the neurosurgery service or the cardiothoracic surgery service increase substantially. Alternatively, the infection control program could survey common operative procedures or operative procedures that previously have been associated with high infection rates. Hospitals that limit SSI surveillance to the surgical intensive care unit (SICU) will miss many infec-

tions, because the average SSI occurs 7 to 10 days postoperatively, and most patients leave the SICU within a few days of surgery. Infection control programs that sequentially rotate surveillance for SSIs on different surgical wards will underestimate the SSI rates and also may miss problems or epidemics that occur when a unit is not under surveillance.

Risk Indices to Direct Surgical Site Infection Surveillance

Another way to perform targeted surveillance is to stratify patients according to their risk of developing an SSI and then survey the group of selected patients.

The ideal risk index would be a simple additive scale that could be calculated at the end of surgery and that would predict the patients who are at high risk of SSIs. In addition, the risk index should be validated prospectively on specific services or in individual hospitals to document that it predicts a patient's risk accurately. Furthermore, it might be helpful if the index also could predict patients' risk of having postoperative pneumonia, urinary tract infections, or bloodstream infections, because patients who undergo operative procedures have higher rates of other infections. Such an index, however, would need to include variables considered to be primary risk factors for these infections, such as exposure to mechanical ventilation, urinary catheters, or intravenous lines. Although such an index could be developed, we question whether it would be sensitive or specific.

The idea of controlling for intrinsic risk is far from new. In 1964, the National Research Council's study of ultraviolet light in the operating room led to the development of the traditional wound-classification scheme (see Table 11-2).[24] The traditional wound classification, the primary method of risk stratification used in many hospitals, stratifies wounds by level of intraoperative contamination. The traditional wound classification has limited ability to stratify patients, because infection rates vary substantially within each group.[25] For example, SSI rates in the clean-wound category vary from 1% to 16%. Therefore, investigators have developed risk indices that include other variables (eg, the type of operative procedure, duration of the procedure, the patient's characteristics) to predict better which patients are at highest risk of developing SSIs. In 1985, Haley et al published the SENIC risk index (Table 11-3),[26] which included measures of wound contamination and a proxy for the patient's susceptibility to infection. Although the SENIC risk index predicted the risk of SSI twice as well as the traditional wound classification, its major weakness was that one of the index components, discharge diagnoses, must be obtained retrospectively. Therefore, when Culver et al adapted the SENIC risk index, they assessed host susceptibility with the ASA score, which reflects the patient's overall preoperative physical status. This risk index, now known as the "NNIS risk index," (see Table 11-3), also included a component that accounted for the expected variability in the duration of the operative procedure.[27] Instead of using the constant 2-hour cut point for length of surgery as used by the SENIC index, the NNIS index defined "T time" as the 75th percentile of the duration for each operative procedure. These three variables are easy to find, because they usually are included in the anesthesia record.

The NNIS risk index is a simple additive scale; scores range from 0 to 3. In the CDC's study, the SSI rates increased from 1.5%, for a score of 0, to 13.0%, for a score of 3. The NNIS index rarely has been validated in populations other than in the NNIS participating hospitals or compared with other risk indices. As individual hospitals try to use the NNIS risk index, some are reporting that the NNIS risk index does not stratify patients accurately by their risk of SSIs. In particular, the NNIS risk index does not discriminate well when applied to patients undergoing certain procedures, such as cesarean sections, craniotomies, and ventricular shunt placements.[28] We

TABLE 11-3

RISK INDICES FOR SSI SURVEILLANCE: THE SENIC[26] AND NNIS[27] RISK INDICES

Risk Factors	Score
SENIC Risk Index*	
Intra-abdominal procedure	1
Operative procedure lasting longer than 2 hours	1
Operative procedure classified as either contaminated or dirty by the traditional wound classification system	1
Patient with three or more discharge diagnoses	1
NNIS Risk Index†	
ASA preoperative assessment score of 3, 4, or 5	1
Operative procedure lasting longer than "T" hours‡	1
Operative procedure classified as either contaminated or dirty by the traditional wound classification system	1

SENIC = Study on the Efficacy of Nosocomial Infection Control; NNIS = National Nosocomial Infections Surveillance; ASA = American Society of Anesthesiologists.
*To calculate total score, sum factors present. Total score ranges from 0 to 4.
†To calculate total score, sum factors present. Total score ranges from 0 to 3.
‡"T" depends on the procedure being performed.

have shown that the NNIS risk index had a low sensitivity (24%) and poor predictive power (predictive value positive, 43%) for identifying SSIs after cardiothoracic operative procedures.[22] Hence, we have chosen not to use the NNIS risk index for SSI surveillance on our cardiothoracic surgery service.

A general risk index such as the NNIS risk index may predict poorly, because the procedures and the patients are too diverse. Procedure-specific risk indices may solve the problems encountered with the NNIS risk index or its predecessors.[29-31] For example, Nichols et al published a risk index that accurately predicted postoperative septic complications in a subset of patients who underwent operations after penetrating abdominal trauma.[29] In validating this risk index in a new population, they showed that the risk factors included in the index could identify high-risk patients who benefited from prolonged (5 days) antibiotic therapy and from delayed wound closure, and low-risk patients who did well with short-term (2 days) antibiotic therapy and primary wound closure.[30] Thus, this risk index not only stratifies patients by their risk of infection but also helps staff predict which patients will benefit from costly preventive strategies and help them limit this intervention to only a subgroup of patients at high risk of SSIs.

Postdischarge Surveillance

In a recent study, nearly half (46.3%) of the SSIs were detected after discharge.[32] Sands et al found even more alarming results when they evaluated 5,572 nonobstetric operative procedures in adult patients who were members of Harvard Pilgrim Health Care. Of 132 SSIs, 84% became apparent after the patients were discharged.[5] Thus, when choosing which populations to survey for SSIs, infection control personnel must decide whether or not they will conduct postdischarge surveillance. The CDC recommends that discharged patients be contacted 30 days after the procedure to determine whether an SSI has occurred.[33] We agree that infection control programs will need to develop strategies that identify SSIs after discharge. However, there is no standard method for conducting surveillance outside the hospital. The census approach, surveying each patient or physician for a defined period, is the method used in several studies that measured nosocomial infection rates during the postdischarge recovery period.[32] Telephone surveys and questionnaires sent to patients or physicians also have been used.[5,34,35] Seaman and Lammers found that patients, despite using verbal or printed instructions,[34] were unable to recognize infections. They concluded that "reliance on printed instructions, telephone interviews, or any other means of patient self-evaluation may not allow early recognition of infection" and therefore should not be used for clinical investigations of wound healing. Similarly, Sands et al found that questionnaires sent to patients and to surgeons had sensitivities of 28% and 15%, respectively.

These investigators also evaluated several other types of data that were available in computerized databases. Several variables had relatively high sensitivity, but none of them had a high predictive value positive.[5] (See discussion under "Other Methods.")

Investigators have not determined which, if any, method provides the best response rate and the most accurate data.[32-35] In addition, the cost and the time required to do postdischarge surveillance prohibit many infection control programs from instituting such systems. Few studies have compared the benefits gained by postdischarge surveillance with the costs associated with such a process. Consequently, none of the methods of postdischarge surveillance have been accepted widely.

On the basis of the literature, we do not advocate adopting any of the methods described above. Rather, we suggest that infection control programs consider linking with home healthcare agencies or other agencies that provide care for patients at home to develop mechanisms by which SSIs can be identified. In addition, as infection control programs wait for data delineating which postdischarge surveillance strategies are most productive, accurate, and economical, they must acknowledge that inpatient surveillance alone will underestimate the actual rates of SSI. Furthermore, they must not conclude prematurely that same-day surgeries and endoscopic surgeries are not complicated by SSIs.

In the future, the severity of illness among surgical patients will increase, the operative procedures will become more sophisticated, the average length of stay after surgery will decrease, and more patients will have operative procedures in the outpatient setting. The ultimate irony is that these dramatic shifts in patient populations, operative techniques, and healthcare delivery may increase the need for outpatient surveillance, but also increase the difficulty of performing surveillance and obtaining accurate data. Unfortunately, surveillance methodology and operative technology are not changing at the same pace.

Tabulation, Analysis, and Reporting of Data

Once data are collected and, if possible, entered into a computerized database, one can tabulate SSI rates. The following formulas may help the beginner to calculate different SSI rates. To calculate the rate of the outcome (ie, SSI) in a clearly delineated population, for a given time (eg, 1 month, 1 quarter, or 1 year), divide the numerator (the number of patients with SSI) by the denominator (all patients at risk for developing an SSI), and then multiply the result by 100 to obtain a percentage. Some examples follow.

1. Service-specific rates:

$$\frac{\text{Number of SSIs in patients on the neurosurgery service}}{\text{Number of patients who had a neurosurgical procedure}} \times 100$$

2. Surgeon-specific rates:

$$\frac{\text{Number of SSIs in patients who were operated on by a particular surgeon}}{\text{Number of patients operated on by that same surgeon}} \times 100$$

3. Procedure-specific rates:

$$\frac{\text{Number of SSIs occurring after a specific procedure (eg, cholecystectomy)}}{\text{Number of procedures (eg, cholecystectomies)}} \times 100$$

4. Risk-specific rates:

$$\frac{\text{Number of SSIs in patients with an NNIS risk index score of 2}}{\text{Number of patients with an NNIS risk index score of 2}} \times 100$$

Once infection control staff identify the population to be surveyed, they easily can identify the proper denominator by searching the operating room logbook or the hospital's computerized database. All of the patients in the defined population are followed throughout the time frame designated by the definition of SSI (ie, 30 days postoperatively or 1 year postoperatively if an implant was inserted). Each patient who develops an SSI is included in the numerator. If the denominator is too broad (eg, all surgical patients in a large hospital), the group then becomes very heterogeneous, and the calculated infection rate probably will be falsely low. Consequently, infection control personnel may not identify clusters of SSIs or other problems. Surgeon-specific or procedure-specific rates more closely reflect true SSI rates.

The infection control program should stratify rates by the type of procedures or by specific risk indices to allow intersurgeon or interhospital comparisons. The traditional wound classification[24] has served this purpose for a quarter of a century, but it has some limitations, as mentioned earlier. The NNIS risk index, advocated by the CDC, is used widely today, but it does not perform well in certain circumstances.[22,28] Despite these limitations, it may be to a hospital's advantage to stratify the patients' risk by one of the available indices, particularly if the patients have numerous severe underlying illnesses or the operative procedures performed in the hospital are quite complex.

The infection control program should report SSI rates to surgeons, because they are the clinicians who could alter the outcomes. SSI rates should be sent to the chief of surgery, and individual surgeons should receive their own rates. Confidentiality is of utmost importance in such a process. Therefore, codes should be used instead of names if surgeons are allowed to compare their rates with the rates of other surgeons or if surgeon-specific rates are reported to the infection control committee. Reporting SSI rates to practicing surgeons has been shown to reduce rates by the so-called Hawthorne Effect (ie, the effect due to having one's performance observed).[6-8] However, one must interpret the conclusions with caution as most studies have included confounding factors.

Busy surgeons may ignore written reports. Therefore, infection control personnel should periodically meet with the surgeons to discuss rates, clusters, and specific SSI cases. These discussions could improve communication and cooperation between the infection control and the surgical teams. During these discussions, infection control personnel might learn ways to make the data more useful to the surgeons. The infection control staff also could use these feedback sessions as a means to introduce the surgical team to the state-of-the-art preventive measures that might reduce the risk of SSIs.

The infection control program should report SSI rates, costs, lengths of stay associated with SSIs, and the effects of preventive measures to the hospital's administrators. Several investigators have demonstrated that SSIs are the primary independent determinant of hospital costs and length of stay after operative procedures.[36,37] Moreover, Olson and Lee demonstrated a $3 million cost savings in a 10-year wound surveillance program.[7] The hospital administration may be more likely to provide infection control personnel with resources if they can demonstrate that their programs decrease the rate of SSIs and decrease costs and lengths of stay attributable to SSIs.

Finally, infection control personnel periodically should review their data to determine whether they should change their priorities or focus their energy on specific problems. For example, if a program analyzes their data and finds, after a few months, that the sensitivity of the case-finding method used for postdischarge surveillance is very low (eg, only 2% of SSIs are identified by this method), epidemiology staff may change their case-finding method instead of spending time and energy for a year or more before realizing that the method was not effective.

Interventions to Reduce SSI

Once data are collected, tabulated, and analyzed, the infection control program can develop and implement interventions to reduce SSI rates. These interventions will be dictated largely by the problems that have been identified through surveillance and data analysis. Epidemiology staff should ask a number of questions including:

- Could the problems encountered or the high SSI rates be explained by failure to apply infection-reducing adjuncts?
- Were parenteral prophylactic antibiotics indicated, and, if so, were they properly chosen and administered?
- Was mechanical bowel preparation performed properly before colon surgery?
- Was preoperative skin preparation adequate?
- Was hair removed from operative sites? If yes, what method was used?
- Was elective surgery delayed if an infection was identified preoperatively?
- Does the implicated surgeon use specific techniques that might increase the rate of infection?

Infection control personnel could institute interventions in three time periods: the preoperative period, the perioperative and intraoperative period, and the postoperative period. Before developing interventions for the preoperative period, one must ask whether the risk of SSI can be decreased by manipulating one or more host risk factors before the operation. Unfortunately, some variables cannot be modified (eg, age, gender); others can be modified (eg, diabetes, steroid therapy), but we lack evidence that stabilizing these conditions reduces SSI rates. Several interventions, such as minimizing the duration of preoperative hospital stay and eradicating remote infections, do reduce SSI rates. These measures are reviewed elsewhere.[19]

Perioperative and intraoperative risks may not be amenable to change, but several interventions during this period have reduced SSI rates. If infection control personnel find unusually high SSI rates for clean procedures or increased rates of *Staphylococcus aureus* or polymicrobial wound infections, they may want to review procedures in the operating room, such as the hair removal technique, the antiseptics used to prepare the operative site and for surgical hand scrubs, the timing of antibiotic prophylaxis, and the operative technique, to ensure that practices deviating from standard guidelines are not contributing to elevated rates.

If an epidemiologic investigation suggests that the source of the outbreak might be healthcare workers who carry the organism, infection control personnel should obtain appropriate cultures from the implicated individuals (eg, cultures of nares and skin lesions for *S aureus,* cultures of the throat, skin lesions, and, if necessary, the vagina and rectum for *Streptococcus pyogenes). S pyogenes* SSI infections usually are related to a healthcare worker who carries this organism. Therefore, even one case should prompt an immediate investigation. Healthcare workers also can carry unusual organisms, such as *Rhodococcus* species, that cause individual cases or outbreaks of SSI.

Perioperative antibiotic prophylaxis is of particular importance. Pathogens that infect wounds during the operative procedure can be acquired from the patient, the hospital environment, or the personnel. The patient's endogenous flora is the source of most infections, especially if clean-wound infections are excluded. Antibiotic prophylaxis has been shown to reduce SSIs for operative procedures in which the gastrointestinal, respiratory, genital, and urinary tracts are sources of contamination. Antibiotic prophylaxis still is controversial for many clean-wound procedures, but experts suggest that prophylactic antibiotics should be used when an implant is inserted or if an infection would be associated with severe or life-threatening consequences (eg, endocarditis after valve replacement). To be effective, prophylactic antibiotics must be given during the appropriate time interval. The patient's skin and anterior nares may be a source of contam-

ination in the clean-wound category, and much research is underway to determine whether eradicating endogenous sources reduces SSI rates.[38,39]

Because most contamination happens during the operation through contact or airborne transmission, events that occur during the postoperative period (eg, improper dressing changes or isolation techniques) are less likely to contribute to SSIs. If epidemiological data indicate that postoperative care may be associated with increased SSI rates, the infection control staff may need to investigate practices during this period.

How to Survive

In the following paragraphs, we will offer a few suggestions that the new hospital epidemiologist or ICP might find useful when implementing or improving an SSI surveillance program.

The ICP is a very important component of any surveillance program. The ICP should have personality traits that facilitate a good working relationship with the surgeons. The ICP needs training, feedback on performance, and time to attend conferences on nosocomial infections. The ICP also should be an active member of the infection control committee. Finally, in programs that use direct wound examination to identify SSIs, a surgeon should train the ICPs, so that they can evaluate subtle nuances of a wound's appearance.

Most importantly, the infection control program must involve the surgical staff, so that they take the responsibility for controlling SSIs. To achieve this goal, infection control staff should:

- Review the definitions of SSI with the surgeons, so they understand and accept the criteria.
- Ask the surgeons what data should be included in their infection control reports and whether they prefer a report with surgeon-specific or procedure-specific SSI rates.
- Confidentially report personal SSI rates to all staff surgeons and possibly to fellows and residents.

- Meet with surgeons and surgical nurses on a regular basis to build trust and to discuss issues such as surveillance methods.
- Visit the operating room routinely and during outbreaks to identify potential problems and to develop rapport and mutual respect.
- Encourage a surgeon or a surgical nurse to join the infection control committee.
- Join the Surgical Infection Society and attend its annual meeting in order to understand the surgeons' perspective on SSIs.
- Discuss protocols and goals for studies of SSIs with surgical staff and encourage them to participate.
- Attempt to develop creative strategies for identifying SSIs as the medical environment changes.
- Publish results of studies in surgical journals.

In addition, the infection control program needs adequate resources to conduct effective surveillance. Clerical support, computerized databases, such as fully computerized operating room logs, and medical records personnel contribute significantly to the SSI surveillance program.

Conclusion

Surveillance for SSIs is an important component of any infection control program, and it is a special form of continuous quality assurance in which the ultimate benefactors of control efforts are the patients. Therefore, the infection control program should define clear objectives, write precise definitions, and meticulously implement a surveillance system. Although methods of case-finding are hard to choose, the infection control team should focus on patients or procedures at high risk of infection if their resources are limited. Collecting data and calculating rates are useless if epidemiology and surgical staff do not use the data to reduce SSI rates. To succeed in such an effort, infection control personnel must collaborate with the surgical team.

As healthcare delivery shifts to the outpatient setting, numerous aspects of SSI surveillance must change, because many factors that influence the risk of SSI also will change. Surveillance methods that worked well in the past, and that were supported by well-designed studies, no longer will be efficacious. Unfortunately, few data exist to guide us as we endeavor to develop appropriate methods.[40] We desperately need creative research to determine how we should develop and apply risk indices and to identify which methods we should use for postdischarge surveillance. Indeed, exciting opportunities are open to those willing to accept the challenges.

References

1. Vicary T. The English-man's treasure. With the true anatomie of man's body. In: Sabiston DC Jr, ed. Textbook of Surgery. Philadelphia, Pa: WB Saunders; 1977.
2. Emori TG, Gaynes RP. An overview of nosocomial infections, including the role of the microbiology laboratory. Clin Microbiol Rev. 1993;6:428-442.
3. Leape LL, Brennan TA, Laird N, et al. The nature of adverse events in hospitalized patients: results of the Harvard medical practice study II. N Engl J Med. 1991;324:377-384.
4. Brachman PS, Dan BB, Haley RW, Hooton TM, Garner JS, Allen JR. Nosocomial surgical infections: incidence and cost. Surg Clin North Am. 1980;60:15-25.
5. Sands K, Vineyard G, Platt R. Surgical site infections occurring after hospital discharge. J Infect Dis. 1996;173:963-970.
6. Haley RW, Culver DH, White JW, et al. The efficacy of infection surveillance and control programs in preventing nosocomial infections in US hospitals. Am J Epidemiol. 1985;121:182-205.
7. Olson MM, Lee JT Jr. Continuous, 10-year wound infection surveillance: results, advantages, and unanswered questions. Arch Surg. 1990;125:794-803.
8. Cruse PJ, Foord R. The epidemiology of wound infection: a 10-year prospective study of 62,939 wounds. Surg Clin North Am. 1980;60:27-40.
9. Ehrenkranz NJ, Richter EI, Phillips PM, Shultz JM. An apparent excess of operative site infections: analyses to evaluate false-positive diagnoses. Infect Control Hosp Epidemiol. 1995;16:712-716.

10. Horan TC, Gaynes RP, Martone WJ, Jarvis WR, Emori TG. CDC definitions of nosocomial surgical site infections, 1992: a modification of CDC definitions of surgical wound infections. *Infect Control Hosp Epidemiol.* 1992;13:606-608.

11. Wenzel RP, Osterman CA, Hunting KJ, Gwaltney JM Jr. Hospital acquired infections, I: surveillance in a university hospital. *Am J Epidemiol.* 1976;103:251-260.

12. Perl TM. Surveillance, reporting and the use of computers. In: Wenzel RP, ed. *Prevention and Control of Nosocomial Infections.* 2nd ed. Baltimore, Md: Williams & Wilkins; 1993:139-176.

13. Lee JT Jr. Wound infection surveillance. *Infect Dis Clin North Am.* 2nd ed. 1992;6:643-656.

14. Cardo DM, Falk PS, Mayhall CG. Validation of surgical wound surveillance. *Infect Control Hosp Epidemiol.* 1993;14:211-215.

15. Haley RW, Schaberg D, McClish D, et al. The accuracy of retrospective chart review in measuring nosocomial infection rates: results of validation studies in pilot hospitals. *Am J Epidemiol.* 1980;111:516-533.

16. Manian FA, Meyer L. Comprehensive surveillance of surgical wound infections in outpatient and inpatient surgery. *Infect Control Hosp Epidemiol.* 1990;11:515-520.

17. Broderick A, Mori M, Nettleman MD, Streed SA, Wenzel RP. Nosocomial infections: validation of surveillance and computer modeling to identify patients at risk. *Am J Epidemiol.* 1990;131:734-742.

18. Hirschhorn LR, Currier JS, Platt R. Electronic surveillance of antibiotic exposure and coded discharge diagnoses as indicators of postoperative infection and other quality assurance measures. *Infect Control Hosp Epidemiol.* 1993;14:21-28.

19. Mayhall CG. Surgical infections including burns. In: Wenzel RP, ed. *Prevention and Control of Nosocomial Infections.* 2nd ed. Baltimore, Md: Williams & Wilkins; 1993:614-664.

20. Kernodle DS, Kaiser AB. Postoperative infections and antimicrobial prophylaxis. In: Mandell GL, Bennett JE, Dolin R, eds. *Principles and Practice of Infectious Diseases.* 4th ed. New York, NY: Churchill Livingstone; 1995:2742-2756.

21. Nagachinta T, Stephens M, Reitz B, Polk BF. Risk factors for surgical-wound infection following cardiac surgery. *J Infect Dis.* 1987;156:967-973.

22. Roy M-C, Herwaldt LA, Embrey R, Kuhns K, Wenzel RP, Perl TM. Does the NNIS risk index predict which patients are at high risk of wound infections after cardiothoracic surgery? Thirty-fourth Interscience Conference on Antimicrobials Agents and Chemotherapy; September 1994; Orlando, Fla. Abstract.

23. Haley RW. Surveillance by objective: a new priority-directed approach to the control of nosocomial infections. The National Foundation for Infectious Diseases Lecture. *Am J Infect Control.* 1985;13:78-89.

24. National Academy of Sciences—National Research Council. Postoperative wound infections: the influence of ultraviolet irradiation of the operating room and of various other factors. *Ann Surg.* 1964;160(suppl 2):1-132.

25. Ferraz EM, Bacelar TS, Lamartine De Andrade AJ, Ferraz AAB, Pagnossin G, Batista JEM. Wound infection rates in clean surgery: a potentially misleading risk classification. *Infect Control Hosp Epidemiol.* 1992;13:457-462.

26. Haley RW, Culver DH, Morgan WM, White JW, Emori TG, Hooton TM. Identifying patients at high risk of surgical wound infection: a simple multivariate index of patient susceptibility and wound contamination. *Am J Epidemiol.* 1985;121:206-215.

27. Culver DH, Horan TC, Gaynes RP, et al. Surgical wound infection rates by wound class, operative procedure, and patient risk index. National Nosocomial Infectious Surveillance System. *Am J Med.* 1991;91(suppl 3B):152S-157S.

28. Horan TC, Gaynes R, Culver D. Development of predictive risk factors for nosocomial surgical site infections. The Fourth Annual Meeting of the Society for Healthcare Epidemiology of America; March 1994; New Orleans, La. Abstract.

29. Nichols RL, Smith JW, Klein DB, et al. Risk of infection after penetrating abdominal trauma. *N Engl J Med.* 1984;311:1065-1070.

30. Nichols RL, Smith JW, Robertson GD, et al. Prospective alterations in therapy after penetrating abdominal trauma. *Arch Surg.* 1993;128:55-63.

31. Richet HM, Chidiac C, Prat A, et al. Analysis of risk factors for surgical wound infections following vascular surgery. *Am J Med.* 1991;91(suppl 3B):170S-172S.

32. Burns SJ, Dippe SE. Postoperative wound infections detected during hospitalization and after discharge in a community hospital. *Am J Infect Control.* 1982;10:60-65.

33. Garner JS. Guideline for prevention of surgical wound infections, 1985. *Am J Infect Control.* 1986;14:71-80.

34. Seaman M, Lammers R. Inability of patients to self-diagnose wound infections. *J Emerg Med.* 1991;9:215-219.

35. Rosendorf LL, Octavio J, Estes JP. Effect of methods of postdischarge wound infection surveillance on reported infection rates. *Am J Infect Control.* 1983;11:226-229.

36. Weintraub WS, Jones EL, Craver J, Guyton R, Cohen C. Determinants of prolonged length of hospital stay after coronary bypass surgery. *Circulation.* 1989;80:276-284.

37. Taylor GJ, Mikel FL, Moses HW, et al. Determinants of hospital charges for coronary artery bypass surgery: the economic consequences of postoperative complications. *Am J Cardiol.* 1990;65:309-313.

38. Perl TM, Roy M-C. Postoperative wound infections: risk factors and role of *Staphylococcus aureus* nasal carriage. *J Chemother.* 1995;7:29-35.

39. Wenzel RP, Perl TM. The significance of nasal carriage of *Staphylococcus aureus* and the incidence of postoperative wound infection. *J Hosp Infect.* 1995;31:13-24.

40. Meier PA. Same-day surgery care issues. In: Wenzel RP, ed. *Prevention and Control of Nosocomial Infections.* 3rd ed. Baltimore, Md: Williams & Wilkins; 1997:261-282.

41. Eickhoff TC, Brachman PW, Bennett JV, Brown JF. Surveillance of nosocomial infections in community hospitals, I: surveillance methods, effectiveness, and initial results. *J Infect Dis.* 1969;120:305-317.

42. Laxson LB, Blaser MJ, Parkhurst SM. Surveillance for the detection of nosocomial infections and the potential for nosocomial outbreaks, I: microbiology culture surveillance is an effective method of detecting nosocomial infection. *Am J Infect Control.* 1984;12:318-324.

43. Yokoe DS, Platt R. Surveillance for surgical site infections: the uses of antibiotic exposure. *Infect Control Hosp Epidemiol.* 1994;15:717-723.

CHAPTER 12

Surveillance for Infections Associated With Vascular Catheters

Robert J. Sherertz, MD

Abstract

Intravascular devices are the source of most primary bloodstream infections. Unfortunately, there are few studies that demonstrate how surveillance for catheter-related infection should be done. This chapter attempts to provide infection control personnel with information necessary to develop such surveillance.

Introduction

In the most recent data summary from the National Nosocomial Infections Surveillance (NNIS) System, primary bloodstream infection is the fourth most common site (13%) of nosocomial infection after urinary tract infection (33%), pneumonia (16%), and surgical site infection (15%).[1] Intravascular devices are the source of most primary bloodstream infections.[2] Dennis Maki has estimated that 90% of intravascular-device–related bloodstream infections are secondary to central venous catheters.[2] Surveillance data from NNIS show that, in intensive-care units (ICUs), primary bloodstream infection rates are twofold to 30-fold higher in patients with central lines than in patients without them.[3] The magnitude of this problem is substantial in the United States, where it is conservatively estimated that 50,000 to 100,000 catheter-related bloodstream infections occur each year.[2] In addition to causing substantial morbidity, catheter-related infections prolong hospitalization and lead to excess cost.[2]

Thus, catheter-related infection in the hospital setting is an important problem worthy of monitoring by surveillance. Unfortunately, there are few studies that demonstrate how surveillance of catheter-related infection should be performed. Most investigators who study catheter-related infection feel that quantitative culture techniques are optimal for making the diagnosis of catheter-related infection. However, investigators have yet to determine whether one technique is better than another or whether different methods give comparable results. Despite these uncertainties, there is enough information to guide infection control personnel as they begin surveillance of catheter-related infections. This chapter attempts to provide infection control personnel with information necessary to institute such surveillance.

Case Finding

The biggest problem in surveillance for vascular catheter infections is that investigators have not identified a gold standard for diagnosing catheter-related infections. Most studies use the criteria being investigated to determine sensitivity and specificity. This circular reasoning makes it difficult to compare different criteria. There are significant problems with both clinical criteria and microbiologic criteria that are used to diagnose catheter-related infections. Thus, infection control personnel should choose diagnostic criteria that reflect the goals of their surveillance. Epidemiology staff who plan to compare infection rates with those of other institutions should use the criteria used by those institutions. If the hospital epidemiology staff investigate a problem, they may include other criteria that may help them identify the source of the problem.

Clinical Diagnosis of Catheter-Related Infection

The clinical diagnosis of catheter-related infection is insensitive and not very specific. Erythema may suggest which peripheral catheters are infected[4]; however, it is an unreliable indicator of central catheter infection.[5] Purulence around the catheter exit site is thought to be unequivocal evidence of catheter-related infection; however, it also is too insensitive (in both retrospective and prospective studies) to be useful by itself in surveillance for catheter-related infections.[5,6]

Microbiologic Diagnosis of Catheter-Related Infection

Many studies have demonstrated that broth culture of vascular catheters is quite sensitive, but not adequately specific. In the first report of this type by Maki et al,[4] broth cultures were 100% sensitive at detecting catheter-related bloodstream infection, but only 50% specific. Quantitative cultures of vascular catheters offer much greater specificity in the diagnosis of catheter-related bloodstream infection.

The best-studied quantitative culture method is the roll-plate semiquantitative culture technique developed by Dennis Maki.[4] This technique was 100% specific (compared with itself) in diagnosing catheter-related bloodstream infection, with twice the specificity of broth culture. The predictive value positive of the roll-plate method for catheter-related bloodstream infection increased with duration of catheterization, from a low of approximately 10% (mean catheter duration 3 to 5 days) to a high of 75% (mean catheter duration 24 days).[7,8]

Clinical trials have validated additional quantitative catheter culture methods including broth flush,[9] centrifugation,[10] vortexing,[11] and sonication.[6,12] Few studies have been done comparing the relative diagnostic accuracy of these various techniques. Linares et al studied 135 central catheters removed from patients receiving hyperalimentation. The broth flush method was more sensitive (subcutaneous segment 75%, tip segment 100%) than the roll-plate method (subcutaneous segment 56.6%, tip segment 87.5%)[13] when used to assess patients who had catheter-related bloodstream infection secondary to catheter hub contamination (n=16). Also, when used to assess patients with catheter-related bloodstream infection secondary to skin contamination (n=2), they found that the roll-plate method was more sensitive (subcutaneous segment 100%, tip segment 100%) than the broth flush method (subcutaneous segment 50%, tip segment 50%). Although the numbers were small, the data simplistically suggested that infection can be confined to either the lumen or the external surface of the catheter and that culture methods that only sample the lumen (broth flush) or the external surface (roll plate) would give false-negative results when used alone. Conversely, these data suggested that culture methods such as centrifugation, vortexing, or sonication, which theoretically could remove organisms simultaneously from the catheter lumen and external surface, might be more sensitive than either the roll-plate or broth technique.

Raad et al obtained cultures of 177 catheter tips by two methods and found that the roll-plate method was less sensitive (78%) than the sonication method (93%) at detecting catheter-related bloodstream infection.[14] Pittet et al obtained cultures of 22 central venous catheters by these two methods and found that vortexing and sonication had similar sensitivities, and both were better than the roll-plate method for evaluating catheter tips (personal communication, 1991, Didier Pittet).[15] Sherertz et al, in a prospective, multicenter study, evaluated 191 triple-lumen catheters. Sonication and roll-plate cultures were obtained from each tip and subcutaneous segment, and cultures of all three lumens were obtained by either aspirated blood or broth flush.[16] The relative sensitivity of the seven cultures for diagnosing significant catheter colonization in comparison to a composite index were as follows: tip sonication, 56%; subcutaneous sonication, 55%; tip roll plate, 46%; subcutaneous roll plate, 38%; and catheter lumens, 36%, 30%, and 20%. The difference between tip sonication and tip roll plate was statistically significant (P=.004). This study demonstrated a high correlation between tip and subcutaneous segment cultures (r >0.7), suggesting that contamination at these sites was related. The study also found a low correlation between either tip or subcutaneous cultures and lumen cultures (r <0.4), providing further evidence that contamination of the catheter lumen and the external surface of the catheter usually were independent events.

Widmer et al recently challenged the traditional view by stating that cultures of central venous catheters should not be obtained at all.[17] These investigators obtained cultures of 157 consecutive catheters from patients in a surgical ICU, and only 4% of the culture results altered patient care. Notably, 81% of all central venous catheters, however, in that ICU were sent for culture, which is not standard practice. Many cultures were performed for surveillance or research reasons, not for clinical indications. Until studies are done that evaluate many patients with catheter-related infections, one cannot conclude that quantitative catheter cultures are of no benefit.

A number of studies used quantitative paired blood cultures to diagnose vascular catheter infections. Wing et al, who originally described this approach, diagnosed a catheter-related bloodstream infection if blood drawn through the catheter had more colony-forming units (CFU) per mL than did blood drawn from a peripheral vein.[18] The major limitation of this technique is that many microbiology laboratories do not perform quantitative blood cultures routinely. Investigators at a number of institutions have used this technique successfully to study catheter-related infections in adults and children.[19-25]

When Weightman et al performed both quantitative catheter hub cultures and paired blood cultures, they found that if the number of CFU in the catheter blood exceeded that in the peripheral blood, 80% (8 of 10) of hubs were contaminated with the same organism; if not, only 13.6% (24 of 177) of hubs were contaminated.[21] Two prospective studies in which the investigators obtained roll-plate cultures of the catheter tips and paired blood cultures showed that when the number of CFU in catheter blood exceeded (at least greater than or equal to twofold, usually 10-fold) that in the peripheral blood, the roll-plate cultures frequently (18 of 38, 47.4%) were negative.[24,25] These findings suggest that when a contaminated hub allows the catheter lumen to become colonized, one should find higher numbers of organisms in the blood culture drawn through the catheter than in a culture obtained from a peripheral vein. The ratio of the number of CFU in the catheter blood to CFU in the peripheral blood can be used to help diagnose catheter-related bloodstream infections. Although investigators have not identified the ideal ratio, one can conclude relatively safely that the patient has a catheter-related bloodstream infection if the catheter blood has five times more CFU than the peripheral blood. However, when the number of CFU in the catheter blood is >0 and that in the peripheral blood = 0, one should not diagnose a catheter-related bloodstream infection.

Microscopic methods for identifying catheter colonization or infection appear to have good sensitivity and specificity when compared with the roll-plate culture method. Gram's stain examination of catheter tips was 100% sensitive and 97% specific,[26] and fluorescence microscopy with acridine orange was 84% sensitive and 99% specific,[27] in comparison to the roll-plate method. Most laboratories have been unwilling to adopt either of these methods because they require too much time.

Recommendations for Catheter Cultures

When infection control or laboratory personnel choose a vascular catheter culture methodology, they must remember that most investigators (including those in the NNIS System) who have published infection rates used the roll-plate method. The sonication and vortex methods appear to be more sensitive, but they are slightly more labor intensive.

I would recommend the following principles to infection control programs and laboratories that perform cultures of intravascular catheters:

- Unless they are conducting research or investigating a problem, physicians should obtain catheter cultures only when clinically indicated.
- The laboratory should use the roll-plate method for peripheral catheters.
- The laboratory can use various culture methods for removable central venous catheters: roll plating, vortexing, or sonication.
- Paired blood cultures obtained through the catheter and from a peripheral vein can help clinicians decide whether to remove an implanted central venous catheter.
- The laboratory should culture the tip segment of central venous catheters because:

a) Cultures of this segment are more cost-effective than cultures of other segments.

b) Cultures of this segment have the highest predictive value positive in patients who have long-term catheters.

Unless they are conducting research or investigating a problem, clinicians should send for culture only one catheter segment (the tip) per episode.

Surveillance Definitions of Catheter-Related Complications

Larson and colleagues' recent survey of 297 randomly chosen hospitals in the United States revealed that 78.1% used the Centers for Disease Control and Prevention's (CDC) definitions for surveillance purposes.[28] The most recent version of the CDC's surveillance definitions,[29] published in 1988, defines intravascular-device–related infection as either purulence at the vascular site or as a positive semi-quantitative catheter culture (≥15 colonies)[4] plus either fever (>38°C), pain, erythema, or heat at the vascular site. In addition to the CDC's definition, a number of other methods for diagnosing vascular catheter infection have been established, as discussed above. The definitions proposed below consider the newer methods.

Phlebitis is defined as inflammation, induration, and tenderness around a vascular catheter inserted in a peripheral vein, with or without associated thrombosis. The article by Maki and Ringer discusses in detail the diagnosis of phlebitis.[30]

Catheter colonization is defined as:
- Positive quantitative culture of the catheter, catheter lumen, or catheter hub **and**
- Both of the following:
1. No evidence of local catheter infection (see the following paragraphs).
2. No evidence of catheter-related bloodstream infection (see the following paragraphs).

Local catheter infection is defined as:
- One of the following criteria:

1. Purulence at the catheter exit site.
2. Cellulitis overlying the catheter.
3. Positive quantitative catheter culture and either phlebitis or fever (≥38°C).
4. Positive blood culture drawn through a catheter and either phlebitis or fever (≥38°C) **and**

- Negative or no peripheral blood culture.

Catheter-related bloodstream infection is defined as meeting one or more of the following criteria:

- Catheter exit site purulence and peripheral blood culture growing the same organism.
- Peri-catheter cellulitis and primary bacteremia (CDC surveillance definition).[29]
- Positive quantitative culture of the catheter plus a peripheral blood culture growing the same organism.
- Paired quantitative blood cultures with the number of CFUs from the culture drawn through the catheter being at least five times greater than the number of CFUs from the peripheral blood culture.

In hospitals where quantitative catheter culture methods are not available, a surrogate measure of catheter-related bacteremia may be catheter-associated bacteremia. Although this approach has not been validated, existing data suggest that up to 90% of primary bacteremias probably are catheter-related infections (see introductory discussion above).

Central catheter-associated bloodstream infection is defined as:

- Primary bacteremia (CDC surveillance definition)[29] **and**
- Central catheter present at the time the blood culture was obtained.[3]

Infusate-related bloodstream infection is defined as:

- Cultures obtained simultaneously from infusate and peripheral blood yield the same organism **and**

- No other identifiable source for the bacteremia.

Quantitative cultures of the catheter usually are negative if the bloodstream infection is caused by contaminated infusate. However, positive quantitative catheter cultures do not exclude contaminated infusate as the source of a bacteremia, because the infusate could contaminate the catheter. Most infection control programs culture infusate only when investigating a problem or when conducting research. If the cultures indicate that infusate is contaminated, and if the product might have been contaminated during its manufacture, the hospital must notify both the manufacturer and the CDC.

Recommendations for Definitions

After extensively reviewing the literature, I would offer the following suggestions to infection control personnel who choose to do surveillance for intravascular-catheter–related bloodstream infections.

- Local catheter infections and catheter-related bloodstream infections provide the most meaningful data at most institutions.
- If quantitative cultures are not available, the infection control staff should consider catheter-associated bloodstream infection as an alternative definition.
- To determine whether poor technique is a problem, infection control personnel should assess catheter colonization, as it is the most sensitive endpoint.

Surveillance

Target Population

Although central catheters make up a small percentage of the total number of vascular catheters, they are associated with 90% of catheter-related bloodstream infections.[2] Thus, most infection control programs should focus their surveillance efforts on patients who have central venous catheters, including patients receiving home infusion therapy, inpatients receiving hyperalimentation, hematology-oncology patients with central venous catheters, and patients in ICUs. The epidemiology staff may choose to evaluate additional patient groups based on their clinical suspicions, such as a high rate of peripheral catheter infections on a particular hospital ward.

Goals

At most institutions and with most patient populations, the primary goal of vascular catheter surveillance is to monitor the endemic catheter-related or catheter-associated infection rate and to determine whether these rates are within an acceptable range. To do this, infection control personnel can compare their rates with those published by programs that use the same methods. This means that both laboratories use the same culture method (eg, both use the roll-plate method) or at least similar culture methods (eg, both institutions use quantitative methods such as roll-plate and sonication). More importantly, the case definition and case-finding methods should be the same. Many published infection rates were determined by investigators who prospectively obtained cultures of all catheters. This approach is more sensitive than the usual clinical approach in which catheter cultures are obtained when the patient's condition warrants. Thus, if infection control personnel compare the rate of catheter-related infections in their hospital with rates summarized in several recent chapters on catheter-related infection, they may conclude falsely that their rates are substantially lower than the published rates.[2,8,31] Remember, you must read the study methods to reach accurate conclusions.

For hospitals in which quantitative catheter culture methods are not routinely available, infection control personnel could use rates of primary bacteremia in patients who have central venous catheters as a surrogate measure of catheter-related

infections in ICUs. The CDC recently published such rates for ICUs within the NNIS hospital system: 2.1 per 1,000 catheter days in respiratory ICUs, 4.5 in neurosurgical ICUs, 5.1 in medical-surgical ICUs, 5.8 in trauma ICUs, 5.8 in surgical ICUs, 6.9 in medical ICUs, 7.0 in coronary ICUs, 11.4 in pediatric ICUs, and 30.2 in burn units.[3]

If infection control personnel identify a cluster of vascular catheter-related infections due to the same organism, they should investigate it immediately. The epidemiology staff first should review the medical charts of the patients involved, searching for commonalties. The investigators must determine whether the problem is caused by contaminated infusate, devices such as pressure monitors that are used improperly, intrinsic contamination of the catheter itself, or personnel who use poor technique. If necessary, infection control personnel can conduct a case-control study to narrow the focus of their investigation. The investigators may need to obtain cultures of infusate or other fluids that might be reservoirs. Of note, these outbreaks often are caused by Gram-negative bacteria and involve a "wet reservoir."[2] Occasionally, they involve Gram-positive organisms[32] or yeasts.[33] Additional information about how to investigate such an outbreak may be found in a recent book chapter written by Dennis Maki.[2]

Surveillance for vascular catheter-related infection can be used to evaluate whether certain devices or techniques are better than others. Infection control personnel can use surveillance and retrospective chart reviews to answer several important questions. Such studies can:

• Determine the risk of catheter-related infections in AIDS patients requiring long-term venous access in comparison to other patients.[34]

• Determine whether removing central venous catheters reduces recurrence of catheter-related coagulase-negative staphylococcal bacteremia.[35]

- Compare infections in Hickman versus implanted-port catheters in adult solid-tumor patients.[36]

In addition, investigators may need to conduct prospective studies to confirm conclusions based on retrospective studies. Prospective studies are necessary, because certain key data elements are missing in retrospective reviews. Prospective studies can:

- Determine whether training staff or modifying infection control policy changes the risk of catheter-related infection.[37,38]
- Evaluate whether care of catheter hubs changes the risk of catheter-related infection.[39]
- Evaluate whether the results of quantitative catheter cultures alter patient management.[17]
- Determine the rates of infection by type of intravascular device.[40]
- Determine whether particular intravascular devices are associated with higher rates of infection.[40]

Surveillance Recommendations

Surveillance for intravascular catheter-related infections is still an inexact science. Despite these limitations, infection control personnel can design effective surveillance systems. For infection control programs that wish to begin surveillance for these infections, I would offer the following recommendations:

- Begin with a single ICU or other well-defined patient population, and determine the endemic rate of catheter-related or catheter-associated infection.
- Once the surveillance methodology is working well, the epidemiology staff can use the surveillance data to answer important questions or to evaluate the effect of interventions designed to reduce infections.

The Hospital Infection Control Practices Advisory Committee of the CDC recently issued its recommendations for the prevention of vascular catheter-related infection.[41] Infection control personnel must read these recommendations, because they contain information that may help the hospital reduce the risk of catheter-related infections. Epidemiology programs that wish to compare their rates with NNIS data must implement most of the CDC's recommendations.

References

1. Emori TG, Gaynes RP. An overview of nosocomial infections, including the role of the microbiology laboratory. *Clin Microbiol Rev.* 1993;6:428-442.
2. Maki DG. Infections due to infusion therapy. In: Bennett JV, Brachman PS, eds. *Hospital Infections.* Boston, Mass: Little, Brown, and Co; 1992:849-898.
3. Jarvis WR, Edwards JR, Culver DH, et al. Nosocomial infection rates in adult and pediatric intensive care units in the United States. *Am J Med.* 1991;91(suppl 3B):185S-191S.
4. Maki DG, Weise CE, Sarafin HW. A semi-quantitative culture method for identifying intravenous-catheter-related infection. *N Engl J Med.* 1977;296:1305-1309.
5. Maki DG, Cobb L, Garman JK, Shapiro JM, Ringer M, Helgerson RB. An attachable silver-impregnated cuff for prevention of infection with central venous catheters: a prospective randomized multicenter trial. *Am J Med.* 1988;85:307-314.
6. Sherertz RJ, Raad II, Belani A, et al. Three-year experience with sonicated vascular catheter cultures in a clinical microbiology laboratory. *J Clin Microbiol.* 1990;28:76-82.
7. Sitges-Serra A, Linares J. Limitations of semiquantitative method for catheter culture. *J Clin Microbiol.* 1988;26:1074-1075.
8. Widmer AF. IV-related infections. In: Wenzel RP, ed. *Prevention and Control of Nosocomial Infections.* 2nd ed. Baltimore, Md: Williams & Wilkins; 1993:556-579.
9. Cleri DJ, Corrado ML, Seligman SJ. Quantitative culture of intravascular catheters and other intravascular inserts. *J Infect Dis.* 1980;141:781-786.
10. Bjornson HS, Colley R, Bower RH, Duty VP, Schwartz-Fulton JT, Fischer JE. Association between microorganism growth at the catheter insertion site and colonization of the catheter in patients receiving total parenteral nutrition. *Surgery.* 1982;92:721-727.
11. Brun-Buisson C, Abrouk F, Legrand P, Huet Y, Larabi S, Rapin M. Diagnosis of central venous catheter-related sepsis. Critical level of quantitative tip cultures. *Arch*

Intern Med. 1987;147:873-877.

12. Heard SO, Davis RF, Sherertz RJ, et al. Influence of sterile protective sleeves on the sterility of pulmonary artery catheters. *Crit Care Med.* 1987;15:499-502.

13. Linares J, Sitges-Serra A, Garau J, Perez JL, Rogelio M. Pathogenesis of catheter sepsis: a prospective study with quantitative and semiquantitative cultures of catheter hub and segments. *J Clin Microbiol.* 1985;21:357-360.

14. Raad II, Sabbagh MF, Rand KH, Sherertz RJ. Quantitative tip culture methods and the diagnosis of central venous catheter-related infections. *Diagn Microbiol Infect Dis.* 1992;15:13-20.

15. Pittet D, Lew PD, Auckenthaler R, Waldvogel FA. Bacterial spread as a pathogenic factor in catheter-related infections. Presented at the 30th Interscience Conference on Antimicrobial Agents and Chemotherapy; October 1990; Atlanta, Ga. Abstract.

16. Sherertz R, Heard S, Raad I, Gentry L. Culturing catheter tips is an insensitive method for diagnosing triple lumen vascular catheter infection. Presented at the 32nd Interscience Conference on Antimicrobial Agents and Chemotherapy; October 1992; Anaheim, Calif. Abstract.

17. Widmer AF, Nettleman M, Flint K, Wenzel RP. The clinical impact of culturing central venous catheters. A prospective study. *Arch Intern Med.* 1992;152:1299-1302.

18. Wing EJ, Norden CW, Shadduck RK, Winkelstein A. Use of quantitative bacteriologic techniques to diagnose catheter-related sepsis. *Arch Intern Med.* 1979;139:482-483.

19. Raucher HS, Hyatt AC, Barzilai A, et al. Quantitative blood cultures in the evaluation of septicemia in children with Broviac catheters. *Pediatrics.* 1984;104:29-33.

20. Flynn PM, Shenep JL, Barrett FF. Differential quantitation with a commercial blood culture tube for diagnosis of catheter-related infection. *J Clin Microbiol.* 1988;26:1045-1046.

21. Weightman NC, Simpson EM, Speller DCE, Mott MG, Oakhill A. Bacteraemia related to indwelling central venous catheters: prevention, diagnosis and treatment. *Eur J Clin Microbiol Infect Dis.* 1988;7:125-129.

22. Ruderman JW, Morgan MA, Klein AH. Quantitative blood cultures in the diagnosis of sepsis in infants with umbilical and Broviac catheters. *J Pediatr.* 1988;112:748-751.

23. Fan ST, Teoh-Chan CH, Lau KF. Evaluation of central venous catheter sepsis by differential quantitative blood culture. *Eur J Clin Microbiol Infect Dis.* 1989;8:142-144.

24. Paya CV, Guerra L, Marsh HM, Farnell MB, Washington J, Thompson RL. Limited usefulness of quantitative culture of blood drawn through the device for diagnosis of intravascular-device-related bacteremia. *J Clin Microbiol.* 1989;27:1431-1433.

25. Capdevila JA, Planes AM, Palomar M, et al. Value of differential quantitative blood cultures in the diagnosis of catheter-related sepsis. *Eur J Clin Microbiol Infect Dis.* 1992;11:403-407.

26. Cooper GL, Hopkins CC. Rapid diagnosis of intravascular catheter-associated infection by direct Gram staining of catheter segments. *N Engl J Med.* 1985;312:1142-1147.

27. Zufferey J, Rime B, Francioli P, Bille J. Simple method for rapid diagnosis of catheter-associated infection by direct acridine orange staining of catheter tips. *J Clin Microbiol.* 1988;26:175-177.

28. Larson E, Horan T, Kotilainen HR, Landry S, Terry B. Study of the definitions of nosocomial infections. *Am J Infect Control.* 1991;19:259-267.

29. Garner JS, Jarvis WR, Emori TG, Horan TC, Hughes JM. CDC definitions for nosocomial infections, 1988. *Am J Infect Control.* 1988;16:128-140.

30. Maki DG, Ringer M. Risk factors for infusion-related phlebitis with small peripheral catheters. *Ann Intern Med.* 1991;114:845-854.

31. Hamory BH. Nosocomial bloodstream and intravascular device-related infections. In: Wenzel RP, ed. *Prevention and Control of Nosocomial Infections.* Baltimore, Md: Williams & Wilkins; 1987:283-319.

32. Centers for Disease Control. Postsurgical infections associated with an extrinsically contaminated intravenous anesthetic agent—California, Illinois, Maine, and Michigan, 1990. *MMWR.* 1990;39:426.

33. Sherertz RJ, Gledhill KS, Hampton KD, et al. Outbreak of Candida bloodstream infections associated with retrograde medication administration in a neonatal intensive care unit. *J Pediatr.* 1992;120:455-461.

34. Raviglione MC, Battan R, Pablos-Mendez A, Aceves-Casillas P, Mullen MP, Taranta A. Infections associated with Hickman catheters in patients with acquired immunodeficiency syndrome. *Am J Med.* 1989;86:780-786.

35. Raad I, Davis S, Khan A, Tarrand J, Elting L, Bodey GP. Impact of central venous catheter removal on the recurrence of catheter-related coagulase negative staphylococcal bacteremia. *Infect Control Hosp Epidemiol.* 1992;13:215-221.

36. Pegues D, Axelrod P, McClarren C, et al. Comparison of infections in Hickman and implanted port catheters in adult solid tumor patients. *J Surg Oncol.* 1992;49:156-162.

37. Puntis JWL, Holden CE, Smallman S, Finkel Y, George RH, Booth IW. Staff training: a key factor in reducing intravascular catheter sepsis. *Arch Dis Child.* 1990;65:335-337.

38. Selva J, Toledo A, Maroney A, Forlenza S. The value of participation in the CDC-National Nosocomial Infection Surveillance in a large teaching hospital. *Am J Infect Control.* 1989;17:117.

39. Weightman NC, Simpson EM, Speller DCE, Mott MG, Oakhill A. Bacteraemia related to indwelling central venous catheters: prevention, diagnosis and treatment. *Eur J Clin Microbiol.* 1988;7:125-129.

40. Sherertz, RJ, Falk RJ, Huffman KA, Thomann CA, Mattern WD. Infections associated with subclavian Uldall catheters. *Arch Intern Med.* 1983;143:52-56.

41. Pearson ML, Hospital Infection Control Practices Advisory Committee. Centers for Disease Control and Prevention. Guideline for prevention of intravascular device-related infections. *Am J Infect Control.* 1996;24:262-293.

CHAPTER 13

Designing Surveillance for Noninfectious Outcomes of Medical Care

R. Michael Massanari, MD, MS, Kim Wilkerson, ART,
Sheri Swartzendruber, RN, BS

Abstract

We present basic information that a hospital epidemiologist needs when designing a surveillance system for noninfectious adverse outcomes of care. Specific topics reflect key characteristics of such a surveillance system: the purpose, rationale, priorities, definitions, data collection tools, data collection, analysis and reporting, and validation.

Introduction

Purpose

The measurement of outcomes of medical care has attracted considerable attention in initiatives to reform the US healthcare system. Outcomes assessment provides a method for evaluating and managing the quality and efficiency of healthcare. While outcomes assessment and management are new concepts for many in healthcare, hospital epidemiologists have worked to monitor and prevent adverse outcomes—nosocomial infections—for decades. In this chapter, we share our experiences with designing and implementing surveillance for noninfectious adverse outcomes of healthcare at the University of Iowa Hospitals and Clinics (UIHC).[1] We identify and discuss important issues that epidemiologists should consider when developing and implementing surveillance programs for noninfectious outcomes of medical care.

Rationale

The rationale for expanding the scope of outcomes surveillance is multifactorial. First, studies of outcomes enable healthcare providers to assess and improve the quality of care. For example, the New York Hospital Study reported that adverse events complicated 3.7% of hospitalizations in 1984, and 16% of the events caused permanent disability or mortality.[2] At least 27% of the adverse events could have been prevented. The authors suggested that epidemiologic principles, used successfully to reduce the risk of nosocomial infections, should be employed to study and manage other adverse outcomes of medical care. Second, studies of outcomes enable healthcare providers to evaluate long-held, and often poorly substantiated, assumptions regarding the effectiveness of medical and surgical technologies.[3] Finally, studies of out-

TABLE 13-1
MEASURABLE DIMENSIONS OF THE QUALITY OF MEDICAL CARE

Clinical Outcomes of Medical Care

    Beneficial outcomes

    Adverse outcomes

Patient Perceptions of Medical Care

    Patient satisfaction with treatment

    Health status following treatment

Appropriateness of Medical Care

    Too little (access)

    Too much (inappropriate care)

Economic Impact of Medical Care

    Cost of medical care

    Value of medical care

comes are mandated by purchasers and regulators of healthcare, including the Joint Commission on Accreditation of Healthcare Organizations and the National Committee for Quality Assurance.

What to Measure

Outcomes

The literature describing healthcare outcomes and tools for measuring these outcomes is expanding. Table 13-1 summarizes several categories of outcomes that have been proposed or that are under development, including positive and negative outcomes of care, the appropriateness of clinical decision making, the value of medical care, and patients' perceptions of outcomes. In this chapter, we focus on measurement of adverse outcomes of care; however, the principles that we present apply across the spectrum of outcomes measurement.

We must consider two caveats. First, we know little about the association between technical quality in the process of rendering care and clinical outcomes. Therefore, hospital epidemiologists should not assume that any measure independently assesses the quality of care. Rather, when examining a specific outcome, one should aim to describe variation and to explain sources of the variation. Second, assessing outcomes of care and assessing the process of care are two different aspects of quality assessment. In this chapter, we discuss measurement of outcomes and not assessment of processes. By excluding process measurement, we are not minimizing the importance of quality improvement initiatives that assess processes. In the authors' opinion, these methodological approaches evaluate different dimensions of quality and can be used synergistically. For example, if issues of quality of care are identified by outcomes studies, quality improvement tools could be used to assess, improve, and monitor the associated processes of care.

Priorities

The spectrum of outcomes that can be included in surveillance programs is very broad. Because resources for surveillance are limited, one must select a manageable subset of outcomes that can be monitored and reported. The epidemiologist should review the literature to identify outcomes for which risk factors have been identified or for which an association between the quality of care and outcome has been established. Such data will help the epidemiologist set priorities and design surveillance. The following criteria may help epidemiologists select outcomes that will provide the most value for the effort expended:

- The outcomes should be important to patients and/or providers.
- The outcomes should reflect processes that can be managed by providers. For example, one should not monitor adverse outcomes experienced by neonates born to mothers who use drugs in order to measure the quality of obstetric care, because many of these outcomes may be related to the mother's drug use and not to poor medical care.
- Monitoring outcomes of high volume procedures may be most efficient.

- The outcomes monitored should not be limited to those recommended by external regulators, but should be guided by the needs and objectives of each institution.

Defining Criteria for Surveillance and Measurement

After hospital epidemiologists decide which outcomes to include in the surveillance program, they must define the criteria by which they will identify the outcomes. Well-developed, explicit definitions provide the foundation for consistent measurement across time, place, or other referents. Therefore, this step will determine, in part, the success of the program. The following are attributes of effective criteria[4]:

Explicit Definitions

The definitions for outcomes indicators should be succinct, unambiguous, and constant over time. Such definitions are not designed as diagnostic tools and will not account for all contingencies. Rather, explicit definitions that are constant over time will allow the epidemiologist to analyze aggregate data and to study variation across different referents.

Validity

Criteria or outcomes must accurately reflect reality or truth. The best criteria are those that are validated scientifically and reported in peer-reviewed literature. The Centers for Disease Control and Prevention (CDC) definition of surgical site infection is an example of a validated criterion. Some investigators have tried to assess quality of care by assessing mortality associated with hospitalization. However, mortality rates do not effectively monitor adverse outcomes because they lack sensitivity and specificity.

Unfortunately, investigators have not validated many of the criteria used to assess noninfectious adverse outcomes of medical care. Therefore, when hospital epidemiologists develop new criteria, they may need to obtain consensual validation. Consensual validation is obtained when experts agree that a criterion reasonably reflects reality. The "Delphi Technique" is a formal method used by healthcare researchers to obtain consensual validation. Hospital epidemiologists are more likely to reach consensus, or "buy-in" by less formal methods, such as soliciting the opinions of clinical leaders and important committees before starting surveillance.

Importance

The criteria should measure outcomes that are of clinical significance and that can be changed by clinical intervention.

Recordability

Data required for analysis of outcomes criteria should be reported consistently and should be readily accessible. The source of data usually is the written medical record. However, surveillance will be most efficient when data are obtained from an electronic medical record (information systems).

Reflects Variation

The surveillance system should evaluate events or outcomes that vary among patients. Indicators are most useful if a substantial proportion of the variation is attributable to differences in the quality of care. In other words, differences in the quality of care should cause differences in the outcomes.

Stability

The best indicators are those that can be evaluated over time. If the surveillance program changes criteria and definitions, hospital epidemiologists cannot accurately assess the trends. Therefore, criteria should be stable over time.

Screening Efficiency

Screening efficiency includes descriptive characteristics of the criteria, such as sensitivity, specificity, and predictive value. For a more comprehensive description of these characteristics, readers should refer to standard textbooks of clinical epidemiology. With few exceptions, information describing screening efficiency will not be published for indicators of noninfectious adverse outcomes.

A brief example will illustrate the significance of these attributes. Healthcare researchers often use "readmissions" to hospitals as outcome criteria or indicators of quality of care. Although it is not unreasonable to assume that substandard care may result in readmissions (consensual validity), there is minimal scientific validation for this conclusion. The criterion has the advantage of being both explicit and readily accessible through most hospital information systems. But "readmissions" has exceedingly low sensitivity and low specificity. Most readmissions are determined by the patient's underlying condition and cannot be controlled by the healthcare provider.

Selection of Criteria for Surveillance of Noninfectious Adverse Outcomes

Most clinicians agree that particular outcomes of medical care are undesirable. Therefore, hospital epidemiologists may more easily identify, define, and obtain consensus on criteria for adverse outcomes of medical care than on criteria for expected benefits of care.

The surveillance program for noninfectious adverse events at UIHC focused on five major categories:

1. *Events related to medication administration.* This category included events related to drug errors (eg, wrong drug, wrong dose, wrong patient, drug omitted), drug toxicity, allergic reactions, or idiosyncratic reactions.
2. *Events related to procedures.* This category included any noninfectious complication associated with diagnostic or therapeutic procedures.
3. *Accidents.* This category included falls, burns, or other events.
4. *New conditions not present on admission.* This category included nosocomial deep venous thrombosis, pulmonary emboli, decubitus ulcer, and myocardial infarctions that could not be linked to procedures or medications.
5. *Events related to equipment.* This category included equipment defects, malfunctions, or user-related errors.

A hospital epidemiologist and personnel from the Quality Assessment Support Service developed explicit definitions for each outcome. When possible, we used definitions published in the medical literature to ensure scientific and consensual validity. To obtain informal consensual validation, we asked clinical leaders to review and critique the criteria. We modified many definitions in response to reviews. If a proposed criterion was so controversial that clinicians did not agree, we deleted the criterion from the program.

Data Gathering

The process for data gathering will be determined by the outcomes that one wants to evaluate. The data collected and the processes for collecting the data must be consistent across patients or other referents. This objective can be accomplished by using a standardized data collection tool. When developing a data collection tool, the quality assessment team should consider what data to collect, which sources to survey, how to structure (layout) the tool, and how to store and retrieve data.

What Data to Collect

The objectives of the surveillance program should guide quality assessment personnel in deciding which data elements should be collected. In general, the primary objective should be to identify accurately and efficiently those patients with specific adverse outcomes. Therefore, the program should collect sufficient data to achieve these ends.

On the other hand, collecting unnecessary data leads to inefficient use of the data collectors' time and inefficient use of data storage.

The data should be collected in a concise format that will minimize transcribing errors and facilitate easy data entry and analysis. Clinical variables such as age, hemoglobin, or serum creatinine can be collected as numerics. If clinical variables are collected serially during the course of care, decision rules must specify which data point to record. Some data, such as surgical wound class, can be reduced easily to a simple numerical format. Categorical variables, such as gender, drug errors, or postoperative pulmonary embolus, can be classified as dichotomous variables. For example, either the patient has a condition ("Yes" or "1") or doesn't have the condition ("No" or "0"). Alternatively, one can assign categorical data-specific numeric codes (eg, pulmonary embolism = 827). Although in some instances one may need more than one category, one should not attempt to account for every contingency or rare event. Usually four or five categories will account for 75% to 90% of the clinically important circumstances. The remainder can be listed under "other," followed by a single line of free text to identify the category for future reference.

Hospital epidemiologists must avoid two pitfalls when developing a data collection tool. First, one must minimize the entry of free text. Recording data as text or statements is labor intensive and increases opportunity for error. Second, one should not expect data collectors to judge whether an outcome meets the criteria or whether an outcome was iatrogenic. These judgments are subjective. Causation is better determined through scientific studies.

The data collection tool should include the following categories:

- *Demographic data.* These data include variables that describe the subject (eg, age, gender, mobility, and socioeconomic status).
- *Environmental data.* These data should

include information describing where, when, and how the event of interest occurred. When appropriate, data collectors should include the identification number of the healthcare workers involved in the processes related to the event. These data may be most important for procedure-related adverse events.

- *Risk factors.* Other investigators may have identified risk factors for some adverse outcomes (ie, preexisting neurological deficits or poor vision increase the risk of falls). Categorical information describing risk factors should be included because the data will be important in analysis or in generating intervention strategies.
- *Outcomes.* The tool should include lists of all outcomes selected for surveillance.
- *Sequelae of adverse outcomes.* Although not imperative, the epidemiologist may choose to collect categorical data describing sequelae of adverse outcomes, including no sequelae, reversible injury, irreversible injury, or death.

Sources of Data

After deciding what data to collect, the epidemiologist should identify the source of the data for each element. One should prospectively identify the data sources to ensure that the data are available. Furthermore, this process will help the epidemiologist plan the format of the data collection tool, understand the limitations of the data collected, and train personnel to collect data.

The epidemiologist should identify and evaluate several possible sources of pertinent data. First, one must decide whether to abstract data concurrently from the evolving medical record or retrospectively from the discharge abstract. The latter has the advantage of being accessible on electronic information systems. However, the discharge abstract contains limited information, is subject to coding and recording errors, and only provides access to data retrospectively. Second, if data are obtained from the medical record, one must decide whether to use the written medical record or the electronic medical record. As clinical data become increasingly available in electronic records, the computer should become the principle source of data. Electronic access to data increases the efficiency of data collection and decreases recording and transcribing errors. However, for the foreseeable future, much information will not be available through information systems and will be found only in the written record. Finally, some data may be available only through incident reports or by interviews with patients or healthcare workers.

Optimal sources of data might include one or all of the sources described above. For example, the medical record provides data on nosocomial renal failure. However, the best source of information regarding drug errors may be incident reports or personal interviews with nurses responsible for managing patient units.

Structure of the Data Tool

The data collection tool should enable the data collector to record data easily, efficiently, and accurately. Therefore, data collectors should help design the tool.

The design of the tool should account for sources of data. For example, if demographic data are available on patient identification cards, the card should be used to imprint the data directly onto the form. If the hospital has an electronic medical record, the computer system could identify patients who meet particular criteria and then generate preliminary data forms that are completed by technical staff after they review the medical records.

The data collection tool will be easier to manage if it is only a single page or card. To minimize the amount of data that technical staff must write, the tool could have check boxes or check lists for categorical data.

Figure 13-1 shows a data collection tool that we designed for the surveillance program at the UIHC.

Data Storage and Retrieval

Data must be stored in an easily retrievable format or the entire surveillance effort will be thwarted. Although data can be stored in hard copy (eg, data cards, paper), inexpensive personal computing systems have made these methods obsolete. Even individuals who have minimal computer skills can develop programs for storing, analyzing, and reporting data if they use commercially available database packages. We used a commercial database program to develop the database that supports the surveillance program at the UIHC.[5] Epi Info is an inexpensive software database available from CDC that novices can use to store, analyze, and report surveillance data.

Reporting Information

Goals

The principal goals in reporting surveillance data are twofold. First, the information should report variation in indicators (eg, postoperative hemorrhage rates) across referents (eg, surgeon or procedure) of interest. Second, the information should enable clinicians to compare current data with those trended over time (ie, internal comparisons) or with data (ie, standards, benchmarks) generated from comparable institutions by similar methods (external comparisons). Therefore, the surveillance program must convert event-specific data into rates. Accurate rates are essential if the epidemiologist and the clinicians want to assess the effectiveness of interventions designed to improve quality of care. To compare outcomes across institutions or across other referents, one must risk-adjust the data. We will not discuss the details of risk adjustment. Rather, we will describe briefly how event-focused data can be converted into rates that can be reported to clinical departments and followed over time.

PT NAME: _____

HOSP. NO: ___ - ___ ___ ___ - ___   SEX: M F   D.O.B.:

ADM/OPV:_____ DC:_____ AO DATE:_____ PROC DATE:_____ TIME: _____

UNIT:_____ SERV:_____ CLDIV:_____ NDIV:_____ SHIFT: 0 1 2 3

■STAFF: NA Unk #_____ ■CONTACT: NA Unk #_____ INDICATOR: 11 12 13 14 15

BOC: A = Acute R = Recovery O = Observation C = Custodial OP = Outpatient

CASE #: __ __ __ __ __ __

UIHC/Quality Assessment Support Service
RISK CONTROL SURVEILLANCE

CONFIDENTIAL

This material has been prepared for use by a University Hospitals Staff Committee investigating ways to reduce morbidity and mortality.

Dx/Comments:_____
RC24Form.doc   04/01/95 kj

OCCURRENCES (Select 1)

MEDICATIONS

_____
(Specify Medication [30])

Doses
Affected #_____ or UNK

Route Given:

IM IV NG PO SQ OTH

_____
(Specify Other Only [30])

■ 701 Allergic Reaction
■ 702 Anesthesia Related
■ 703 Contraindication
704 Discontinued
■ 705 IV Site Related
706 Duplication
707 Omission
708 Wrong Route
■ 709 Adverse Effect
711 Wrong Dose
712 Wrong Med Admin
713 Wrong Patient
714 Wrong Rate of Flow
715 Wrong Time
746 Transcription Error
■ 747 Wrong Med Ordered
748 Other

_____
(Specify Other only [30])

Med Error Consequence:

NA or _____
(e.g., omitted [30])

PROCEDURE RELATED

_____
(Specify Procedure [30])

PROC AREA: OR OTH
■ 716 Complication
■ 718 Performance
■ 722 Wrong Patient
■ 723 Wrong Proc/Test
■ 752 Return to OR/DR

■ 724 NEW CONDITIONS ✳
● 728 FALL

EQUIPMENT RELATED

_____
(Specify Equipment/Device [30])
736 Complication
737 Defect
738 Malfunction
739 Improper Set-up
740 Wrong Setting
741 Removed by Patient
742 Unplanned Removal
744 Struck by Equipment
■ 745 Missing Equipment
■ 753 Counts off/Item Found
■ 754 Counts off/Item Not Found
743 Equipment Other

_____
(Specify Other only [30])

READM./SPEC. CARE UNITS
749 Return ≤ 24 hrs
750 Return > 24 hrs ≤ 48 hrs
751 Return > 48 hrs ≤ 72 hrs

735   OTHER OCCURRENCES

_____
(Specify Other only [30])

● **FALLS ONLY**

RESTRAINTS
(Select 1)
601 No Data
602 No Factor
604 Ineffective
605 Defective
607 Other

_____
(Specify Other only [30])

● ● ● ● ● ● ● ● ●

● **FALL**
BED RAILS

01 Up
02 Down
03 No Data
04 No Factor

● ● ● ● ● ● ● ● ●

● **FALL**
PROTOCOL

Yes No Unk

● ● ● ● ● ● ● ● ●

● **FALL**
LOCATION

(Be Very Specific [30])

● ● ● ● ● ● ● ● ●

● **FALL**
ELIMINATION

Yes No Unk

801 No Data
802 None
812 Death ✳
818 Ileus
823 Hepatic Failure
824 Renal Failure
831 Hypotension
852 Bowel Obs
837 Other

_____
(Specify Other only [30])

CARDIAC
804 Acute MI ✳
865 Recurrent MI ✳
810 Cardiac Arrest ✳
866 Rec. Cardiac Arrest ✳
819 EP Changes
822 Cardiac Failure

NEONATAL
839 Stillbirth
856 ROP
858 IVH w/Hydrocephalus
860 IVH w/o Hydrocephalus

NEUROLOGIC
811 Change in Mentation
821 N/S Loss

_____
(Specify N/S only [30])
830 Seizures
834 Stroke
857 Hearing Loss
859 Sight Loss

RESPIRATORY
806 Aspiration ✳
825 Respiratory Failure
◆ 827 PE ✳
828 Respiratory Arrest ✳
867 Rec. Resp. Arrest ✳
841 Resp. Compromise

OUTCOMES (Select 1-3)

SKIN

_____
(Specify Site for All [30])
832 Skin Rash
862 Extravasation
◆ 813 Breakdown I ✳
◆ 853 Breakdown II ✳
◆ 854 Breakdown III ✳
◆ 855 Breakdown IV ✳
◆ 870 Eschar ✳

Adm Braden:_____ ND NA
PreSB Braden: ___ ND NA
PreSB Date:_____
Mo/Day/Yr

SURGICAL WOUND
814 Dehiscence
842 Disruption

TRAUMA/HEMORRHAGE

_____
(Specify Site for All [30])
803 Abrasion
808 Bruise
809 Burn
815 Fracture ✳
817 Hemorrhage
820 Laceration
868 Laceration-3
869 Laceration-4
■ 829 Retained FB
848 Coagulopathy
849 Dislocation
851 Phlebitis
863 Thrombus
◆ 864 DVT ✳

PROC. RELATED T/O INJ.
836 T/O Injury
(Proc. Related Only)

_____
(Specify Type & Site [30])

FACTORS (Select 1-6)

PERSONNEL
(Select 1-3)
200 No Data
201 No Factor
206 Nursing
■ 211 Clinical
213 Dietary
216 Lab
219 Pharmacy
220 Physical Therapy
223 Respiratory Care
229 Other

_____
(Specify Other Only [30])

GENERAL FACTORS
401 No Data
402 No Factor
403 Confused/Disoriented
412 Previous Adm
413 Surgery
414 Transfer to ICU
418 Transfer to Clin
         Dept/Div
419 DNR
420 Baby (OB Only)
411 Other

_____
(Specify Other Only [30])

STOCKINGS ◆
421 Teds
422 Kendalls
423 Teds/Kendalls

ACTIVITY ◆
424 Bedrest
425 Chair
426 PT
427 Up Ad Lib
428 Up/Assisted

SPECIAL BED ◆
429 Bariatric
430 Biodyne
431 Kinair
432 Pediacare/Kinair
433 Rotokinetic
434 Other Special
         Bed

_____
(Specify Other Only)

435 ANTI-
       COAGULATION ◆

436 CAST/FIXATOR ◆

DIAGNOSIS ◆
437 Hemorrhage
438 Paralysis
439 Stroke
440 Trauma
441 Tumor
___ None of the Above

REFERRED:

Y   N

SS: _____

TECH:

_____

■ Report Staff/
    Contact physician
    codes
◆ PE/DVT/SB Factors
● Patient Falls
✳ New Condition/
    Housewide

FIGURE 13-1. Example of a standardized data collection tool for adverse outcomes.

Denominator Data

Separate processes are necessary for gathering data on subjects at risk for specific adverse outcomes (denominator data). These data should include number of admissions (or discharges) by patient unit, clinical service, or hospital; number of patient-days by unit or hospital; number of patients undergoing a procedure of interest; or number of medication doses administered. Unless one is conducting an analytical study that requires more detailed clinical data, the information required for subjects at risk is minimal and may be available from hospital information systems.

Rates

Several different rates can be used to report adverse outcomes of medical care. The frequency of new conditions or accidents can be reported as cumulative incidence (event of interest per 100 admissions per unit of time [month, year]) or reported as incidence density (event of interest per 1,000 patient-days).

To facilitate internal comparisons and analyses of patterns, statistical control limits, calculated using data from the previous 20 time intervals, can be included on the graphic display. Rates of procedure-related adverse events or outcomes can be reported as cumulative incidence and reported as postoperative surgical site infection rates:

events/100 procedures/unit of time

(month, year)

Basic reports should use the total number of procedures performed by the service per unit of time as the denominator. However, for more detailed reports, the program could stratify the data by procedure or physician. If physician-specific rates are reported, data should be coded to maintain confidentiality.

The rates of medication-related adverse outcomes can be reported as cumulative incidence or incidence density. Because each medication dose could cause an adverse event, we recommend using as the demoninator the number of doses per unit during a specific time period. This denominator controls for the frequency of administration:

event of interest/10,000 doses administered/ unit of time

If pharmacy data are accessible, one could report drug-specific rates of adverse events. However, epidemiologists may not be able to calculate these rates if denominator data are not available on computers.

Communicating With Customers of the Report

The principle objective of surveillance reports is to improve the quality of medical care. However, if the epidemiologist wants the recipients of the data to accept the data and to change their practice, the quality assessment team must consider seriously the manner in which they present the data. Hard experience has demonstrated that chastising a presumed outlier is almost never successful. Surveillance data are intimidating and potentially threatening. Furthermore, variation in surveillance data is not necessarily caused by actual changes in the frequency of particular outcomes, but may be caused by surveillance artifacts. Therefore, the better short-term strategy is to present the reports and simply to raise unthreatening questions. Confronted with an attitude of open inquiry, recipients of surveillance reports will find it less threatening to examine the processes that may have contributed to adverse outcomes.

Who Should Receive Reports

Managers of surveillance programs should identify clinical and administrative staff who should receive periodic surveillance reports. Recipients will include the hospital epidemiologist who manages the surveillance program, the institutional committee that provides authoritative oversight for surveillance, and the hospital's legal advisors. However, the most important recipients of the information are the clinical leaders (nurses and physicians) and administrators who manage the clinical processes and outcomes that are being surveyed. In addition, special reports may be generated for other committees, operating boards, and regulatory agencies, or they may be published in the scientific literature.

What Should Be Reported

The importance of transforming surveillance data into comprehensible information cannot be overstressed. Periodic reports of information describing adverse outcomes should include rates over time for the events of interest. Graphs will help personnel review and analyze the data quickly.

When problems are identified through surveillance, the epidemiologist may need to produce additional ad hoc reports that are tailored to the problem under investigation. Ad hoc reports usually summarize the results of analytic epidemiologic studies, such as case-control or cohort studies, conducted to assess the problem. In the authors' experience, the paper trail of ad hoc reports should be supplemented with periodic face-to-face discussions with clinical managers. These discussions facilitate communication and reduce impediments to improving quality of care.

How Often to Report

The frequency of periodic reports should be determined by the needs of managers who use the information, the frequency of the outcomes of interest, and the capacity of the surveillance program to produce accurate, valid information. Departmental and unit-specific outcomes reports can be generated monthly. Because provider-specific events (ie, physician-specific outcomes) are infrequent, reports should not be generated more than once per year. Special ad hoc reports can be generated as needed.

The surveillance program should assist the hospital in traditional risk management. To do this, the personnel from the surveillance program could report particularly serious adverse events directly to the hospital's legal staff.

Evaluating Interventions

A successful surveillance program will identify opportunities for improving medical care. The tools of total quality management or continuous quality improvement are particularly apropos at this juncture. Teams of clinicians and support personnel who are responsible for processes of care should review information describing the problem and then formulate hypotheses and possible interventions. One or two of the strategies should be selected and implemented.

Surveillance data also enable healthcare providers to evaluate intervention strategies. Furthermore, if the intervention study includes two or more alternative strategies and is coupled with data on costs, the outcomes surveillance program can study the cost-effectiveness of alternative interventions. Thus, a successful outcomes assessment program is not simply one that identifies problems, but one that helps users choose solutions and provides to users data on the effectiveness and cost-effectiveness of alternative strategies.

Resources Supporting the Surveillance Program

Surveillance programs are labor intensive; therefore, the principle resources will be personnel. Capital needs for the surveillance program alone are relatively small. However, a strong hospital information system will increase efficiency and reduce the number of personnel required to support the program.

Support Staff

The UIHC surveillance program is integrated so that surveillance staff assigned to specific units gather data for risk control, infection control, utilization review, and transfusion review. Of the 10 surveillance technicians, three to four full-time equivalents are required to do surveillance for non-

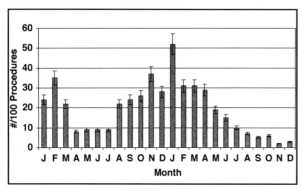

FIGURE 13-2. Postoperative hemorrhage on a surgical service. This graph illustrates how a surveillance program can report data on outcomes associated with procedures. In this hypothetical example, the rates of hemorrhage varied over time. In September, the surveillance program noted a substantial increase in the rate of hemorrhage. They informed the department chair of the increased rates. Because the rates remained high, the surveillance program conducted a case-control study. The study revealed an association between the intraoperative use of a particular drug and the adverse outcome. The surveillance program reported this result to the department chair, to the pharmacy, and to the quality assessment committee. The surgical service stopped using the drug in March, and the rates of hemorrhage decreased.

infectious adverse events in this 800-bed tertiary-care hospital. Management of the program includes a nurse manager (1.0 full-time equivalent [FTE]), a data analyst (1.0 FTE), and a senior programmer analyst (0.5 FTE).

Validating and Measuring the Efficacy of Surveillance Programs

Epidemiologists who direct nontraditional surveillance programs should include two additional long-range objectives in their planning. First, the epidemiologist should design studies to validate the surveillance program (Figure 13-2).[6] These studies assess the validity, sensitivity, specificity, and predictive value of indicators and the consistency of data collection across surveillance staff. In addition, the epidemiologist must demonstrate that the program is cost-effective and that it improves the

quality and decreases the cost of healthcare.[7] Epidemiologists can accomplish this objective by documenting that the costs saved by reducing adverse outcomes exceeds the cost of the surveillance program.

Conclusion

The basic epidemiologic methods that should undergird surveillance for noninfectious adverse outcomes of care have been well established by individuals practicing infection control. However, healthcare researchers are still identifying the definitions, indicators, and the case-finding methods appropriate for such surveillance systems. In addition, they are attempting to determine whether the processes of care are associated with the outcomes of care. Hospital epidemiologists have the opportunity and responsibility to help establish these programs on sound epidemiologic principles.

References

1. Massanari RM. Quality improvement: controlling the risk of adverse events. In: Wenzel, RP, ed. *Assessing Quality Health Care*. Baltimore, Md: Williams & Wilkins; 1992.

2. Brennan TA, Leape LL, Laird NM, et al. Incidence of adverse events and negligence in hospitalized patients. *N Engl J Med*. 1991;324:370-376.

3. Ellwood PM. Outcomes management: a technology of patient experience. *N Engl J Med*. 1988;318:1549-1556.

4. Donabedian A. *The Definition of Quality and Approaches to Its Assessment*. Ann Arbor, Mich: Health Administration Press; 1980.

5. Streed SA, Massanari RM. Data Management System for Evaluating Complications of Health Care. Proceedings of the 12th Annual Symposium on Computer Applications in Medical Care. 1988;(November):874-876.

6. Nettleman MD, Nelson AP. Adverse occurrences during hospitalization on a general medicine service. *Clinical Performance and Quality Health Care*. 1994;2:67-72.

7. Nettleman MA, Bock MJ, Nelson AP, Fieselmann J. Impact of procedure-related complications on patient outcome on a general medicine service. *J Gen Intern Med*. 1994;9:66-70.

CHAPTER 14

Outbreak Investigations

Consuelo Beck-Sague, MD, William R. Jarvis, MD,
William J. Martone, MD

Abstract

Epidemic nosocomial infections are defined as hospital-acquired infections that represent an increase in incidence over expected rates. Epidemic-associated infections usually are clustered temporally or geographically, suggesting that the infections are from a common source or are secondary to increased person-to-person transmission. Epidemics are important because they account for a substantial percentage of nosocomial infections. Furthermore, if infection control personnel thoroughly investigate outbreaks of nosocomial infections, they may identify new agents, reservoirs, or modes of transmission.

Introduction

Epidemic nosocomial infections are defined as hospital-acquired infections that represent an increase in incidence over expected rates. Epidemic-associated infections usually are clustered temporally or geographically, suggesting that the infections are from a common source or are secondary to increased person-to-person transmission. Often, outbreaks are associated with specific procedures or devices. Although epidemic nosocomial infections occur infrequently, in some settings, such as intensive care units (ICUs), they account for a substantial percentage of hospital-acquired infections.[1] Among hospitals in the National Nosocomial Infections Surveillance System, approximately 5% of nosocomial infections occur in epidemics. Most of these infections occur in small clusters of two to three patients.[2] However, many outbreaks, particularly those caused by common pathogens, are unrecognized. Thus, the published data may underestimate the frequency of outbreaks substantially.

If infection control personnel thoroughly investigate nosocomial epidemics, they may identify new agents, reservoirs, or modes of transmission.[3] To accomplish these goals, infection control personnel must evaluate data obtained from epidemiologic studies and from microbiologic and molecular studies. In this chapter, we will describe briefly how to recognize, investigate, and control outbreaks in healthcare settings, including hospitals and outpatient facilities.

TABLE 14-1
IDENTIFIED CAUSES OF VARIOUS TYPES OF NOSOCOMIAL OUTBREAKS, CENTERS FOR DISEASE CONTROL AND PREVENTION, 1978 TO 1993

Outbreak	Cause
Group A streptococcal surgical site infections	Healthcare worker who carries the organism
Pyrogenic reactions or BSIs in hemodialysis units	Use of contaminated water for disinfecting dialyzers or preparing dialysate
BSIs in intensive care units	Contaminated pressure transducers
Pseudomonas cepacia pseudo-infections	Contaminated povidone iodine
BSIs caused by *Candida* species	Contaminated total parenteral nutrition solutions
BSIs caused by *Yersinia enterocolitica*	Contaminated packed red blood cells
Gram-negative pneumonia, common source	Contaminated respiratory therapy equipment, eg, nebulizers
Gram-negative infections at sterile sites	Contaminated multidose vials
TB, including multidrug-resistant	Exposure of immunosuppressed patients to TB patients in absence of adequate source or engineering controls
Legionnaire's disease	Contaminated potable water or water in a cooling tower

BSIs = bloodstream infections; TB = tuberculosis.

Recognizing Outbreaks

Tips for Identifying Outbreaks

Hospitals must have reliable, sensitive surveillance systems that allow infection control personnel to detect increased infection rates in a defined time period and geographic area, suggestive of epidemic transmission.[4] Sometimes outbreaks are easy to recognize. For example, even one episode of an uncommon infection, such as a group A streptococcal surgical site infection, can indicate an outbreak. In other cases, an increased incidence of infection caused by unusual organisms, such as *Ewingella* species, or by unusual strains, such as multidrug-resistant *Mycobacterium tuberculosis*, indicate epidemic transmission (Table 14-1).[5]

Even if pathogens or anatomic sites are not unusual, increased numbers of infections in specific hospital units may indicate epidemic transmission. This is true particularly of units caring for highly vulnerable patients such as ICUs, units for human immunodeficiency virus-infected patients, organ transplant units, and hemodialysis units.[6] Similarly, abrupt temporal increases over well-established baseline rates usually result from epidemic spread. In exceptional cases, increased rates may occur when the number of high-risk patients increases (eg, when a new oncology ward opens). Even if increased rates of nosocomial infections appear to be consistent with recognized secular trends, infection control personnel should investigate such increases to rule out the possibility of epidemic transmission. For example, rates of nosocomial bloodstream infections and fungal infections are increasing nationally. Thus, increased rates of these infections could be consistent with the national trends or could represent an outbreak.

Some procedures, vehicles, and technical errors repeatedly are associated with hospital outbreaks (see Table 14-1). Infection control personnel will be able to investigate outbreaks more efficiently if they are aware of these associations. For example, inappropriate disinfection of reusable pressure transducers has caused numerous epidemics of bloodstream infections in ICUs. When investigating an outbreak of bloodstream infections, infection control personnel should evaluate this procedure promptly. Likewise, improperly reprocessed hemodialyzers and inadequately processed water used to mix dialysate or to reprocess dialyzers have caused epidemics of pyrogenic reactions or bacteremia in hemodialysis units. Thus, infection control personnel should review procedures for reprocessing hemodialyzers and for water treatment early in the management of such outbreaks.

The First Few Steps

Once the infection control team suspects that an outbreak exists, they should take steps to confirm whether an outbreak actually is occurring (Table 14-2). Infection control personnel should review some or all medical records from putative case-patients to provide the basis for a preliminary case definition. A case definition states who (person) had the symptoms or findings, delineates a finite time period (time) during which the symptoms began or were recognized, and specifies the location (place) in which transmission occurred. A case definition may be based on clinical, laboratory, radiologic, or pathologic data, and the definition may change, becoming broader or more specific, as additional information becomes available. The following statement is an example of a case definition: "A case of *Acinetobacter baumanii* bloodstream infection was defined as a patient who was in the surgical intensive care unit between January 1, 1994, and May 3, 1994, and who had symptoms suggestive of sepsis and a blood culture positive for *A baumanii* after January 1, 1994."

Infection control personnel can identify additional cases by searching in a variety of sources for persons who meet the case definition, including records from infection control, microbiology, pathology, radiology, surgery, and pharmacy. After identifying all suspected case-patients, infection control personnel can chart an epidemic curve and

TABLE 14-2
STEPS IN OUTBREAK INVESTIGATIONS

Preliminary Investigation and Descriptive Study
- Review existing information
- Determine the nature, location, and severity of the disease problem
- Verify the diagnosis
- Establish a case definition
- Find and ascertain case-patients
- Request that the laboratory save isolates from affected patients and from suspected sources or vehicles
- Draw an epidemic curve
- Summarize data in a line-listing
- Establish the existence of an outbreak
- Institute or assess adequacy of emergency control measures

Comparative Study and Definitive Investigations
- Review records of existing case-patients
- Develop hypotheses
- Test hypotheses in comparative (case-control or cohort) studies
- Conduct microbiologic or other laboratory studies and surveys
- Conduct additional studies, including observational studies, surveys, or experiments, to confirm the mode of transmission

calculate rates of infection during the preoutbreak and outbreak periods. The shape of the epidemic curve may suggest the possible source and mode of transmission of the etiologic agent. Statistical analysis of rates during the outbreak and preoutbreak periods will determine whether the observed rate increase is unlikely to be due to chance.

At this point, infection control personnel should begin a thorough investigation. Infection control personnel should review carefully records of patients identified as case-patients to produce a line-listing. The line-listing enumerates all affected patients, and displays characteristics of the patients that may be important to the investigation (Tables 14-3 and 14-4).

TABLE 14-3

A LINE-LISTING FROM AN OUTBREAK OF SURGICAL SITE INFECTIONS CAUSED BY GROUP A STREPTOCOCCI, 1980

Case	Age	Gender	Ward	Type of Surgery	Date of Surgery	Operating Room	Parenteral Antibiotic Prophylaxis	Duration of Surgery (Min)	Wound Drain	Fever (> 101°) Hrs After Surgery	Date of Wound Inflammation	Culture Date	Culture Site
1	46	F	5NW	TAH, BSO	4/23	A	No	100	No	17	4/29	4/30	Wound
2	77	M	3C	Cholecystectomy, choledocholithotomy	5/2	F	No	150	Yes	32	5/4	5/6	Wound
3	47	M	5SW	Laminectomy	5/6	C	No	120	Yes	24	5/9	5/9	Wound
												5/8,5/10	Blood
4	55	F	3C	Lobar resection and pleural stripping	5/8	D	No	120	Yes	17	5/12	5/16	Wound
5	84	F	2SE	Pyelolithotomy	5/14	C	No	60	Yes	36	5/17	5/21	Wound
												5/21,5/24	Blood
6	55	M	3C	Sigmoid resection	5/20	F	No	105	Yes	48	5/23	5/23	Wound
7	22	F	5SW	ORIF-ankle	7/6	A	No	150	No	20	7/7	7/8	Wound
8	65	F	5SW	Bunionectomy	7/21	F	No	45	No	18	7/23	7/23	Wound
9	40	F	4SW	Melanoma resection with skin graft	7/21	A	No	145	Yes	99	7/25	7/25	Wound
10	37	F	5NW	TAH, BSO	7/30	A	No	105	No	32	8/1	8/4	Wound

TAH = total abdominal hysterectomy; BSO = bilateral salpingo-oophorectomy; ORIF = open reduction, internal fixation. Revised from Berkelman RL et al.[11]

Because impressions and recollections change rapidly during times of stress, infection control personnel should interview staff and review procedures immediately after they recognize a potential epidemic. The epidemiology staff also should review relevant policies and procedures and verify compliance or noncompliance. In addition, infection control staff should review the literature to identify the source and mode of transmission in similar outbreaks. On the basis of all available data, infection control personnel should develop a hypothesis to explain how the epidemic developed. They also can use these data to plan rational emergency control measures.

Infection control personnel should immediately request that the clinical laboratories save all isolates and relevant specimens from patients possibly related to the outbreak. Likewise, infection control personnel should remove suspected sources or vehicles from the clinical areas to prevent healthcare workers from using or discarding these items.

Epidemiology staff who are calm and systematic can avert an atmosphere of fear and can investigate the outbreak effectively. If staff panic, they may discard vital materials inadvertently, introduce various procedural changes, or disinfect possible reservoirs before appropriate samples are obtained. Interventions that are not chosen on a rational basis may impair or impede the investigation.

Emergency Measures

If infection control personnel confirm that an epidemic has occurred or is occurring, they must decide immediately whether to:

- Conduct a full epidemiologic study.
- Obtain cultures from equipment or suspected

TABLE 14-4
A Line-Listing of Exposures for Patients Affected in an Outbreak of Group A Streptococcal Surgical Site Infections

Patient	Operating Room	Surgeon	Surgical Assistant	Nurse Anesthetist	Scrub Nurse	Circulating Nurse
1	A	E, K	—	E	e, f	F, G, I, K
2	F	F	b	C	d	I, J
3	G	B, L	—	A	f	I, L
4	D	A	a	A	b, c	D, I
5	C	C, I	—	B	b	D, E
6	F	D	a	D	f	I, J
7	A	G	—	A	—	D, I
8	F	G	—	E	d	I, M
9	A	F	c	D	g	J
10	A	H, J	—	B	a	D, I

Revised from Berkelman RL et al.[11]

vehicles.
- Call local, state, or federal agencies.
- Institute emergency control measures.

When making these decisions, infection control personnel should consider the following factors:
- The mortality associated with the epidemic.
- The public health importance of the outbreak.
- The frequency of infection versus colonization.
- The possibility of a common source.
- The size of the outbreak.
- The characteristics of the pathogen.
- Local and state regulations that may require healthcare facilities to report epidemics.

The healthcare facility should identify a spokesperson who will update appropriate internal (eg, staff or patients) and external constituencies (eg, regulatory and advisory governmental agencies) regularly. The spokespersons should present enough data to assure these parties that the facility is investigating the problem thoroughly and carefully. However, the spokesperson should not divulge prematurely the hypotheses that the epidemiology program is testing.

Closing the Ward

The epidemiology staff must weigh carefully the benefit of closing a ward or unit against the risk of decreased access to care. There are no laws or regulations dictating when a ward should be closed. In general, a healthcare facility should close wards only for conditions that cause high mortality or permanent disability, that had a clear onset, and that continue despite infection control precautions. Before deciding to close the ward or to discontinue surgery or specific procedures, the epidemiology program should determine what criteria must be met before the suspended activities may be resumed.

Reporting Outbreaks

State and federal laws require that healthcare facilities notify public health authorities of certain conditions.[7] Infection control personnel should consult their state's laws. However, at a minimum, epidemiology programs should report to the coun-

TABLE 14-5
SOURCES OF INFORMATION

- Log books
   - Operating room or delivery room
   - Emergency room
   - Nursing unit
   - Intensive care unit
   - Procedure room
- Microbiology records
- Employee health records
- Infection control surveillance data
- Medical records
- Operative notes
- Pathology reports
- Pharmacy records
- Radiology reports
- Hospital billing records
- Central-service records
- Purchasing records

ty and state health departments all outbreaks that have potential public health implications at the state or national level. In addition, infection control personnel should report suspected intrinsic contamination of sterile products, fatal blood transfusion reactions, infections caused by contaminated blood products, and infections associated with defective devices to both the Hospital Infections Program, Centers for Disease Control and Prevention (404-639-6413), and the Food and Drug Administration's MED WATCH Program (1-800-FDA-1088). Hospitals that report outbreaks to state and national agencies may benefit by receiving help as they evaluate and control the problem. The Hospital Infections Program receives numerous calls each day from infection control personnel who request either advice on managing outbreaks or on-site assistance.

Conducting an Epidemiologic Study

Reviewing the Line-Listing

Before conducting a comprehensive epidemio-

logic study, infection control personnel should review the line-listing and the epidemic curve, because these tools may suggest the cause of the outbreak. This is true particularly if the problem is an acute, self-limited, one-time incident, such as those associated with a recognized contamination.

Comparative Studies

Infection control personnel usually must review the patients' medical records to determine which exposures might be significant. Hospitalized patients usually do not know or recall details essential to the investigation. Moreover, patients may be too ill to answer questions. Infection control personnel may learn important information from short, open-ended interviews with patients. In general, the medical and laboratory records and other documents will provide the most information (Table 14-5). Epidemiology staff should design a standardized abstracting form on which they collect demographic data, information about exposures, and other data regarding the study subjects. The abstracting form ensures that personnel will collect data uniformly and that they will not need to review records repeatedly to find missed items.

In many outbreaks, a putative risk factor can be confirmed only if it meets certain criteria. First, the risk factor must have been present before the onset of the disease. Second, the risk factor generally will be associated with the condition statistically. To confirm the latter point, epidemiology staff must either compare affected patients with patients who did not acquire the condition ("controls") or compare the rate of the condition among patients with a certain putative risk factor to the rate among patients without the risk factor. Infection control personnel can use a case-control study to make the former comparison and a cohort study to make the latter comparison.

The epidemiology staff should consider several factors, including what resources are available, before they decide to conduct a comparative study. Ongoing outbreaks generally deserve to be evaluated by a comparative study. This is true particularly of outbreaks that could cause high mortality or severe disease, that might be caused by a new or unusual agent, or that have new reservoirs or modes of transmission. Because epidemics of pseudoinfections or other nonfatal conditions also may affect patient care negatively, infection control personnel may need to evaluate such clusters with comparative studies.

Case-control studies, which compare case-patients with controls, cannot always quantify the extent to which exposure to a factor increases risk. Case-control studies establish only that case-patients were more likely to have been exposed to the putative risk factor than were controls. Case-control studies also provide an odds ratio, which measures the strength of the association between the condition and exposure to the risk factor.[8] In contrast, cohort studies, which evaluate all patients during a defined time period in a specific setting, can quantify the extent to which the exposure increases the risk of developing the condition (the "relative risk").

Nosocomial outbreaks with very high attack rates lend themselves to retrospective cohort studies, especially when the population is small (<100) and clearly defined. Conversely, outbreaks that have low attack rates and affect large patient populations are better suited for retrospective case-control studies. An advantage of case-control studies is that they require less time to complete than do cohort studies. A cohort study may take months if the susceptible population is very large, whereas a typical case-control study may be completed in a few days.

Each variable that is evaluated as a possible risk factor will increase the time and expense required for the outbreak investigation. Furthermore, each additional variable increases the likelihood that a characteristic entirely unrelated to the outbreak will appear to be a risk factor (ie, statisti-

cally significant by chance alone). To avoid these pitfalls, infection control personnel should include few, if any, characteristics that are not biologically plausible risk factors. Similarly, epidemiology staff would be wise to avoid investigating characteristics that would be "interesting" but are unlikely, according to the literature, the line-listing, or expert advice, to be related to the outbreak.

Infection control personnel should consider carefully whether or not to perform a matched study. Variables on which case-patients and controls are matched cannot be evaluated as potential risk factors. Furthermore, matching may make controls and case-patients so similar that the investigators would miss all but the most obvious risk factors. Matching is very useful when numerous characteristics are associated with the epidemic condition, but are not the real cause(s) ("confounders"). These confounders can obscure the real causative factors. Many investigators choose not to match, but to control for confounding variables by either stratifying the analysis by possible confounders or by using multivariate analysis.

In small outbreaks or clusters, the causative factor may not achieve statistical significance. If the power of the study is low, infection control personnel should explore any factor with an odds ratio or relative risk that suggests an association, even if the *P* value does not achieve statistical significance.

EPI INFO is a software package that allows infection control personnel to analyze data generated in their epidemiologic investigations.[9] The program enables the investigator to do the statistical analysis easily and to calculate odds ratios, relative risks, 95% confidence intervals, chi-squares, and *P* values.[9]

Observational Studies

Infection control personnel should observe healthcare workers perform procedures, particularly patient-care techniques, that might be related to the outbreak. Observational studies help the epidemiology staff generate hypotheses regarding the origin of the outbreak and confirm findings in the comparative study. For example, if an epidemiologic study suggests that a vehicle is associated with the epidemic, an observational study allows infection control personnel to determine how the etiologic agent was transmitted from the contaminated source. Epidemiology staff also should review written protocols, interview supervisory staff, and identify procedural changes implemented before, during, or after the epidemic. However, infection control personnel also must observe implicated procedures and must question personnel who perform these techniques directly. Epidemiology staff may obtain valuable information by observing different personnel on the same shift and personnel on different shifts as they perform these procedures.

Culture Surveys

Experts disagree about the value of obtaining cultures from staff and the environment as a means of identifying the source of an outbreak. Organisms that cause nosocomial outbreaks (eg, Gram-negative water organisms; fungi, including *Aspergillus* species; and Gram-positive cocci, including *Staphylococcus aureus*) can be isolated frequently from nonsterile environmental sources or from staff. However, in our experience, culture results are only rarely helpful in the absence of epidemiologic data linking these sources to the outbreak.[7] In fact, random culture surveys may increase the cost of an investigation substantially and may identify the wrong source.[7]

For example, some staff may become transiently colonized with the epidemic strain after working with infected or colonized patients, but may not transmit the organism to other patients.[6] Thus, infection control personnel generally should obtain cultures from staff members who are linked epidemiologically to the epidemic and should compare results to those staff who are not implicated, instead of using the culture results to determine who is

linked to the epidemic. Likewise, we recommend that infection control personnel obtain cultures only from environmental sources implicated by epidemiologic data. Culture surveys of nonsterile areas (eg, floors, sinks, walls), which do not have plausible connections to the outbreak, waste valuable resources and frequently yield uninterpretable data.

Conversely, infection control personnel should not abandon their hypothesis if cultures do not recover the organism from a source or reservoir that was implicated strongly in the epidemiologic study. For example, only a small proportion of the individual units of a commercially prepared medication may be contaminated. Similarly, individuals who disseminate the epidemic strain may shed the organism only intermittently, may be colonized intermittently, or colonized in an unusual site.[10,11] Thus, infection control personnel never should vindicate a source, which was identified by a well-designed epidemiologic study, solely on the basis of negative cultures.

Techniques for obtaining cultures vary considerably by organism and source. Infection control personnel can save time and resources if they consult with a microbiologist before they collect specimens or consume a limited supply of the suspected vehicle. For example, settle plates or devices such as the Anderson® or Reyneirs® air sampler can help identify the source of some airborne infections. In some outbreaks (eg, outbreaks associated with hemodialysis fluid), the laboratory may need to use special techniques for obtaining cultures of large volumes of fluid.[12]

Demonstrating Biological Plausibility

Because many epidemics in hospitals are caused by hitherto unappreciated events, infection control personnel must prove conclusively that the event can happen. Thus, the investigators should design and conduct additional studies to confirm that the reservoir and the mode of transmission are biologically plausible. The epidemiology staff should use data gathered from procedure reviews, staff interviews or questionnaires, and observational studies to generate a possible scenario for how the organism was transmitted. Then, the staff should simulate the implicated procedure to establish that the organism could be transmitted in the postulated manner. Infection control personnel can simulate some procedures on-site, but may use in-vitro laboratory studies to simulate others. Settle plates may confirm that a staff member's activities in an area can disseminate the organism. In outbreaks of airborne diseases, such as tuberculosis or aspergillosis, infection control personnel may need chemical smoke tubes to evaluate the direction of air flow.[13]

In many instances, infection control personnel will want to confirm that the outbreak-associated isolates are identical to each other and to those recovered from the implicated source. Molecular typing techniques are available for evaluating a wide variety of nosocomial organisms, including typical bacterial pathogens, *Mycobacteria* species, fungi, and viruses.[14]

Acting on Results

Infection control personnel should focus their interventions on the immediate cause of an outbreak and should institute the simplest measures that will correct the problem. The more focused the control measures, the more likely healthcare workers will comply. Infection control personnel should emphasize the specific measures required to stop the outbreak and also should encourage staff to comply with routine infection control procedures. Sometimes, during an investigation, infection control personnel will identify numerous deficiencies other than those directly associated with transmission of the epidemic strain. The epidemiology staff may be tempted to use the epidemic as an opportunity to revamp the entire infection control program; however, this may be counterproductive.

Infection control personnel should develop a plan and timeline for implementing the control

measures. After implementing the control measures, the epidemiology staff should continue to work closely with the staff in the affected area to ensure that they understand the recommendations, that they efficiently implement the recommendations, and that they continue to comply with the recommendations over time.

Infection control personnel must determine whether the measures are effective. Often, infection control personnel can prove that the interventions were effective by demonstrating that no new cases occurred after the control measures were implemented. If the pathogen causes endemic infections (eg, methicillin-resistant *S aureus* or vancomycin-resistant enterococci), the epidemiology program may need to conduct prospective surveillance to ensure that the outbreak has been terminated.

Conclusion

Most nosocomial infections are endemic, and epidemics are relatively infrequent. However, in some settings, such as ICUs, outbreaks account for a substantial percentage of hospital-acquired infections. Outbreaks can cause substantial morbidity and mortality and can increase the cost of medical care significantly. Infection control personnel who identify outbreaks quickly and investigate them thoroughly and systematically can improve medical care and advance medical knowledge.

References

1. Wenzel RP, Thompson RL, Landry SM, et al. Hospital-acquired infections in intensive care unit patients: an overview with emphasis on epidemics. *Infect Control.* 1983;1:371-375.

2. Doebbeling BN. Epidemics: identification and management. In: Wenzel RP, ed. *Prevention and Control of Nosocomial Infections.* 2nd ed. Baltimore, Md: Williams & Wilkins; 1992:177-206.

3. Jarvis WR. Nosocomial outbreaks: the Centers for Disease Control's Hospital Infections Program Experience, 1980-1990. *Am J Med.* 1991;91(suppl 3B):101S-106S.

4. Beck-Sague CM, Jarvis WR. The epidemiology and pre-

vention of nosocomial infections. In: Block SS, ed. *Disinfection, Sterilization and Preservation*. 4th ed. Philadelphia, Pa: Lea & Febiger; 1991:663-675.

5. Haley RW, Gaynes RP, Aber RC, Bennett JV. Surveillance of nosocomial infections. In: Bennett JV, Brachman PS, eds. *Hospital Infections*. 3rd ed. Boston, Mass: Little, Brown and Co; 1992:79-108.

6. Dixon RE. Investigation of endemic and epidemic nosocomial infections. In: Bennett JV, Brachman PS, eds. *Hospital Infections*. 3rd ed. Boston, Mass: Little, Brown and Co; 1992:109-113.

7. Garner JS, Favero MS. Guideline for handwashing and hospital environmental control, 1985. In: *Guidelines for the Prevention and Control of Nosocomial Infections*. Atlanta, Ga: Centers for Disease Control; 1985:4-18.

8. Rotham KJ. Types of epidemiologic study. In: Rotham KJ, ed. *Modern Epidemiology*. Boston, Mass: Little, Brown and Co; 1986:51-76.

9. Dean AG, Dean JA, Burton AD, Dicker RC. *Epi Info, Version 5: A Word Processing, Database and Statistics Program for Epidemiology on Microcomputers*. Stone Mountain, Ga: USD, Inc; 1990.

10. Mastro TD, Farley TA, Elliott JA, et al. An outbreak of surgical wound infection due to group A streptococcus carried on the scalp. *N Engl J Med*. 1990;323:368-372.

11. Berkelman RL, Martin D, Graham DR, et al. Streptococcal wound infections caused by a vaginal carrier. *JAMA*. 1982;247:2680-2682.

12. Association for the Advancement of Medical Instrumentation: *American National Standard for Hemodialysis Systems*. Arlington, Va: AAMI; 1981.

13. Centers for Disease Control and Prevention. Guidelines for preventing the transmission of *Mycobacterium tuberculosis* in health-care facilities. *MMWR*. 1994;43:1-19.

14. Pittet D, Monod M, Filthuth I, Frenk E, Suter PM, Auckenthaler R. Contour-clamped homogeneous electric field gel electrophoresis as a powerful epidemiologic tool in yeast infections. *Am J Med*. 1991;91(suppl 3B):256S-263S.

CHAPTER 15

Exposure Workups

Loreen A. Herwaldt, MD, Jean M. Pottinger, RN, MA, CIC,
Cheryl D. Carter, RN, BSN, Brenda A. Barr, RN, MS, CIC,
Elyse D. Miller, MA

Abstract

Exposure workups are an important responsibility for infection control personnel. A well-designed plan for investigating exposures, which includes appropriate algorithms, will enable infection control personnel to evaluate exposures rapidly and consistently so that nosocomial transmission is minimized. Infection control personnel should use their own data to develop policies and procedures that suit the needs of their facility. After they have implemented the plan, infection control personnel should continue to collect data on exposures so they can continuously improve their performance.

Introduction

It is 5:25 on Friday afternoon. Everyone else in the infection control program has gone home already, but you stayed late to organize your desk. You have just finished filing the last paper when the telephone rings. Thinking that the caller is your husband, you pick up the telephone and greet the caller eagerly. But the voice is not your husband's.

It takes you a minute to realize that the caller is John Smith, the head nurse on the pediatric hematology and oncology inpatient unit. He is talking very rapidly about a child on his unit. When you get him to slow down, you learn that a 6-year-old patient, who has been in the hospital for 5 days, broke out with chicken pox this afternoon. This child has been in the playroom with numerous immunocompromised children. He also was in the waiting rooms of the pediatric clinic and the radiology department. To make matters worse, a nurse on the unit is 2-months' pregnant, and she is not sure whether she has had chicken pox.

You ask Mr. Smith to start making a list of all unit staff who worked during the time this patient has been hospitalized and to ask the healthcare workers whether or not they have had chicken pox. You tell him that you will come out to the unit in approximately 20 minutes, after you have had a chance to call radiology and several other departments whose staff might have been exposed. After hanging up the telephone, you sink back into your chair, groan, and berate yourself for not insisting that the hospital develop a computer database of the employees' immune status. You then pick up the telephone to call your husband and ask him to cancel your long-planned dinner reservations.

This fictional scenario actually comes close to the experience of many infection control staff who have practiced for any length of time. The scenario illustrates several axioms about exposures in the hospital. First, they always come at inconvenient times. There is no good time for an exposure even if it's not Friday. The corollary to this axiom is that exposure workups always interrupt other important infection control activities. The second axiom is that exposures usually involve more than one department and that at least one of the affected areas will be a large open room in which many persons congregate who may be very difficult to identify. The third axiom is that exposures almost always will involve the most vulnerable patients or healthcare workers. The corollary to this axiom is that exposures are guaranteed to cause great anxiety among patients and staff.

Infection control personnel define *exposures* as events in which persons were exposed to infectious microorganisms or ectoparasites. The goals of an exposure workup are to prevent disease, if possible, in the persons who were exposed to the agent, and to prevent further transmission if exposed persons become ill. To achieve this goal, infection control personnel must identify all patients, visitors, and staff who might have been exposed and then determine whether these persons are susceptible or immune. If the exposed persons are immune to the etiologic agent, they do not require further investigations or interventions. If exposed persons are not immune to the etiologic agent or do not know their immune status, infection control personnel may need to obtain further data, prescribe prophylactic treatment, and institute work restrictions. In this chapter, we will describe exposure workups for a number of important pathogens.

Many nosocomial exposures do not cause sec-

ondary cases of infection, or, if secondary cases occur, they are often mild. However, on occasion, patients, visitors, or healthcare workers acquire infections that cause serious short- or long-term consequences, including prolonged absence from work, exposure to toxic treatments, incurable chronic illness, irreversible disability, or death.[1] Regardless of the ultimate consequences, exposure workups consume considerable time, money, and other resources.[2-4] Therefore, infection control staff should strive to prevent exposures with the following measures:

- Implementing policies that reduce the number of susceptible persons exposed (eg, requiring all healthcare workers to be immune to measles, mumps, and rubella or requiring all clinics to screen patients for symptoms consistent with communicable diseases).
- Teaching healthcare workers to recognize when they should stay home to prevent the spread of infectious agents.
- Teaching healthcare workers to institute isolation precautions properly.

Given the serious consequences that can result from exposures, healthcare facilities must manage exposures in a systematic and consistent manner. Many healthcare facilities assign this responsibility to infection control personnel. In this chapter, we have described the steps in exposure investigations and provided decision algorithms that infection control personnel could use to manage exposures in their institutions. The decision algorithms can help infection control staff identify exposed persons who are susceptible to infection, implement control measures, provide susceptible persons with appropriate prophylactic treatment, and follow susceptible exposed persons for signs and symptoms of infection. The algorithms provide basic information that we think is relevant to most healthcare facilities. However, infection control personnel may need to adapt the algorithms to suit the unique characteristics of their healthcare facilities.

Personnel in the Program of Hospital Epidemiology at the University of Iowa Hospitals and Clinics have developed numerous algorithms over the years for use in our hospital. Staff from our program have previously published algorithms for chicken pox,[5] scabies,[5] lice,[5] *Mycobacterium tuberculosis*,[6] *Neisseria meningitidis*,[6] measles virus,[6] and mumps virus.[7] In this chapter, we have included substantially revised and updated versions of those algorithms, and we have added algorithms for rubella virus, parvovirus B19, hepatitis A virus, influenza virus, Creutzfeldt-Jakob agent, and *Bordetella pertussis.* When developing the new and revised algorithms, we used the format described by the Agency for Health Care Policy and Research[8] and the basic information and recommendations published in the *1994 Red Book.*[9] We used *Control of Communicable Diseases Manual*[10] and *Principles and Practice of Infectious Diseases*[11] as additional references. Infection control personnel who prefer the recommendations published in other references will need to modify the algorithms appropriately. We have excluded bloodborne pathogens from this discussion.

General Recommendations Regarding Exposure Workups

Obtain Mandate From the Administration

If the hospital administration assigns the responsibility for doing exposure workups to the infection control program, the administrators also must define the scope of that responsibility and delegate the authority for the associated activities to staff in the infection control program. The hospital administration must define prospectively what tests and prophylactic treatments the hospital will provide. In addition, the hospital administration must specify if exposed healthcare workers will be granted administrative leave, leave with pay, or leave without pay or if they will be allowed to work in nonpatient-care areas during the period in which they might be infectious.[12,13]

Develop Policies and Procedures

Once the infection control program has been given the authority to do exposure workups, the staff must develop specific policies that define exposures to various bacterial and viral pathogens and to ectoparasites and describe the investigative and preventive measures that should be undertaken for exposures caused by each agent. The staff also should develop general policies and procedures that define what tasks should be undertaken and who will do them.

Collaborate With Employee Health

In many institutions, the infection control staff initiate the exposure workup and recommend the prophylaxis and work restrictions for exposed healthcare workers. However, staff in the employee health service actually evaluate whether the employee was exposed and susceptible, examine the healthcare worker, enforce work restrictions, and give permission for healthcare workers to return to work. Thus, as they develop policies and procedures, infection control personnel must collaborate extensively with staff in employee health.

Develop a Database on the Immune Status of Healthcare Workers

Infection control personnel will save countless hours if they have a database in which they store information on the immune status of all healthcare workers. The most important data are the employee's immune status to chicken pox, measles, mumps, rubella, and hepatitis B. The employee's tuberculosis skin-test results also should be recorded in the database. The database also could store information on the employee's immunity to diphtheria, tetanus, and hepatitis A. Baseline data should be obtained from all new healthcare workers before they start working in the institution. If the hospital is establishing a new database, the same data should be obtained from all current employees.

In small hospitals, the database could be a paper line-list or a card file. The infection control staff or the staff in various departments or units could maintain the file or list. In large hospitals, the database should be computerized. The persons who develop and maintain the database could be in the hospital's information management group, in the infection control program, or in the employee health service. Regardless of who manages the database, the persons investigating exposures must have unobstructed access to the database so that they can use the data regardless of when the exposure occurs. One of the authors previously worked in a hospital in which the database was stored on a secretary's computer. If the secretary was not there, other staff did not have access to the data.

Develop a Data Collection Form

Infection control staff must investigate exposures in a consistent fashion. Therefore, in addition to developing the appropriate policies and procedures, infection control staff should design a form (either paper or electronic) with which they can collect the necessary data for each exposure. For most exposures, we currently use the hospital's mainframe computer to generate a list of healthcare workers who were in the affected areas and, as appropriate, either the immune status of these employees or the date of their last tuberculin skin test. For small exposures and exposures that involve visitors, we currently use a paper form that has four carbonless copies. Once the forms are completed, we distribute copies to the departments that must be informed of the exposure. Hospitals that have an institution wide information system could implement a computerized form that staff on each affected unit could access, complete, and send electronically to the infection control program.

Educate Staff

As noted in the introduction, infection control staff can prevent exposures by educating healthcare workers appropriately. For example, healthcare workers should know the modes of transmission for common communicable pathogens and basic infection control precautions that limit the spread of microorganisms. In addition, exposure workups will go more smoothly if infection control personnel prospectively educate healthcare workers about exposure workups in general and about the specific steps taken during common exposure workups. Infection control staff also will need to educate and calm the staff while doing many exposure workups, because staff who think they have been exposed to *N meningitidis* or to lice frequently panic and act irrationally.

Collect and Evaluate Data on Exposures

Infection control personnel should collect data on the exposure workups that they conduct. They can tabulate the data on paper, or they can develop a computer database in which to store the information. At least once per year infection control staff should assess the following:

- The number of exposures.
- The etiologic agents.
- The affected locations.
- The number of susceptible healthcare workers, patients, and visitors exposed.
- The number of secondary cases.
- The number of healthcare workers who were placed on leave.
- The number of leave days.
- The breaks in infection control technique that led to the exposures.
- The prophylactic treatments given.
- The cost in time and dollars.

Infection control personnel should report these data to the infection control committee and should use these data to do the following:

- Document their effort to the administration.

- Identify topics for in-service educational programs.
- Identify appropriate interventions (eg, require all healthcare workers to be immune to measles, mumps, and rubella).
- Identify areas for collaboration with other departments (eg, work with staff in other departments to develop methods for screening, triage, and isolation).
- Identify areas for improvement.
- Document quality improvement efforts required for accreditation.

Disease-Specific Exposure Workups

Viral Diseases

Varicella-zoster Virus

Varicella-zoster virus (VZV) causes a primary infection, chicken pox, and a recrudescent infection, herpes zoster, or shingles. VZV can be transmitted through the air by persons with chicken pox or through direct contact with fresh chicken pox or herpes zoster lesions. Thus, patients with chicken pox or disseminated zoster should be placed on airborne and contact precautions until all lesions are crusted to prevent exposures within hospitals.[14] Nonimmune patients who have been exposed to chicken pox should be placed on airborne precautions between days 8 and 21 after their exposure (day 28 if the person is immunocompromised or received varicella-zoster immune globulin [VZIG]). Because VZV rarely is spread through the air from persons with localized herpes zoster, patients, visitors, and healthcare workers with this entity do not need to be restricted if their lesions can be covered.

VZV is one of the most common communicable agents causing exposures at the University of Iowa Hospitals and Clinics. However, we have been fortunate, because very few of the exposures have caused secondary cases. Five or fewer health-care workers acquire chicken pox each year, and most of them acquire their infections in the community. Some healthcare facilities have not been as fortunate and have experienced large nosocomial outbreaks affecting numerous healthcare workers.

Currently, 2% to 5% of all healthcare workers are not immune to VZV,[15,16] and 28% of those with no known history of chicken pox are susceptible to this virus.[15] Approximately 4% to 15% of susceptible healthcare workers will develop chicken pox each year.[15] Nonimmune healthcare workers who have been exposed to a person with chicken pox could be incubating the infection. To prevent the spread of VZV, infection control personnel must identify those healthcare workers and restrict their work during the incubation period. Santa Clara Valley Medical Center allows exposed healthcare workers to continue direct patient-care activities if they wear masks.[17] However, this approach is not standard. Most healthcare facilities do not allow susceptible, exposed healthcare workers to continue their patient-care duties during the incubation period. Some healthcare facilities place such staff on leave,[12,13] and other facilities reassign exposed susceptible staff to nonpatient-care areas if all the employees in that area are immune.[18] Exposed staff who are permitted to work must take care not to expose persons as they enter and exit the building. At the University of Iowa Hospitals and Clinics, we have used the latter approach since 1977 without difficulty. We require those healthcare workers to use the most direct route to the area in which they will work (ie, excluding the main entrances), and we do not allow them to be in areas in which many people congregate (eg, waiting areas, lobbies, lounges, gift shop, cafeteria, etc). Staff who develop active disease must not work until all lesions are crusted.

Infection control personnel should work with employee health staff, expert clinicians, pharmacists, and hospital administrators to determine whether exposed persons will be offered the chicken pox vaccine (Varivax, Merck & Co, West Point,

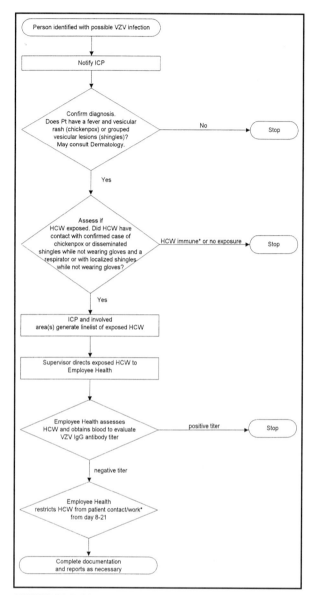

FIGURE 15-1. Managing chicken pox or shingles exposures. The diagnostic criteria listed are meant to be helpful guides and are not all-inclusive. Abbreviations: HCW = healthcare worker; ICP = infection control professional; IgG = immunoglobulin G; Pt = patient; VZV = varicella-zoster virus. *See Table 15-1 for further information.

PA) or VZIG. If the healthcare facility provides one or both of these agents, this group should decide prospectively which persons will be offered either agent. In addition, this group should decide whether their healthcare facility will offer the chicken pox vaccine to all nonimmune healthcare workers. This decision may not be a simple one for the following reasons:

- Five percent of healthcare workers who receive the vaccine will develop a varicella-like rash that will require them to miss work, because transmission of the vaccine virus has been documented.

- For approximately 6 weeks after receiving the vaccination, healthcare workers should not care for susceptible, high-risk persons, including immunocompromised persons, pregnant women who do not have a history of chicken pox or detectable antibody to VZV, and newborns of such women.

- According to the Varivax package insert, up to 27% of vaccinated persons will have subclinical or breakthrough varicella infection after close exposure to a person with chicken pox.

Figure 15-1 and Table 15-1 outline the approach to managing healthcare workers who have been exposed to chicken pox.[5,9,19] Infection control personnel who want additional information about chicken pox exposures should consult the appropriate references.[10,11,15,16,18]

Measles Virus

Measles is a febrile illness that is characterized by Koplik's spots on the buccal mucosa and by an erythematous rash. The measles rash starts on the face and spreads to the trunk and extremities and also progresses from maculopapular to confluent. Measles virus, which is highly communicable, is spread by airborne transmission. Despite sensitivity to acid, strong light, and drying, the measles virus can remain viable in airborne droplets for hours, especially if the relative humidity is low. Consequently, outbreaks have occurred in healthcare facilities when the index patient was no longer present.[20,21] To prevent the spread of measles virus within healthcare facilities, patients with measles should be placed on airborne precautions.[14]

Before the measles vaccine was licensed in 1963, 500,000 cases of measles occurred in the United States each year.[9,15] Subsequently, the number of measles cases in the United States declined dramatically, reaching a nadir in 1983. Thereafter, the incidence of measles increased for several years.[9] More recently, increased immunization rates and routine use of two doses of the vaccine have helped decrease the number of measles cases. Measles now occurs most frequently in preschool children, many of whom are too young to be vaccinated.

However, despite the declining incidence of measles, outbreaks and nosocomial transmission continue to occur.[20-36] For example, of the 22,384 cases of measles reported to the Centers for Disease Control and Prevention (CDC) between 1980 and 1984, 241 cases (1.1%) probably were acquired in medical settings.[22] Of those cases, 104 (46.6%) were acquired in hospitals, 79 (35.4%) were acquired in physicians' offices, and 33 (14.8%) were acquired in nonhospital outpatient clinics.[22] Data published by Istre et al are more impressive.[23] They evaluated 33 cases of measles reported to the Oklahoma State Department of Health between September 1981 and August 1985.[23] Nine persons (27%) acquired measles in a medical office or clinic waiting room, and six (18%) acquired measles from persons who were exposed in a medical setting. Thus, 45% of persons with measles acquired the infection directly or indirectly from exposures in a medical setting.[23]

At present, 5% to 10% of healthcare workers are susceptible to measles,[15] including 4.7% of those born before 1957, 16% of those born in the 1960s, and 34% of those born in the 1970s.[35] In fact, healthcare workers are the source of 5% to 10% of all measles cases and account for 28% of measles cases acquired in medical settings in the United States.[15] A recent case in South Dakota demonstrates that healthcare workers still acquire measles while caring for patients. A 37-year-old nurse acquired measles from a patient who may have been exposed to the virus while in an airplane (*Huron Daily Plainsman.* May 1, 1997).

Measles exposures are relatively uncommon in many hospitals. At the University of Iowa Hospitals and Clinics, we have not had a patient with the diagnosis of measles admitted in the last 2 years. However, a representative from a specialty bed company became ill with measles 1 day after delivering beds to five patient-care areas. Fifteen healthcare workers were possibly exposed, but 13 of these employees were born before 1957, and 2 were vaccinated 3 to 4 years before the exposure. Three patients were possibly exposed, but 2 were born before 1957, and the third had detectable antibody.

Although measles exposures are infrequent, infection control personnel still must develop policies that will limit the spread of measles if it is introduced into the hospital. A study conducted by Enguidanos et al suggests that infection control programs may be ignoring measles because the incidence is low.[36] These investigators noted that 74 adults employed in acute-care hospitals acquired measles during a community-wide outbreak in 1987 through 1989. The investigators surveyed all 102 infection control professionals in the acute-care hospitals in Los Angeles County to determine whether infection control policies were adequate. Only 17% of the hospitals required healthcare workers to document immunity to measles, and only 4% had policies that covered students or volunteers. The investigators also surveyed the healthcare workers who became ill. Of these 74 persons, 46% worked in hospitals that did not have measles infection control policies, 43% were born before 1957, and 31% were working in jobs that have not been considered to increase the risk of measles exposure.[36]

As discussed previously, infection control personnel should work with employee health to develop a database that has each healthcare worker's history of measles vaccination. If such a database is not available and a person with measles comes to the hospital, the infection control staff must identi-

TABLE 15-1
Basic Information Regarding Agents that Cause Most Nosocomial Exposures[9]

Etiologic Agent	Incubation Period	Exposure Criteria	Period of Communicability	Employee Health	Work Restrictions	Prophylaxis
Varicella-zoster virus	Usually 14-16 d Range 10-21 d Up to 28 d in persons who received VZIG	**Chicken pox or disseminated zoster** Continuous household contact ≥5 min face-to-face contact with infected person without wearing a respirator Direct contact with vesicle fluid without wearing gloves **Shingles** Direct contact with vesicle fluid without wearing gloves	**Chicken pox** Most contagious 1-2 d before and shortly after rash appears Transmission can occur up to 5 d after onset of rash Immunocompromised persons may be contagious as long as new lesions are appearing **Shingles** 24 h before the first lesion appears and up to 48 h after final lesion appears	Assess immunity HCW susceptible unless he or she has history of chicken pox, or has serologic evidence of immunity Consider obtaining varicella IgG antibody titer to determine immune-status before HCW is exposed	**Exposed** Days 1-7, no restrictions Days 8-21 for a single exposure, or day 8 of first exposure through day 21 of last exposure, HCW either must not work or have no direct patient contact and work only with immune persons away from patient-care areas Restrict HCW who received VZIG through day 28 **Infected** May return to work after all lesions are crusted	Consider giving VZIG to nonimmune, immuno-compromised persons within 96 h of exposure

| Measles virus | Usually 8-12 d Range 7-18 d | Spent time in a room with an infected person without wearing a respirator If air is recirculated, spent time in the area supplied by the air-handling system while infected person was present or within 1 h after the person's departure Contact with nasal or oral secretions from an infected person or items contaminated with these secretions without wearing gloves | 3-5 d before rash to 4-7 d after rash appears, but transmission is minimal by 2-4 d after rash appears | Assess immunity HCW susceptible unless he or she was born before 1957,* or provides serologic evidence of immunity, or has two documented doses of measles vaccine Obtain blood for IgG antibody titers as needed; for staff who have not received two doses of measles vaccine, consider initiating or completing the vaccine series | **Exposed** Days 1-4, no restrictions Days 5-21 for a single exposure, or day 5 of first exposure through day 21 of last exposure, HCW either must not work or have no direct patient contact and work only with immune persons away from patient-care areas **Infected** May return to work 4 d after developing rash | Consider giving susceptible HCW vaccine within 3 d or IG within 6 d of exposure to modify infection Vaccine or IG given after exposure does not change work restrictions |

TABLE 15-1 (continued)
BASIC INFORMATION REGARDING AGENTS THAT CAUSE MOST NOSOCOMIAL EXPOSURES[9]

Etiologic Agent	Incubation Period	Exposure Criteria	Period of Communicability	Employee Health	Work Restrictions	Prophylaxis
Rubella virus	Usually 16-18 d Range, 14-21 d	Contact within 3 ft of infected person without wearing a mask Contact with naso-pharyngeal secretions from an infected person or items contaminated with these secretions without wearing gloves Contact with naso-pharyngeal secretions or urine from infant with congenital rubella without wearing gloves	7 d before rash to 7 d after rash appears Up to 1 y for infants with congenital rubella	Assess immunity HCW susceptible unless he or she was born before 1957, or provides serologic evidence of immunity, or has one documented dose of rubella vaccine Obtain blood for IgG antibody titers as needed; for staff who have not received two doses of rubella vaccine, consider initiating or completing the vaccine series	**Exposed** Days 1-6, no restrictions Days 7-21 for a single exposure, or day 7 of first exposure through day 21 of last exposure, HCW either must not work or have no direct patient contact and work only with immune persons away from patient-care areas **Infected** May return to work 7 d after developing rash	None Rubella vaccine does not prevent infection after exposure IG does not prevent infection

| Mumps virus | Usually 14-16 d Range 12-25 d | Contact within 3 ft of infected person without wearing a mask

Contact with saliva or items contaminated with saliva from an infected person without wearing gloves | Most communicable 48 h before onset of illness, but may begin as early as 7 d before onset of overt parotitis and continue 5-9 d (average 5) thereafter | Assess immunity

HCW susceptible unless he or she was born before 1957, or provides serologic evidence of immunity, or has one documented dose of mumps vaccine

Obtain blood for IgG antibody titers as needed; for staff who have not received two doses of mumps vaccine, consider initiating or completing the vaccine series | **Exposed**

Days 1-10, no restrictions

Days 11-26 for a single exposure, or day 11 of first exposure through day 26 of last exposure, HCW either must not work or have no direct patient contact and work only with immune persons away from patient-care areas

Infected

May return to work 9 d after onset of parotid gland swelling | None

Mumps vaccine not proven to prevent infection after exposure

Mumps IG does not prevent infection |

TABLE 15-1 (continued)
BASIC INFORMATION REGARDING AGENTS THAT CAUSE MOST NOSOCOMIAL EXPOSURES[9]

Etiologic Agent	Incubation Period	Exposure Criteria	Period of Communicability	Employee Health	Work Restrictions	Prophylaxis
Parvovirus B19	Usually 4-14 d Range up to 20 d Rash and joint symptoms occur 2-3 wk after acquisition	Criteria have not been defined but probably include close person-to-person contact (within 3 ft) with infected person without wearing a mask; contact with respiratory secretions from an infected person or items contaminated with these secretions without wearing gloves	Transmission decreases significantly after rash appears Immunocompromised persons can have chronic infections and can shed virus for prolonged periods	Assess immunity Obtain blood for IgG antibody titers as needed Describe signs and symptoms and inform exposed HCWs that they should not work if these symptoms occur; refer a pregnant HCW to her obstetrician	Have not been defined; we recommend that, during the incubation period, an exposed HCW should not work with patients at high risk of complications	None
Hepatitis A virus	Usually 25-30 d Range 15-50 d	Contact with stool of infected person without wearing gloves Consuming uncooked food prepared by an infected person	Viral shedding in stool lasts 1-3 wk Highest viral titers are found in stool 1-2 wk before onset of symptoms Risk of transmission is minimal 1 wk after onset of symptoms	Assess immunity Obtain blood for IgG antibody titers as needed Describe signs and symptoms, and ask exposed HCW to return to the employee health department if these occur	**Exposed** None **Infected** May return to work 7 d after onset of jaundice or other clinical symptoms	Consider giving exposed HCW IG within 2 wk of exposure

Agent	Incubation period	Period of infectiousness / type of exposure	Management of HCW	Work restrictions	Prophylaxis
Influenza virus	Usually 1–3 d	Most infectious 24 h before onset of symptoms. Viral shedding usually ceases within 7 d but can persist longer in children. Contact within 3 ft of infected person without wearing a mask. Direct contact with secretions from respiratory tract of infected person or items contaminated with these secretions without wearing gloves	Assess immunization status. Discuss risks and benefits of chemoprophylaxis. Describe signs and symptoms, and inform HCWs that they should not work if these symptoms occur	**Exposed** Have not been defined for nonimmune HCW exposed to persons with influenza. **Infected** Ill HCW should not work	Consider vaccinating exposed nonimmune HCW. Amantadine or rimantadine 100 mg to 200 mg per day for adults exposed to influenza A only
Creutzfeldt-Jakob Agent[†]	15 mo to >30 y	Unknown, but probably during symptomatic illness and an undetermined period before symptoms appear. Criteria have not been defined but probably include the following if patient diagnosed with CJD or has risk factors for CJD[‡]: puncture or cut with instruments contaminated with patient's blood or cerebrospinal fluid; handling cerebrospinal fluid or tissue from brain, spinal cord, or eye without gloves; HCWs working in the operating room, autopsy suite, ophthalmology department, pathology laboratory, or microbiology laboratory have the highest risk of exposure	Educate employee about CJD and risk of transmission. Counsel employee using data from the literature indicating that the risk of transmission is very low	None	None

TABLE 15-1 (continued)
BASIC INFORMATION REGARDING AGENTS THAT CAUSE MOST NOSOCOMIAL EXPOSURES[9]

Etiologic Agent	Incubation Period	Exposure Criteria	Period of Communicability	Employee Health	Work Restrictions	Prophylaxis
		Routine patient care poses a very low risk to HCW				
Mycobacterium tuberculosis	2-10 wk from exposure to detection of positive TST. Risk of developing active disease is greatest in first 2 y after infection	Spent time in a room with a person who has active disease without wearing a respirator. Packing or irrigating wounds infected with *M tuberculosis* without wearing a respirator	Persons are infectious until they have taken 2-3 wk of effective antituberculosis chemotherapy. Persons whose smears are AFB-positive are 20 times more likely to cause secondary infection than persons who are smear-negative. Children with primary pulmonary TB are rarely contagious	Obtain baseline TST if not done recently and if HCW previously negative. Perform postexposure TST at 12 wk. Prescribe prophylaxis if postexposure TST is positive	**Exposed** None for persons whose TST becomes positive. **Infected** Restrict HCWs with active TB until after they have taken 2-3 wk of effective antituberculosis chemotherapy	Isoniazid 300 mg daily for 6 mo, or 12 mo for HIV-infected persons and pyridoxine 25-50 mg daily
Neisseria meningitidis	Usually ≤4 days. Range, 1-10 days	Extensive contact with respiratory secretions from an infected person without wearing a mask, particularly during suctioning, resuscitation, intubation	Persons are infectious until they have taken 24 h of effective antibiotic therapy	Prescribe prophylaxis. Educate exposed HCW about signs and symptoms of meningitis	**Exposed** None	Rifampin 600 mg every 12 h for 2 d (contraindicated in pregnancy). Ciprofloxacin 500 mg, single dose (contraindicated in pregnancy). Ceftriaxone 250 mg IM, single dose (safe during pregnancy)

Organism	Incubation period	Period of communicability / mode of transmission	Management	Work restrictions	Recommended therapy/prophylaxis
Bordetella pertussis	Usually 7-10 d Range, 6-20 d	Most contagious during the catarrhal stage Communicability diminishes rapidly after onset of cough, but can persist as long as 3 wk. Unprotected (ie, no mask), face-to-face contact for 10 min or spending 1 hr in a room with a confirmed case [4] Direct contact with respiratory tract secretions from infected persons or items contaminated with these secretions without wearing gloves	If HCW has no symptoms, begin prophylaxis and return to work If HCW symptomatic, begin therapy and relieve from work until test results are available	**Exposed** No restrictions **Infected** HCW may return to work after taking at least 5 d of therapy	Recommended drug is erythromycin 40 mg/kg/d in 4 divided doses (maximum 2 gm/d) for 14 d (estolate preparation preferred) Azithromycin or clarithromycin may be tolerated better than erythromycin. If person is allergic to macrolide, consider trimethopriam-sulfamethoxazole DS, 1 tablet twice daily for 14d, or azithromycin 500 mg once daily for 5d.
Lice	6-10 d	As long as lice or eggs remain alive on infested person, clothing, or personal items Survival time for lice away from the host: 10 d for head lice, 10 d for body lice, 2 d for pubic lice Nits ≥10 mm from scalp have been present ≥2 wk and may not be viable. Head lice: hair-to-hair contact with infested person Body lice: contact with linen or clothes of infested person without wearing gloves Pubic lice: sexual contact	Treat HCW only if infested	**Exposed** No restrictions **Infested** Immediate restriction until 24 h after treatment	Not recommended

TABLE 15-1 (continued)
BASIC INFORMATION REGARDING AGENTS THAT CAUSE MOST NOSOCOMIAL EXPOSURES[9]

Etiologic Agent	Incubation Period	Exposure Criteria	Period of Communicability	Employee Health	Work Restrictions	Prophylaxis
Scabies	4-5 wk if no previous infestation; 1-4 d if previous infestation	Direct skin-to-skin contact; Minimal direct contact with crusted scabies can result in transmission	Transmission can occur before the onset of symptoms; Person remains contagious until treated	Prescribe scabicide for all exposed HCW; Pregnant women should not use lindane	**Exposed** No restriction after scabicide used; **Infested** Immediate restriction until 24 h after treatment	Drug of choice: 5% permethrin; Alternative drugs, lindane, crotamiton

AFB = acid-fast bacilli; CJD = Creutzfeldt-Jakob disease; HCW = healthcare worker; HIV = human immunodeficiency virus; IgG = immunoglobulin G; IG = immune globulin; IM = intramuscular; TB = tuberculosis; TST = tuberculin skin test; VZIG = varicella-zoster immune globulin.

*A small percentage of HCWs born before 1957 will not be immune to measles.[35] Infection control personnel should determine whether this criterion is appropriate for the staff in their hospital.

†These precautions should be used for persons who have CJD, progressive dementia, or have a family history of prion disease, CJD, Gerstmann-Sträussler-Scheinker syndrome, or fatal familial insomnia. The precautions should also be used for patients who have received gonadotropin or human growth hormone extracted from cadaveric pituitary glands.

‡ Data from a study with mice suggest that prions might be transmitted by contact of infected blood or cerebrospinal fluid with mucous membranes.[121] No data are available with humans to support or refute the data from mice.

fy exposed personnel and then determine whether these persons are immune. Nonimmune patients who have been exposed to measles should be placed on airborne precautions between day 5 and day 21 after their exposure.[14] Nonimmune family members and friends who have been exposed to a person with measles should not come to the hospital during the incubation period. Figure 15-2 and Table 15-1 illustrate a systematic approach to a measles exposure.[6,9]

Rubella Virus

Rubella (German measles) is an acute exanthematous viral infection that affects children and adults. Postnatal rubella, which resembles a mild case of measles, is characterized by rash, fever, and lymphadenopathy. In contrast, rubella acquired in pregnancy can cause fetal death, premature labor, and severe congenital defects. Consequently, it is very important to prevent the spread of rubella in healthcare facilities. However, the mild clinical symptoms associated with rubella have, at times, facilitated nosocomial spread of rubella virus because healthcare workers have continued to work while they were ill. The literature documents numerous outbreaks of rubella in medical settings, some of which affected many susceptible pregnant women.[37-45] Furthermore, these institutions had to invest large amounts of time and money to control the outbreaks.[41,43,45]

Rubella virus is spread in droplets that are shed from the respiratory secretions of infected persons. Persons with rubella are most contagious when the rash is erupting. In addition, persons with subclinical illness also may transmit the virus. To prevent nosocomial spread, patients with rubella should be placed on droplet precautions until 7 days after the onset of the rash. Infants with congenital rubella shed large quantities of virus for many months, despite having high titers of neutralizing antibody. Such patients should be isolated each time they are admitted during the first year of life unless

nasopharyngeal and urine cultures after 3 months of age are negative.

Nonimmune patients who have been exposed to rubella should be placed on droplet precautions between days 7 and 21 after their exposure.[14] Nonimmune family members and friends who have been exposed to a person with rubella should not come to the hospital during the incubation period.

Despite vaccination campaigns, 10% to 20% of hospital personnel are susceptible to rubella.[15] Given the adverse effects of rubella virus on the fetus, many healthcare facilities require employees, especially those working in obstetrics, to be immune to rubella.[24,37]

Figure 15-3 and Table 15-1 illustrate how infection control personnel could evaluate an exposure to a person with rubella.[8,9] Infection control personnel will be able to investigate such exposures more readily if the healthcare facility maintains a computer database that includes information about the employees' immune status.

Mumps Virus

Mumps is characterized by fever and parotitis. In postpubertal men, mumps virus also can cause orchitis, which can be the primary manifestation of the infection. The mumps virus is transmitted through direct contact with contaminated respiratory secretions, inhalation of droplet nuclei, or through contact with fomites contaminated by respiratory secretions. Transmission of mumps virus requires more intimate contact with the infected person than does transmission of either measles virus or VZV. To prevent exposures in healthcare facilities, persons with mumps should be placed on droplet precautions until 9 days after parotid (or other glandular) swelling began.[14]

The incidence of mumps decreased substantially in the United States after the vaccine was licensed in 1967.[9,11,24] Consequently, exposures to persons with mumps and nosocomial transmission of mumps are rare.[46,47] In fact, we have not had a mumps exposure at the University of Iowa Hospitals and Clinics for over 5 years.

As discussed previously, a computerized database that includes the healthcare workers' immune status for mumps will help infection control personnel if an exposure to mumps occurs in their hospital. If a database is not available, infection control personnel will need to determine whether healthcare workers have had either mumps or the mumps vaccine. Most adults are immune to mumps, and approximately 90% of adults who have no history of mumps have antibody to the virus.[9] Thus, only a small proportion of healthcare workers will be susceptible to mumps. For example, Nichol and Olson found that 6.7% of the medical students they studied were nonimmune.[48] Consequently, it might be cost-beneficial to assess antibody titers of exposed persons who have no history of mumps and who have not received the mumps vaccine. Only those who are seronegative would be excluded from patient care during the incubation period (days 11 through 26). Figure 15-4 and Table 15-1 illustrate an approach to a mumps exposure.

Nonimmune patients who have been exposed to mumps should be placed on droplet precautions between days 11 and 26 after their exposure.[14] Nonimmune family members and friends who have been exposed to a person with mumps should not come to the hospital during the incubation period.

Parvovirus B19

Erythema infectiosum, or fifth disease, is a common manifestation of acute parvovirus B19 infection. Fifth disease acquired its name because common childhood exanthems were numbered in the late 19th century. The first three illnesses were scarlet fever, rubeola, and rubella, and the fourth was a variation of scarlet fever known as Filatov-Dukes Disease. Erythema infectiosum was the fifth disease, and roseola infantum was the sixth. Erythema infectiosum is characterized by mild systemic symptoms (fever in 15% to 30%), followed

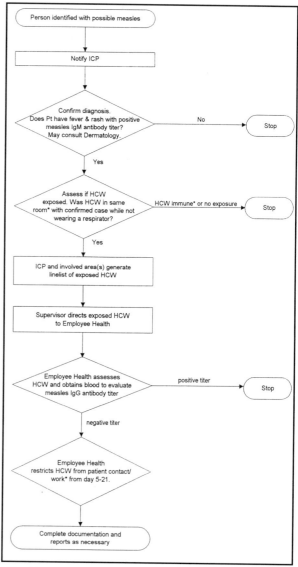

FIGURE 15-2. Managing measles exposures. The diagnostic criteria listed are meant to be helpful guides and are not all-inclusive. Abbreviations: HCW = healthcare worker; ICP = infection control professional; IgG = immunoglobulin G; IgM = immunoglobulin M; Pt = patient.
*See Table 15-1 for further information.

in 1 to 4 days by an erythematous rash on the cheeks, the "slapped cheek" appearance. Subsequently, an asymmetric macular or maculopapular, lace-like erythematous rash can involve the trunk and extremities.

Parvovirus B19 has a predilection for infecting rapidly dividing cells, especially rapidly dividing

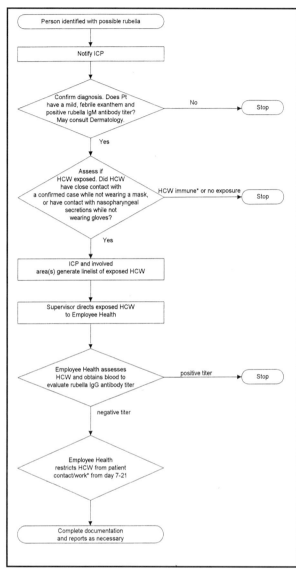

FIGURE 15-3. Managing rubella exposures. The diagnostic criteria listed are meant to be helpful guides and are not all-inclusive. Abbreviations: HCW = healthcare worker; ICP = infection control professional; IgG = immunoglobulin G; IgM = immunoglobulin M; Pt = patient.
*See Table 15-1 for further information.

red blood cells. Thus, persons with sickle cell disease, hereditary spherocytosis, pyruvate kinase deficiency, and other hemolytic anemias can develop transient hemolytic crises. Parvovirus B19 can cause severe chronic anemia associated with red cell aplasia in persons who are on maintenance chemotherapy for acute lymphocytic leukemia,

who have congenital immunodeficiencies, or who have acquired immunodeficiency syndrome. Parvovirus B19 also can cause hydrops fetalis. However, most parvovirus B19 infections during pregnancy do not affect the fetus adversely. Several studies indicate that the risk of fetal death is less than 10% in infected fetuses.[9]

Transmission of parvovirus B19 is common in the community.[49] Outbreaks have occurred in day-care centers and in elementary and junior high schools. Secondary spread to susceptible household contacts also is frequent. Documented transmission within hospitals has been uncommon.[50-53] However, when transmission occurs, a high proportion (13% to 47%) of susceptible persons may be infected.[51,52,54]

Parvovirus B19 DNA has been found in the respiratory secretions of viremic patients, but most persons are no longer viremic when the rash appears. Persons with transient hemolytic crises and babies with hydrops fetalis can remain viremic for prolonged periods. These patients can be the source of infection for susceptible patients or healthcare workers and thus should be placed on droplet precautions while they are hospitalized to prevent spread of parvovirus B19.[14] In general, routine infection control precautions should minimize nosocomial transmission of this virus.[55] A study by Cartter et al of risk factors for parvovirus B19 infection in pregnant women demonstrated that the rate of infection was highest among nurses who cared for patients before they were isolated.[56] These results suggest that isolation precautions can prevent nosocomial spread of this virus from infected patients. Figure 15-5 and Table 15-1 illustrate how infection control personnel could evaluate an exposure to parvovirus B19.[8,9]

Persons with fifth disease usually are not infectious shortly after they develop the rash. Thus, healthcare workers with parvovirus B19 infection usually do not need to be removed from patient care. Some hospitals might choose to restrict healthcare workers from caring for patients at high risk of complications until the healthcare worker's symptoms have resolved.

Hepatitis A Virus

Hepatitis A is transmitted primarily by the fecal-oral route, but, in hospitals, hepatitis A virus also can be transmitted by blood transfusions. Infected persons excrete the highest concentration of virus in their stools during the 2 weeks before their symptoms begin. Most persons are no longer shedding the virus 1 week after they become jaundiced. However, infants can shed the virus in their stools for months.

Nosocomial transmission of hepatitis A is relatively uncommon. Most nosocomial outbreaks have occurred after an infant or a young child has received blood from a viremic but asymptomatic donor. The child often has an asymptomatic infection,[57-62] and unsuspecting healthcare workers become infected when they handle the patient's stool without using proper precautions. In one such incident, a neonate transmitted hepatitis A virus to 10 of 61 susceptible nurses.[57] In another outbreak, a child with an immunodeficiency and negative antibody titers transmitted hepatitis A virus to 15 of 102 staff.[63] Occasionally, nosocomial outbreaks have occurred when healthcare workers cared for an older child or an adult who had vomiting, diarrhea, or fecal incontinence.[64-69]

Healthcare workers who are exposed to the stool of infected patients are at greatest risk for acquiring hepatitis A infection. Occasionally, patients, visitors, and healthcare workers could be at risk of acquiring hepatitis A if they eat uncooked food prepared by a food handler who is shedding the virus. Several food-related nosocomial epidemics have been reported.[70,71]

The University of Iowa Hospitals and Clinics experienced an outbreak of hepatitis A in which 11 healthcare workers and 1 patient became ill after a man, who subsequently became jaundiced, and his

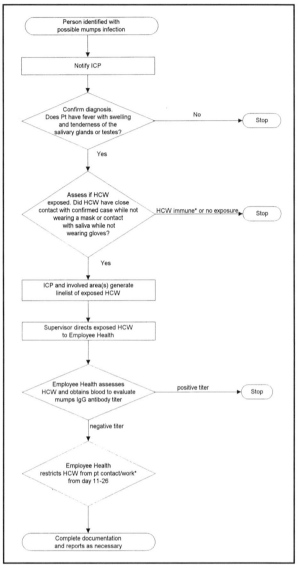

FIGURE 15-4. Managing mumps exposures. The diagnostic criteria listed are meant to be helpful guides and are not all-inclusive. Abbreviations: HCW = healthcare worker; ICP = infection control professional; IgG = immunoglobulin G; Pt = patient.
*See Table 15-1 for further information.

asymptomatic 8-month-old son, whose hepatitis A IgM was positive, were admitted to the burn unit.[72] Risk factors for illness included caring for either the infant or the father during the week before the father became ill and eating on the hospital ward.[72]

To prevent nosocomial transmission of hepatitis A virus, healthcare workers should wear gowns

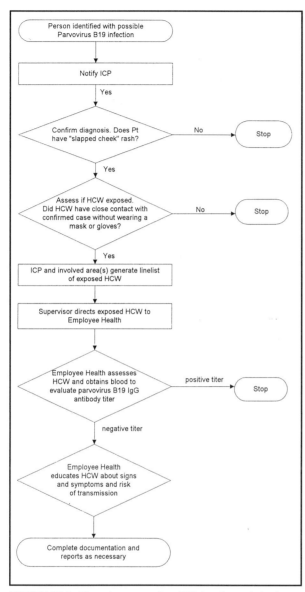

FIGURE 15-5. Managing parvovirus B19 (erythema infectiosum, fifth disease) exposures. The diagnostic criteria listed are meant to be helpful guides and are not all-inclusive. Abbreviations: HCW = healthcare worker; ICP = infection control professional; IgG = immunoglobulin G; Pt = patient.

and gloves whenever they might contaminate their hands or clothes with a patient's stool. Healthcare workers must wash their hands after performing any patient-care activities or after removing their gloves. Adult patients with hepatitis A who are continent do not require private rooms, but diapered or incontinent persons should be placed in

private rooms.[14] Healthcare workers who cared for patients with hepatitis A do not need to be restricted from work unless they develop hepatitis, because the risk of acquiring hepatitis from a patient is low, and the risk of transmission from infected healthcare workers to patients also is low. Healthcare workers with hepatitis A infection should not work during the first 7 days of their symptomatic illnesses. Figure 15-6 and Table 15-1 illustrate how infection control personnel could evaluate an exposure to hepatitis A.[8,9]

The CDC does not recommend routine postexposure prophylaxis for healthcare workers in the absence of an outbreak. However, we think that healthcare workers who are directly exposed to the stools of patients with serologically confirmed hepatitis A should be offered immune globulin (0.02 mg/kg IM) as postexposure prophylaxis. If given within 2 weeks of exposure, immune globulin prevents disease or diminishes the severity of clinical illness with 80% to 90% efficacy. The hepatitis A vaccine has helped terminate outbreaks in the community, but its role in hospitals has not been determined.

Influenza Virus

Transmission of influenza virus usually occurs in the community. However, patients, visitors, and healthcare workers can spread this virus in healthcare facilities.[73-77] In fact, Pachucki et al reported an outbreak in which 118 workers were affected, including 8% of the nurses and 3% to 6% of the doctors.[74] However, nosocomial influenza probably goes unrecognized in many instances. Clinicians and infection control personnel should consider this diagnosis when staff or hospitalized patients develop symptoms of influenza during the appropriate season. Figure 15-7 and Table 15-1 describe how infection control personnel might work up nosocomial exposures to influenza.[8,9]

Influenza increases absenteeism among staff and increases the costs associated with sick leave.

In addition, the Advisory Committee on Immunization Practices has recommended that the following persons be vaccinated: physicians, nurses, and other personnel in both inpatient- and outpatient-care settings who have contact with high-risk persons.[78] Thus, many healthcare facilities offer their employees the influenza vaccine free of charge to protect the staff and to prevent spread of influenza within the healthcare facility.

Creutzfeldt-Jakob Agent

Creutzfeldt-Jakob agent, a prion, has been transmitted in the healthcare setting by brain-to-brain inoculation (eg, through contaminated instruments) and by contaminated tissues or tissue extracts. To date, there have been no documented instances of transmission to healthcare workers, and the incidence of Creutzfeldt-Jakob disease is not higher in healthcare workers than it is in the general population.[79,80] Berger and Noble reported that 24 healthcare workers have been identified as having Creutzfeldt-Jakob disease.[81] These authors provided five case reports of healthcare workers (one neurosurgeon, one pathologist, one internist who did autopsies for 1 year during his training, and two histopathology technicians) who developed Creutzfeldt-Jakob disease.[81] However, none of these persons had documented exposures to the agent.

Criteria for defining exposures to the Creutzfeldt-Jakob agent have not been developed. Blood, cerebrospinal fluid, brain tissue, spinal cord tissue, and eye tissue from patients who have Creutzfeldt-Jakob disease, or tissues from the central nervous system (ie, cerebrospinal fluid) can contain the etiologic agent. Thus, persons who have unprotected exposures to these fluids or tissues should be considered exposed. Persons who perform lumbar punctures, neurosurgery, and autopsies are at highest risk of exposure. High-risk areas in the hospital include the operating and autopsy suites.

If an exposure occurs, infection control personnel should create a list of all exposed staff, which should be saved indefinitely in case anyone develops the disease (Figure 15-8). Staff from infection control and the employee health service also should counsel healthcare workers, because they most likely will be very distraught and angry. In addition, infection control staff should work with staff from the operating suite and central sterile supply to ensure that, if possible, the reusable surgical instruments used on the index case are recalled and reprocessed properly and that all contaminated equipment in other departments (eg, pathology) is properly cleaned and disinfected.

The best exposure management for Creutzfeldt-Jakob agent is to prevent exposures from occurring. Therefore, infection control staff would be wise to work with persons from the operating suite, the neurosurgery department, the ophthalmology department, the pathology department, the laboratory, central sterile supply, and the morgue to develop policies that prevent exposures. These precautions should be used for all persons who undergo invasive procedures or ophthalmologic exams and who are known to have Creutzfeldt-Jakob disease or a progressive dementia or who have a family history of prion disease, Creutzfeldt-Jakob disease, fatal familial insomnia, or Gerstmann-Sträussler-Scheinker disease.[82,83] The precautions also should be used for patients who have received gonadotropin or human growth hormone extracted from cadaveric pituitary glands.[83]

At the University of Iowa Hospitals and Clinics, we developed and implemented a Creutzfeldt-Jakob policy. The first policy covered only patients with known Creutzfeldt-Jakob disease. Soon after we implemented this policy, a patient who had a progressive dementia underwent a diagnostic brain biopsy. The clinicians were surprised and dismayed when the histopathology revealed spongiform degeneration. The subsequent exposure workup involved 62 personnel from the Department of Pathology, the

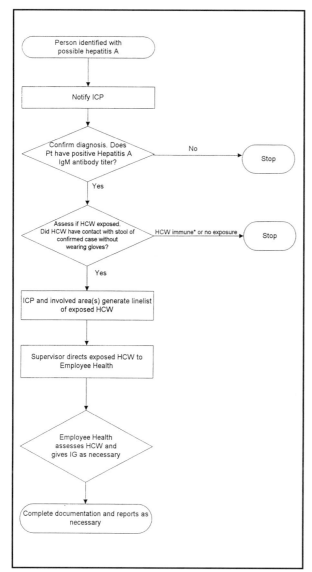

FIGURE 15-6. Managing hepatitis A exposures. The diagnostic criteria listed are meant to be helpful guides and are not all-inclusive. Abbreviations: HCW = healthcare worker; ICP = infection control professional; IgG = immunoglobulin G; IgM = immunoglobulin M; Pt = patient.

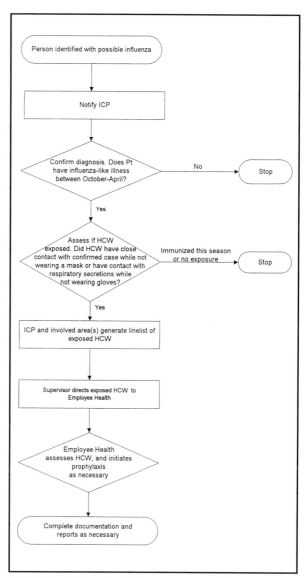

FIGURE 15-7. Managing influenza exposures. The diagnostic criteria listed are meant to be helpful guides and are not all-inclusive. Abbreviations: HCW = healthcare worker; ICP = infection control professional; Pt = patient.

operating suite, and central sterile supply. In addition, personnel in the Department of Pathology spent numerous hours and approximately $1,200 disinfecting the laboratory and equipment that might have been contaminated by the tissues. Thereafter, we expanded our policy to include the conditions, treatments, and family histories listed above.

Infection control personnel who are developing

these policies should review recommendations written by Steelman[82,83] and by Rutala.[84] These documents recommend methods for protecting staff from exposure to potentially infectious tissues, limiting contamination of equipment and the environment, and effectively eradicating the organism from surgical equipment. The guidelines on the care of surgical equipment are extremely important, because the Creutzfeldt-Jakob agent is not killed by routine chemical and physical means of sterilization, including routine steam sterilization, ethylene oxide sterilization, and dry heat sterilization; processes using peracetic acid, hydrogen peroxide, ultraviolet light, radiation, freezing, drying, or hot bead glass; and any level of cleaning and disinfection with glutaraldehyde, dry heat radiation, detergents, or formaldehyde. Of note, some of the recommendations differ between the documents developed by Steelman and Rutala.

Bacterial Diseases

Mycobacterium tuberculosis

M tuberculosis is an acid-fast bacillus that is spread through the air. This organism causes a primary infection that, in normal hosts, usually is not manifested as clinical disease and recrudescent pulmonary or disseminated disease. Persons who are infected with *M tuberculosis* have positive tuberculin skin tests but are not contagious. Those who have active pulmonary disease are infectious and are the persons who cause most nosocomial exposures. On occasion, patients who have active infections at other sites also can cause exposures. For example, a patient with a large soft-tissue abscess underwent incision, drainage, and irrigation in the operating suite.[85] Because he continued to have copious drainage, the wound was cleaned with a pressurized irrigation system. Subsequently, 59 employees were identified who converted their tuberculin skin tests, and 9 persons acquired active tuberculosis (5 employees, 2 patients, and 2 family members of the index patient).

Persons are considered exposed to *M tuberculosis* if they were not wearing an N95 or better respirator and they shared air space with a patient who had active pulmonary tuberculosis or who had an extrapulmonary site of infection from which *M tuberculosis* was aerosolized. Data indicate that, during outbreaks, a large proportion (3.6% to

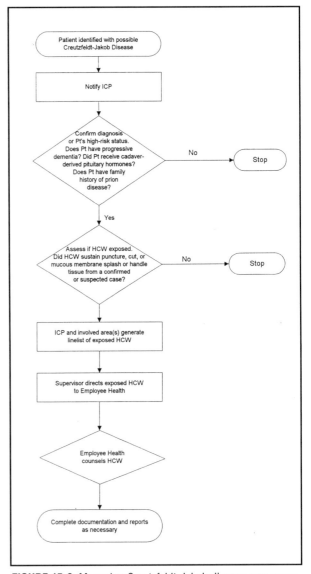

FIGURE 15-8. Managing Creutzfeldt-Jakob disease exposures. The diagnostic criteria listed are meant to be helpful guides and are not all-inclusive. Abbreviations: HCW = healthcare worker; ICP = infection control professional; Pt = patient.

100%) of exposed persons may become tuberculin skin-test positive.[85-88] In general, approximately 30% of persons will become infected when they are exposed to a patient whose sputum contains acid-fast bacilli, whereas only 10% of persons will become infected when they are exposed to an infected patient whose sputum does not contain visible acid-fast bacilli.[89]

As with the other airborne infections—measles and chicken pox—it is best to prevent exposures by appropriately screening patients in clinics and on admission for symptoms and signs of tuberculosis. However, screening can be difficult, because patients can present with tuberculosis at unusual sites and immunocompromised patients can have atypical signs and symptoms. For example, during a 2-month period in 1993, two patients were seen at the University of Iowa Hospitals and Clinics who had unusual presentations of tuberculosis. One patient was a 28-year-old man who had a testicular mass that was found to be an abscess during an operation. Subsequently, drainage from the abscess, his urine, and lung tissue all were found to contain *M tuberculosis*.

The second patient was a 57-year-old woman whose tuberculin skin test was negative before she underwent a bilateral lung transplant. The patient was seen several times after the transplant for complaints of decreasing exercise tolerance, fever, and right shoulder pain. Twelve weeks after the transplant, she was admitted with fever, continued right shoulder pain, and cavitary lesions in her lungs.[90] Material from a lung cavity contained acid-fast bacilli, and she was begun on isoniazid, ethambutol, and pyrazinamide. However, she developed renal failure, progressive liver-function abnormalities, a coagulopathy, and respiratory distress. Despite receiving supportive care, including mechanical ventilation, the patient died. An autopsy identified an ill-defined abscess of the subscapularis muscle and numerous abscesses caused by *M tuberculosis* in the lungs, liver, spleen, pancreas, and small intestine.

During the course of their care, the two patients described above exposed 150 persons (48 and 102, respectively). Five employees (3.3%) became tuberculin skin-test positive, including two persons in the Department of Pathology who had handled tissues from the patients.

The goal of an exposure workup is to identify all patients, visitors, and healthcare workers who were exposed, so that those who become infected are given prophylactic antimicrobial agents (Figure 15-9). This task can be very difficult if, before being diagnosed, the person visited many clinics and diagnostic laboratories or was hospitalized in an open bay of an intensive care unit. All persons who meet the criteria for exposure should have baseline tuberculin skin testing if they have not had a recent skin test (within 6 weeks in a high-prevalence area or 1 year in a low-prevalence area). Healthcare workers should be seen in the employee health service. Patients and visitors should be notified about the exposure and told to contact their own physician. In addition, the patients' primary physicians should receive letters informing them of the exposure. Twelve weeks after the exposure, exposed persons should have another skin test. If that skin test is positive, they should receive the appropriate prophylactic antimicrobial treatment.[87]

Neisseria meningitidis

N meningitidis is a Gram-negative diplococcus that causes meningitis and septicemia. Household contacts of persons with invasive meningococcal disease are at 500 to 800 times greater risk of acquiring meningococcal infection than are members of the general public.[91] Other semiclosed or closed populations, such as persons living in college dormitories, chronic-care hospitals, nursery schools, and military barracks, also are at high risk of infection.[92] Despite caring for patients with meningococcal infection, healthcare workers are not at higher risk than members of the general population for acquiring this infection.[92]

N meningitidis is transmitted by respiratory droplets. Thus, patients with meningococcal infections should be placed on droplet precautions for the first 24 hours of treatment.[14] Nosocomial transmission of *N meningitidis*, which has occurred rarely, may be more likely to occur from patients who have meningococcal pneumonia than from patients with meningitis or septicemia.[93,94] We conducted a computerized literature search of reports published between 1975 and 1997 and identified only two papers reporting on healthcare workers who acquired meningococcal infection after nosocomial exposure.[95] Four of the five affected healthcare workers did mouth-to-mouth resuscitation on patients with meningococcal disease,[96] and one was a nurse who did not receive a prophylactic antimicrobial agent after she helped intubate and suction an infected patient.[95]

Persons are considered exposed to *N meningitidis* if they did not wear a mask and had either prolonged close contact with a person who had meningococcal disease or had contact with the patient's respiratory secretions. Exposed persons should begin prophylactic treatment within 24 hours of their exposure.[9] Thus, immediately upon identifying a patient with meningococcal disease, infection control personnel must determine whether any healthcare workers met the criteria for exposure (Figure 15-10). Staff who met criteria for exposure must be sent to the employee health service at once to receive the appropriate antimicrobial agent. If the employee health service is not open, infection control staff should ensure that the healthcare workers receive the prophylactic agent.

Despite the very low risk of transmission to healthcare workers, staff often react irrationally when they learn that a patient with meningococcal disease has been admitted to their unit. Staff who do not meet the criteria for exposure frequently demand prescriptions for prophylactic antimicrobial agents. If infection control personnel refuse to oblige them, these staff members often have another physician write a prescription for them. However, prophylactic treatment is not without complications. In fact, one of the authors investigated an exposure to *N meningitidis* in which the hospital had to replace two sets of contact lenses because rifampin turned them orange.

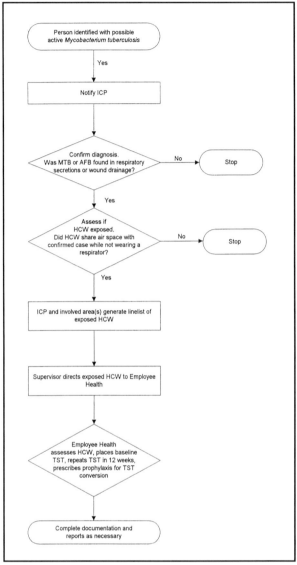

FIGURE 15-9. Managing *Mycobacterium tuberculosis* exposures. The diagnostic criteria listed are meant to be helpful guides and are not all-inclusive. Abbreviations: AFB = acid-fast bacilli; HCW = healthcare worker; ICP = infection control professional; MTB = *M tuberculosis;* TST = tuberculin skin test.

Bordetella pertussis

The whole-cell pertussis vaccines dramatically altered the epidemiology of pertussis. Before the vaccines were introduced, most adults were immune to pertussis because they had the disease during childhood. However, most adults are now susceptible to pertussis because vaccine-induced immunity disappears within 12 years after the last vaccination.[97] Consequently, the incidence of pertussis in adults is now increasing,[98-102] and adults have become the primary source of infection for susceptible young children.[101]

Pertussis has been transmitted in the hospital by patients, visitors, and healthcare workers.[103-106] In one nosocomial outbreak, a nurse's aide suggested that a pediatric resident might have pertussis, but the physicians discounted her astute diagnosis as a joke.[103] Outbreaks also have occurred in other healthcare institutions, including homes for handicapped persons[107-109] and a nursing home.[102] During the outbreak in the nursing home, 11 (10%) of 107 residents and 17 (14%) of 116 employees developed clinical or laboratory-confirmed pertussis infection.[102] The mean age of persons with clinical infection was 75 years for residents and 34 years for employees.

Most adults with pertussis experience persistent and perhaps severe cough. These adults frequently are diagnosed as having bronchitis. Thus, many exposures are not identified. Several studies indicate that erythromycin treatment early in the course of illness decreases the frequency of secondary spread.[108-110] However, physicians rarely see adult patients early in their illness.

Several communities have experienced outbreaks of pertussis in the last few years.[4] Patients involved in these outbreaks have caused exposures when they were evaluated in clinics or were admitted to a hospital. We think that more exposures will occur in the future unless a pertussis vaccine for adults becomes available. Figure 15-11 and Table 15-1 illustrate how infection control personnel could evaluate an exposure to a person with whooping cough.[8,9,111]

Ectoparasites

Infection control personnel also must investigate exposures to ectoparasites such as lice and scabies.[112] We have found that healthcare workers often react more hysterically to these exposures than they do to exposures involving infectious agents. In fact, healthcare workers frequently demand prophylactic treatment when it is not appropriate. One of the authors remembers a nurse who did not meet the criteria for exposure to lice. When infection control personnel refused to recommend a pediculicide, the nurse had her private physician prescribe Kwell (Reedco, Inc, Humacao, Puerto Rico). The nurse subsequently developed a severe cutaneous allergic reaction that took weeks to resolve.

Lice

Pediculus humanus capitis, Pediculus humanus corporis, and *Phthirus pubis* are found not infrequently on patients who have been admitted to healthcare facilities. These ectoparasites are transmitted by direct contact with infested persons or their clothing. Persons infested with lice should be placed on contact precautions until they have been treated appropriately.[14,113] All clothing, bedding, hats, and other personal-care items should be washed in hot water and dried on the hot cycle, because lice and their eggs cannot survive temperatures above 53.5°C.[9] Clothes that cannot be washed should be dry cleaned or placed in a plastic bag for 2 weeks.[9] Brushes and combs should be soaked in a pediculicide shampoo.[9] Healthcare workers who have had direct contact with the patient's head (head lice) or clothes (body lice) should be evaluated by personnel in the employee health clinic (Figure 15-12).[5] Because the risk of acquiring lice in a healthcare facility is very low, only staff members who become infested should be treated with a pediculicide.

Scabies

In contrast to lice, *Sarcoptes scabiei* can be transmitted easily within healthcare facilities, especially if the index case has crusted (Norwegian) scabies.[114-120] Such exposures can be quite expensive. For example, an outbreak of scabies occurred in an extended-care unit that was attached to an acute-care hospital. To terminate the outbreak, 78 residents and over 100 staff and family members were treated at a cost of more than $20,000.[120] Scabies spread within the unit, in part because the protocol for control of this ectoparasite was inadequate. The policy was based on the assumption that all staff would know what to do, because they would have had previous experience with scabies exposures.[120]

Persons with scabies should be placed on contact isolation precautions until they are treated appropriately.[14] Personnel who have cared for patients with scabies should be evaluated in the employee health clinic, and those who had contact with the patient's skin should be treated (Figure 15-13).[5] If two or more persons who live or work in a long-term care facility acquire scabies, all residents and employees should be treated to prevent further spread. Persons receiving effective therapy may have pruritus for up to 2 weeks after therapy. Thus, infection control personnel should not interpret pruritus that occurs within this time period as treatment failure.

The index patient's bedding and the clothes that contacted the patient's skin should be washed in hot water and dried on the hot cycle.[9] Clothes that cannot be washed can be stored for several days to a week, because the mite cannot survive more than 3 to 4 days in the environment.[9]

Conclusion

Exposure workups are an important responsibility for infection control personnel. If they evaluate exposures promptly and effectively, infection control staff can prevent transmission of infectious agents or ectoparasites to numerous healthcare workers, patients, and visitors. Exposure workups consume much time and money. In addition, many exposures could be averted if healthcare workers were immune to vaccine-preventable infections and if staff used isolation precautions appropriately. Thus, wise infection control staff learn from their own experience and develop policies and procedures to limit the

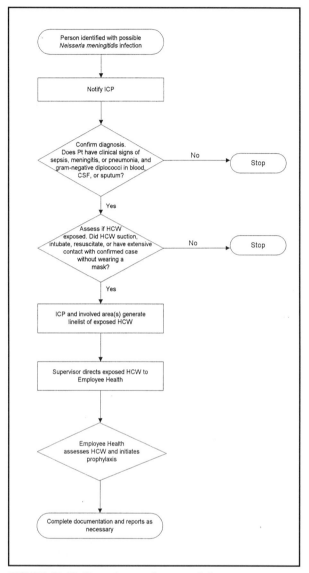

FIGURE 15-10. Managing meningococcal disease exposures. The diagnostic criteria listed are meant to be helpful guides and are not all-inclusive. Abbreviations: CSF = cerebrospinal fluid; HCW = healthcare worker; ICP = infection control professional; Pt = patient.

number of exposures in their institutions.

Acknowledgments

The authors thank the previous and current staff of the Program of Hospital Epidemiology at the University of Iowa Hospitals and Clinics who helped develop our approach to exposure workups and the algorithms published in this manuscript:

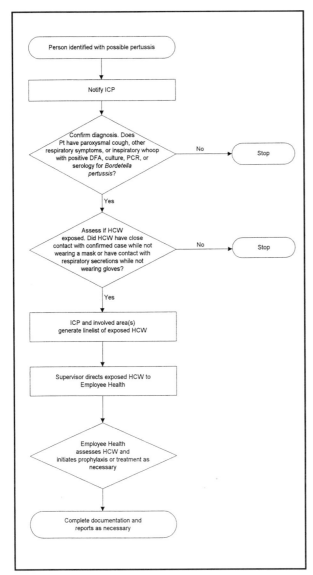

FIGURE 15-11. Managing pertussis exposures. The diagnostic criteria listed are meant to be helpful guides and are not all-inclusive. Abbreviations: DFA = direct fluorescent antibody; HCW = healthcare worker; ICP = infection control professional; PCR = polymerase chain reaction; Pt = patient.

Walter Hierholzer, Dorothy Rasley, Michael Massanari, Stephen Streed, Richard Wenzel, Jeanne Lyons, Sandra Blake, Marlene Schmid, and J. Robert Adams. In addition, the surveillance technicians have helped us conduct numerous exposure workups: Linda Gorsh, Sandy Huedepohl, Kristin Kuhns, Melody Schwenke, Joan Barr, Nancy Jones, Lisa Washington, Mary Kistler, Donna Divishek, Ethel Bontrager, Sarah Wallace, Gatana Stoner, and Jeanne Bock.

Note

The recommendations in Chapters 26 and 15 vary slightly because different sources were used to formulate them. Infection control staff should evaluate the recommendations and apply those that best suit their institution.

References

1. Weltman AC, DiFerdinando GT, Washko R, Lipsky WM. A death associated with therapy for nosocomially acquired multidrug-resistant tuberculosis. *Chest.* 1996;110:279-281.

2. Weber DJ, Rutala WA, Parham C. Impact and costs of varicella prevention in a university hospital. *Am J Public Health.* 1988;78:19-23.

3. Faoagali JL, Darcy R. Chicken pox outbreak among the staff of a large, urban adult hospital: costs of monitoring and control. *Am J Infect Control.* 1995;23:247-250.

4. Christie CDC, Glover AM, Willke MJ, Marx ML, Reising SF, Hutchinson NM. Containment of pertussis in the regional pediatric hospital during the greater Cincinnati epidemic of 1993. *Infect Control Hosp Epidemiol.* 1995;16:556-563.

5. Schmid MW, Barr BM, Adams JR, Rasley DA, Yank TJ, Streed SA. Assistive algorithms for exposure management, part I: chicken pox, scabies, and lice. *Clinical Performance and Quality Health Care* 1993;1:152-154.

6. Barr BM, Adams JR, Schmid MW, Rasley DA, Yank TJ, Streed SA. Assistive algorithms for exposure management, part II: *Mycobacterium tuberculosis,* meningococcemia, and measles. *Clinical Performance and Quality Health Care.* 1994;2:33-36.

7. Schmid MM, Miller ED. Managing exposures to infections. In: Wenzel RP, ed. *Prevention and Control of Nosocomial Infections.* 3rd ed. Baltimore, Md: Williams & Wilkins; 1997:437-460.

8. Appendix D. Constructing algorithm flowcharts for performance measure evaluation. In: *Using Clinical Practice Guidelines to Evaluate Quality of Care. Volume 2: Methods.* Rockville, Md: US Department of Health and Human Services, Public Health Service, Agency for Health Care Policy and Research; 1995:109-115.

9. Committee on Infectious Diseases, American Academy of Pediatrics. *1994 Red Book: Report of the Committee on*

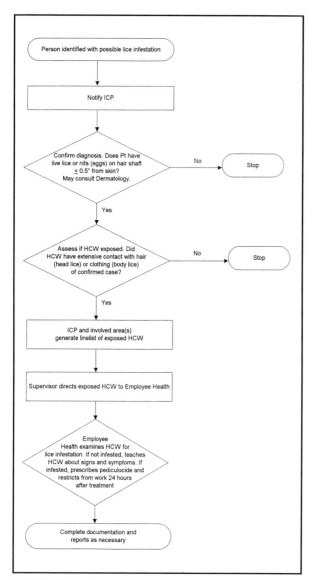

FIGURE 15-12. Managing lice exposures. The diagnostic criteria listed are meant to be helpful guides and are not all-inclusive. Abbreviations: HCW = healthcare worker; ICP = infection control professional; Pt = patient.

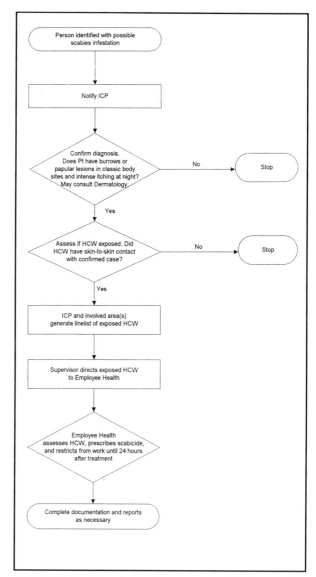

FIGURE 15-13. Managing scabies exposures. The diagnostic criteria listed are meant to be helpful guides and are not all-inclusive. Abbreviations: HCW = healthcare worker; ICP = infection control professional; Pt = patient.

Infectious Diseases. 23rd ed. Elk Grove Village, Ill: American Academy of Pediatrics; 1994.

10. *Control of Communicable Diseases Manual.* 16th ed. In: Benenson AS, ed. Washington, DC: American Public Health Association; 1995.

11. Mandell GL, Douglas RG, Bennett JE, eds. *Principles and Practice of Infectious Diseases.* 3rd ed. New York, NY: Churchill Livingstone; 1990.

12. Valenti WM. Employee work restrictions for infection control. *Infect Control.* 1984;5:583-584.

13. Meyers MG, Rasley DA, Hierholzer WJ. Hospital infection control for varicella-zoster virus infection. *Pediatrics.* 1982;70:199-202.

14. Garner JS. Hospital Infection Control Practices Advisory Committee. Guideline for isolation precautions in hospitals. *Infect Control Hosp Epidemiol.* 1996;17:53-80.

15. Sepkowitz KA. Occupationally acquired infections in healthcare workers. Part I. *Ann Intern Med.* 1996;125:826-834.

16. McKinney WP, Horowitz MM, Battiola RJ. Susceptibility

of hospital-based health care personnel to varicella-zoster virus infections. *Am J Infect Control.* 1989;17:26-30.

17. Haiduven DJ, Hench CP, Stevens DA. Postexposure varicella management of nonimmune personnel: an alternative approach. *Infect Control Hosp Epidemiol.* 1994;15:329-334.

18. Hayden GF, Meyers JD, Dixon RE. Nosocomial varicella. part II: suggested guidelines for management. *West J Med.* 1979;130:300-303.

19. Weitekamp MR, Schan P, Aber RC. An algorithm for the control of nosocomial varicella-zoster virus infection. *Am J Infect Control.* 1985;13:193-198.

20. Bloch AB, Orenstein WA, Ewing WM, et al. Measles outbreak in a pediatric practice: airborne transmission in an office setting. *Pediatrics.* 1985;75:676-683.

21. Remington PL, Hall WN, Davis IH, Herald A, Gunn RA. Airborne transmission of measles in a physician's office. *JAMA.* 1985;253:1574-1577.

22. Davis RM, Orenstein WA, Frank JA, et al. Transmission of measles in medical settings. 1980 through 1984. *JAMA.* 1986;255:1295-1298.

23. Istre GR, McKee PA, West GR, et al. Measles spread in medical settings: an important focus of disease transmission? *Pediatrics.* 1987;79:356-358.

24. Williams WW, Atkinson WL, Holmes SJ, Orenstein WA. Nosocomial measles, mumps, rubella, and other viral infections. In: Mayhall CG, ed. *Hospital Epidemiology and Infection Control.* Baltimore, Md: Williams & Wilkins; 1996:523-535.

25. Edmonson MB, Addiss DG, McPherson Berg JL, Circo SR, Davis JP. Mild measles and secondary vaccine failure during a sustained outbreak in a highly vaccinated population. *JAMA.* 1990;263:2467-2471.

26. Atkinson WL, Markowitz LE, Adams NC, Seastrom GR. Transmission of measles in medical settings—United States, 1985-1989. *Am J Med.* 1991;91(suppl 3B):320S-324S.

27. Raad II, Sherertz RJ, Rains CS, et al. The importance of nosocomial transmission of measles in the propagation of a community outbreak. *Infect Control Hosp Epidemiol.* 1989;10:161-166.

28. Sienko DG, Friedman C, McGee, et al. A measles outbreak at university medical settings involving health care providers. *Am J Public Health.* 1987;77:1222-1224.

29. Rivera ME, Mason WH, Ross LA, Wright HT. Nosocomial measles infection in a pediatric hospital during a community-wide epidemic. *J Pediatr.* 1991;119:183-186.

30. Rank EL, Brettman L, Katz-Pollack H, DeHertogh D,

Neville D. Chronology of a hospital-wide measles outbreak: lessons learned and shared from an extraordinary week in late March 1989. *Am J Infect Control.* 1992;20:315-318.

31. Farizo KM, Stehr-Green PA, Simpson DM, Markowitz LE. Pediatric emergency room visits: a risk factor for acquiring measles. *Pediatrics.* 1991;87:74-79.

32. Weber DJ, Rutala WA, Orenstein WA. Prevention of mumps, measles and rubella among hospital personnel. *J Pediatr.* 1991;119:322-326.

33. Subbarao EK, Andrews-Mann L, Amin S, Greenberg J, Kumar ML. Postexposure prophylaxis for measles in a neonatal intensive care unit. *J Pediatr.* 1990;117:782-785.

34. Ammari LK, Bell LM, Hodinka RL. Secondary measles vaccine failure in healthcare workers exposed to infected patients. *Infect Control Hosp Epidemiol.* 1993;14:81-86.

35. Wright LJ, Carlquist JF. Measles immunity in employees of a multihospital healthcare provider. *Infect Control Hosp Epidemiol.* 1994;15:8-11.

36. Enguidanos R, Mascola L, Frederick P. A survey of hospital infection control policies and employee measles cases during Los Angeles County's measles epidemic, 1987 to 1989. *Am J Infect Control.* 1992;20:301-304.

37. Greaves WL, Orenstein WA, Stetler HC, Preblud SR, Hinnman AR, Bart KJ. Prevention of rubella transmission in medical facilities. *JAMA.* 1982;248:861-864.

38. Polk BF, White JA, DeGirolami PC, Modlin JF. An outbreak of rubella among hospital personnel. *N Engl J Med.* 1980;303:541-545.

39. Centers for Disease Control and Prevention. Rubella in hospitals—California. *MMWR.* 1983;32:37-39.

40. Poland GA, Nichol KL. Medical students as sources of rubella and measles outbreaks. *Arch Intern Med.* 1990;150:44-46.

41. Storch GA, Gruber C, Benz B, Beaudoin J, Hayes J. A rubella outbreak among dental students: description of the outbreak and analysis of control measures. *Infect Control.* 1985;6:150-156.

42. Strassburg MA, Stephenson TG, Habel LA, Fannin SL. Rubella in hospital employees. *Infect Control.* 1984;5:123-126.

43. Fliegel PE, Weinstein WM. Rubella outbreak in a prenatal clinic: management and prevention. *Am J Infect Control.* 1982;10:29-33.

44. Strassburg MA, Imagawa DT, Fannin SL, et al. Rubella outbreak among hospital employees. *Obstet Gynecol.* 1981;57:283-288.

45. Gladstone JL, Millian SJ. Rubella exposure in an obstetric clinic. *Obstet Gynecol.* 1981;57:182-186.

46. Wharton M, Cochi SL, Hutcheson RH, Schaffner W. Mumps transmission in hospitals. *Arch Intern Med.* 1990;150:47-49.

47. Fischer PR, Brunetti C, Welch V, Christenson JC. Nosocomial mumps: report of an outbreak and control. *Am J Infect Control.* 1996;24:13-18.

48. Nichol KL, Olson R. Medical students' exposure and immunity to vaccine-preventable diseases. *Arch Intern Med.* 1993;153:1913-1916.

49. Dowell SF, Torok TJ, Thorp JA, et al. Parvovirus B19 infection in hospital workers: community or hospital acquisition? *J Infect Dis.* 1995;172:1076-1079.

50. Bell LM, Naides SJ, Stoffman P, Hodinka RL, Plotkin SA. Human parvovirus B19 infection among hospital staff members after contact with infected patients. *N Engl J Med.* 1989;321:485-491.

51. Seng C, Watkins P, Morse D, et al. Parvovirus B19 outbreak on an adult ward. *Epidemiol Infect.* 1994;113:345-353.

52. Ray SM, Erdman DD, Berschling JD, Cooper JE, Torok TJ, Blumberg HM. Nosocomial exposure to parvovirus B19: low risk of transmission to healthcare workers. *Infect Control Hosp Epidemiol.* 1997;18:109-114.

53. Shishiba T, Matsunaga Y. An outbreak of erythema infectiosum among hospital staff members including a patient with pleural fluid and pericardial effusion. *J Am Acad Dermatol.* 1993;29:265-267.

54. Lohiya GS, Stewart K, Perot K, Widman R. Parvovirus B19 outbreak in a developmental center. *Am J Infect Control.* 1995;23:373-376.

55. Centers for Disease Control and Prevention. Risks associated with human parvovirus B19 infection. *MMWR.* 1989;38:81-88, 93-97.

56. Cartter ML, Farley TA, Rosengren S, et al. Occupational risk factors for infection with parvovirus B19 among pregnant women. *J Infect Dis.* 1991;163:282-285.

57. Noble RC, Kane MA, Reeves SA, Roeckel I. Posttransfusion hepatitis A in a neonatal intensive care unit. *JAMA.* 1984;252:2711-2715.

58. Azimi PH, Roberto RR, Guralnik J, et al. Transfusion-acquired hepatitis A in a premature infant with secondary nosocomial spread in an intensive care nursery. *Am J Dis Child.* 1986;140:23-27.

59. Giacoia GP, Kasprisin DO. Transfusion-acquired hepatitis A. *South Med J.* 1989;82:1357-1360.

60. Seeberg S, Brandberg A, Hermodsson S, Larsson P, Lundgren S. Hospital outbreak of hepatitis A secondary to blood exchange in a baby. *Lancet.* 1981;1:1155-1156. Letter.

61. Klein BS, Michaels JA, Rytel MW, Berg KG, Davis JP. Nosocomial hepatitis A. A multinursery outbreak in Wisconsin. *JAMA.* 1984;252:2716-2721.

62. Rosenblum LS, Villarino ME, Nainan OV, et al. Hepatitis A outbreak in a neonatal intensive care unit: risk factors for transmission and evidence of prolonged viral excretion among preterm infants. *J Infect Dis.* 1991;164:476-482.

63. Burkholder BT, Coronado VG, Brown J, et al. Nosocomial transmission of hepatitis A in a pediatric hospital traced to an anti-hepatitis A virus-negative patient with immunodeficiency. *Pediatr Infect Dis J.* 1995;14:261-266.

64. Drusin LM, Sohmer M, Groshen SL, Spiritos MD, Senterfit LB, Christenson WN. Nosocomial hepatitis A infection in a pediatric intensive care unit. *Arch Dis Child.* 1987;62:690-695.

65. Reed CM, Gustafson TL, Siegel J, Duer P. Nosocomial transmission of hepatitis A from a hospital-acquired case. *Pediatr Infect Dis J.* 1984;3:300-303.

66. Krober MS, Bass JW, Brown JD, Lemon SM, Rupert KJ. Hospital outbreak of hepatitis A: risk factors for spread. *Pediatr Infect Dis J.* 1984;3:296-299.

67. Orenstein WA, Wu E, Wilkins J, et al. Hospital-acquired hepatitis A: report of an outbreak. *Pediatrics.* 1981;67:494-497.

68. Edgar WM, Campbell AD. Nosocomial infection with hepatitis A. *J Infect.* 1985;10:43-47.

69. Goodman RA, Carder CC, Allen JR, Orenstein WA, Finton RJ. Nosocomial hepatitis A transmission by an adult patient with diarrhea. *Am J Med.* 1982;73:220-226.

70. Eisenstein AB, Aach RD, Jacobsohn W, Goldman A. An epidemic of infectious hepatitis in a general hospital: probable transmission by contaminated orange juice. *JAMA.* 1963;185:171-174.

71. Meyers JD, Romm FJ, Tihen WS, Bryan JA. Food-borne hepatitis A in a general hospital: epidemiologic study of an outbreak attributed to sandwiches. *JAMA.* 1975;231:1049-1053.

72. Doebbeling BN, Li N, Wenzel RP. An outbreak of hepatitis A among health care workers: risk factors for transmission. *Am J Public Health.* 1993;83:1679-1684.

73. Weingarten S, Friedlander M, Rascon D, Ault M, Morgan M, Meyer RD. Influenza surveillance in an acute-care hospital. *Arch Intern Med.* 1988;148:113-116.

74. Pachucki CT, Pappas SA, Fuller GF, Krause SL, Lentino JR, Schaaff DM. Influenza A among hospital personnel and patients. Implications for recognition, prevention, and control. *Arch Intern Med.* 1989;149:77-80.

75. Berlinberg CD, Weingarten SR, Bolton LB, Waterman SH. Occupational exposure to influenza—introduction of an index case to a hospital. *Infect Control Hosp Epidemiol.* 1989;10:70-73.

76. Centers for Disease Control and Prevention. Suspected nosocomial influenza cases in an intensive care unit. *MMWR.* 1988;37:3-4, 9.

77. Adal KA, Flowers RH, Anglim AM. Prevention of nosocomial influenza. *Infect Control Hosp Epidemiol.* 1996;17:641-648.

78. Centers for Disease Control and Prevention. Prevention and control of influenza: recommendations of the Immunization Practices Advisory Committee (ACIP). *MMWR.* 1992;41(no. RR-9):1-14.

79. Will RG. Epidemiology of Creutzfeldt-Jakob disease. *Br Med Bull.* 1993;49:960-970.

80. Harries-Jones R, Knight R, Will RG, Cousens S, Smith PG, Matthews WB. Creutzfeldt-Jakob disease in England and Wales, 1980-1984: a case-control study of potential risk factors. *Journal of Neurology, Neurosurgery and Psychiatry.* 1988;51:1113-1119.

81. Berger JR, Noble JD. Creutzfeldt-Jakob disease in a physician: a review of the disorder in health care workers. *Neurology.* 1993;43:205-206.

82. Steelman VM. Creutzfeldt-Jakob disease: recommendations for infection control. *Am J Infect Control.* 1994;22:312-318.

83. Steelman VM. Creutzfeldt-Jakob disease: decontamination issues. *Infection Control and Sterilization Technology.* 1996;2:32-39.

84. Rutala WA. APIC guideline for selection and use of disinfectants. *Am J Infect Control.* 1996;24:313-342.

85. Hutton MD, Stead WW, Cauthen GM, Block AB, Ewig WM. Nosocomial transmission of tuberculosis associated with a draining abscess. *J Infect Dis.* 1990;161:286-295.

86. Bowden KM, McDiarmid MA. Occupationally acquired tuberculosis: what's known. *Journal of Occupational Medicine.* 1994;36:320-325.

87. Stead WW. Management of health care workers after inadvertent exposure to tuberculosis: a guide for the use of preventive therapy. *Ann Intern Med.* 1995;122:906-912.

88. Templeton GL, Illing LA, Young L, Cave D, Stead WW, Bates JH. The risk for transmission of *Mycobacterium tuberculosis* at the bedside and during autopsy. *Ann Intern Med.* 1995;122:922-925.

89. Sepkowitz KA, Raffalli J, Riley L, Kiehn TE, Armstrong D. Tuberculosis in the AIDS era. *Clin Microbiol Rev.* 1995;8:180-199.

90. Miller RA, Lanza LA, Kline JN, Geist LJ. *Mycobacterium tuberculosis* in lung transplant recipients. *Am J Respir Crit Care Med.* 1995;152:374-376.

91. The Meningococcal Disease Surveillance Group. Analysis of endemic meningococcal disease by serogroup and evaluation of chemoprophylaxis. *J Infect Dis.* 1976;134:201-204.

92. Apicella MA. *Neisseria meningitidis.* In: Mandell GL, Douglas RG, Bennett JE, eds. *Principles and Practice of Infectious Diseases.* 3rd ed. New York, NY: Churchill Livingstone; 1990:1896-1909.

93. Rose HD, Lenz IE, Sheth NK. Meningococcal pneumonia. A source of nosocomial infection. *Arch Intern Med.* 1981;141:575-577.

94. Cohen MS, Steere AC, Baltimore R, et al. Possible nosocomial transmission of group Y *Neisseria meningitidis* among oncology patients. *Ann Intern Med.* 1979;91:7-12.

95. Centers for Disease Control. Nosocomial meningococcemia—Wisconsin. *MMWR.* 1978;27:358, 363.

96. Feldman HA. Some recollections of the meningococcal diseases. *JAMA.* 1972;220:1107-1112.

97. Lambert HJ. Epidemiology of a small pertussis outbreak in Kent County, Michigan. *Public Health Rep.* 1965;80:365-369.

98. Bass JW, Stephenson SR. The return of pertussis. *Pediatr Infect Dis J.* 1987;6:141-144.

99. Mortimer EA Jr. Pertussis and its prevention: a family affair. *J Infect Dis.* 1990;161:473-479.

100. Mink CM, Cherry J, Christenson P. A search for *B pertussis* infection in college students. *Clin Infect Dis.* 1992;14:464-471.

101. Nelson JD. The changing epidemiology of pertussis in young infants: the role of adults as reservoirs of infection. *Am J Dis Child.* 1978;132:371-373.

102. Addiss DG, Davis JP, Meade BD, et al. A pertussis outbreak in a nursing home. *J Infect Dis.* 1991;164:704-710.

103. Linnemann CC Jr, Nasenbeny J. Pertussis in the adult. *Annu Rev Med.* 1977;28:179-185.

104. Kurt TL, Yeager AS, Guenette S, Dunlop S. Spread of pertussis by hospital staff. *JAMA.* 1972;221:264-267.

105. Linnemann CC Jr, Ramundo N, Perlstein PH, et al. Use of pertussis vaccine in an epidemic involving hospital staff. *Lancet.* 1975;2:540-543.

106. Valenti WM, Pincus PH, Messner MK. Nosocomial pertussis: possible spread by a hospital visitor. *Am J Dis Child.* 1980;134:520-521.

107. Steketee RW, Burstyn DG, Wassilak SGF, et al. A comparison of laboratory and clinical methods for diagnosing pertussis in an outbreak in a facility for the developmentally disabled. *J Infect Dis.* 1988;157:441-449.

108. Steketee RW, Wassilak SGF, Adkins WN, et al. Evidence for a high attack rate and efficacy of erythromycin prophylaxis in a pertussis outbreak in a facility for the developmentally disabled. *J Infect Dis.* 1988;157:434-440.

109. Fisher MC, Long SS, McGowan KL, Kaselis E, Smith DG. Outbreak of pertussis in a residential facility for handicapped people. *J Pediatr.* 1989;114:934-939.

110. Biellik RJ, Patriarca PA, Mullen JR, et al. Risk factors for community- and household-acquired pertussis during a large-scale outbreak in central Wisconsin. *J Infect Dis.* 1988;157:1134-1141.

111. Weber DJ, Rutala WA. Management of healthcare workers exposed to pertussis. *Infect Control Hosp Epidemiol.* 1994;15:411-415.

112. Lettau LA. Nosocomial transmission and infection control aspects of parasitic and ectoparasitic diseases, part III: ectoparasites/summary and conclusions. *Infect Control Hosp Epidemiol.* 1991;12:179-185.

113. Meinking TL, Taplin D, Kalter DC, Eberle MW. Comparative efficacy of treatments for *Pediculosis capitis* infestations. *Arch Dermatol.* 1986;122:267-271.

114. Degelau J. Scabies in long-term care facilities. *Infect Control Hosp Epidemiol.* 1992;13:421-425.

115. Pasternak J, Richtmann R, Ganme APP, et al. Scabies epidemic: price and prejudice. *Infect Control Hosp Epidemiol.* 1994;15:540-542.

116. Yonkosky D, Ladia L, Gackenheimer L, Schultz MW. Scabies in nursing homes: an eradication program with permethrin 5% cream. *J Am Acad Dermatol.* 1990;23:1133-1136.

117. Clark J, Friesen DL, Williams WA. Management of an outbreak of Norwegian scabies. *Am J Infect Control.* 1992;20:217-220.

118. Corbett EL, Crossley I, Holton J, Levell N, Miller R, De Cock KM. Crusted ("Norwegian") scabies in a specialist HIV unit: successful use of ivermectin and failure to prevent nosocomial transmission. *Genitourin Med.* 1996;72:115-117.

119. Sirera G, Rius F, Romeu J, et al. Hospital outbreak of scabies stemming from two AIDS patients with Norwegian scabies. *Lancet.* 1990;335:1227.

120. Jack M. Scabies outbreak in an extended care unit—a positive outcome. *Journal of Infection Control.* 1993;8:11-13.

121. Scott JR, Foster JD, Fraser H. Conjunctival instillation of scrapie in mice can produce disease. *Vet Microbiol.* 1993;34:305-309.

CHAPTER 16

Isolation

Michael Edmond, MD, MPH

Abstract

Patients infected or colonized with certain microorganisms must be placed in isolation while hospitalized to prevent nosocomial transmission of these pathogens. Isolation systems enable healthcare workers to identify patients who need to be isolated and to institute the appropriate precautions. This chapter presents an overview of isolation precautions, emphasizing the latest guidelines from the Centers for Disease Control and Prevention.

Introduction

The goal of isolation is to prevent transmission of microorganisms from infected or colonized patients to other patients, hospital visitors, and healthcare workers. Personal protective equipment (eg, masks, eyewear, gloves, and gowns) and specific room requirements help to accomplish this goal.

The importance of appropriate isolation cannot be overstated. The medical literature is replete with examples of nosocomial outbreaks of influenza, tuberculosis, varicella, and even hepatitis A, all of which could have been prevented if isolation techniques had been optimal. Isolation efforts may be costly, but the direct and indirect costs of nosocomial outbreaks is often substantial. Appropriate isolation remains the cornerstone of infection control and is assuming ever-greater importance as the number of multiply antibiotic-resistant organisms increases.

The ideal isolation system is described in Table 16-1. While no system meets all of these standards, infection control personnel should consider these ideals when designing and implementing a system.

The Centers for Disease Control and Prevention (CDC) has led the effort to formalize guidelines for isolation. They published their first guidelines in 1970. Subsequently, the CDC has modified and streamlined these guidelines several times to address emerging problems in infectious diseases, such as multidrug-resistant *Mycobacterium tuberculosis* and vancomycin-resistant enterococci, and to incorporate an increased understanding about the mechanisms of transmission for some diseases.

For the past several years, most hospitals employed disease-specific, category-specific, or

TABLE 16-1
CHARACTERISTICS OF THE IDEAL ISOLATION SYSTEM

- Uses current understanding of the mechanisms for transmitting infectious pathogens

- Requires isolation precautions for all patients with infectious diseases that may be transmitted nosocomially (ie, eliminates nosocomial transmission of infection)

- Avoids isolation of patients who do not require it ("over-isolation")

- Is understood easily by all members of the healthcare team

- Is implemented easily

- Encourages compliance

- Avoids unnecessary use of disposable products

- Is inexpensive

- Interferes minimally with patient care

- Minimizes patient discomfort

body substance isolation. The CDC and the Hospital Infection Control Practices Advisory Committee (HICPAC) issued a guideline in 1996 for a new system of isolation. This system replaces the previous category and disease-specific systems and integrates universal precautions and body substance isolation. Still, individual healthcare institutions may find it necessary to modify these basic guidelines.

This chapter presents an overview of isolation so that infection control personnel can implement an appropriate system. Infection control personnel also should consult the detailed guidelines for implementing isolation precautions that are referenced at the end of this chapter.

Previous Isolation Systems

Category-Specific and Disease-Specific

Category-specific isolation grouped all infectious diseases into six categories based on their mechanism of transmission.[1] These categories included strict, contact, respiratory, tuberculosis, enteric, and drainage-secretion precautions. In the

disease-specific isolation method, isolation requirements were individualized for each infectious disease.[1] One disadvantage of this kind of isolation was that it offered no protection against undiagnosed cases, because a disease process must be suspected or documented before the isolation precautions are instituted. Another disadvantage was that disease-specific isolation was complex because it required healthcare workers to acquire considerable clinical data and to use their judgment. Furthermore, a patient's initial differential diagnosis could be broad. Therefore, healthcare workers would need to implement precautions appropriate for all of the diseases being considered to ensure that nosocomial transmission did not occur. However, tailoring the isolation precautions to the individual patient does prevent unnecessary use of disposable products and conserves financial resources.

Universal Precautions

Universal precautions were designed as a supplement to disease-specific and category-specific isolation. The intent of universal precautions was to protect healthcare workers from infection by preventing contact with blood and certain body fluids (ie, amniotic fluid, pericardial fluid, peritoneal fluid, pleural fluid, cerebrospinal fluid, semen, vaginal secretions, and any body fluid visibly contaminated with blood) of all patients.[2] Universal precautions did not apply to saliva, feces, nasal secretions, sputum, sweat, tears, urine, or vomitus, unless visibly bloody. Universal precautions required healthcare workers to:

- Use barrier precautions when they might contact blood or the specified body fluids.
- Wear gloves for contact with blood and designated body fluids, mucous membranes, and nonintact skin, for venipuncture and all invasive procedures, and for touching items contaminated with blood or body fluids.
- Wash hands immediately after removing gloves.

- Immediately wash skin contaminated by blood and body fluids.
- Avoid recapping used needles.
- Discard used needles in puncture-resistant containers.

Body Substance Isolation

In the late 1980s, Lynch and Jackson proposed an alternative to the category- and disease-specific systems, which they called body substance isolation.[3,4] It was based on the premise that all moist body sites and substances potentially were infectious. Unlike category- and disease-specific isolation designed for patients with documented or suspected disease, body substance isolation was appropriate for all patients and therefore protected healthcare workers from acquiring pathogens from undiagnosed patients. It was similar to universal precautions in that both systems protected healthcare workers. However, body substance isolation also was designed to prevent nosocomial transmission of organisms from patient to patient via healthcare workers.

Body substance isolation stipulated that healthcare workers use barrier precautions (ie, gloves always; masks, protective eyewear, and gowns as needed) to avoid contact with blood, secretions, mucous membranes, nonintact skin, and all moist body substances. For those illnesses spread by the airborne route, additional precautions were necessary. As originally proposed, handwashing was deemed unnecessary unless the hands were visibly soiled due to a glove puncture. Subsequently, it was shown that organisms adhering to the surface of gloves may contaminate healthcare workers' hands even when the gloves appear to be intact. Another disadvantage of body substance isolation was that it did not specify precautions for contact with dry skin and environmental sources that may have been contaminated with epidemiologically important organisms (eg, *Clostridium difficile,* methicillin-resistant *Staph-*

ylococcus aureus, and vancomycin-resistant enterococci).

New CDC Guidelines

The CDC and HICPAC recently proposed a new system for isolation that has two levels of precautions: standard precautions, which apply to all patients, and transmission-based precautions, employed for patients with documented or suspected colonization or infection with certain microorganisms.

Standard Precautions

Standard precautions synthesize the advantages of universal precautions and body substance isolation.[5] Standard precautions apply to blood; all body fluids, secretions, excretions except sweat, whether or not they are visibly bloody; nonintact skin; and mucous membranes. Requirements for standard precautions are outlined in Table 16-2.

Transmission-Based Precautions

While standard precautions apply to all patients, transmission-based precautions apply to selected patients, based on either a suspected or confirmed clinical syndrome or specific diagnosis.[5] Transmission-based precautions (Table 16-3) are divided into three categories that reflect the major modes of transmission of infectious agents within the healthcare setting: airborne, droplet, and contact. Some diseases require more than one isolation category.

Airborne Precautions

Airborne precautions prevent diseases transmitted by droplet nuclei or contaminated dust particles.[5] Droplet nuclei are less than 5 μm in size and may remain suspended in the air, allowing them to migrate for long periods of time. Patients with suspected or confirmed tuberculosis (pulmonary or laryngeal), measles, varicella, or disseminated zoster should be placed on airborne precautions. In

TABLE 16-2
REQUIREMENTS FOR STANDARD PRECAUTIONS[5]

Handwashing

- After touching blood, body fluids, secretions, excretions, contaminated items

- Immediately after removing gloves

- Between patient contacts

Gloves

- For touching blood, body fluids, secretions, excretions, contaminated items

- For touching mucous membranes, nonintact skin

Mask, Eye Protection, Face Shield

- To protect mucous membranes of the eyes, nose and mouth during procedures and patient-care activities likely to generate splashes or sprays of blood, body fluids, secretions, excretions

Gown

- To protect skin and prevent soiling of clothing during procedures and patient-care activities likely to generate splashes or sprays of blood, body fluids, secretions, excretions

Patient Care Equipment

- Soiled patient-care equipment should be handled in a manner to prevent skin and mucous membrane exposures, contamination of clothing, and transfer of microorganisms to other patients and to the environment

- Reusable equipment must be cleaned and reprocessed before use in the care of another patient

Environmental Control

- Develop procedures for routine care, cleaning, and disinfection of patient furniture and the environment

Linen

- Soiled linen should be handled in a manner to prevent skin and mucous membrane exposures, contamination of clothing, and transfer of microorganisms to other patients and to the environment

Sharps

- Avoid recapping used needles

- Avoid removing used needles from disposable syringes by hand

- Avoid bending, breaking, or manipulating used needles by hand

- Place used sharps in puncture-resistant containers

Patient Resuscitation

- Use mouthpieces, resuscitation bags, or other ventilation devices to avoid mouth-to-mouth resuscitation

Patient Placement

- Patients who contaminate the environment or cannot maintain appropriate hygiene should be placed in private rooms

addition, human immunodeficiency virus-infected patients with cough, fever, and unexplained pulmonary infiltrates in any location should be placed empirically on airborne precautions until tuberculosis can be ruled out. Appropriate isolation requires a private room with negative air pressure and at least six air exchanges per hour. Air from the room should be exhausted directly to the outside or through a high-efficiency filter. The door to the room must be closed at all times.

If the patient must be transported from the isolation room to another area of the hospital, the patient should put on a mask before leaving the isolation room. All persons entering the room should

wear repirators. The repirator must meet the following CDC performance criteria:

- Filters 1 μm particles with an efficiency of at least 95%.

- Fits different facial sizes and characteristics.

- Can be fit tested to obtain a leakage of ≤10%.

- Can be checked for fit each time the health-care worker puts on the mask.[6]

Currently, 13 repirators have been certified by the National Institute for Occupational Safety and Health to meet the N-95 standard, and more than 100 repirators await approval.

Patients with suspected or confirmed tubercu-

TABLE 16-3
Transmission-Based Precautions[5]

	Airborne Precautions	Droplet Precautions	Contact Precautions
Room	Negative-pressure private room, >6 air changes/hr, exhaust to outside or use high-efficiency filter; keep door closed Private room for patients who contaminate the environment or cannot maintain appropriate hygiene	Private room (may cohort if necessary); door may remain open	Private room (may cohort if necessary); dedicate use of noncritical patient-care items to a single patient (or a cohort of patients colonized or infected with the same organism)
Masks	For entering room	Within 3 feet of patient or when entering the room	Not required
	To protect oral and nasal mucosa during procedures and activities likely to generate splashes or sprays of blood, body fluids, secretions, or excretions		
Face shield/eye protection	To protect mucosa of eyes, nose, and mouth during procedures and activities likely to generate splashes or sprays of blood, body fluids, secretions, or excretions		If clothing contacts patient, surfaces, items in room; if patient has diarrhea, ileostomy, colostomy, uncontained wound drainage
Gowns	To protect skin and clothing during procedures and activities likely to generate splashes or sprays of blood, body fluids, secretions, or excretions		When entering room
Gloves	When touching blood, body fluids, secretions, excretions, contaminated items, mucous membranes, or nonintact skin		Use medicated handwashing agent
Handwashing	After touching blood, body fluids, secretions, excretions, contaminated items; immediately after glove removal; between patients		
Diseases/pathogens	Measles Tuberculosis, pulmonary or laryngeal Varicella* Zoster (disseminated or immunocompromised patient)*	Adenovirus (infants, children)* Diphtheria, pharyngeal Group A streptococcal pharyngitis, pneumonia, scarlet fever (infants and young children) *Haemophilus influenzae* meningitis, epiglottitis *H influenzae* pneumonia (infants, children) Influenza Meningococcal infections Mumps *Mycoplasma* pneumonia Parvovirus B19 Pertussis Plague, pneumonic Rubella	Adenovirus (infants, children)* *Clostridium difficile* enterocolitis Congenital rubella Diphtheria, cutaneous *Escherichia coli* O157:H7 colitis (diapered or incontinent patients) Enteroviral infections (infants, young children) Furunculosis (infants, young children) Group A streptococcal major skin, burn, or wound infection Hemorrhagic fevers (Lassa, Marburg, Ebola) Hepatitis A (diapered or incontinent patients) Herpes simplex (neonatal; disseminated; severe primary mucocutaneous) Impetigo Major (noncontained) abscess, cellulitis, or decubitus ulcers Multidrug-resistant bacteria (eg, methicillin-resistant *Staphylococcus aureus*, vancomycin-resistant Enterococcus) infection or colonization Parainfluenza infection (infants, children) Pediculosis, scabies Rotavirus (diapered/incontinent patients) Respiratory syncytial virus infection (infants, children, immunocompromised) *Staphylococcus aureus* major skin, wound, or burn infection *Shigella* (diapered or incontinent patients) Varicella* Viral conjunctivitis Zoster (disseminated or immunocompromised patient)*

Shaded areas denote standard precautions.
Condition requires two types of precautions.

losis should be instructed to cover their mouth and nose with a tissue when coughing or sneezing. Those with suspected tuberculosis should remain in isolation until tuberculosis can be ruled out. Patients with confirmed tuberculosis who are receiving effective anti-tuberculous treatment can be moved out of the negative-pressure rooms when they are improving clinically and when three consecutive sputum smears collected on separate days have no detectable acid-fast bacilli. Patients with multidrug-resistant tuberculosis may need to be isolated for the duration of their hospital stay.

If the patient has suspected or confirmed measles, varicella, or disseminated zoster, nonimmune individuals should not enter the room. If a nonimmune healthcare worker must enter the room, he or she should wear a respirator (described above). Persons immune to measles or varicella do not need to wear a respirator when entering the room.

Droplet Precautions

Droplet precautions prevent the transmission of microorganisms by particles larger than 5 μm.[5] These droplets are produced when the patient talks, coughs, or sneezes. Droplets also may be produced during some procedures. Some illnesses that require droplet precautions include bacterial diseases, such as invasive *Haemophilus influenzae* type B infections, meningococcal infections, multidrug-resistant pneumococcal disease, pharyngeal diphtheria, *Mycoplasma* pneumonia, and pertussis. Some viral diseases, including influenza, mumps, rubella, and parvovirus infection, also require these precautions.

Droplet precautions require patients to be placed in a private room or cohorted with another patient who is infected with the same organism. The door to the room may remain open. Healthcare workers should wear masks when within 3 feet of the patient; some hospitals may require healthcare workers to wear a mask when entering the room.

When transported out of the isolation room, the patient should wear a mask.

Contact Precautions

Contact precautions prevent transmission of epidemiologically important organisms from an infected or colonized patient through direct (touching the patient) or indirect (touching surfaces or objects in the patient's environment) contact.[5] Contact precautions require patients to be placed in a private room or cohorted with another patient who is infected with the same organism. Healthcare workers should wear gloves when entering the room. They should change the gloves while caring for the patient if they touch materials containing high concentrations of microorganisms. While still in the isolation room, healthcare workers should remove their gloves and wash their hands with a medicated handwashing agent; they must take care not to contaminate their hands before leaving the room. Healthcare workers should wear gowns if they may have substantial contact with the patient or the patient's environment. They should also wear gowns in situations where there is an increased risk of contact with potentially infective material (eg, the patient is incontinent, has diarrhea, a colostomy, ileostomy, or has wound drainage that is not contained by a dressing). Healthcare workers should remove gowns while in the isolation room, and they should avoid contaminating their clothing before leaving the room. Noncritical patient care items (eg, stethoscopes, bedside commodes, etc) that are used for the patients in contact isolation should not be used for other patients. If such items must be shared, they should be cleaned and disinfected before reuse. Patients should leave the isolation room infrequently.

Contact isolation is indicated for patients infected or colonized with multidrug-resistant bacteria (eg, methicillin-resistant *S aureus* and vancomycin-resistant enterococci). It also is indicated for patients

TABLE 16-4

CLINICAL SCENARIOS REQUIRING ASSIGNMENT OF EMPIRIC ISOLATION PRECAUTIONS[5]

Airborne Precautions	Droplet Precautions	Contact Precautions
• Vesicular rash*	• Meningitis	• Acute diarrhea with infectious etiology; patient incontinent or diapered
• Maculopapular rash with coryza and fever	• Petechial or ecchymotic rash with fever	• Diarrhea in an adult with a history of recent antibiotic use
• Cough, fever, upper lobe pulmonary infiltrate	• Paroxysmal or severe, persistent cough during periods of pertussis activity	• Vesicular rash*
• Cough, fever, pulmonary infiltrate in any location in an HIV-infected patient (or patient at risk for HIV infection)		• Respiratory infections, particularly bronchiolitis and croup, in infants and young children
		• History of infection or colonization with MDR organisms (except MDR *Mycobacterium tuberculosis*)
		• Skin, wound, or urinary tract infection in a patient with a recent hospital or nursing home stay in a facility where MDR organisms are prevalent
		• Abscess or draining wound that cannot be covered

HIV = human immunodeficiency virus; MDR = multidrug-resistant.
*Condition requires two types of precautions.

with *C difficile* enteritis and for patients who have other agents transmitted by the oral-fecal route (eg, *Escherichia coli* O157:H7, *Shigella,* rotavirus, and hepatitis A) and who are diapered or incontinent. Infants and young children with respiratory syncytial virus, parainfluenza, or enteroviral infections also require contact isolation, as do patients with herpes simplex virus infections (ie, neonatal, disseminated, or severe primary mucocutaneous disease), impetigo, scabies, and pediculosis. Patients with varicella or disseminated zoster infections require both contact and airborne precautions. Infants and children with adenovirus infection require both contact and droplet precautions.

Instituting Empiric Isolation Precautions

Frequently, patients are admitted to the hospital without a definitive diagnosis. However, they may have an infectious process that may place other patients and healthcare workers at risk.

Therefore, patients with certain clinical syndromes should be isolated while a definitive diagnosis is pending. Table 16-4 delineates appropriate empiric isolation precautions for various clinical syndromes based on the potential mechanisms of transmission.

Special Considerations for Vancomycin-Resistant Organisms

Over the last several years, vancomycin-resistant enterococci have become important nosocomial pathogens. Appropriate isolation for patients colonized or infected with vancomycin-resistant enterococci can be implemented by following the guidelines for contact isolation.[5,7] The experimental transfer of vancomycin resistance from enterococci to *S aureus* and the increasing prevalence of vancomycin resistance among the enterococci have caused concern that vancomycin-resistant *S aureus* will emerge as a nosocomial pathogen. Given the

TABLE 16-5

ISOLATION PRECAUTIONS FOR PATIENTS INFECTED OR COLONIZED WITH VANCOMYCIN-RESISTANT *STAPHYLOCOCCUS AUREUS*[8]

- Standard and contact precautions apply.
- After gloves are removed, handwashing with 4% chlorhexidine or 60% isopropyl alcohol is required.
- Consider placing a monitor at the door to the patient's room 24 hours per day to prevent unauthorized access and to assess compliance with handwashing and barrier precautions.
- Record the names of all persons entering the room for future use if nasal surveillance cultures become necessary.
- Place a filter or condensate trap on the expiratory-phase tubing of the mechanical-ventilator circuit for patients with VRSA pneumonia requiring mechanical ventilation.
- If patient requires oxygen therapy by nasal cannula, all persons entering the room should wear a standard surgical mask.
- Patients who have VRSA in their nares should be treated with mupirocin.
- Infectious disease consultants should review the patient's antimicrobial therapy to reduce the selection of VRSA by eliminating or substituting antibiotics.
- Limit the number of healthcare workers who come into contact with the VRSA-infected or -colonized patient. To the greatest extent possible, limit care of the patient to one nurse and one physician per shift. The primary nurse or primary physician should perform phlebotomy and other ancillary services.
- Until more is learned about the epidemiology of VRSA, all healthcare workers caring for the patient should have nasal surveillance cultures for VRSA performed every 2 weeks.
- Healthcare workers known to be at higher risk for staphylococcal colonization (eg, those with exfoliative dermatitis or diabetes mellitus requiring treatment with insulin) should not care for patients with VRSA colonization or infection.
- Instruct housekeeping personnel to clean all horizontal surfaces in the patient's immediate vicinity on a daily basis with a quaternary ammonium compound. Cleaning cloths used in the room should not be used to clean other patients' rooms and equipment, but should be discarded carefully.
- Continue isolation precautions for the duration of the hospital stay.
- After the infected or colonized patient is discharged and housekeeping personnel have terminally disinfected the room, obtain environmental cultures. The room should remain closed to new admissions until negative cultures have been reported. Disinfect all equipment used in the room.
- Before discharging the patient, affix an epidemiology alert sticker to the cover of the medical chart, and make a notation in the hospital's information system.
- If a patient with previous VRSA infection or colonization is readmitted, place the patient into isolation immediately. The patient should remain in isolation until surveillance cultures of the nares and any previously infected, open sites have been obtained and are negative.
- If nosocomial transmission is documented on a hospital unit, close the unit to new admissions. If a previously uninfected patient from the unit requires transfer to another hospital unit, isolate the patient in the receiving unit until two nasal cultures separated by 48 hours are negative.
- When possible, postpone diagnostic and therapeutic procedures that require the patient to leave the isolation room.
- When diagnostic tests are performed at the bedside (eg, portable radiography, electrocardiography), wipe equipment with a disinfectant when the tests are complete.
- Collect microbiologic and other specimens for clinical testing in the patient's room.
- Keep clinical specimens from colonized or infected patients in a leak-proof plastic bag for transport. Do not place laboratory forms in the bag with the specimen. Make every attempt to prevent contamination of the outside of the bag. Take the specimen to the laboratory immediately; it should not be sent through a pneumatic tube system.

VRSA=vancomycin-resistant Staphylococcus aureus.

virulence of *S aureus* and the frequency with which it causes nosocomial infections, the emergence of vancomycin resistance in this organism would have a devastating effect on institutions where this organism was found. Guidelines for controlling vancomycin-resistant *S aureus* have been proposed based on knowledge regarding transmission and control of *S aureus* (Table 16-5).[8]

References

1. Garner JS, Simmons BP. Guideline for isolation precautions in hospitals. *Infect Control.* 1983;4:245-325.

2. Centers for Disease Control. Update: Universal precautions for prevention of transmission of human immunodeficiency virus, hepatitis B virus, and other bloodborne pathogens in health-care settings. *MMWR.* 1988;37:377-388.

3. Lynch P, Jackson MM, Cummings J, Stamm WE. Rethinking the role of isolation practices in the prevention of nosocomial infections. *Ann Intern Med.* 1987;107:243-246.

4. Jackson MM, Lynch P. An attempt to make an issue less murky: a comparison of four systems for infection precautions. *Infect Control Hosp Epidemiol.* 1991;12:448-450.

5. Garner JS, Hospital Infection Control Practices Advisory Committee. Guideline for isolation precautions in hospi-

tals. *Infect Control Hosp Epidemiol.* 1996;17:53-80.

6. Centers for Disease Control and Prevention. Guidelines for preventing the transmission of *Mycobacterium tuberculosis* in health-care facilities, 1994. *MMWR.* 1994;43(RR-13):1-132.

7. Hospital Infection Control Practices Advisory Committee. Recommendations for preventing the spread of vancomycin resistance. *Infect Control Hosp Epidemiol.* 1995;16:105-113.

8. Edmond MB, Wenzel RP, Pasculle AW. Vancomycin-resistant *Staphylococcus aureus:* perspectives on measures needed for control. *Ann Intern Med.* 1996;124:329-334.

Recommended Reading

American Academy of Pediatrics. In: Peter G, ed. *1994 Red Book: Report of the Committee on Infectious Diseases.* 23rd ed. Elk Grove Village, Ill: American Academy of Pediatrics; 1994.

Boyce JM, Jackson MM, Pugliese G, et al. Methicillin-resistant *Staphylococcus aureus* (MRSA): a briefing for acute care hospitals and nursing facilities. *Infect Control Hosp Epidemiol.* 1994;15:105-115.

Edmond MB, Wenzel RP. Isolation. In: Mandell GL, Bennett JE, Dolin R, eds. *Principles and Practice of Infectious Diseases.* 4th ed. New York, NY: Churchill Livingstone; 1995:2575-2579.

Larson EL. APIC guideline for handwashing and hand antisepsis in health care settings. *Am J Infect Control.* 1995;23:251-269.

CHAPTER 17

Basics of Stratifying for Severity of Illness

Peter A. Gross, MD

Abstract

Conventional wisdom suggests that those who assess healthcare processes and outcomes should always stratify cases by severity of illness; however, infection control personnel should analyze each quality assessment tool with and without severity adjustment and determine whether such adjustment is necessary. I will briefly review severity adjustments for both diseases or procedures involving specific organ systems and those for all diseases, including the commercially available systems. I will also discuss whether and how these various systems for adjusting for severity can be compared. Finally, the chapter will provide selected references for individuals who will use these scoring systems and need more information.

Introduction

The conventional wisdom suggests that severity stratification is always necessary when assessing healthcare processes and outcomes. However, stratifying for severity of illness may or may not be the most essential correction. For example, adjusting for physician practice patterns may account for much of the variation among outcomes. Thus, the investigator should analyze data with and without severity adjustment to determine whether the adjustment is necessary.

Stratification is defined as placing patients in different levels or categories of risk. Risk, in turn, identifies the odds of suffering harm or loss. When the likelihood of a poor outcome has been associated with a specific risk factor, then a patient needs to be placed or stratified into a particular category that reflects the level of risk. This placement process is called risk adjustment. A severity of illness indicator or indicator of risk is comprised of one or more risk factors that are likely to affect the process or outcome being studied. Before selecting a particular severity of illness indicator, the investigator must be assured that the indicator has been tested or validated and that the indicator reliably and reproducibly predicts the outcome in question. "Ay, there's the rub!"[1] Unfortunately, many investigators have not approached validation with the necessary vigor.

A study by Localio and colleagues illustrates why severity of illness indicators must be carefully validated.[2] These investigators stratified in-hospital mortality for adult patients with pneumonia by the MedisGroups admission severity group and by model-based standardization. The mortality rates in the "worst" hospital as assessed by the admission severity group did not, when assessed by model-based standardization method, differ significantly from the mortality rates in the other 21 hospitals. The authors concluded that "simplistic methods applicable to large samples fail when applied to outcomes of typical patients, such as those admitted for pneumonia."[2] Unfortunately, incorrect risk assessments themselves have not only theoretical but also very concrete adverse outcomes. In the case described by Localio and colleagues, a managed care program hired a consultant to assess the quality of care given by hospitals in central Pennsylvania. The consultant adjusted the rates of in-hospital deaths only by the admission severity rate. Partly on the basis of these data, the managed care company ranked the hospitals and selected 10 of 22 for its program.[2]

As you examine different measures of risk adjustment described in this chapter, note that the measures define outcomes differently. For example, some measures define mortality as in-hospital deaths and other measures define mortality as deaths that occur 30 days or 180 days after hospital admission.[3] Furthermore, different investigators may use different definitions of risk to study the same outcome. Thus, the results of different studies may be difficult to compare. Moreover, Iezzoni and associates found that different severity of illness indicators predict in-hospital mortality with variable accuracy.[4]

Investigators can measure numerous outcomes, including mortality, complications of disease, complications of medical care, resource utilization, cost of care, quality of life, and functional status.[3] There are also numerous dimensions of risk to consider.[3] Examples include age, gender, principal diagnosis, comorbid diagnoses, severity of underlying diseases, clinical stability, functional stability, socioeconomic factors, and patient preferences for outcomes.[3]

This chapter examines some of the common or important areas in which investigators may adjust for severity of illness, although this is not a comprehensive review. Rather, it briefly reviews severity adjusters from two points of view. First, some methods used to adjust for the severity of diseases or procedures involving specific organ systems will be reviewed, discussing both infectious diseases and non-infectious diseases. Second, severity adjustment schemes that have been tested for all diseases will be examined. The commercially available systems are in the latter category. Selected references have been included for individuals who will use these scoring systems and need more information.

Stratification for Severity Within a Disease Group

Cardiac Disease

Functional Classification

The New York Heart Association (NYHA) scoring system is the most widely used method for predicting the functional status of patients with heart disease (Table 17-1).[5] However, some consider the newer classification system developed by the Canadian Cardiovascular Society (CCS) to be superior (Table 17-2).[6] More recently, Goldman et al developed a more specific and sensitive system, the Specific Activity Scale (SAS) (Table 17-3).[7]

Goldman et al compared the three scoring systems for reproducibility (defined as interobserver agreement or disagreement on the assessment of functional class) and validity (defined as agreement or disagreement on the functional classification estimates with the patient's true functional class determined by objective exercise test).[7] They found that the reproducibility of the NYHA, CCS, and SAS systems was 56%, 73%, and 73%, respectively; and that the validity was 51%, 59%, and 68%, respectively. A scoring system based on medical history will not be perfectly reproducible or valid because the way questions are asked will vary and

TABLE 17-1

NEW YORK HEART ASSOCIATION CLASSIFICATION FOR SEVERITY OF CARDIAC DISEASE

- Class I: Patients with cardiac disease but without resulting limitations of physical activity. Ordinary physical activity does not cause undue fatigue, palpitation, dyspnea, or anginal pain.

- Class II: Patients with cardiac disease resulting in slight limitation of physical activity. They are comfortable at rest. Ordinary physical activity results in fatigue, palpitation, dyspnea, or anginal pain.

- Class III: Patients with cardiac disease resulting in marked limitation of physical activity. They are comfortable at rest. Less than ordinary physical activity causes fatigue, palpitation, dyspnea, or anginal pain.

- Class IV: Patients with cardiac disease resulting in inability to carry on any physical activity without discomfort. Symptoms of cardiac insufficiency or of the anginal syndrome may be present even at rest. If any physical activity is undertaken, discomfort is increased.

TABLE 17-2

CANADIAN CARDIOVASCULAR SOCIETY CLASSIFICATION FOR SEVERITY OF CARDIAC DISEASE

- Class I: Ordinary physical activity, such as walking and climbing stairs, does not cause angina. Angina with strenuous or rapid or prolonged exertion at work or recreation.

- Class II: Slight limitation of ordinary activity. Walking or climbing stairs rapidly, walking uphill, walking or stair climbing after meals, or in cold, or in wind, or under emotional stress, or only during the few hours after awakening. Walking more than two blocks on the level and climbing more than one flight of ordinary stairs at a normal pace and in normal conditions.

- Class III: Marked limitation of ordinary physical activity. Walking one to two blocks on the level and climbing one flight of stairs in normal conditions and at normal pace.

- Class IV: Inability to carry on any physical activity without discomfort — anginal syndrome may be present at rest.

because some patients give contrary responses to repeated questions. Even responses that are reproducible do not always predict the patient's response to the exercise test accurately.

Angioplasty Risk

Bergelson analyzed risk factors for hemodynamic compromise during percutaneous transluminal coronary angioplasty (PTCA).[8] They examined three factors. Left ventricular ejection fraction less than 35% was 13% sensitive and 95% specific. Greater than 50% of the myocardium at risk was associated with a sensitivity of 31% and a specificity of 85%. The angiographer's subjective assessment of which patients were at high risk for hemodynamic compromise had the highest sensitivity (56%) and a specificity of 86%. Because the sensitivity of the three factors was low, the investigators performed a multivariate analysis of 28 variables and found that multivessel disease, diffuse disease, percent myocardium at risk, and stenosis before PTCA independently

predicted which patients developed hemodynamic compromise. They used the regression coefficients to develop a 13-point weighted scoring system (Table 17-4).

The authors validated their scoring system in another population. In this study, they defined patients at high risk of hemodynamic compromise as those with scores of 4 or greater. The sensitivity and specificity of this scoring system were both 92%. Ryan et al have also published additional data on risk factors for complications during PTCA.[9]

Cardiac Surgery Mortality Risk

O'Connor and associates used logistic regression analysis to predict in-hospital mortality following coronary artery bypass graft surgery (CABG).[10] The following variables were significantly associated with in-hospital death: age, gender, body surface area, presence of comorbid disease as identified by the Charlson comorbid index, history of CABG, left ventricular end-diastolic pressure, ejection fraction score, and priority of

TABLE 17-3
SPECIFIC ACTIVITY SCALE CLASSIFICATION FOR SEVERITY OF CARDIAC DISEASE

	Yes	No
1. Can you walk down a flight of steps without stopping? (4.5-5.2 mets*)	Go to #2	Go to #4
2. Can you carry anything up a flight of steps without stopping (5-5.55 mets) or can you:	Go to #3	Class III
(a) have sexual intercourse without stopping (5-5.5 mets)		
(b) garden, rake, weed (5.6 mets)		
(c) roller skate, dance the fox-trot (5-6 mets)		
(d) walk at a 4 miles-per-hour rate on level ground (5-6 mets)		
3. Can you carry at least 24 pounds up 8 steps or can you:	Class I	Class II
(a) carry objects that are at least 80 pounds (8 mets)		
(b) do outdoor work—shovel snow, spade soil (7 mets)		
(c) do recreational activities such as skiing, basketball, touch football, squash, handball (7-10 mets).		
(d) jog/walk 5 miles per hour (9 mets)		
4. Can you shower without stopping (3.6-4.2 mets) or can you:	Class III	Go to #5
(a) strip and make bed (3.9-5 mets)		
(b) mop floors (4.2 mets)		
(c) hang washed clothes (4.4 mets)		
(d) clean windows (3.7 mets)		
(e) walk 2.5 miles per hour (3-3.5 mets)		
(f) bowl (3-4.4 mets)		
(g) play golf (walk and carry clubs) (4.5 mets)		
(h) push power lawn mower (4 mets)		
5. Can you dress without stopping because of symptoms? (2-2.3 mets)	Class III	Class IV

Mets = metabolic equivalents of activity.

surgery. The degree of left main coronary artery stenosis and the number of diseased coronary vessels did not improve the model's ability to predict death. For the entire study population, the area under the receiver operator curve (ROC) was 0.76, indicating that the observed and expected mortality were highly correlated. The ROCs for a few subgroups were not as high as that for the whole group. Persons interested in learning more about ROCs are encouraged to read the article by O'Connor and colleagues.[10]

In New York, a lawsuit mandated that the state disseminate to hospitals and the public reports describing hospital-specific and physician-specific outcomes after CABG.[11] Many leading cardiologists and cardiac surgeons in New York supported the program. Healthcare institutions and physicians increased their efforts to improve quality measures after the surgeon-specific mortality data were published. Some hospitals identified emergency cases as a subgroup with particularly poor outcomes and changed the processes of care to better stabilize the patients before surgery. Other hospitals altered referral patterns to funnel the most difficult cases to surgeons with the best results. Hospitals also stopped referring patients to surgeons who performed too few operations or had consistently poor results. Subsequently, risk-adjusted mortality after CABG decreased by 41%, from 4.17% in 1989 to 2.45% in 1992.

Infectious Diseases

Surgical Site Infections

Altemeier and colleagues popularized the first method for predicting the risk of a surgical site infection. These investigators classified wounds as clean, clean-contaminated, contaminated, and dirty or infected and they documented that the wound infection rate increased as the level of wound contamination increased.[12] In the 1970s, researchers conducting the Study on the Efficacy of Nosocomial Infection Control (SENIC) analyzed risk factors for surgical site infections. They used stepwise multiple logistic regression to develop a more sophisticated method for predicting the risk of surgical site infection.[13] The clinician could calculate the patient's risk of wound infection by adding one point for each of the following factors:

- Abdominal operations.
- Operations lasting longer than 2 hours.
- Wounds classified by the traditional method as contaminated, dirty, or infected.
- Patients having three or more different underlying diagnoses at discharge.

Although the average surgical site infection rate increased stepwise from 2.9% for clean to 12.6% for dirty wounds, the SENIC investigators noted a wide range of infection rates within each category: 1.1% to 15.8% for patients with clean wounds, 0.6% to 17.7% for patients with clean-contaminated wounds, 4.5% to 23.9% for patients with contaminated wounds, and 6.7% to 27.4% for patients with dirty wounds.

In the early 1990s, investigators from the Centers for Disease Control (CDC) developed a new composite risk index, the Surgical Site Infection Risk Index, that included three risk fac-

TABLE 17-4

WEIGHTED SCORING SYSTEM TO PREDICT WHICH PATIENTS WILL DEVELOP HEMODYNAMIC COMPROMISE DURING PTCA*

Angiographic Characteristic	Score
Myocardium at risk (%)	
6-14	-2
15-23	-1
24-32	0
33-41	1
42-50	2
51-59	3
60-69	4
Multivessel disease	3
Pre-PTCA stenosis (%)	
50-57	3
58-65	2
66-73	1
74-81	0
82-89	-1
90-97	-2
98-100	-3
Diffuse disease	3

PTCA = percutaneous transluminal coronary angioplasty.

tors.[14] Clinicians could calculate the patient's risk of surgical site infection by adding one point for each of the following risk factors:

- American Society of Anesthesiology (ASA) score of 3, 4, or 5.
- Duration beyond the procedure-specific cutpoint (T-time).
- Wounds classified by the traditional method as contaminated, dirty, or infected.

These researchers noted that surgical site infection rates doubled for each additional point in the risk index. The infection rate varied from 1.5% when no risk factors were present to 13.0% when all three risk factors were present. The infection rates within each risk level did not vary substantially.

Ventilator-Associated Pneumonia

Kollef studied risk factors for ventilator-associated pneumonia (VAP) and its associated mortality.[15] He found four factors that were independently associated with VAP: an organ system failure index of 3 or greater, age 60 years or older, prior antibiotic administration, and supine head position during the first 24 hours of mechanical ventilation. Mortality from VAP was associated with an organ system failure index of 3 or greater, a premorbid lifestyle score of 2 or greater, and supine head position during the first 24 hours of mechanical ventilation.

Community-Acquired Pneumonia

Researchers have identified a number of factors that predict death from pneumonia, for example, advanced age, absence of chest pain, tachypnea, diastolic hypotension, confusion, elevated blood urea nitrogen, leukocytosis, and leukopenia.[16] Other investigators have noted that several factors predict a complicated course of pneumonia: age 65 years or older, a comorbid illness, temperature above 38°C, immunosuppression, and nontypical etiologic agents.[17] Chassin and associates developed an index, which includes six factors, to predict the likelihood of death from pneumonia: patient age older than 65 years, chest pain on inspiration, a vital sign abnormality, altered mental status, neoplastic disease, and the etiologic agent.[18] Subsequently, Pine et al examined whether severity of illness explained differences in mean length of stay for pneumonia at four hospitals.[19] The individual hospital means were 9.3, 12.1, 9.1, and 6.6 days. Chassin and associates' pneumonia prognostic index accounted for 7% of the variation in length of stay, eight other patient variables explained another 7% of the variation, and 86% of the variation was unexplained. The

authors surmised that physicians' practice patterns and hospital factors may have accounted for much of the remaining variation.

Sepsis

Many investigators have identified factors that are associated with survival following sepsis and have developed models to predict survival.[20,21] Despite these sophisticated efforts, McCabe and Jackson's simple method for assessing the risk of death associated with sepsis is the most generally accepted method.[21] McCabe and Jackson predicted that underlying host illness determined survival following Gram-negative sepsis. They divided cases into those with nonfatal (NF), ultimately fatal (UF), and rapidly fatal (RF) underlying disease. The worse the underlying disease category, the higher the predicted mortality. Setia and Gross used the McCabe and Jackson criteria to stratify mortality from Gram-negative sepsis and Gram-positive sepsis.[21] They noted that the mortality for patients with Gram-negative sepsis increased from 13% for patients with nonfatal diseases to 42% and 82%, respectively, for patients with ultimately fatal and rapidly fatal diseases. Mortality rates for Gram-positive sepsis within each category were even higher than those noted for Gram-negative sepsis: 37% for nonfatal diseases, 56% for ultimately fatal diseases, and 100% for rapidly fatal diseases.

The McCabe and Jackson classification has been very useful. However, researchers need more refined prognostic instruments to assess accurately whether the new cytokines and monoclonal antibodies affect the course of the sepsis syndrome and decrease its associated mortality.

AIDS Outcome Prediction Tools

The commonly used case definitions and other classification systems such as those from the CDC (Table 17-5) and Walter Reed Medical Center

TABLE 17-5
CDC 1993 REVISED CLASSIFICATION SYSTEM FOR HIV INFECTION

CD4 Cell Count X 10⁹/L	Asymptomatic, Acute HIV or PGL	Symptomatic, but not A or C	AIDS Conditions
>0.50	A1	B1	C1
0.20-0.49	A2	B2	C2
<0.20	A3	B3	C3

CDC = Centers for Disease Control and Prevention; HIV = human immunodeficiency virus; PGL = persistent generalized lymphadenopathy.

TABLE 17-6
WALTER REED STAGING CLASSIFICATION FOR HIV INFECTION*

Stage	HIV Antibody or Virus Detected	Chronic Adenopathy	CD4 Cells/mm³	DHS	Oral Thrush	OI
WR0	-	-	>400	NL	-	-
WR1	+	-	>400	NL	-	-
WR2	+	±	>400	NL	-	-
WR3	+	±	<400	NL	-	-
WR4	+	±	<400	P	-	-
WR5	+	±	<400	C	+	-
WR6	+	±	<400	P/C	+	+

DHS = delayed hypersensitivity; NL = normal; OI = opportunistic infections; P = partial; C = complete.

(Table 17-6) do not include disease severity and do not account for functional status.[22] Furthermore, the CDC's classification system is not intended for prognostic purposes, and the Walter Reed system excludes a proportion of the HIV-infected patient population such as men who had CD4 counts that were greater than 400 and who were anergic.[23,24] Researchers have developed illness severity scales, which have varying degrees of complexity, to predict the likelihood of progression to AIDS and of mortality. For example, the proportion of patients who progress to AIDS within 4 years increases as the CD4 count decreases (Table 17-7). Rabeneck and Wray added clinical parameters and assigned numerical scores to three factors:

- Thrush present (1 point).
- Night sweats present (1 point).
- CD4 count 0.5 × 10⁹/L (0 points), 0.50 to 0.20 (1 point), and <0.20 (2 points).[22]

Using this scoring system, they described three stages of HIV infection in which the risk of progression to AIDS varied significantly (Table 17-8). In addition, the World Health Organization used clinical findings, laboratory data, and functional status to develop a complex method for predicting mortality in AIDS patients.

Some of these systems have important deficiencies. For example, some investigators failed to include the 95% confidence intervals for their scoring systems. Other investigators did not demonstrate that the risk factors included in the scores were independently associated with the out-

TABLE 17-7
4-YEAR CUMULATIVE AIDS INCIDENCE

CD4 Cell Count X 10⁹/L	Percent
>0.40	18
0.30-0.39	25
0.20-0.29	41
<0.20	84

TABLE 17-8
PROPORTION OF HIV-INFECTED PATIENTS PROGRESSING TO AIDS IN 3-YEAR PERIOD[18]

Stage	Point Score	Percent
I	0	15
II	1-2	29
III	3-4	55

come of interest. Furthermore, no one has compared these systems.

Cancer

Colorectal Cancer

Dukes described the most frequently used staging system for colorectal cancer. Kirklin, Astler, and Coller and others subsequently modified Dukes' staging system (Table 17-9).[25] As most recurrences of colorectal cancer appear within 3 to 4 years, the 5-year survival rate estimates the cure rate. Although the death rate has remained constant, the 5-year survival rate for colorectal cancer has improved in recent decades (see Table 17-9). This difference may be due to more meticulous staging at the time of surgery.

Lung Cancer

The TNM staging system describes the anatomic features of lung cancer: T for primary tumor, N for lymph nodes, and M for metastases. The TNM staging system graded tumors as I, for localized; II, for regional spread; or III, for distant spread. However, Feinstein and Wells found that adding clinical severity scores, which included designated signs and symptoms of disease, increased the accuracy of their ability to predict survival and response to different forms of therapy.[26] These investigators observed a consistent prognostic gradient based on clinical severity.

Other

Pancreatitis Risk Adjusters

Ranson and associates developed criteria for predicting mortality associated with pancreatitis and for predicting whether pancreatitis would be complicated by pancreatic abscess.[27] The Ranson criteria were designed to help clinicians predict, within the first 48 hours after admission, whether the patient would die in the hospital (Table 17-10).[28] Clinicians could apply these criteria on admission or within the first 48 hours after admission. Mortality increased as the number of risk factors increased. Less than 1% of patients with one to two risk factors died compared with 15% of those with three to four risk factors and 100% of those with six to seven risk factors.

Severity of Illness Indicators for All Disease Groups

In 1986, the US Congress mandated that Medicare incorporate severity of illness and case-mix adjusting methods into its prospective payment system that is based on diagnosis-related groups (DRGs). Investigators thought that one third of the variation in the average cost per case under DRGs could be explained by severity of illness and case mix. Hence, the mandate to develop an accurate system for characterizing case-mix and severity.

Comorbidity Indicatorc

Comorbidity is an important predictor of outcome that is independent of the disease stage. This association is clearly shown in a study of survival among women with primary breast cancer.[29]

TABLE 17-9
STAGING SYSTEM FOR COLORECTAL CANCER

Stage	Description	5-Year Survival % (1940s and 1950s)	5-Year Survival % (1960s and 1970s)
A	Infiltration only to submucosa	80	>90
B1	Infiltration of muscularis	60	85
B2	Extension through colonic wall	45	70-75
C1	Infiltration of muscularis*	15-30 (C1&C2)	35-65 (C1&C2)
C2	Extension through colonic wall*		
D	Distant metastases*	<5	<5

*With lymph node involvement.

Comorbidity indices, in general, are simpler to use than the commercial systems that are described below. However, investigators often overlook comorbidity indices when they risk adjust their data. Rohrer has described an approach to developing a risk-adjusting system.[30] Tobacman reviewed 11 different studies that describe methods by which comorbidities have been defined, scored, and validated.[31] The studies evaluated various outcomes including mortality, length of hospital stay, development of complications, and resource use. Tobacman noted that the investigators awarded points indifferently. Some awarded points for the total number of comorbid conditions; others awarded a specific number of points for individual comorbid diseases.

Physiologic Indicators

The simplified acute physiology score (SAPS II) includes 12 physiologic variables (heart rate, systolic blood pressure, temperature, PaO_2/FiO_2, urine output, serum levels of urea nitrogen, potassium, sodium, bicarbonate, bilirubin, Glasgow Coma Score, and white blood cell count), age, type of admission (scheduled surgical, unscheduled surgical, or medical), and three underlying disease variables (acquired immunodeficiency syndrome, metastatic cancer, and hematologic malignancy).

SAPS II can be used to estimate the risk of death regardless of the primary diagnosis. LeGall and colleagues have proposed that investigators use SAPS II to evaluate the efficiency of care in intensive care units.[32]

Commercial Systems

Diagnosis-Related Groups (DRGs)

DRGs have been modified substantially over the years and now incorporate adjustments for severity of illness through an expanded number of DRGs.[33] In addition, comorbidities and complications have been added for many DRGs. Moreover, formal checks of ICD-9 coding have improved the accuracy of these data. Thus, if used correctly, the International Classification of Diseases, 9th revision, Clinical Modification (ICD-9-CM) can estimate the severity of illness.

APACHE (Acute Physiology, Age, and Chronic Health Evaluation)

Knaus and Wagner developed the APACHE to predict the intensity of service and likelihood of death in an intensive care unit (ICU).[34] They revised the original version in 1985 and produced the popular APACHE II, in which the final score is the sum of scores in the three eponymous cate-

TABLE 17-10
CRITERIA FOR ASSESSING RISK OF DEATH

Pancreatitis Not Due to Gallstones

On admission:

Age >55 years

White-cell count >16,000/mm³

Glucose >200 mg/dL

Lactic dehydrogenase >350 U/L

Aspartate aminotransferase >250 U/L

Within 48 hours of hospitalization:

Decrease in hematocrit >10 points

Increase in blood urea nitrogen >5 mg/dL

Serum calcium <8 mg/dL

Partial pressure of oxygen <60 mm Hg

Base deficit >4 mmol/L

Fluid deficit >6 L

Gallstone-Induced Pancreatitis

On admission:

Age >70 years

White-cell count >18,000/mm³

Glucose >220 mg/dL

Lactic dehydrogenase >400 U/L

Aspartate aminotransferase >250 U/L

Within 48 hours of hospitalization:

Decrease in hematocrit >10 points

Increase in blood urea nitrogen >2 mg/dL

Serum calcium <8 mg/dL

Base deficit >5 mmol/L

Fluid deficit >4 L

gories. Up to 60 points come from the acute physiologic measurements: pulse rate, mean blood pressure, temperature, respiratory rate, PaO_2 or $P(A-a)O_2$, hematocrit, white blood cell count, creatinine with or without renal failure, sodium, potassium, arterial pH, and Glasgow coma score. Relative age contributes up to six points, and chronic health status contributes up to five points. Although the highest possible score is 71, most

scores are below 30 because the relative disability in each category determines the score.

Because the APACHE II score uses primarily physiologic variables, some authors developed a simplified physiologic score (SAPS, described above) that includes age, acute physiologic signs, and mechanical ventilation needs.[35] Others have developed and tested further variations on APACHE.[36] Knaus and Wagner and other researchers have validated APACHE II in ICUs; other investigators have evaluated its use in units other than ICUs. Some researchers have found APACHE II to be useful, but others found that it predicted survival in the ICU no better than did the clinicians caring for the patients.[37] Some investigators have stated that APACHE II's predictive accuracy is diminished because the score does not include disease-specific factors.

To address these concerns, an expanded team of developers updated all scoring system components and provided more disease categories to create APACHE III.[38] The team added physiologic variables, gave more weight to extreme physiologic values, accounted for interactions among some of the physiologic variables (eg, serum creatinine and urine output), modified the Glasgow coma scoring, and included coefficients for up to 78 major disease categories in the final risk equation. Specific diseases affect the score most when it falls between 20 and 140. In this most recent version, the score can go up to 299, but the mean score in a large study population was 50.[39] Of the 299 points, up to 192 come from physiologic variables, 12 from acid-base disturbances, 48 from the Glasgow coma score, 24 from age, and 23 from seven comorbid conditions that are statistically associated with death. In the first 24 hours after admission, ICU staff can calculate the probability that adult patients in medical and surgical ICUs will die in the hospital. Staff can update the prediction thereafter. The APACHE III developers studied its reliability,[39] and other researchers have reviewed the ethical problems of using probability estimates of mortality risk for medical decision making.[40]

MedisGroups (Medical Illness Severity Grouping System)

The original developers of the system, Brewster and Karlin, based it on a list of key clinical findings (KCFs).[41] They assigned each KCF a score between 0 and 3 based on the likelihood of organ failure resulting from that KCF. The following are examples of KCF scores:

- A history of diabetes and a potassium level above 2.4 meq/L are both assigned a score of 0.
- A defect on a ventilation perfusion scan and a temperature above 101°F are both assigned a score of 1.
- Spinal cord obstruction documented on myelogram and a potassium level above 6.9 meq/L are both assigned a score of 2.
- Coma and a systolic blood pressure of <60 mm Hg are both assigned a score of 3.

To calculate a patient's score, a clinician or an investigator must review the patient's medical record for 260 different KCFs, although, on average, patients will have only 5 to 10 KCFs. On admission, staff can assign patients to an admission severity group based on data collected in the first 48 hours. Between the third and seventh hospital day, staff can classify a patient's status further as nonmorbid, morbid, or major morbid.

Despite the complexity of the MedisGroups admission scoring, it explains only 3% of costs not accounted for by DRGs.[42] MedisGroups is widely used despite this limitation and despite the high cost of collecting the required data. In addition, the MedisGroups Comparative Hospital Database, which comprises more than 60 million severity-adjusted patient records, has been used to compare rates among physicians and hospitals and to study morbidity, mortality, length of stay, and changes in various severity-adjusted expected rates. However,

Iezzoni suggests that this database is not sufficiently refined to predict mortality or to assess quality of care.[43]

Computerized Severity Index (CSI)

Susan Horn and her colleagues at The Johns Hopkins University developed the Severity of Illness Index to explain variation in resource use that was not explained by DRGs. Their initial index, the Severity of Illness Index, evaluated principal diagnoses, complications, comorbidities, dependency on nursing and ancillary staff, nonoperative procedures, treatment response, and residual disease at discharge. These investigators subsequently simplified the index and developed a computerized scoring method. The new index, called CSI, evaluates only the principal diagnoses, complications, and comorbidities, because the additional dimensions of care accounted for little variation.[44,45]

The CSI system adds a sixth digit to the five digit ICD-9-CM diagnostic code. This sixth digit records illness severity on a scale of 1 to 5, in which 5 represents death. Staff can calculate the score at admission or discharge, or can calculate a maximum (ie, the highest score for the admission). The developers found that the same level of a single clinical factor (ie, signs and symptoms of disease, or laboratory and radiographic findings) may signify different severity of illness in different settings. For example, pneumonia with fever of 102°F is scored as a 2 in a normal host, but as a 3 in an immunocompromised host.

The developers have conducted several validation studies. When they studied differences between resource use as predicted by DRGs and actual resource use, they found that CSI explained most differences of more than $10,000. When they studied variation in length of stay, the maximum CSI score at 7 days explained the greatest variation. Moreover, the admission CSI score predicted death better than the method used by the Health Care Financing Administration (HCFA) to predict death.

Disease Staging

Gonella and associates[46] based this severity scoring system on the oncology staging concept. They defined four stages:

1. Disease with no complications or a problem of minimal severity.
2. Disease with local complications (ie, limited to an organ or system) or a problem of moderate severity.
3. Disease with numerous, systemic complications or a problem of extreme severity.
4. Death.

Within each stage, substages are designated by a number to the right of the decimal point. For example, simple appendicitis would be stage 1.0, appendicitis with perforation causing localized peritonitis and/or peritoneal abscess would be stage 2.1, and appendicitis with perforation causing generalized peritonitis would be stage 2.2.

With more than one ICD-9-CM code, a Disease Staging Unrelated Comorbidity Algorithm is used to convert them to a smaller number of Staging Disease Categories. The initial format uses the required extraction of data from the medical record and is called Clinical Staging. The latter format uses the computerized Uniform Hospital Discharge Data Set (UHDDS) and is called Coded Staging. Gonella et al validated the concept that increasing severity of illness increases the length of hospital stay.[47]

Coding staging has been modified and is currently marketed by Health Care Investment Analyst (HCIA). They also sell The Guide to Hospital Performance, which catalogues hospital pricing policies, lengths of stay, and other utilization patterns, as well as risk-adjusted mortality rates for over 5,600 hospitals in the United States.[48] Independent reviewers have not evaluated the usefulness of these products.

Patient Management Categories (PMCs)

Wanda Young and associates, now located at the Pittsburgh Research Institute, developed this system to replace DRGs.[49] They designed it to compare use of resources and cost of treating similar patients with similar diagnoses at the same hospital or different hospitals. Using PMC software, staff download a UHDDS abstract to assign a patient to one or more PMCs. The developers designated patient management paths for the diagnostic and treatment services required for each PMC, and they assigned relative cost weights for services ordered by physicians. The system is marketed as useful for quality improvement programs, but the developers have conducted most of the published studies.

Acuity Index Method

Mohlenbrock and colleagues developed the Acuity Index Method (AIM) scoring system and Iameter of San Mateo, California, now markets the AIM. It uses information from the UHDDS and derives an acuity rating or severity score between 1 (least ill) to 5 (most ill) for each DRG. Using a database comprising 30 million cases, they calculated normative severity-adjusted values for all DRGs that can be used as benchmarks for length of stay, charges, and mortality. The acuity index method has been used in a few metropolitan areas to compare performance among hospitals.[50]

Other Severity Scoring Systems

Many other scoring systems are available, including the Medicare Mortality Predictor System, the Refinement Grouper Number, Body Systems Count, Trauma Score, Nursing Intensity, and Therapeutic Intervention Scoring System. These scoring systems have been discussed elsewhere.[33,51]

Comparison of Severity Scoring Systems

Developers and vendors have prepared most of the reports on the validity of the commercial severity scoring systems. Few independent investigators have assessed or compared these products.[33] Thomas and Ashcraft compared APACHE II, MedisGroups, CSI, Coded Disease Staging, PMCs, and AIM to assess the ability of the systems to explain variations in costs not explained by an early DRG system.[52] The researchers divided the six systems into those that used data from the discharge abstract (ie, Disease Staging, PMCs, AIM) and those that required additional clinical data beyond that in the discharge abstract (ie, APACHE II, MedisGroups, and CSI). Relative performance of all six systems varied greatly across adjacent DRG groups. Scoring systems that provided a maximum (Max.) score (ie, Max. MedisGroups and Max. CSI) explained more cost variation than systems scored at the time of hospital admission (Adm.) (ie, Adm. MedisGroups, Adm. CSI, and Adm. APACHE II). Two systems based on the discharge abstract (ie, Disease Staging and PMCs) fell in between; they explained cost variation better than the admission scores but worse than the maximum scores.

Mackenzie and colleagues reviewed several severity scoring systems.[53] All systems predicted cost more accurately than did DRGs. The Refined Grouper Number (RGN) for DRGs, however, was the best and most efficient because it was based on the automated discharge abstract. APACHE, MedisGroups, CSI, and RGN predicted death at 30 and 60 days post discharge most accurately. All systems improved hospital payments by anywhere from <5% to >15%.

The time required to calculate a score with each of the systems correlates with the clinical data that has to be extracted from the medical record beyond that which appears in the automated discharge abstract. Systems that use additional clinical data require 5 to 30 more minutes per chart.

It is difficult to say which systems are best for assessing the quality of care. Again, they have not been compared side-by-side for this purpose. HCFA is collecting the Uniform Clinical Data Set (UCDS) to assess the quality of care in America's hospitals. Some states have mandated that hospitals use a severity scoring system to assess quality. Iezzoni and associates used CSI and MedisGroups to assess the

quality of care following acute myocardial infarction and coronary artery bypass graft surgery.[54] They identified a worsening condition when the maximum severity score exceeded the admission severity score, and they identified substandard care by explicit and implicit criteria. With CSI, 49% of the patients who worsened had 71% of the potentially substandard care. With MedisGroups, 35% of the patients who worsened had 71% of the potentially substandard care. Moreover, Hayward et al have questioned the value of implicit review itself.[55] In short, general statements cannot be made regarding the usefulness of these scoring systems.

In summary, we may be focusing excessively on severity of illness. While it no doubt explains a part of variation in cost and quality, other factors may be even more critical, including small area variation. Small area variation is the term used to describe the wide variation in costs or utilization rates found among healthcare delivery systems in different geographic areas.[56] For example, Wennberg found lower rates of hospital use in New Haven than in Boston. Other factors may also account for variation such as differences in physician practice patterns, difficulty in clinical management, inaccuracies in diagnostic coding, and recording errors in the medical record, to name only a few. For example, McMahon and Newbold, who used Disease Staging to evaluate variations in length of stay, found that physician practice patterns explained more of the variation in length of stay than did severity of illness.[57] Moreover, the latest versions of DRGs provide a more comprehensive assessment of illness severity and a more accurate estimate of resource use. Thus, groups most interested in cost may be able to use DRGs without adding further adjustments for severity of illness.

For the present and near future, investigators will use severity adjustment systems and risk adjustment models more to assess the quality of healthcare delivery than to analyze variations in cost. Insurance companies and other payers will select hospitals based on the lowest cost, while they will begin to look at severity and risk-adjusted outcomes as a surrogate of quality. They, however, cannot put too much faith in the outcomes data for quality assessment because they too realize that the science of evaluating the quality of care is in its infancy.

References

1. Shakespeare W. *Hamlet* III, 1,59.

2. Localio AR, Hamory BH, Sharp TJ, Weaver SL, TenHave TR, Landis JR. Comparing hospital mortality in adult patients with pneumonia: a case study of statistical methods in a managed care program. *Ann Intern Med.* 1995;122:125-132.

3. Iezzoni LI. Risk and outcomes & dimensions of risk. In Iezzoni LI, ed. *Risk Adjustment for Measuring Health Care Outcome.* Ann Arbor, Mich: Health Administration Press; 1994:1-118.

4. Iezzoni LI, Ash AS, Schwartz M, Daley J, Hughes JS, Mackiernan YD. Predicting who dies depends on how severity is measured: Implications for evaluating patient outcomes. *Ann Intern Med.* 1995;123:763-770.

5. The Criteria Committee of the New York Heart Association, Inc. *Diseases of the Heart and Blood Vessels; Nomenclature and Criteria for Diagnosis.* 6th ed. Boston, Mass: Little Brown; 1964.

6. Lemmedu DK, Kemp JW, Judkins HG Gosselin AJ, Killp T. Complications of coronary arteriography from the Collaborative Study of Coronary Artery Surgery (CASS). *Circulation.* 1979;59:11-15.

7. Goldman L, Hashimoto B, Cook FD, Loscalzo A. Comparative reproducibility and validity of systems for assessing cardiovascular functional class: advantages of a new specific activity scale. *Circulation.* 1981;64:1227-1234.

8. Bergelson BA, Jacobs AK, Cupples LA, et al. Prediction of risk for hemodynamic compromise during percutaneous transluminal coronary angioplasty. *Am J Cardiol.* 1992;70:1540-1545.

9. Ryan TJ, Baumn WB, Kennedy JW. ACC/AHA Task Force Report. Guidelines for percutaneous transluminal coronary angioplasty—a report of the American College of Cardiology/American Heart Association Task Force on Assessment of Diagnostic and Therapeutic Cardiovascular Procedures (Committee on Percutaneous Transluminal Coronary Angioplasty). *J Am Coll Cardiol.* 1993;22:2033-2052.

10. O'Connor GT, Plume SK, Olmstead EM, et al. Multivariate prediction of in-hospital mortality associated with coronary artery bypass graft surgery. In-hospital mortality and CABG. *Circulation.* 1992;85:2110-2118.

11. Hannan EL, Kilburn H, Racz M, Shields E, Chassin MR. Improving the outcomes of coronary artery bypass surgery in New York state. *JAMA.* 1994;271:761-766.

12. Altemeier WA, Burke JF, Pruitt BA, Sandusky WE, eds. *Manual on Control of Infection in Surgical Patients.* Philadelphia, Pa: JB Lippincott; 1976.

13. Haley RW, Culver DH, Morgan WM, et al. Identifying patients at high risk of surgical wound infection. A simple multivariate index of patient susceptibility and wound contamination. *Am J Epidemiol.* 1985;121:206-215.

14. Culver DH, Horan TC, Gaynes RP, et al. Surgical wound infection rates by wound class, operative procedure, and patient risk index. *Am J Med.* 1991;91(suppl 3B):152S-157S.

15. Kollef MH. Ventilator-associated pneumonia. A multivariate analysis. *JAMA.* 1993;270:1965-1970.

16. Marie TJ. Community-acquired pneumonia. *Clin Infect Dis.* 1994;18:501-515.

17. Fine MJ, Smith DN, Singer DE. Hospitalization decision in patients with community-acquired pneumonia: a prospective cohort study. *Am J Med.* 1990;89:713-721.

18. Chassin MR, Park RE, Lohr KN, et al. Differences among hospitals in Medicare patient mortality. *Health Serv Res.* 1989;24:1.

19. Fine MJ, Singer DE, Phelps AL, Hanusa BH, Kapoor WN. Differences in length of hospital stay in patients with community-acquired pneumonia: a prospective four-hospital study. *Med Care.* 1993;31:371-380.

20. McCabe WR, Jackson GG. Gram-negative bacteremia, II: clinical, laboratory and therapeutic observations. *Arch Intern Med.* 1962:110-856.

21. Setia U, Gross PA. Bacteremia in a community hospital. Spectrum and mortality. *Arch Intern Med.* 1977;137:1698-1701.

22. Rabeneck L, Wray NP. Predicting the outcomes of human immunodeficiency virus infection. *Arch Intern Med.* 1993;153:2749-2755.

23. Centers for Disease Control and Prevention. Revised classification system for HIV infection and expanded surveillance case definition for AIDS among adolescents and adults. *MMWR.* 1992;41(No. RR-17).

24. MacDonell KB, Chimel JS, Goldsmith J, et al. Prognostic usefulness of the Walter Reed staging classification for HIV infection. *J Acquir Immune Defic Syndr.*

1988;1:367-374.

25. Rubenstein E, Federman DD, eds. Gastrointestinal cancer. In: Mayer RJ, ed. *Scientific American Medicine*. New York, NY: Scientific American Medicine Inc; 1986;VIII:1-18.

26. Feinstein AR, Wells CK. A clinical-severity staging system for patients with lung cancer. *Medicine*. 1990;69:1-33.

27. Steinberg W, Tenner S. Acute pancreatitis. *N Engl J Med*. 1994;330:1198-1210.

28. Ranson JHC, Rifkind KM, Roses DF, Fink SD, Eng K, Spencer FC. Prognostic signs and the role of operative management in acute pancreatitis. *Surg Gynecol Obstet*. 1974;139:69-81.

29. Satariano WA, Ragland DR. The effect of comorbidity on 3-year survival of women with primary breast cancer. *Ann Intern Med*. 1994;120:104-110.

30. Tobacman JK. Assessment of comorbidity: a review. *Clinical Performance and Quality Health Care*. 1994;2:23-32.

31. Roher JE. Developing risk-adjusted monitoring systems: illustration of an approach. *Clinical Performance and Quality Health Care*. 1994;2:84-91.

32. LeGall JR, Lemeshow S, Saulnier F. A new simplified acute physiology score (SAPS II) based on a European/North American multicenter study. *JAMA*. 1993;270:2957-2964.

33. Gross PA. Use of severity of illness indices. In: Mayhall G, ed. *Hospital Epidemiology and Infection Control*. Baltimore, Md: Williams & Wilkins; 1996.

34. Knaus WA, Draper EA, Wagner DP, Zimmerman JE. APACHE II: a severity of disease classification system. *Crit Care Med*. 1985;9:591-597.

35. Moreau R, Soupison T, Vauquelin P, Derrida S, Beaucur H, Sicto C. Comparison of two simplified severity scores SAPS and APACHE (II) for patients with acute myocardial infarction. *Crit Care Med*. 1989;17:409-413.

36. McMahon LF, Hayward RA, Bernard AM, Rosevear JS, Weissfeld LA. Apache-L: A new severity of illness adjuster for impatient medical care. *Med Care*. 1992;30:445-452.

37. Kruse JA, Thil-Baharozian MC, Carlson RW. Comparison of clinical assessment with APACHE II for predicting mortality risk in patients admitted to a medical intensive care unit. *JAMA*. 1988;260:1739-1742.

38. Zimmerman JE, ed. APACHE III study design: analytic plan for evaluation of severity and outcome in intensive care units. *Crit Care Med*. 1988;17:169S-221S.

39. Knaus WA, Douglas PW, Draper EA, et al. Clinical investigations in critical care: the APACHE III prognostic system. Risk prediction of hospital mortality for critically ill hospitalized adults. *Chest*. 1991;100:1619-1636.

40. Knaus WA, Wagner DP, Lynn J. Short-term mortality predictions for critically ill hospitalized adults: science and ethics. *Science*. 1991;254:345-488.

41. Brewster AC, Karlin BG, Hyde LA, et al. MedisGroups: a clinically based approach to classifying hospital patients at admission. *Inquiry*. 1985;12:377-387.

42. Iezzoni LI, Ash AS, Cobb JL, Moskowitz MA. Admission Medis-Groups score and the cost of hospitalizations. *Med Care*. 1988;26:1068-1080.

43. Iezzoni LI, Hotchkin EK, Ash AS, Schwartz M, Mackiernan Y. MedisGroups data bases: the impact of data collection guidelines on predicting in-hospital mortality. *Med Care*. 1993;31:277-283.

44. Horn SD, Sharkey PD, Buckle JM, Backofen JE, Averill RF, Horn RA. The relationship between severity of illness and hospital length of stay and mortality. *Med Care*. 1991;29:305-317.

45. Averill RF, McGuire TE, Manning BE, Fowler DA, Horn SD, Dickson PS. A study of the relationship between severity of illness and hospital cost in New Jersey hospitals. *Health Services Research*. 1992;27:587-606.

46. Coffee RM, Goldfarb MKG. DRGs and disease staging for reimbursing Medicare patients. *Med Care*. 1986;24:814-829.

47. Gonnella JS, Hornbrook MC, Louis DZ. Staging of disease. A case-mix measurement. *JAMA*. 1984;251:637-646.

48. *The Guide to Hospital Performance*. Baltimore, Md: HCIA Inc; 1993.

49. Young WW, Macioce DP. Product line analyses using PMCs versus DRGs. *Public Budgeting & Fin Mngmt*. 1992;4:83-106.

50. Kenkel PJ. Projects serving up a data smorgasbord. *Modern Healthcare*. April 12, 1993.

51. Gross PA. Severity of illness and other confounders of quality measurement. In: Wenzel R, ed. *Assessing Quality Health Care: A Perspective for Clinicians*. Baltimore, Md: Williams & Wilkins; 1992:101-123.

52. Thomas JW, Ashcraft MLF. Measuring severity of illness: six severity systems and their ability to explain cost variations. *Inquiry*. 1991;28:39-55.

53. Patient classification systems: an evaluation of the state of the art. Vol 1. *Case Mix Research*. Kingston, Ontario: Queen's University; 1991.

54. Iezzoni LI, Hotchkin EK, Ash AS, Schwartz M, Mackiernan Y. MedisGroups databases: the impact of data collection guidelines on predicting in-hospital mortality. *Med Care*. 1993;31:277-283.

55. Hayward RA, McMahon LF, Bernard AM. Evaluating the care of general medicine inpatients: how good is implicit review? *Ann Intern Med*. 1993;118:550-556.

56. Wennberg JE. Future directions for small area variations. *Med Care*. 1993;31:YS75-YS80.

57. McMahon LF, Newbold R. Variation in resource use within diagnosis-related groups: the effect of severity of illness and physician practice. *Med Care*. 1986;24:388-397.

CHAPTER 18

Quantitative Epidemiology

Jonathan Freeman, MD, ScD

Abstract

We provide guidance for new practitioners in the vocabulary of modern epidemiology and the application of quantitative methods. Most hospital epidemiology involves surveillance (observational) data that were not part of a planned experiment, so the rubric and logic of controlled experimental studies cannot be applied. Forms of incidence and prevalence often are confused. The names "cohort study" and "case-control study" are unfortunate, as cohort studies rarely involve cohorts and case-control studies allow no active control by the investigator. Either type of study can be prospective or retrospective. Results of studies with discrete outcomes (infected or not, lived or died) often are represented best by a form of the risk ratio with 95% confidence intervals. The potential distorting effects of selection bias, misclassification and confounding need to be considered.

Introduction

Epidemiology is the study of the occurrence of illness in human populations. The logic and definitions in this chapter generally come from four sources, cited here in increasing order of difficulty.[1-4] Out of the confusion resulting from conflicts in traditional use, there recently has emerged a set of definitions that have specific mathematical formulations and interrelations.

Types of Epidemiologic Studies

All epidemiologic studies are described in terms of exposures and outcomes. In simple terms, the exposure is the putative "cause" under study, and the outcome is the disease or other event that may result from the exposure.

Experimental Studies or Intervention Trials

The closest we come to a standard experiment in bench biology is in the conduct of experimental studies. In bench biology, the experimenter has control of the process and can create controls for the experiment, which usually lack one ingredient or another. Similarly, in an experimental study, the investigator also can assign the exposure (or non-exposure) according to some scheme, such as randomization. During intervention trials, the experimenter can deal out the exposures in much the same way that a bench biologist allocates contrasting parts of an experiment to different vessels. The word "control" appropriately is used for a nonexposed vessel or subject in experimental studies. Experimental studies only occasionally are relevant to situations in the hospital. They are mentioned here for contrast to the more usual observational studies, in which the investigator is allowed only a relatively passive role. Surveillance data, thus, are observational data.

Nonexperimental or Observational Studies

During surveillance, we are not allowed to assign the exposures, so the epidemiologist is merely the professional witness to what happens. Patients, physicians, nurses, and random processes all play a part in assigning exposures in the hospital—only the hospital epidemiologist is left out. The major contrast between experimental studies and observational studies is simply that the experimenter has no control over who gets what in an observational study (eg, surveillance). For this reason, I will not use the word "control" in the remainder of this chapter; instead, I will use the terms "comparison subjects" or "referents" to remind readers that observers have no control over the assignment of exposure in observational studies.

The goal of observational studies is to simulate the results of an experiment, had one been possible, as in an "experiment of nature." John Snow's study of cholera in London is the most famous observational imitation of a community intervention trial, but even John Snow had no control over the water supply. In hospital epidemiology, we have many fewer subjects in a much more complicated situation, and the analogy to an experimental study becomes strained. I have put this notice up front to remind all of us that observational studies in epidemiology are only very distant relatives of experiments in bench biology. Observational studies are, however, the primary sources of information for hospital epidemiologists.

Cohort Studies

In a cohort, follow-up, or incidence study, the investigator compares the occurrence of a given outcome (usually a disease) in two or more groups of people who initially are free of the outcome and who differ in their exposure to a potential cause of the outcome. The investigator may select subjects randomly or according to exposure, but the crucial distinction here is that a cohort study is defined by the comparison of outcomes. The label is an unfortunate choice, because cohort studies usually do not use cohorts in the epidemiologic sense, such as birth cohorts. In old-fashioned terminology, cohort studies sometimes were called prospective studies, but this is misleading, as a cohort study may also be retrospective. *If one is comparing outcomes, one is doing a cohort study.*

What has not been specified is the timing of the cohort study. In a prospective cohort study, the investigator may enroll exposed and nonexposed subjects before the outcome is apparent. In a retrospective cohort study, the investigator may assemble subjects according to exposure, after the outcome already has taken place. It does not matter whether the study was conceived and carried out before or after the outcomes became apparent; if one is comparing outcomes, one is doing a cohort study. The primary advantages of the cohort study are its intuitive appeal and the fact that absolute population rates of exposure and outcome (disease) usually are available. That is, in a cohort study, one usually can observe the frequency of the exposures and the outcomes in a defined group, as well as the time course over which they occur. One can determine, for example, the absolute proportion of all patients admitted to a certain ward who had indwelling bladder catheters (the exposure) and those in whom, with or without a catheter, urinary tract infections developed (the outcome). The forms of the risk ratio (defined later) that arise from cohort studies are incidence density ratios or cumulative incidence ratios.

Case-Referent (Case-Control) Studies

The case-referent study has no real parallel in bench biology. Cases and noncases of a given outcome are entered into the study, and then compared for their exposures. If one is comparing exposures, one is doing a case-referent study. Note that the traditional name "case-control study" mistakenly implies that the investigator has some control over the process. This unfortunate name became commonplace before the important distinction between experimental studies and observational studies was recognized and before the total lack of control by the investigator was fully appreciated. In old-fashioned terminology, case-referent studies sometimes were called retrospective studies. However, this is misleading, because a case-referent study may be done prospectively. For example, we can plan to study some events that have not yet happened, such as the deaths in a community next year. If a disease is rare, a case-referent study is much more efficient and economical than a cohort study, because one may choose all or most of the cases of the rare disease. Even if a large cohort is available, it may be more economical to conduct a small case-referent study within the cohort. As such, a "nested" case-referent study may produce the same information as the larger cohort study at a fraction of the cost. To repeat, *if one is comparing exposures, one has a case-referent study*, and the form of the risk ratio (discussed later) that arises from the case-referent study is the exposure odds ratio. Under some conditions, the exposure odds ratio is identical to the incidence density ratio.

Cross-Sectional or Prevalence Studies

If an entire population is enrolled irrespective of exposure and outcome (disease), and if the exposure and outcome are ascertained at the same time in this population, then the study is cross-sectional. Depending on the nature of the population, a cross-sectional study may be analyzed as a cohort study or a case-referent study.

Definitions of Prospective and Retrospective

The above definitions have included the terms "prospective" and "retrospective," and these terms now will be defined. There still is not complete agreement on these definitions, but the most common functional definition of a prospective study is one in which the observer plans the study (and possibly records exposures) before the outcome is apparent. The sense of this schedule is that the observer cannot be influenced by an outcome that has not yet occurred. A case-referent study can be prospective in this sense, because one can plan now to enroll deaths and nondeaths from hospital discharges next year. A retrospective study, in contrast, is one in which the outcome has taken place already. Thus, a cohort study can be retrospective if one plans to study deaths that took place last year.

The word "retrospective" often has been used in a pejorative way in epidemiology, which is justified only sometimes. The crucial question in hospital epidemiology is "When does this distinction matter?" If one wants data on length of stay or death in the hospital, this information usually is available from the administration, with similar accuracy, no matter whether patients are followed prospectively or looked up years later. In contrast, if one wants data on the occurrence of nosocomial infection, medical records are notoriously incomplete in this regard. A retrospective record review might miss the majority of nosocomial infections, whereas continuous prospective surveillance at the bedside presumably would identify most nosocomial infections.

Measures of Disease Frequency

Measures of disease frequency arc of three general types: rates, proportions, and ratios. A rate has two different units in the numerator and denominator, as in 55 miles per hour or 20 first nosocomial infections per 1,000 observed patient-days. A rate can have any value from zero to infinity.

A proportion is a special type of ratio that often may be taken as a probability. The denominator of a proportion includes all individuals in the numerator or eligible to be in the numerator. A proportion is unitless, because it has the same units in the numerator and denominator, and has bounds of zero and unity. If 15% of patients in a certain group acquire nosocomial infections, this "attack rate" is the proportion, or probability 0.15. We speak of disease frequency when probabilities are applied to populations, but the same probability applied to an individual is called a risk.

All proportions also are ratios, but not all ratios are proportions. There also are ratios, similar to betting odds, that are used to approximate proportions. Odds have a numerator with a given attribute and a denominator without the attribute, but do not contain a quantity that includes the sum of all individuals. Odds also are unitless, but have bounds of zero and infinity. Odds are not used alone in epidemiology, but they appear in ratios, as will be described later. The textbook by Fleiss is the classic reference on rates and proportions.[5]

Measures of Incidence

Incidence measures the number of new disease onsets or incident cases during a time period. The interval may be explicit or implied, but time is an essential feature of incidence, because time determines how rare an event really is. We all have one death per lifetime; it may be unavoidable, but it matters very much just when that death occurs.

Incidence Density (Incidence Rate)

Incidence density is the number of new events (disease onsets) in a specified quantity of person-time (hospital days) in the population at risk. Incidence density usually is restricted to first events, for example, first nosocomial infections. It is standard to consider only first events, for second events (second infections or second malignancies) are not statistically independent from

first events in the same individuals.[1-3] All those who have not yet suffered a first event compose the population at risk. After a patient acquires a first nosocomial infection, that patient then is withdrawn and would not be a part of the population still at risk for a first event. Each patient who never acquired a nosocomial event would contribute all hospital days to the pool of days at risk for a first event, but a patient who became infected would contribute only those hospital days before the onset of the infection.

$$\textbf{Incidence Density} = \frac{\textbf{Number of First Events}}{\substack{\textbf{Observed Time at} \\ \textbf{Risk for a First Event}^{1\text{-}4}}}$$

Because the number of first events is just a number, incidence density has the unlikely units of events divided by time (1/time), which makes the interpretation less than intuitive. Incidence density is the instantaneous rate of change, or what used to be called the force of morbidity. For convenience in hospital epidemiology, nosocomial infection rates usually are expressed as the number of first events in 1,000 hospital days, because this usually produces a small single- or double-digit number.

The basic value of this measure can be seen when comparing nosocomial infection rates in short-stay patients versus long-stay patients, or infection rates with peripheral venous catheters versus Hickman catheters. When the time at risk in one group is tenfold the time at risk in another, the incidence density, or risk per day, is the most convenient way to correct for time and, thus, separate the effect of time (duration of exposure) from the effect of daily risk.

Incidence Density When There Are Multiple Events in the Same Individual

Every study that has looked at multiple nosocomial infections in the same individual has found that patients with a first event are more likely to suffer a second, indicating that multiple infections in the same patients are not statistically independent.[6-10] For quantitative analyses, these nonindependent events cannot simply be summed and placed over a denominator. Furthermore, a first nosocomial infection itself becomes a risk factor for a second, and risk factors for multiple infections are different from the risk factors for a first infection. The most common way to cope with multiple incident events in the same individual is to restrict quantitative analyses to first events.

If one desires to include both first events and multiple events in a study, then multiple events and the time the patient spends at risk for each of these multiple events must be enumerated separately and kept in a separate stratum.[10-12] The risk per day for multiple events generally will be much higher than the risk per day for first events.[10,12] I will describe later the manner in which data from different strata (first events over time at risk for first events, second events over time at risk for second events) can be combined.

Cumulative Incidence

A more intuitive measure is the cumulative incidence or the proportion of all those at risk who ultimately suffered a first event. In infectious disease epidemiology, this traditionally has been termed the "attack rate." Note that an attack rate is a proportion, not a rate. Cumulative incidence is derived from incidence density and may be thought of as the sum of all of the incidence densities for first events over all of the person-time at risk for a first event. This proportion, like all proportions, is unitless or is expressed as a percentage. For the overall cumulative incidence of nosocomial infections, the time implied is the course of hospitalization until a first event or until discharge without a first event. However, patients do not all stay in hospitals and remain at risk for exactly the same period of time. Furthermore, most nosocomial infections are time related, and comparing over-

all attack rates of nosocomial infection among patient groups with differing lengths of stay can be very misleading.

When one compares proportions such as attack rates or cumulative incidences of nosocomial infections, classifying patients as ever infected or never infected is the same as analyzing only first infections. Remember that cumulative incidence is a measure of incidence with an implied duration of time. In this setting, the implied average time is the average duration of hospitalization until first infection, which is different from total hospital stay. Total length of stay includes duration of hospital stay associated with the underlying disease plus the added stay engendered by the nosocomial infections.[7,13]

By contrast, if one looks at events that come from a point source, such as gastroenteritis caused by eating vanilla ice cream at a church supper, or events that are not time related, such as tuberculosis acquired from a contaminated bronchoscope, then the attack rate, or cumulative incidence, is an excellent measure of incidence. Surgical wound infections (site infections) usually are thought of as having a point source, the operation.

In the past, nosocomial infection rates sometimes were reported as a quantity related to cumulative incidence, the number of infections per 100 discharges. This definition had no unique quantitative meaning, as it did not separate first infections from multiple infections in the same patient, and allowed undefined multiple counting of individuals. The biological and statistical import of five infections per 100 discharges would be entirely different, depending on whether it represented five sequential infections in a single moribund patient or five first infections in five different but healthy patients, such as women with normal deliveries. Also, when one patient is included multiple times in the same calculation, the lack of statistical independence would render quantitative comparisons uninterpretable.

TABLE 18-1

	Exposed	Unexposed	Totals
Outcome (1)	a	b	a+b
Outcome (2)	c	d	c+d
Total	a+c	b+d	a+b+c+d

Measures of Prevalence

Prevalence is a measure of the presence of a disease, but not the first occurrence of the disease. The prevalence of a disease is also related to time—the duration of the disease—so that for a given incidence, the longer the duration of disease, the higher the prevalence. The prevalence of congenital abnormalities or arthritis always will be high for this reason.

Point Prevalence

The only useful measure of prevalence is point prevalence, which is the proportion of individuals with a disease or condition at one point in time. Point prevalence also is a unitless proportion. Prevalence can be derived from incidence density and distributions of durations of disease. Historically, there was a quantity called period prevalence, but this contained an undefined mixture of both prevalent and incident cases, and has no quantitative use.

Interconvertibility of Prevalence and Incidence

Point prevalence and incidence density are linked mathematically; and, in a steady-state or dynamic population, one can be derived from the other. Prevalence can be derived from incidence density and distributions of durations of disease, and incidence density can be derived from prevalence and distributions of durations-to-date of disease.[13-16]

Measures of Size of Effect

In cohort studies, case-referent studies, and prevalence studies, we basically compare two mea-

sures of incidence or two measures of prevalence, which are loosely termed "risks." The most intuitive measure of effect for categorical data (infected versus not infected or lived versus died) is the risk ratio, in which the risk among the cases or the exposed is compared with the baseline risk taken from the reference group of noncases or unexposed.

General Definition of a Risk Ratio or Relative Risk

The risk ratio may be thought of as the ratio of two probabilities: the probability of the outcome among the exposed divided by the probability of the outcome in the unexposed. If the probability is the same in both groups, then the ratio of relative risks is unity. A risk ratio of 1.0 is called the value of no effect or the null value. A risk ratio of 5.0 means that the exposed were five times as likely to have the outcome in question, as might happen with indwelling bladder catheters as a cause of nosocomial urinary tract infections. On the other hand, a risk ratio of 0.5, or a halving of the risk with the exposure, would indicate a preventive effect, as might result from a vaccine trial. In actual practice, depending on the type of study, risk ratios can be ratios of incidence densities, ratios of cumulative incidences, ratios of prevalences, or ratios of the prevalence odds or exposure odds. There are important differences among these estimates of the risk ratio, but a detailed description is beyond the scope of this chapter.

The intuitive accessibility of the risk ratio has made this a central concept in epidemiology. The generic term, risk ratio, can be understood equally well in relation to individuals or to groups (in the latter case, they are termed rate ratios). In each setting, risk ratios have the same intuitive meaning, which is their appeal.

Risk Ratios from Cohort Studies

In a cohort study, one enrolls all subjects, or selects groups of exposed and unexposed subjects, and then compares the outcomes of the two groups. If one conducts a cohort study, then one usually can derive population-based rates or proportions. One may have the number of events, for example, the number of first urinary tract infections, and the amount of person-time for those exposed and unexposed to bladder catheters, which can be used to calculate the absolute incidence densities for each group (catheterized or not) and also the incidence density ratio form of the risk ratio. With this same group, one also would be able to compute the cumulative incidences and the cumulative incidence ratio. From a cohort study, one usually can calculate both absolute and relative risks.

For example, one might find that, in a specific group of patients, 10% of those with bladder catheters acquired nosocomial urinary tract infections, which is an absolute cumulative incidence, or attack rate. When one compares the absolute rate of nosocomial urinary tract infection in these catheterized patients with the absolute rate during a similar time period for patients who never had bladder catheters, the cumulative incidence of urinary tract infection for the catheterized group might be 20 times as high as the cumulative incidence among those without catheters, which represents a rate ratio or relative risk of 20.

Risk Ratios from Case-Referent Studies

In a case-referent study, one enrolls a group who have experienced a given outcome and another group without the outcome, then compares them for prior exposures. In this setting, without additional information, one has no idea how common the outcomes or the exposures are in the entire study population. The magic of the case-referent study is that, even without knowing any absolute rates or proportions, one can compute accurate risk ratios by comparing the relative frequencies of various exposures among cases and referents. That is, one can measure the relative risk without knowing the absolute risks.

TABLE 18-2

	Exposed	Unexposed	Totals
Outcome (+)	a	b	a+b
Person-time	N_1	N_0	T

In a steady-state population (one in which the distributions of exposure and disease remain constant), the exposure odds ratio from a case-referent study is identical to the incidence density ratio that would have been computed from a population-based cohort study in the same steady-state population. In a steady-state population, in general, it is possible to calculate one type of prevalence or incidence risk ratio from another, given certain distributions of time.[13-16]

General Form of the Fourfold Table for Count Data for Both Cohort and Case-Referent Studies

Categorical count data in epidemiologic studies are displayed most conveniently in fourfold tables like Table 18-1. These are termed count data, because each cell contains a number representing a count of individuals. Complex data sets may produce several, or even hundreds, of fourfold tables, but each table will have the same general form. Data from cohort, case-referent, or prevalence studies are displayed in the same type of table, but how the subjects were enrolled determines which measures of effect are applicable.

Measure of Effect for a Cohort Study Using Count Data

The cumulative incidence ratio can be calculated for count data from a cohort study. This ratio of two proportions is called the relative risk.

$$\text{Relative Risk} = \frac{\text{Probability of Outcome (+) Among Exposed}}{\text{Probability of Outcome (+) Among Unexposed}} = \frac{\frac{a}{a+c}}{\frac{b}{b+d}}$$

Form of a Table for a Cohort Study Using Incidence Density Data

Data comprised of incidence densities are termed density data. Incidence densities are constructed of numbers of first events and observed person-time. N_1, N_0, and T represent numbers of person-days (Table 18-2).

Measure of Effect for a Cohort Study Using Density Data

The incidence density ratio can be calculated with density data from a cohort study. This ratio of two incidence densities is called the incidence density ratio or the rate ratio.

$$\text{Relative Risk} = \frac{\text{Incidence of Outcome (+) Among Exposed}}{\text{Incidence of Outcome (+) Among Unexposed}} = \frac{\dfrac{a}{N_1}}{\dfrac{b}{N_0}}$$

Measure of Effect for a Case-Referent Study (Count Data)

Case-referent studies can produce only count data. The exposure odds ratio can be calculated for data from a case-referent study. The lower-case letters refer to the cells in the general fourfold table for count data (see Table 18-1).

$$\text{Exposure Odds Ratio} = \frac{\text{Odds of Exposure Among Outcome (+)}}{\text{Odds of Exposure Among Outcome (-)}} = \frac{\dfrac{a}{b}}{\dfrac{c}{d}} = \frac{ad}{bc}$$

Measures of Strength of Association

The most common method of measuring strength of association in a fourfold table is the calculation of χ^2 on one degree of freedom from the comparison of two binomials. The calculation is relatively simple, and with count data (numbers of individuals exposed or not, numbers of individuals with the outcome or not) is identical for all fourfold tables, and does not matter whether they originate from cohort studies, case-referent studies, or prevalence studies.

For a single fourfold table, the value of χ^2 may be computed as (where n = a+b+c+d):

$$\chi^2 = (ad-bc)^2(n-1)/(a+b)(c+d)(a+c)(b+d)$$

The computation of χ^2 is different for density data. When one has the value for χ^2, one can then look up the associated probability that the observed difference between binomial proportions could have arisen by chance alone.

Worldwide, the conventional interpretation of these probabilities is that a *P* value of <.05, or 1/20, indicates that the observed difference is unlikely to have occurred by chance alone and, thus, somehow must represent a real difference. Another way of stating this is that we are 95% certain that this observed difference could not have arisen by chance alone. The adoption of this arbitrary standard has its unfortunate aspects.

Combining Size of Effect and Strength of Association

After completing the computations above, one has an estimate of the risk ratio and an associated probability that the difference observed could have arisen by chance alone. By calculating 95% confidence intervals for the risk ratio, one can combine these two types of information. The interpretation of these results is that we are 95% certain that the true value for the risk ratio lies within this range.

The simplest way to compute confidence intervals is through the use of the calculated χ^2 above. The square root of χ^2 on one degree of freedom is χ, which is used in the computation below. The distribution of χ is taken as the normal distribution (the distribution of z), and the only other datum required is the value of z for the confidence interval being estimated. For a two-tailed 95% confidence interval, the value of z is the familiar 1.96. Here is one simple method for estimating upper and lower bounds for the 95% confidence interval about a risk ratio:

(Upper Bound)=RR$^{(1+z/\chi^2)}$;
(Lower Bound)=RR $^{(1-z/\chi^2)}$

Note that when the risk ratio is less than unity, the relations above calculate the opposite bounds. The near 95% confidence bound (the lower bound if the risk ratio is greater than unity or the upper bound if the risk ratio is less than unity) provides a clear intuitive message about how close to the null value (RR=1.0) the results of any observational study could be. This is much more informative than simply saying that the associated probability of rejecting the null was 0.01.

Epidemiologic Forms of Bias

There are three forms of systematic distortion or bias distinguished according to the logical flaw: selection bias, misclassification, and confounding. For detailed explanations of these concepts, see Freeman and McGowan[8,9,13] and Freeman, Goldmann, and McGowan.[17]

Note

Sections of this chapter are reprinted with permission from Mayhall GC, ed. *Hospital Epidemiology and Infection Control.* Baltimore, Md: Williams & Wilkins; 1996.

References

1. Hennekens CH, Buring JE. *Epidemiology in Medicine.* Boston, Mass: Little, Brown & Co; 1987.

2. Rothman KJ. *Modern Epidemiology.* Boston, Mass: Little, Brown & Co; 1986.

3. Kleinbaum DG, Kupper LL, Morgenstern H. *Epidemiologic Research: Principles and Quantitative Methods.* Belmont, Calif: Lifetime Learning Publications; 1982.

4. Rothman KJ, Boice JD Jr. *Epidemiologic Analysis With a Programmable Calculator.* Boston, Mass: Epidemiology Resources; 1982.

5. Fleiss JL. *Statistical Methods for Rates and Proportions.* 2nd ed. New York, NY: John Wiley and Sons; 1981.

6. Eickhoff TC, Brachman PS, Bennett JV, Brown JF. Surveillance of nosocomial infections in community hospitals, I: surveillance methods, effectiveness, and initial results. *J Infect Dis.* 1969;120:305-317.

7. Freeman J, Rosner BA, McGowan JE Jr. Adverse effects of nosocomial infection. *J Infect Dis.* 1979;140:732-740.

8. Freeman J, McGowan JE Jr. Methodologic issues in hospital epidemiology, I: rates, case finding, and interpretation. *Rev Infect Dis.* 1981;3:658-667.

9. Freeman J, McGowan JE Jr. Methodologic issues in hospital epidemiology, II: time and accuracy in estimation. *Rev Infect Dis.* 1981;3:668-677.

10. Brawley RL, Weber DJ, Samsa GP, Rutala WA. Multiple nosocomial infections: an incidence study. *Am J Epidemiol.* 1989;130:769-780.

11. Baker CJ, Melish ME, Hall RT, Castro DT, Vasan U, Givner LG. Intravenous immune globulin for the prevention of nosocomial infection in low-birth-weight neonates. *N Engl J Med.* 1992;327:213-219.

12. Doebbeling BN, Stanley GL, Sheetz CT, et al. Comparative efficacy of alternative hand-washing agents in reducing nosocomial infections in intensive care units. *N Engl J Med.* 1992;327:88-93.

13. Freeman J, McGowan JE Jr. Methodologic issues in hospital epidemiology, III: investigating the modifying effects of time and severity of underlying illness on estimates of the cost of nosocomial infection. *Rev Infect Dis.* 1984;6:285-300.

14. Freeman J, Hutchison GB. Prevalence, incidence and duration. *Am J Epidemiol.* 1980;112:707-723.

15. Freeman J, McGowan JE Jr. Day-specific incidence of nosocomial infection estimated from a prevalence survey. *Am J Epidemiol.* 1981;114:888-901.

16. Freeman J, Hutchison GB. Duration of disease, duration indicators, and estimation of the risk ratio. *Am J Epidemiol.* 1986;124:134-149.

17. Freeman J, Goldmann DA, McGowan JE Jr. Methodologic issues in hospital epidemiology, IV: risk ratios, confounding, effect modification, and the analysis of multiple variables. *Rev Infect Dis.* 1988;10:1118-1141.

SUPPORT FUNCTIONS

CHAPTER 19

Microcomputers in Hospital Epidemiology

David R. Reagan, MD, PhD

Abstract

Computers can store, manage, and analyze large quantities of data. Thus, computers are a promising tool for the modern practice of infection control. This chapter provides practical information for infection control personnel who must choose or upgrade a computer system.

Introduction

The personal computer has become ubiquitous in both acute and long-term medical care environments. Some infection control professionals have hailed this relentless encroachment on the paper medical record and infection control data card as the dawn of a new era in which they can gather and analyze data quickly from the entire facility.[1-8] Others, drawn to medicine because they valued the patient-provider relationship, dread a system that is the epitome of an impersonal, inflexible, incomprehensible Big Brother. For some, the phrase "user friendly" is an oxymoron when applied to computers. The epigram, "To err is human, but to really screw up takes a computer" still can be found in many healthcare facilities, though often grainy and distorted from numerous trips through the departmental copier.

Many infection control personnel have good reasons to be wary of computers, having experienced inexplicable hardware or software failures. Despite their misgivings, infection control personnel are having to change their ways and join the move to computerization. The central reason for the move to computerization is that manual systems cannot collect, store, and analyze immense quantities of medical data. With limited human resources, infection control personnel must apportion their time reasonably. They must recognize problems quickly, resolve these problems by thoughtful and directed strategies, and conduct further surveillance to establish the effectiveness of the interventions, all of which demand time. The fundamental strengths of computers are the ability to store, retrieve, and analyze large quantities of data accurately and efficiently. Recently, the ability to interchange computerized information has improved, as have the tools for presenting information in an intelligible format.

In this chapter, I will discuss the use of microcomputers in hospital epidemiology. I specifically will address facilities that do not have a comprehensive, hospital-wide information system. Readers with the resources to implement a comprehensive, hospital-wide system are referred to several recent reviews.[7,9-12]

Strategic Planning

Most people have a strong urge to focus immediately on the newest and best hardware and software when they are considering computers. While equipment and programs are important, the infection control team can choose these items more wisely after they develop a strategic plan. First, epidemiology staff should consider the mission and vision of the institution, both at the present time and for the foreseeable future. Infection control efforts must be part of the institution's strategic plan. For example, in hospitals shifting much of their care to the outpatient setting, epidemiology staff should consider how to identify and prevent infections in patients receiving therapy in ambulatory care clinics or through home health agencies. Second, infection control personnel and the infection control committee should develop a list of strategic issues that reflect the primary infection control issues and problems at their institution. In addition, when evaluating this program or planning for the future, infection control personnel should take into account local, national, and international trends in nosocomial infections.[13] Infection control personnel may need to consult with other institutions of similar size and function. After assessing the institution's priorities and the important infection control issues, the infection control team should formulate specific goals and strategies to address each critical issue. One specific goal may be to establish or improve an infection control data management system that uses microcomputers. However, if infection control personnel first clarify the specific purpose of the data management system, they will be able to choose hardware and software that meet their specific needs. They also will

prevent the computer tail from wagging the infection control dog.

Institutional Resources

The infection control team should identify currently available information resources by surveying numerous areas of the hospital or affiliated institutions. Epidemiology personnel should consult administrators, clinicians, computer personnel, and staff from other departments that have independent information systems, such as the laboratory and radiology, to identify possible sources of information. For example, nearly all healthcare facilities have some information about patients available in computer databases, and some institutions have developed an integrated computerized patient record. While conducting the survey, infection control personnel also may gain perspective on critical issues, goals, strategies, and objectives.

I first will discuss computer resources for infection control programs in institutions that have little current computer support and then will discuss the more common situation, hospitals that have computerized some patient data.

Some facilities have little computer support for infection control and do not see an immediate need for it. A paper-based system may be adequate for small institutions with limited infection control problems. However, infection control personnel in these institutions should reevaluate their needs in light of anticipated growth or increased demands for infection control (such as vancomycin-resistant enterococci [VRE] or increased regulatory demands). Some infection control programs have not used computers because of budgetary constraints or because staff were unfamiliar with programs or software. Such programs should reevaluate the issue, as powerful computer systems are now available for as little as $1,500, and both hardware and software are easier to use now.

Most facilities have computerized some administrative and departmental data, but these systems usually lack a common interface, making data transfer between these diverse systems difficult or impossible. Consequently, in many facilities, infection control personnel have not used data that are computerized already. Computer systems in the hospital's administration, laboratory, radiology, and pharmacy may store information that infection control personnel can use. If the infection control program currently is not using data from these systems, the staff may assume wrongly that these systems cannot provide computer support.

A simple computer-based surveillance system can search departmental databases (eg, radiology) at night and print reports on the infection control program's printer (eg, all patients whose chest radiographs were reported to be consistent with possible or probable pneumonia).[14-16] The next morning, infection control personnel can scan these reports and review other relevant data to identify patients who might have nosocomial infections.

Several groups have produced computer systems that evaluate the microbiology database and help the infection control program conduct surveillance. At Barnes Hospital, an expert system called GERMWATCHER extracts data from the microbiology database and applies culture-based criteria from the Centers for Disease Control and Prevention (CDC)'s definitions to identify patients with a high probability of having a nosocomial infection.[17] Dessau and Steenberg described an automated system that detects potential outbreaks by analyzing a commercial microbiology database to detect changes in the frequency with which specific bacteria are identified.[18]

While the infection control program may benefit from having direct access to departmental databases, incompatible interfaces present substantial difficulty. Hospitals with several departmental computer systems with incompatible interfaces may balk at the expense of developing specialized software that would allow the systems to export data directly to the infection control database.

Because of programming costs and the cost of keeping up with the inevitable changes in individual departmental systems (any upgrade may make the current specialized interface obsolete), epidemiology personnel should limit the data obtained from departmental databases to those that are essential for the infection control program, and, if possible, use a commercial program that helps translate data between mainframe computers and personal computers. One such program is Monarch (Datawatch, Wilmington, Mass), which is widely available, versatile, and relatively inexpensive. Monarch is available in versions for DOS, Windows (Microsoft Corp, Redmond, Wash), and networks. This program captures routine output from a department's system as long as the data are arranged in a columnar format. Selected data then may be exported in one of several formats used by common databases or spreadsheets and can be used directly by a relational database or the infection control database.

Perhaps infection control personnel wish to analyze antibiotic susceptibility patterns in a manner that is more relevant than the laboratory's usual reports. For example, the laboratory output may be difficult to assess by patient location (eg, inpatient unit, intensive care unit, or outpatient clinic), or, the laboratory's system may not be able to exclude duplicate cultures fully. To overcome these limitations, data from the yearly summary are captured in a disk file and then input into Monarch. Monarch retains selected elements, discards unnecessary elements, and outputs the data in a format that is used by a more flexible commercial relational database. Thus, programs like Monarch enable infection control personnel to perform analyses that could not be performed adequately on the departmental system.

There are several advantages to maximizing the use of information that is available in current databases. First, the data already are collected and stored in a database. Second, this method eliminates errors introduced by individuals who transfer data manually. Third, this method can function as a computer-assisted surveillance system, allowing epidemiology staff the freedom to conduct more directed surveillance, to analyze the data, and to design specific interventions. Fourth, it enables infection control personnel to do projects that are too massive for manual systems.

There are several potential disadvantages to moving data across interface incompatibilities. First, the hospital must purchase an independent database (ie, either a commercial relational database or the infection control database). Second, the hospital probably will need an intermediary program. Third, the hospital will need an employee who can use all of these programs.

A few facilities have developed comprehensive hospital information systems (HISs) that take infection control needs into account. To my knowledge, none of these systems are commercially available. One example of such a system is that developed by the Latter Day Saints (LDS) Hospital in Salt Lake City, Utah. This extensive, integrated HIS has enabled the infection control program to conduct computer-assisted surveillance that would be too laborious to do manually.[14,19] At LDS Hospital, information on a patient who requires isolation is entered into a program that determines the appropriate type of isolation, provides instructions to healthcare workers, orders necessary supplies, and notifies infection control personnel.[14,19,20] The computer also reviews each patient's laboratory, pharmacy, and radiology records daily and uses an algorithm to identify patients who might have nosocomial infections. Infection control personnel then review the records of the patients identified by the computer program.[14,19] Rocha et al modified this system so that it can be used in neonatal units.[21]

The computer system at LDS Hospital also assesses use of antimicrobial agents by first linking the pharmacy and microbiology databases. Artificial intelligence routines then assess whether agents are used appropriately and generates an alert if use might be inappropriate.[22-24] In addition, the computer surveys perioperative use of antimicrobial agents and reports to the responsible clinicians use patterns that fall outside accepted ranges.[25,26]

Unfortunately, the integrated HIS is the least common computer system, and artificial intelligence rarely has been applied to infection control issues. Hospitals that purchase a commercial HIS are likely to implement systems that were designed to manage administrative and cost data, not infection control data. Additionally, system managers often put the infection control program's requests to modify the system at the lowest priority. This leads to a paradox: infection control data theoretically are available, but practically absent.

Basic Functions of Computers in Infection Control

Infection control personnel can apply computer technology to data collection, storage, retrieval, analysis, and presentation. Surveillance provides the raw material from which infection control staff can identify problems and can scrutinize the effect of interventions. However, manual surveillance requires many hours,[27,28] limiting the time available for analysis, decision-making, and intervention. The computer can review large data sets efficiently and thoroughly, thus allowing the epidemiology staff to evaluate only a few specific patients and their medical records.

Surveillance data must be stored in an organized form that is easy to retrieve. Computers efficiently store large amounts of data, allowing epidemiology staff to retrieve data rapidly with minimal effort. However, infection control staff still must plan carefully which data to collect so that they do not overwhelm the system with data that they never will use. Computers also allow infection control programs to store important data for long periods of time. For example, an infection control program might want to store some data indefinitely, including basic data on nosocomial infections, data on antibiotic susceptibility, data from outbreak investigations, and data on selected pathogens (eg, methicillin-resistant *Staphylococcus aureus* [MRSA], VRE, and highly antibiotic-resistant *Pseudomonas aeruginosa*).

To assess the infection control problems in their institution, infection control staff often must analyze large amounts of data collected over months or years. Computers efficiently manipulate large data sets, summarize data graphically, perform appropriate statistical tests, and expedite literature review. At a more advanced level, artificial intelligence programs assess automatically the likelihood of nosocomial infection (or many other endpoints). Such arrangements free infection control personnel from repetitively analyzing low-risk patients and allow them to evaluate in depth a smaller patient population at high risk of developing nosocomial infections. Unfortunately, commercial software packages that apply artificial intelligence to infection control are not readily available.

In addition to collecting and analyzing data carefully, infection control personnel also must present their results in a format that other members of the healthcare team can understand easily. Computers can help infection control personnel write reports, produce graphics, and communicate with important constituencies.

Software for Infection Control

The software that the infection control program chooses is clearly important. Infection control personnel will use the software daily. Therefore, it is best to buy a program that is easy to use, powerful, flexible, and efficient. Unfortunately, software programs rarely achieve all of these goals; available programs often provide trade-offs in these areas.[29-33] Each team that develops infection control software leaves their approach to infection control imprinted on their software. Thus, each program has a consistent way of approaching problems and a personality. In the following sections, I will

attempt to characterize the available infection control software programs.

Each software package is designed to run under one or more operating systems. Commercially available infection control programs operate under Microsoft-compatible DOS (Microsoft Corp), Windows (Microsoft Corp), or other operating systems. Infection control personnel must ensure that an infection control software program will run under the operating system used by their facility and also under operating systems that the hospital may use in the future. This consideration is especially important if the infection control program wants to use a network version of the software.

Software requirements dictate hardware requirements. Thus, infection control personnel, when possible, should choose the software before selecting hardware. In addition, when they select software, infection control personnel should consider the time needed to install, learn, initialize, and implement software. They also should investigate the cost of product support and upgrades.

Dedicated Infection Control Databases

Numerous infection control groups have developed software specific to their center. However, I would encourage most infection control staff to suppress the urge to develop new software from scratch, as the time and effort needed for such a task is prodigious. I would encourage infection control programs to buy a program that is commercially available. Four major companies publish comprehensive infection control software. I will discuss their software programs in alphabetical order.

Infection Control and Prevention Analysts, Incorporated ([ICPA] Austin, Texas), publishes several programs relevant to infection control and employee health, most notably AICE Pro5 ($4,750). The company has much experience in the practice of infection control, especially with the "surveillance by objective" model. ICPA currently produces software that runs under Microsoft DOS

(Microsoft Corp) with a consistent, if Spartan, interface. ICPA takes a direct and practical approach to both software development and infection control practice.

AICE Pro5 is easy to use and efficient. The program centers around a main screen that allows access to its basic functions: enter, edit, analyze monitoring data, special functions, and backup utilities. The program uses one data entry form that fills one or two computer screens, depending on the number of variables used. Information is entered for each infection on this form, making manual data entry more efficient. AICE has been upgraded several times in the last few years in response to critiques from users and to changing regulatory demands. The program is quite flexible and is widely applicable to large and small institutions. In addition, the publisher has improved the documentation. The new manual is well illustrated and thoughtfully presents the basic information about the program. AICE's statistical module is very good for routine analyses. If infection control personnel must do complex analyses, AICE users may purchase StatGo ($250) to facilitate exporting data stored in AICE to large statistical packages such as SAS (SAS Institute, Cary, NC) and SPSS (Statistical Package for the Social Sciences, SPSS Inc, Chicago, Ill). However, most users would need to consult a biostatistician when conducting and interpreting more complex statistical analyses. ICPA offers toll-free user support, and the company can create highly customized data entry screens for unusual infection control needs. Continuing telephone support (800-426-8015) is modestly priced ($499 yearly, or a charge per minute). Thus, this program combines desirable features and economy.

Some of AICE's strengths include its clear focus, flexibility, straightforward approach, basic analysis tools, moderately priced ongoing telephone support, a large user base, and continuing innovation.

AICE has several weaknesses. At present, the program does not support use of a mouse. This problem will be remedied in a version for Windows NT (Microsoft Corp). The downloading process (ie, importing data into the program) is complex and limited, and the program processes queries slowly compared with commercial databases such as Paradox (Borland, Scotts Valley, Calif). Queries are more rapid when the program is run on a 486-or-better central processing unit (CPU). The standard AICE program focuses on infection control. However, custom screens can be designed for other applications such as storing and analyzing quality surveillance data. Finally, the program does not implement fully the relational database model.

ICPA also publishes NOVA, a less costly version of AICE Pro5, that has fewer features. This program is designed for smaller institutions such as long-term care facilities that have more limited infection control needs. Characteristics of NOVA include manual data entry, restricted ability to customize the data entry screen (although ICPA can design highly customized screens for NOVA), limited data fields (41), and more basic data analysis and graphics modules than AICE. NOVA ($2,295) is an economical program for managing infection control data in smaller institutions that choose to enter data manually. NOVA users can upgrade to the Pro5 version. Continuing support is equivalent to that for AICE Pro5.

IDEAS

The CDC established the National Nosocomial Infections Surveillance (NNIS) System to survey a representative sample of US hospitals. The NNIS System was designed to identify trends in nosocomial infections and in antibiotic susceptibility of nosocomial pathogens. Hospitals that participate in the NNIS System must have an average census of greater than 100 inpatients, must devote at least 1.5 employees to infection control, and each year must submit at least 6 months of surveillance data from at least one hospital area or body site (eg, intensive care unit [ICU], high-risk nursery, hospital-wide, or surgical site). The NNIS System protocols specify which data are to be collected. For ICU surveillance, requisite data include total patients, patient days, ventilator days, urinary-catheter days, and central-line days. Infection control personnel enter results manually into the Interactive Data Entry and Analysis System (IDEAS) database supplied by the CDC, format the data, and transmit the data to the CDC via modem or floppy diskette. The NNIS System provides benchmark data so that hospitals can compare their infection rates with those of other participating institutions. The CDC returns summary data in approximately 3 weeks and compiles summary reports every 6 months.

The IDEAS software (currently version 6) runs under Microsoft DOS and is free to hospitals that agree to participate in the NNIS System. However, the hospital must purchase a data analysis tool called PRODAS (Conceptual Software, Inc, Houston, Tex), that costs $1,000. Data are easy to enter manually, and preselected analyses can be performed readily. The IDEAS system can be customized to a limited extent. The program allows free-text fields (4), single-character fields (2), three-character fields (4), and five-character fields (2). These fields enable an infection control program to adapt IDEAS to its own needs.

IDEAS has several advantages. First, member hospitals use a capable system. Second, these hospitals contribute data that help the CDC to identify nationwide trends in nosocomial infection. Third, NNIS System hospitals receive benchmark data relevant to their facility. Fourth, the initial purchase price is low. Fifth, the CDC provides a training course and excellent telephone support (404-639-3311).

Some disadvantages include limited flexibility and limited capabilities for producing graphics. In addition, infection control personnel may need to do additional work to conform their data to the CDC's requirements.

QLogic II

Epi-Systematics (Fort Myers, Fla) publishes a series of programs relevant to infection control, including a database, QLogic II, and a program that facilitates data import, QMerge. The company prefers global solutions to data management problems and produces products that have a larger scope, greater complexity, more flexibility, and somewhat higher overall cost than do most competitors.

QLogic II operates under Microsoft DOS and is based on a run-time version of the commercial database Paradox, which allows excellent processing speed and flexibility. QLogic II offers a central screen from which the user can access any system module including data entry, report, and statistics. Paradox provides modest graphics functions. QLogic II implements the relational database model well, but fragments data entry into several screens, making it seem more complex and decreasing the efficiency of data entry. QMerge allows the user to import data directly, but the process can be quite complex. Notably, Epi-Systematics has developed software links by which the user can download data directly from several commercial HIS systems. QLogic II supports very capable data analyses, but it provides only a few ready-made reports, and the learning curve for designing customized reports is steeper than for other products. QLogic II's documentation is only adequate. However, the company provides support by telephone (800-648-8070) and will help users implement complex programs with interdepartmental interfaces. The company offers two levels of ongoing telephone support ($750 and $1500 yearly) and maintains an e-mail site to facilitate support (episys@gate.net).

Epi-Systematics continues to develop its product line. It has announced Windows-based software that is technically more complex, but has a simplified user interface based on Paradox for Windows. The company will customize this product, QLogic III, to meet the institution's needs at the time of purchase, but the hospital will need to purchase ongoing customer support. The new product should be easier to use and will allow infection control personnel to access available computerized data more readily. The increased cost for initial installation and continuing support is a disadvantage of the windows-based program. Epi-Systematics will continue to offer and support QLogic II as a cheaper alternative for smaller institutions.

WHOCARE

The World Health Organization (WHO) has developed a focused software program for infection control called WHOCARE. This program is based on the FoxPro database system, and runs under Microsoft DOS. WHOCARE comes in two versions: the Basic Version ($250), published in 1989, which was designed only for surveillance of surgical site infections,[34,35] and the Comprehensive Version ($500), which tracks other kinds of nosocomial infections. The interface is clean and efficient. The user enters data on a single screen through a series of nested forms boxes. The user can define a limited number of fields and can customize database queries. The program allows the user to perform repetitions quickly. The documentation is well written and reasonably comprehensive.

Some advantages of the WHOCARE system include its low purchase price, efficient approach to manual data entry, good execution speed, and pleasant user interface. A primary drawback with this system is that product support is provided by the WHOCARE Distribution Center in Copenhagen, Denmark (telephone: +45-32-68-33-16, fax: 45-32-68-38-77). In addition, the program has a limited number of data elements, limited formats for data elements, limited ability to customize data entry screens, and no graphics support.

Relational Databases

Any of the infection control software programs discussed above will help the infection control team store and retrieve surveillance data. In contrast, many of these commercial packages do not provide facile analysis of data from some epidemiologic studies. Thus, infection control personnel will gain flexibility if they export data from the infection control package to another database program. Dbase (Borland), Paradox, FoxPro (Microsoft Corp) and Access (Microsoft Corp) are commercial databases used for this purpose. One infection control package that facilitates such analyses is QLogic II, which provides a link to Paradox for queries and graphics. As previously noted, programs that bridge interface incompatibilities, such as Monarch (Datawatch), can be helpful.

Ancillary Software for Infection Control

Infection control teams should have a system that backs up data stored on a hard disk so that they do not lose important information. Modern hard disks last, on average, 20,000 to 60,000 hours between failure. However, hard disks still fail, data sometimes are erased, and computer viruses delete data.[36] Therefore, every computer user should, like the proverbial Boy Scout, always be prepared. Infection control personnel would be wise to back up critical data, such as infection control databases, each time data are entered, or at least daily. They should back up other data, such as word processing files and graphics, daily or at least weekly. While there are several types of backup hardware, the inexpensive nature of tape backup devices makes them the first choice for many infection control programs. A single portable tape backup unit that communicates with the computer via the parallel port can serve several personal computers and can be purchased for $150. Network-based users benefit from the daily backups that such systems usually provide by storing their databases on a network hard drive.

Some general guidelines for selecting software apply to software used to support infection control activities. Graphical interfaces usually are easier to use and may have shorter learning curves than older character-based interfaces. Most currently available infection control software is designed to run under DOS, but can operate in a DOS window under Windows 3.1 (Microsoft Corp), Windows 95 (Microsoft Corp), or Windows NT. In addition, many larger facilities already have chosen software for word processing, graphics, communication, and literature searches. Some infection control personnel may feel that the institution has, thereby, limited their choices. However, if the infection control team chooses the same programs, the institution's computer support group should be able to assist them when questions arise about individual software programs. In addition, the common software will help them exchange data within the institution.

Many capable programs exist. Although many individuals strongly prefer particular programs, these preferences frequently are not justified. In the following paragraphs, I will describe some competent programs that have survived in an extremely competitive marketplace. The observations are not exhaustive. Infection control personnel who want current, comprehensive information about computer software should read publications such as *PC Magazine* (Ziff-Davis Publishers, New York), which publishes critical reviews of software by category.

The local computer support group often dictates which word processing software package is used throughout the institution. Several commercially available word processing programs are capable and easy to use. Market leaders include Word (Microsoft Corp), and WordPerfect (Corel).

An infection control database package may provide statistical analysis for routine infection control purposes. However, several capable programs are available commercially that can supplement the basic statistical functions offered by infection control databases. Infection control personnel should consider Epistat (shareware) and True Epistat (Tracy L. Gustafson, Richardson, Tex), SAS (SAS Institute, Cary, NC), SPSS-PC for Windows (SPSS Inc, Chicago, Ill), and Minitab (Minitab, Inc, State

College, Pa). Epidemiology staff will need to spend time learning these programs. Furthermore, these programs do not replace statisticians; infection control personnel who need to do complex analyses should consult a statistician.[37]

Infection control staff may understand large tables of data; however, members of the infection control committee may grasp the data more readily if presented in a graphical format. The graphics needs of the epidemiology staff may be met by the infection control database. However, some infection control programs will need more sophisticated graphics packages to generate informative graphics. Newer graphics software often allows the user to import data directly from a database and to predefine the types of graphs. Epidemiology personnel should ask staff in the computer support group which graphics packages they support. If the hospital has chosen a graphics package that was designed for business applications, the infection control program may need to evaluate other software programs that can make complex scientific graphics.

Competent communications software abounds. These programs provide connections with e-mail, the internet, MEDLINE, and networks. Infection control personnel could consider Procomm Plus for Windows (Datastorm Technologies, Columbia, Mo), Hyperaccess for Windows (Hilgraeve, Inc, Monroe, Mich), Smartcom for Windows (Hayes Microcomputer Products, Inc, Atlanta, Ga), and Delrina WinComm PRO (Delrina Corp, San Jose, Calif).

Hardware Considerations for Infection Control

In this section, I will discuss computer hardware so that infection control personnel can purchase or upgrade computer hardware without undue anxiety engendered by the myriad choices. In reality, choosing computer hardware is not difficult. I will discuss only IBM-compatible systems. Apple-compatible systems can perform many functions equally well. However, infection control staff may find Apple systems disadvantageous, because comprehensive infection control databases are not commercially available for this hardware.

First, I will discuss a few general principles. Computer components include the CPU class (eg, Pentium Pro, Pentium, 80486, etc [Intel]), data bus architecture, random access memory (RAM), hard disk storage, CD-ROM storage, floppy drive, communications hardware (modem or network card), tape backup unit, and monitor. While this list looks daunting, some companies provide competent systems that optimally integrate these components. Such companies usually offer 3-year warranties and will repair the computer where you work during the first year. Companies with good reputations for reliability and service include AST (Irvine, Calif), Compaq (Houston, TX), Dell (Round Rock, TX), Digital (Maynard, Mass), Hewlett-Packard (Palo Alto, CA), Gateway (N Sioux City, SD), IBM (Armonk, NY), and Micron (Boise, ID). Many companies build and sell computers locally. One of these systems may be less expensive than the nationally known brands, but warranties and service may not be as good.

Prices for new systems have a remarkable propensity to stay fixed in the personal computer industry. However, what you get for the purchase price changes. A complete "entry-level" system that uses last year's technology costs $1,250 to $1,500 (excluding printer). The "value-level" system, which gives the most computing power for the least money, will cost $2,000 to $2,750. The "power-user" system, which incorporates advanced features and high performance, will cost $3,500 to $6,000. Infection control personnel who enjoy deliberating over the intricacies of SRAM, VRAM, PCI, MPEG, EIDE, EDO RAM, and SCSI-2 probably need no advice. However, individuals whose fight-or-flight instincts are triggered by the preceding list should get advice from a computer expert or a friend who loves this stuff. Alternatively, they can

work with one of the previously mentioned companies and buy a preconfigured hardware package.

The Importance of the User

Capable software and hardware can improve the efficiency of infection control processes. However, the persons using the computer system will determine whether it operates well. Knowledgeable people can maximize the capabilities of available hardware and software. Conversely, perfectly capable hardware and software systems can give inadequate or even erroneous output if used improperly. System users must be educated initially and must obtain "continuing computer education" periodically. Wise hospital managers will provide adequate training for persons who operate the system so that they learn to perform the fundamental tasks: backing up the hard disk, organizing databases, analyzing data, and presenting data. Hospitals should consider the cost of education to be an investment in an effective infection control program.

Persons who think the term "user friendly" is an oxymoron when applied to computers, take heart! Computer systems are not nearly as difficult to set up and use as they were just a few years ago. Infection control personnel may doubt initially whether they should invest their limited time and energy setting up a computer system. However, they will be rewarded soon, because data will be readily accessible, and infection control problems will be easier to investigate.

Many groups, including university computing centers and the computer support departments of large facilities, offer basic courses on operating systems, databases, statistical analysis, and graphics software. Software vendors often provide seminars that train purchasers to use the programs. Infection control software programs also provide tutorials that teach the user to perform basic functions. Additionally, the Association for Professionals in Infection Control and Epidemiology (APIC, Mundelein, Ill) and the Society for

Healthcare Epidemiology of America (SHEA, Mt Royal, NJ) often provide workshops for individuals who want to learn about computer programs for infection control. The most cost-effective and most neglected method of improving the quality of system output is to educate the people who manage the infection control information system.

Access to the Medical Literature

Computers can help infection control personnel to search the literature, both to follow advances in their field and solve difficult problems in their institutions. The National Library of Medicine's (NLM) MEDLINE is an indispensable resource. This massive database of medical references and abstracts is widely available in medical libraries on CD-ROM, or can be accessed for free via the World Wide Web (http://www.nlm.nih.gov/; searchers can use either Grateful Med, a simple search tool designed for medical professionals, or PubMed, an even simpler tool designed for the general public). Retrieved information can be printed directly or stored on disk in a database such as Reference Manager (Research Information Systems, Carlsbad, Calif).

Another approach to searching the healthcare epidemiology literature is to use a tool such as Paradigm (Applied Epidemiology, Sidney, BC), which provides a database of high-quality articles with thoughtful annotations. Although such a tool by its nature includes only selected articles, it can be supplemented by a MEDLINE search to produce a well-rounded review.

Conclusion

In summary, computers have become an indispensable part of efficient data management in infection control. Epidemiology staff should understand the strengths and limitations of computerized data already available at their facilities to make optimal use of such data. Computers increasingly allow infection control personnel to monitor clinical practice prospectively and to disseminate data in a time-

ly fashion. Such data will enable providers to make better decisions about the care of individual patients and will allow infection control personnel to make decisions about care in a unit or in an entire facility. While infection control teams may have difficulty instituting global solutions to data acquisition and management, even partial solutions can reduce the workload significantly. In addition, a computer system may help the epidemiology staff substantially reduce rates of nosocomial infections. Therefore, computer systems are worth the time, expense, and effort expended in their implementation.

References

1. McDonald CJ, Tierney WM. Computer-stored medical records: their future role in medical practice. *JAMA.* 1888;259:3433-3440.

2. Korpman RA, Lincoln TL. The computer-stored medical record: for whom? *JAMA.* 1988;259:3454-3456.

3. Wenzel RP, Streed SA. Surveillance and use of computers in hospital infection control. *J Hosp Infect.* 1989;13:217-229.

4. Greenes RA, Shortliffe EH. Medical informatics: an emerging academic discipline and institutional priority. *JAMA.* 1990;263:1114-1120.

5. Gransden WR. Information, computers, and infection control. *J Hosp Infect.* 1990;15:1-5.

6. Shortliffe EH, Tang PC, Detmer DE. Patient records and computers. *Ann Intern Med.* 1991;115;979-981.

7. Classen DC, Pestotnik SL. The computer-based patient record: an essential technology for hospital epidemiology. In: Mayhall CG, ed. *Hospital Epidemiology and Infection Control.* Philadelphia, Pa: Williams & Wilkins; 1996:123-137.

8. Haley RW. The scientific basis for using surveillance and risk factor data to reduce nosocomial infection rates. *J Hosp Infect.* 1995;30(suppl):3-14.

9. Ball MJ, O'Desky RI, Douglas JV. Status and progress of hospital information systems (HIS). *Int J Biomed Comput.* 1991;29:161-189.

10. Collen MF. A brief historical overview of hospital information system (HIS) evolution in the United States. *Int J Biomed Comput.* 1991;29:169-189.

11. Mertens R, Ceusters W. Quality assurance, infection surveillance, and hospital information systems: avoiding the Bermuda Triangle. *Infect Control Hosp Epidemiol.* 1994;

15:203-209.

12. Classen DC. Information management in infectious diseases: survival of the fittest. *Clin Infect Dis.* 1994;19:902-909.

13. Gaynes RP, Horan TC. Surveillance of nosocomial infections. In: Mayhall CG, ed. *Hospital Epidemiology and Infection Control.* Philadelphia, Pa: Williams & Wilkins; 1996:1017-1031.

14. Evans RS, Larsen RA, Burke JP, et al. Computer surveillance of hospital-acquired infections and antibiotic use. *JAMA.* 1986;256:1007-1011.

15. Evans RS, Burke JP, Classen DC, et al. Computerized identification of patients at high risk for hospital-acquired infection. *Am J Infect Control.* 1992;20:4-10.

16. Broderick A, Mori M, Nettleman MD, Streed SA, Wenzel RP. Nosocomial infections: validation of surveillance and computer modeling to identify patients at risk. *Am J Epidemiol.* 1990;131:734-742.

17. Kahn MG, Steib SA, Fraser VJ, Dunagan WC. An expert system for culture-based infection control surveillance. *Proc Annu Symp Comput Appl Med Care.* 1993:171-175.

18. Dessau RB, Steenberg P. Computerized surveillance in clinical microbiology with time series analysis. *J Clin Microbiol.* 1993;31:857-860.

19. Evans RS, Gardner RM, Bush AR, et al. Development of a computerized infectious disease monitor (CIDM). *Comput Biomed Res.* 1985;18:103-113.

20. Classen DC, Burke JP, Pestotnik SL, Evans RS, Stevens LE. Surveillance for quality assessment: IV, surveillance using a hospital information system. *Infect Control Hosp Epidemiol.* 1991;12:239-244.

21. Rocha BH, Christenson JC, Pavia A, Evans RS, Gardner RM. Computerized detection of nosocomial infections in newborns. *Proc Annu Symp Comput Appl Med Care.* 1994:684-688.

22. Pestotnik SL, Evans RS, Burke JP, Gardner RM, Classen DC. Therapeutic antibiotic monitoring: surveillance using a hospital information system. *Am J Med.* 1990;88:43-48.

23. Evans RS, Pestotnik SL, Classen DC, Burke JP. Development of an automated antibiotic consultant. *MD Comput.* 1993;10:17-22.

24. Evans RS, Classen DC, Pestotnik SL, Lundsgaarde HP. Improving empiric antibiotic selection using computer decision support. *Arch Intern Med.* 1994;154:878-884.

25. Larsen RA, Evans RS, Burke JP, Pestotnik SL, Gardner RM, Classen DC. Improved perioperative antibiotic use and reduced surgical wound infections through use of computer decision analysis. *Infect Control Hosp Epidemiol.* 1989;10:316-320.

26. Evans RS, Pestotnik SL, Burke JP, Gardner RM, Larsen RA, Classen DC. Reducing the duration of prophylactic antibiotic use through computer monitoring of surgical patients. *DICP Ann Pharmacother.* 1990;24:351-354.

27. Bjerke NB, Fabrey LJ, Johnson CB, et al. Job analysis 1992: infection control practitioner. *Am J Infect Control.* 1993;21:51-57.

28. Schifman RB, Howanitz PJ. Nosocomial infections. A college of American pathologists Q-probes study in 512 North American institutions. *Arch Pathol Lab Med.* 1994;118:115-119.

29. Gaynes R, Friedman C, Copeland TA, Thiele GH. Methodology to evaluate a computer-based system for surveillance of hospital-acquired infections. *Am J Infect Control.* 1990;18:40-46.

30. LaHaise S. A comparison of infection control software for use by hospital epidemiologists in meeting new JCAHO standards. *Infect Control Hosp Epidemiol.* 1990;11:185-190.

31. Reagan DR. The choice of microcomputer software for infection control. *Infect Control Hosp Epidemiol.* 1990;11:178-179.

32. Zellner S, Polley N. Infection control software. *Infect Control Hosp Epidemiol.* 1990;11:400-401.

33. LaHaise S. Reply to Zellner and Polley on infection control software. *Infect Control Hosp Epidemiol.* 1990;11:404. Letter.

34. Mertens R, Jans B, Kurz X. A computerized nationwide network for nosocomial infection surveillance in Belgium. *Infect Control Hosp Epidemiol.* 1994;15:171-179.

35. Mertens R, Van den Berg JM, Veerman-Brenzikofer ML, Kurz X, Jans B, Klazinga N. International comparison of results of infection surveillance: The Netherlands versus Belgium. *Infect Control Hosp Epidemiol.* 1994;15:574-578.

36. Bailey TC, Reichley RM. Investigation of a computer virus outbreak in the pharmacy of a tertiary care teaching hospital. *Infect Control Hosp Epidemiol.* 1992;13:594-598.

37. Hierholzer WJ Jr. Health care data, the epidemiologists said: comments on the quantity and quality of data. *Am J Med.* 1991;91(suppl 3b):21S-26S.

CHAPTER 20

The Computer-Based Patient Record:
The Role of the Hospital Epidemiologist

David C. Classen, MD, MS, John P. Burke, MD

Abstract

Despite advances in computers and software for data analysis, hospital epidemiologists must still use manual methods for data collection. To fully automate infection control surveillance, healthcare institutions need computerized medical records; however, very few institutions currently have such a system. Healthcare institutions appreciate the need for automation, but frequently do not see a clear path to the desired outcome. In this chapter we outline the important issues that hospital epidemiologists must understand if they wish to help their institutions computerize medical records.

Introduction

Many hospital epidemiologists anticipate a markedly enhanced role with the advent of highly developed clinical computer systems; however, such systems are rare. The systems that currently exist are personal computer-based programs such as Noso 3 and AICE.[1] In addition, the Centers for Disease Control and Prevention offer a program known as IDEAS to facilitate collection of hospital data for the National Nosocomial Infection Surveillance System.[1] Because these systems increase the efficiency of the analysis but not the collection of data, hospital epidemiologists continue to depend on manual methods for effective surveillance.

Several studies document that clinical information systems can facilitate infection control surveillance. Such systems can provide infection control personnel with better methods for detecting nosocomial infections, investigating outbreaks, and identifying patients who might benefit from preventive strategies. Furthermore, the computer can automatically alert clinical staff to initiate isolation protocols.[2-6] With clinical information systems, a user can track the clinical and cost outcomes associated with events such as nosocomial infections. Hospital epidemiologists will find this ability important as they increasingly must document the costs and benefits of programs to reduce nosocomial infections. In the managed care era, institutions cannot recover these costs directly and consequently may look to an effective infection control program for cost containment.

Few hospital epidemiologists would disagree that highly developed clinical computer systems could enhance infection control activities; however, few institutional systems currently provide the support described above. The problem is not that hospital epidemiologists do not appreciate what needs to be done but rather they do not know how to attain these goals. Developing clinical information systems necessitates both a technical revolution, which enables hospitals to develop large and comprehensive medical databases, and a social revolution, which requires healthcare personnel to develop new roles and job descriptions. Unfortunately, institutions often take what they perceive to be the easiest path possible—linking existing departmental computer systems to create a computerized medical record. Hospital epidemiologists can readily see the advantages of this approach: "If I can just link the laboratory and pharmacy computer systems, then I can begin doing active surveillance." However, to do truly effective surveillance and to develop mechanisms for improving patient care, hospital epidemiologists need comprehensive computerized medical records that the hospital develops systematically.

An automated patient record, often known as the computer-based patient record (CPR), is designed to repair the failures of the traditional paper record.[7-10] The CPR could improve the information management problems of healthcare. In 1991, the General Accounting Office (GAO) reported three major ways in which improved patient records could benefit healthcare.[1] First, automated patient records could improve healthcare delivery by allowing numerous individuals to access data at different sites, and by providing faster data retrieval and higher quality data. The CPR also provides decision-support capabilities, provides clinical reminders to assist clinicians as they care for patients, and supports quality improvement activities. Second, computer-stored medical records can enhance outcomes research by automatically capturing clinical information that investigators can evaluate. Third, automated patient

records reduce costs by improving staff efficiency. The GAO reported that a Department of Veterans Affairs hospital used an automated patient record system to decrease the length of hospital stays and reduce hospital costs by $600 per patient.

Unfortunately, administrators, who are primarily interested in financial systems, have directed the acquisition of most clinical computer systems. Physicians are often frustrated because these systems cannot efficiently provide clinically useful data. If physicians help evaluate systems before the hospital chooses one, the institution may acquire a more clinically useful system.

This chapter is divided into two parts: the first part outlines the critical aspects of a clinical information system and the second outlines an institutional process for choosing a clinical information system. In addition, we include a glossary of terms to help the hospital epidemiologist understand this discussion.

Critical Issues and Concepts of Clinical Computerization

The primary function of a clinical information system (CIS) is to communicate data.[11] To perform this function, a CIS must have software and hardware components that allow the computer to acquire, process, store, retrieve, and rearrange data, and then display that data throughout the institution. The premise that underlies this design strategy is that many providers—including the medical staff, nurses, pharmacists, radiologists, laboratory staff, respiratory therapists, physical therapists, occupational therapists, dietary staff—create patient-care data and those providers need ready access to a variety of patient-care data. The key is that the provider-created data must be comprehensive. Within an integrated CIS, patient data should be entered once and then these data should be available to all users. Ideally, data should be entered at the point-of-care. For example, a nurse should enter the patient's temperature into the CIS at the bedside. Point-of-care data entry allows healthcare workers to use patient data fully because the data are now temporally related to the course of hospitalization. This temporal relationship allows providers to analyze the patient's clinical progress and to relate outcomes to specific events during hospitalization. Point-of-care data entry is equally applicable to automated devices and analyzers, such as ventilators or blood chemistry systems. The technology currently exists that allows point-of-care data to be captured automatically.

There are currently four models for information processing in a CIS: the centralized model, the hub-and-spoke model, the network model, and the distributed model.[12-16] The centralized model, also known as a monolithic system, consists of a mainframe computer that contains all the applications. This model achieves a high degree of data integration and a common user interface. There are numerous advantages associated with this architecture. Foremost is the creation of a central CPR with all data elements going into the same file. Coincident with the creation of a CPR is the development and existence of a data dictionary (a standardized scheme for defining medical terms and patient data).[17] Moreover, a centralized database with a data dictionary allows clinicians and epidemiologists to use expert system tools to provide clinical decision-support (see glossary).

Several vendors now offer centralized systems and promise an integrated CPR. Centralized systems have several drawbacks. First, they force the hospital to contract with one vendor. Second, in hospitals that have departmental computer systems, the interface of a mainframe computer with existing clinical support systems (CSS), such as a laboratory information system, is often technically difficult and time consuming. Third, commercially available CIS software often will not support the variety of users in a hospital. The few hospitals that have fully integrated CISs have adopted the centralized model. These hospitals were forced to build their own CIS

because the marketplace was slow to develop a clinically functional and integrated CIS.

The second model of a CIS is the hub-and-spoke configuration that consists of a mainframe computer or hub that is linked to satellite or feeder systems. Typical satellite systems are CSSs, such as a pharmacy information system. The hub-and-spoke model evolved from the centralized model to take advantage of departmental CSSs. Multiple vendors commonly provide these satellite CSSs, which connect individually to the central mainframe. The CSSs maintain their own databases and often the mainframe only stores recent data. However, some of the more advanced hub-and-spoke systems archive and store patient data (including CSS data) on the mainframe. These advanced hub-and-spoke CISs provide a CPR but are the exception rather than the rule. Healthcare workers use "dumb" terminals, which interact primarily with the mainframe, to review data and place orders. These dumb terminals are hard-wired to the mainframe computer in much the same manner as in the centralized system.

The hub-and-spoke model has two major disadvantages: the intrinsic limitations of the interfaces constrain the clinical usefulness of the CSSs, and the intrinsic limitations of each CSS constrain the overall system. Individual departments developed the satellite systems to satisfy their own needs rather than provide for the total care of the patient. As noted, this model of a CIS often lacks a centralized and integrated CPR, and therefore, it does not help healthcare providers process information. If the hospital chooses the design, the system should include an integrated long-term CPR with an attendant data dictionary. If these two elements are in a hub-and-spoke CIS, then users can take full advantage of expert system tools to provide decision support.

The third CIS design is the network model.[16] This model consists of a local area network (LAN) to which various host computers (a CSS or a mainframe can be a host computer) are attached as nodes on the network. Computer-to-computer interfaces, like the hub-and-spoke model, are the mainstay of this system. The healthcare worker uses a terminal or a minicomputer, which is attached to a back-bone LAN, to gain access to host computers (CSSs or the mainframe). The purpose of the back-bone LAN is to connect various host computers. The network model allows high-speed data transfer and access. Another advantage of the network model is that the integrity and usefulness of the host computers are maintained. For example, a healthcare provider could access a laboratory information system (LIS) through the LAN and have some of the flexibility that the LIS allowed.

Like the other models, the network model has disadvantages. First, the user interacts directly with the host computer, and, therefore, does not have an integrated view of patient information. Second, a user can only access one host computer at a time. Third, the user must learn different commands to communicate with the different host computers because this model does not have a uniform user interface. Fourth, the user undertakes the burden of system interaction rather than standardized interface software providing this function. Current versions of this CIS architecture do not provide for an integrated CPR. To date, LAN technology only allows healthcare workers to do simple applications, such as reviewing results or writing rudimentary orders. However, in the future, servers, dedicated computers that are attached as a node on the LAN, may obtain data from host computers and store the data. Server technology will allow patient data to be merged, but will not eliminate the need for interfaces with numerous computers.

The fourth CIS design strategy is known as the distributive model. The model is very similar to the network model in that host computers act as nodes on a LAN. What distinguishes the distributive model from the network model is that the design integrates the system by creating a central database through relational database software. In the distrib-

utive model, relational database software is installed on each host computer and workstation connected to the LAN. This software is not constrained by the type of hardware or the environment of the operating systems. The various heterogenous host computers can be integrated in three different ways. First, because each host computer has a relational database, standard query language (SQL)[16] can be used across the entire system. The original version of SQL was developed at International Business Machines' San Jose Research Laboratory (now the Almaden Research Center). The language was originally known as Sequel and has evolved to become known as SQL. The American National Standards Institute published an SQL standard in 1986. Since then the computer industry has adopted SQL as the primary tool used to query relational databases. Second, the distributive model uses a central patient database that includes a data dictionary to standardize medical terms and to record the location of various data elements in the system. Third, the relational database software can recognize and read file structures from various host computers; the host files can be read as they exist, or the software can convert them to a relational database file format for storage in the central database. This model creates a knowledge base for system-wide decision support. The major advantages of the distributed model are that:

1. Host-computers exchange information without interfaces.
2. The system creates an integrated CPR.
3. A data dictionary standardizes medical terms and a knowledge base.
4. Users can access various patient data from any workstation regardless of where it physically exists in the system.
5. Relational database software can gather all requested patient information simultaneously at the time of inquiry, and once the requester has completed his or her task, the view disappears. Known as assembling

information on-the-fly, the process eliminates the tasks of copying information from a CSS to the mainframe and of processing that information on the mainframe.

6. An integrated CPR provides the environment for decision-support tools (that is, expert systems).

Decision support is the most critical aspect of CISs for infection control programs. Decision support uses patient-specific information and programmed medical logic to make decisions about patient care. Currently hospitals with integrated information systems and attendant CPRs use decision support in six general ways: alerting, interpreting, assisting, critiquing, diagnosing, and managing. Alerting is defined as the automatic notification of appropriate providers of time-critical decisions. Drug-drug interactions, drug-laboratory interactions, drug-disease, adverse drug reactions, and drug allergy alerts are common clinical examples of this type of decision support.[18-20] Warnings are generated at the time of a medication order if alerting criteria are met. Furthermore, a CIS with the alerting function can scan patient data continuously; alerting is said to occur in the "background," and if criteria are met anytime in the course of hospitalization, appropriate personnel can be notified.

Interpreting is decision support in which the computer gathers, arranges, analyzes and interprets patient data so that the clinician can understand the information. One of the earliest clinical applications of interpretive decision support was computer analysis and interpretation of electrocardiograms.[21] Assisting is decision support that is used to maximize and simplify human interaction with a CIS. This model of decision support usually consists of predictive knowledge about a particular problem or task. Computer-assisted physician ordering is an example of this type of decision support.[22-24] Assisting decision support can be as simple as fixed standing order lists or as sophisticated as comput-

er-assisted antibiotic ordering.[25,26] Critiquing is defined as computer-assisted analysis or review of human decisions for appropriateness. This type of decision support merely uses the CIS knowledge base to evaluate human decisions and to report to the user the result of the computer analysis. Investigators have used critiquing decision support to develop protocols for management of ventilators in intensive care units (ICUs)[27] and to determine the appropriateness of blood transfusions.[28] In diagnostic decision support, the computer assesses available clinical data and then generates a differential diagnosis to help the clinician evaluate the patient in a rational and efficient manner. This type of decision support has been the most widely studied of all decision support techniques in medical informatics.[29] Finally, managing decision support is the automatic generation of decisions that are oriented to the total care of the patient. Managing decision support differs from critiquing decision support; in the former, the computer manages patient care and suggests treatments, while in the latter, the computer reacts to treatment plans or orders initiated by the physician. In clinical management decision support, the physician critiques the computer rather than the computer critiquing the physician. Computerized clinical practice guidelines are an example of this model of decision support. Managing decision support techniques are currently being investigated in ICUs to help clinicians manage patients with adult respiratory distress syndrome.[30]

Different institutions will implement these systems in different ways. There are at least three common options: build it locally, purchase an overall system, or link the existing departmental systems. The least effective approach is to build a system from scratch. The most effective way is to purchase an overall system. Linking existing departmental systems is very difficult and to date has been unsuccessful, but it is the most appealing to hospitals because it appears to require the least amount of change. However, there are no examples of effective decision support programs using this model. The distributive model is currently the most favored model, but the institution must still create a central patient database. Any system without this feature is undesirable.

Institutional Approach to Choosing Clinical Information Systems

Institutions that wish to develop a CPR should follow a clear, rational, and responsible process to achieve this end. We recommend that hospitals use a tripartite approach to choosing a computer system.[31] First, the institution must identify its goals, needs, and priorities for information management. Second, a committee of clinicians advises the administration on clinical functions that require computer support and handles the political aspects of choosing a computer system. Third, a clinical information systems committee considers the priorities set by the institution and the clinicians' needs, and then does the actual work required to choose the computer system.

Each institution that considers purchasing a clinical information system needs both a vision and concrete goals for information management. These goals, will develop from the tradition and the mission of the institution, and will determine the hospital's requirements for an information system. The institution also must develop specific criteria for an information system that will enable it to choose among the multitude of systems available. Once the institution has delineated these factors, the medical staff and the administration must agree with the goals and priorities, before the institution can begin the process of selecting a system.

In the past, clinicians have tried to communicate their needs to the information services department, usually with little success. Now physicians must help their institutions shift the priorities of their computer systems from managing financial data to managing clinical data. If clinicians are not involved in choosing a computer system, the final product will not be clinically useful.

The hospital must first identify a physician leader who can ensure the process will bear fruit. A physician leader must see the broad view of clinical computerization, including the institution's needs and goals, and must not have a narrow view that focuses on a few applications. A physician leader must have experience in data collection and analysis to understand the important role these functions will play in any clinical information system. Because clinical epidemiologists collect, analyze, and interpret data, and they conduct focused investigations, these specialists may be able to contribute important expertise.

To help implement the clinical information system, a physician leader should have credibility with the medical staff. The physician leader must take a strong role in setting vision and educating medical staff members about that mission. The physician leader should also establish a task force of physicians that will specify the clinicians' needs and can help address the myriad of political issues that surface during the selection process. Medical staff should be involved at all stages of the process, as no other group can so effectively undermine a clinical information system.

After establishing a medical staff task force, the physician leader should form a clinical information committee of leaders from various departments: the physician leader, the chief financial officer, the chief information officer, the president of the board, the medical staff president, the director of pharmacy, the chief nursing officer, and influential medical staff members. A physician should lead this committee; neither the administrators nor the chief information officer should control the agenda.

The clinical information committee does the actual work of selecting the computer system. The committee must first prioritize the institution's computing needs by considering both the list of goals developed by the institution and the institutions existing resources. Subsequently, the clinical information committee would be prudent to generate a list of basic requirements that will guide its deliberations. Thereafter, the committee can request proposals from vendors. However, the task of reviewing proposals can be quite laborious! Thus, we recommend that the committee request information from possible vendors.[32] After perusing the responses, the committee selects which products it wants to evaluate further. The committee then can request proposals from those vendors.

The clinical information committee must consider the following important issues and questions when reviewing the proposals and throughout the subsequent evaluations: Is the system designed for direct physician use? If so, where are sites of use in the institution? Is there evidence that the system meets clinical needs? What are the speed and flexibility of the system? Have physician suggestions been incorporated into the system? What is the scope and design of the electronic medical record and can the system provide a longitudinal record? Is there a central database and a knowledge base and who will maintain this? What are the methods for data capture? What are the interfacing capabilities and communication protocols in the system? Does this system capture financial data and true cost data? What is the format for a clinical archive and how can it be queried? What is the state of open architecture in the system and is there any distributed computing? Can the system handle electronic mail? (local and national) Does the system offer order entry? What provisions are there for electronic signatures and security?

Next, the clinical information committee lists desirable systems and arranges site visits. This step is vital because often the vendors' demonstrations lead the purchaser to expect performance that cannot be realized at institutions using the vendors' systems. Vendors often boast about programs that do not exist, hence the term "vaporware." Because these vacuous claims are prevalent, the informed consumer should assume that programs do not exist unless they have been personally observed in operation.

The site visit team should include interested clinicians, such as physicians, nurses, and pharmacists, who will use the system. Given the expense of the systems, the team should also include an influential member of the board. The clinical information committee must choose carefully the members of the team because each individual increases the costs incurred by the hospitals.

During the site visits, individuals from the hospital can thoroughly review each system. The site-visitors should develop a list of specific questions akin to the questions outlined above. Site visitors must interview, in a random fashion that is not staged, clinicians who use the system. The team should observe who actually uses the system and identify those departments and groups that don't use the system. The extent to which other methods are used to transmit information (ie, paper transmission, telephone, fax, and electronic mail) indicates whether the system is used regularly. The team should also observe whether physicians use the system, how often clinicians use the system for acute patient care, whether physicians want to use the system in their offices and homes, and whether a computer-generated chart can be used for acute care. The team must ask the current users about maintenance and upkeep and quantify the cost and difficulty of these essential tasks. Finally, the team must compare the visited site and their own institution.

Ultimately, an institution must choose a system by analyzing all the data the clinical information committee and the site-visitors gathered. The institution should only consider systems that are practical and clinically useful and that have a good track record. Selecting systems that are under development and that will be installed gradually is a very risky proposition. Furthermore, institutions should consider the stability of the vendor, because the system will need to be modified when it is installed and it will need to be updated in the future. Thus, a hospital would be wise to choose a stable vendor that is committed to continually developing and improving its product.

In summary, the hospital epidemiologist of the future will have a much broader mission in both inpatient and outpatient settings as healthcare reform moves forward and as clinical information is computerized. Not only will hospital epidemiologists manage infection control issues more quickly and effectively, but they will lead institutions as they design, select, and manage computerized clinical information systems.

References

1. Berg R. Software. *Am J Infect Control.* 1986;14:139-145.
2. Evans RS, Larsen RA, Burke JP, et al. Computer surveillance of hospital-acquired infections and antibiotic use. *JAMA.* 1986;256:1007-1011.
3. Classen DC, Burke JP, Pestotnik SL, Evans RS, Stevens LE. Surveillance for quality assessment: 4. Surveillance using a hospital information system. *Infect Control Hosp Epidemiol.* 1991;12:239-244.
4. Evans RS. The HELP system: a review of clinical applications in infectious diseases and antibiotic use. *MD Comput.* 1991;5:282-315.
5. Classen DC, Pestotnik SL, Evans RS, Burke JP. Computerized surveillance of adverse drug events in hospital patients. *JAMA.* 1991;266:2847-2851.
6. Classen DC, Evans RS, Pestotnik SL, Horn SD, Menlove RL, Burke JP. The timing of prophylactic administration of antibiotics and the risk of surgical-wound infections. *N Engl J Med.* 1992;326:281-286.
7. Ball MJ, Collen MF, eds. *Aspects of the Computer-Based Patient Record.* New York, NY: Springer-Verlag; 1992.
8. Dick RS, Steen EB, eds. *The Computer-Based Patient Record: An Essential Technology For Health Care.* Washington, DC: National Academy Press; 1991.
9. McDonald CJ, Tierney WM. Computer-stored medical records: their future role in medical practice. *JAMA.* 1988;259:3433-3440.
10. Korpman RA, Lincoln TL. The computer-stored medical record: for whom? *JAMA.* 1988;259:3454-3456.
11. Bleich HL, Slack WV. Designing a hospital information system: a comparison of interfaced and integrated systems. *MD Comput.* 1992;9:293-296.
12. Friedman BA, Dieterle RC. Integrating information systems in hospitals: bringing the outside inside. *Arch Pathol Lab Med.* 1990;114:13-16.
13. Shortliffe EH, Perreault LE, eds. *Medical Informatics: Computer Applications in Health Care.* Reading, Pa: Addison-Wesley; 1990.
14. Ball MJ, O'Desky RI, Douglas JV. Status and progress of hospital information systems (CIS). *Int J Biomed Comput.* 1991;29:161-168.
15. Collen MF. A brief historical overview of hospital information system (HIS) evolution in the United States. *Int J Biomed Comput.* 1991;29:169-189.
16. Korth HF, Silberschatz A. *Database System Concepts.* 2nd ed. New York, NY: McGraw-Hill; 1991.
17. Kuperman GJ, Gardner RM, Pryor TA. *HELP: A Dynamic Hospital Information System.* New York, NY: Springer-Verlag; 1991.
18. Gardner RM, Hulse RK, Larsen KG. Assessing the effectiveness of a computerized pharmacy system. *SCAMC.* 1990;14:668-672.
19. Evans RS, Pestotnik SL, Burke JP, Gardner RM, Larsen RA, Classen DC. Reducing duration of prophylactic antibiotic use through computer monitoring of surgical patients. *DICP Ann Pharmacother.* 1990;24:351-354.
20. Pestotnik SL, Evans RS, Burke JP, Gardner RM, Classen DC. Therapeutic antibiotic monitoring: surveillance using a hospital information system. *Am J Med.* 1990;88:43-48.
21. Gardner RM. Computerized data management and decision making in critical care. *Surg Clin North Am.* 1985;65:1041-1051.
22. Tierney WM, Miller ME, McDonald CJ. The effect of test ordering of informing physicians of the charges for outpatient diagnostic tests. *N Engl J Med.* 1990;322:1499-1504.
23. Tierney WM, Miller ME, Overhag JM, McDonald CJ. Physician inpatient order writing on microcomputer workstations: effects on resource utilization. *JAMA.* 1993;269:379-383.
24. Greer ML. RXPERT: a prototype expert system for formulary decision making. *Ann Pharmacother.* 1992;26:244-250.
25. Evans RS, Pestotnik SL, Classen DC, Burke JP. Development of an automated antibiotic consultant. *MD Comput.* 1993;10:17-22.
26. Evans RS, Classen DC, Pestotnik SL, Lundsgaarde HP, Burke JP. Improving empiric antibiotic selection using computer decision support. *Arch Intern Med.* 1994;154:878-884.
27. East TD, Henderson S, Pace NL, Morris AH, Brunner JX.

Knowledge engineering using retrospective review of data: a useful technique or merely data dredging? *Int J Clin Monit Comput.* 1992;8:259-262.

28. Gardner RM, Golubjatnikov OK, Laub RM, Jacobson JT, Evans RS. Computer-critiqued blood ordering using the HELP system. *Comput Biomed Res.* 1990;23:514-528.

29. Barnett OG, Cimino JJ, Hupp JA, Hoffer EP. DXplain: an evolving diagnostic decision-support system. *JAMA.* 1987;258:67-74.

30. East TD, Morris AH, Wallace CJ, et al. A strategy for development of computerized critical care decision support systems. *Int J Clin Monit Comput.* 1992;8:263-269.

31. Bria WF, Rydel RL. *The Physician-Computer Connection.* Chicago, Ill: American Hospital Publishing; 1992.

32. Medical hardware and software buyer's guide. *MD Comput.* 1992;9:339-512.

CHAPTER 21

Basic Microbiologic Support for Hospital Epidemiology

John E. McGowan Jr., MD, Beverly G. Metchock, DrPH

Abstract

The laboratory plays a major role in the epidemiology program's efforts to minimize nosocomial infections in healthcare institutions (HCI). This chapter describes some of the interactions between the laboratory and the epidemiology program, and will identify resources and procedures that the laboratory needs to achieve epidemiologic goals.

Overview: The Role of the Laboratory in Infection Control

The clinical microbiologist has important responsibilities in hospital infection control. These duties include:

- Participating in hospital-wide infection control activities (especially the infection control committee).
- Recovering and identifying accurately the organisms responsible for nosocomial infections.
- Characterizing the antimicrobial susceptibility of many nosocomial pathogens.
- Reporting, in timely fashion, laboratory data relevant to infection control.
- Routinely conducting a few useful microbiologic studies of the hospital environment.
- Supporting investigations of specific hospital infection problems.
- Performing special typing studies, when necessary, to determine whether organisms are similar or different.[1]

In the past decade, changes in laboratory instrumentation and procedures have dramatically improved the laboratory's ability to support infection control efforts. Among these changes are new techniques for more rapid detection and differentiation of organisms and improved systems for both reporting patient data and analyzing trends. Perhaps the most impressive advances have come in special procedures for examining ("typing") hospital organisms to determine whether they are similar or different. Molecular typing methods and other techniques have permitted the laboratory to examine definitively a wider range of organisms than previously was possible.[2]

Role of the Laboratory in Epidemiologic Evaluations

Infection control personnel take several steps when investigating epidemic or endemic nosocomial infections (Table 21-1). The laboratory participates in virtually all of these activities.[3-5]

TABLE 21-1

STEPS IN THE EPIDEMIOLOGIC AND LABORATORY INVESTIGATION OF AN OUTBREAK

Investigative Step	Laboratory Participation
1. Recognize the problem	1. Laboratory surveillance/early warning
a. Case definition	a. Microbiologic confirmation
2. Complete case finding	2. Characterize isolates accurately
a. Assess reliability	a. Search lab database for more cases and review lab methods
b. Assess completeness	b. Availability of records
c. Obtain additional data	c. Do additional testing as needed
3. Define occurrence	3. Provide archival data on occurrence
	a. Store isolates
4. Characterize the outbreak	4. Determine how many strains are involved
a. Patient demography	a. Type isolates
b. Locations	
c. Time	
5. Form hypotheses about causes	5. Conduct supplementary studies as needed
a. Mode of spread	a. Test specimens from the environment
b. Reservoirs	b. Test specimens from personnel or patients
c. Vectors	c. Other studies
6. Initiate control activities	6. Initiate procedural changes as required
7. Continue surveillance	7. Maintain lab surveillance/early warning
a. Evaluate control measures	

Adapted in part from the following: McGowan JE Jr., Metchock BG. Infection control epidemiology and clinical microbiology. In: Murray PR, Baron EJ, Pfaller MA, Tenover FC, Yolken RH, eds. Manual of Clinical Microbiology. *6th ed. Washington, DC: American Society for Microbiology; 1995:182-189. McGowan JE Jr. Laboratory approach to an outbreak of nosocomial infection: systems and techniques for investigation. In: Cundy KR, Kleger B, Hinks E, Miller LA, eds.* Infection Control: Dilemmas and Practical Solutions. *New York, NY: Plenum Press; 1990:21-31. McGowan JE Jr., Weinstein RA. The role of the laboratory in control of nosocomial infection. In: Bennett JV, Brachman PS, eds.* Hospital Infections. *3rd ed. Boston, Mass: Little Brown and Co; 1992:187-220.*

Laboratory Surveillance: An Early Warning System

Perhaps the most important phase in an epidemiologic investigation is the initial step of realizing that a problem exists and defining it precisely. Infection control personnel may become aware of a problem through direct contact with the clinical services, through surveillance conducted on inpatient units or in follow-up clinics, or through another HCI in the region. On occasion, however, the laboratory may report a problem first. Thus, laboratory workers must be taught to recognize findings or situations that may interest the infection control team. Laboratory workers must report any of these events to the epidemiology staff in a timely fashion.

One of the laboratory's crucial responsibilities is to serve as an early warning system for infection control problems.[6] The laboratory should design their reporting system to ensure that all relevant data are reported to infection control personnel as soon as a problem is recognized. The laboratory must save all potentially relevant organisms during the investigation and perhaps longer, if storage facilities allow.

The epidemiologist and the microbiologist must ascertain whether the laboratory's data is reliable and whether the laboratory has sufficient experience and expertise to recognize the microbiologic entity under investigation. This is the stage in which the epidemiologist or microbiologist must distinguish "pseudo-outbreaks" or "pseudoproblems" from true epidemics (see below).

The epidemiologist must understand the limitations of laboratory data and consider the effect of using these data to identify cases.[7] Many nosocomial infections manifest themselves while the afflicted patient is still in the HCI, but some appear only after the patient has been discharged. For example, about half of all surgical wound infections become manifest after the patient has left the hospital.[8] These infections may first be recognized in a clinical setting where microbiologic testing is rarely employed; this is likely to be even more true as healthcare systems evolve. Thus, laboratory results cannot be used as the sole basis for surveillance. Conversely, infections with onset during the patient's stay in the HCI sometimes were acquired in the community and were incubating in the period after admission. Thus, some infections documented by laboratory testing during a patient's hospital stay may be community-acquired. For these reasons, laboratory data alone cannot be used to identify nosocomial infections, and surveillance programs must use other sources of data as well.

In addition to the limitations noted above, laboratory records may not include basic demographic information needed to identify a problem. For example, at Grady Memorial Hospital, our laboratory requisition includes the ward on which the patient is hospitalized, but not the clinical service caring for the patient. Thus, our laboratory would be unlikely to recognize a service-specific outbreak or endemic problem.

Accurate Microbiologic Characterization

Perhaps the laboratory's most important role is to identify organisms accurately and to test the antimicrobial susceptibility of suspected nosocomial pathogens. The spectrum of organisms causing infectious diseases has changed dramatically in the recent past.[3,9,10] A special concern is the increasing frequency with which fungi such as *Candida, Aspergillus, Fusarium*, and *Trichosporon*,[11] and viruses such as respiratory syncytial virus and rotavirus, cause nosocomial infections.[12] Despite the changing spectrum of nosocomial pathogens, the hospital's laboratory should be able to identify most organisms that cause outbreaks or endemic nosocomial infections.

The infection control program's ability to determine the etiology of an infection problem will depend on both special circumstances during each outbreak and the extent to which the laboratory routinely characterizes organisms. For example, if the laboratory does not identify the individual species of *Klebsiella* but instead groups them as "*Klebsiella* species," then the infection control program will not recognize increased rates of nosocomial infection caused by a particular species of this organism.[13,14] Likewise, some laboratories may perform only susceptibility tests that group pneumococcal isolates as susceptible or resistant. Unless they periodically assess the minimum inhibitory concentration (MIC) of all pneumococcal isolates, infection control personnel would not learn that the MICs of *Streptococcus pneumonia* isolates are gradually increasing within the susceptible range.[15]

Fortunately, technologic developments have increased the laboratory's ability to keep pace with changes in etiologic agents and antimicrobial susceptibilities.[1] The advances have occurred in three major categories. First, new instruments and devices have become widely available. This equipment permits the laboratory to detect organisms in blood cultures more readily, identify organisms to genus and species level, and test antimicrobial susceptibility. Some of these devices are automated, permitting laboratories to improve their services without adding personnel. Many instruments are cost-effective even if the laboratory processes only a limited number of specimens. Thus, both small and large hospital laboratories can use these methods. Moreover, these instruments have helped standardize basic microbiologic methods throughout the country. Second, newer non-culture tests have permitted the laboratory to identify organisms that would not have been recovered by traditional microbiologic methods. For example, immunologic methods and nucleic acid testing have improved our ability to detect viruses and other organisms that are difficult or impossible to grow in standard cultures[16]; some of these organisms cause important nosocomial infections. In addition, new amplification techniques such as the polymerase chain reaction may increase the laboratory's ability to identify nosocomial pathogens.[17] Third, the newer tests and instruments allow the laboratory to identify both new and old pathogens more rapidly. Speedier testing should enable the laboratory and the infection control program to recognize outbreaks earlier and to handle endemic nosocomial pathogens more efficiently. Furthermore, these rapid tests may reduce the likelihood that community-acquired organisms will spread in the hospital.

Laboratories in some HCIs do not have the resources to isolate some organisms or to identify routinely certain organisms to species level. At the time that an epidemiologic investigation begins, these laboratories may need to change their procedures so that they can recover and identify relevant isolates fully. At a minimum, the laboratory should be capable of isolating and identifying Gram-positive cocci and Gram-negative aerobic bacilli to the species level when special or recurring cross-infection problems make this necessary.[3]

Providing Archival Information: Storing Data and Isolates

The laboratory must maintain archival information to establish the baseline frequency with which specific organisms of episodic or continuing interest cause infections. The microbiologist and epidemiologist should periodically assess which data will be saved. These individuals should consider both the needs of the infection control program and the laboratory's resources. Since the advent of electronic data processing systems, information (eg, biochemical reactions), which was traditionally saved on the laboratory's worksheets, may not be maintained on the modern laboratory information system.[4] Therefore, the laboratory may have more difficulty retrieving archival information required for epidemiologic investigations.

The laboratory will only be able to test isolates of possible epidemiologic importance if these isolates have been saved systematically. However, the resources for storing organisms vary markedly among HCIs. Laboratory and infection control personnel should regularly discuss which isolates should be saved routinely and which should be saved during special investigative situations.[6] The source of the isolate and the specific organism are important factors to consider. For example, isolates from blood should be held longer than those from urine specimens. Likewise, it might be more desirable to store isolates of *Mycobacterium tuberculosis* than routine isolates of *Escherichia coli*.

Typing: Establishing Microbiologic Similarity or Difference

The laboratory must frequently determine whether individual strains are related or unrelated to define the features of an epidemiologic problem or to test certain hypotheses about the reservoir or mode of spread. A number of typing systems have been designed to determine whether organisms are similar or different.[2] A full discussion of typing methods is beyond the scope of this chapter (see Chapter 22). However, if the laboratory uses phenotypic characteristics such as susceptibility patterns ("antibiogram") or biochemical markers ("biotype") to determine whether organisms are similar or different, laboratory personnel should test all relevant strains in parallel. The laboratory also must test outbreak-associated isolates with control isolates. These steps are essential precautions because the expression of pheonotypic characteristics can be quite variable.[2] If test results vary from day to day or batch to batch, the epidemiologist could arrive at erroneous conclusions.

Supplementary Studies

In the course of an investigation, the hospital epidemiologist may need to identify patients and personnel who are colonized with the implicated strain. In response, the laboratory must process supplementary cultures or immunologically test specimens from patients, personnel, or the environment. The laboratory must assess carefully the sites to be cultured and must choose the appropriate culture media and techniques.[5] The laboratory may require special techniques to accomplish such projects. For example, during an outbreak of *Salmonella* in a nursery, the laboratory might use selective media to enhance the sensitivity of cultures. Likewise, the laboratory might need to process environmental cultures by several methods depending on the source and likely organism involved. We have described previously specific culture techniques for a wide variety of substances and inanimate items.[5]

We recommend that epidemiologists in HCIs refrain from routinely obtaining environmental cultures.[3,5] However, in specific instances, culture surveys help the epidemiologist identify the reservoir and mode of spread. Thus, targeted culture surveys contribute substantially to epidemiologic investigations.[18] The HCI should consider cultures of the environment or personnel as a cost of the infection

control program and should not bill individual patients for these studies.

Change Procedures as Needed

Clinicians must occasionally alter or eliminate specific practices to solve a problem. Similarly, the laboratory may need to alter its routine procedures. For example, increased rates of nosocomial tuberculosis during the 1990s have forced laboratories to alter dramatically their methods for identifying *M tuberculosis* and for evaluating the antimicrobial susceptibility of those isolates.[19]

Potential Problems Related to Laboratory Activities in Epidemiologic Investigations

The laboratory's critical role in epidemiologic investigations is underscored by both its successes and failures. We will discuss some common problems in the laboratory that hamper epidemiologic activities.[3,4]

Misdiagnosis of Outbreak ("Pseudo-outbreak")

On occasion, the epidemiologist will falsely conclude that an epidemic exists when none is actually present.[20] These episodes involve clusters of "false" infections or false clusters of true infections. Spurious outbreaks of nosocomial infection have been traced to a variety of sources (Table 21-2). For example, at our hospital, a pseudo-outbreak of *Serratia marcescens* bacteremia finally was attributed to healthcare workers who transferred blood from nonsterile specimen containers to blood culture vials.[21] Inaccurate or inconsistent microbiologic procedures, another source of pseudo-outbreaks, are especially important as a source of pseudoinfection. For example, one hospital falsely identified 23 patients as being infected with *Legionella pneumophila*. The laboratory used a new probe technique that had poor specificity to identify *Legionella*. Thus, many false-positive tests were recorded before the laboratory identified the

TABLE 21-2

SOURCES OF PSEUDO-OUTBREAKS OF NOSOCOMIAL INFECTION

A. Related to the clinical entity or to the clinician

  1. Wrong diagnosis of clinical entity

  2. Positive cultures represent colonization rather than infection

  3. Failure to distinguish community-acquired from nosocomial infections

  4. Contamination during specimen collection

B. Related to laboratory

  1. Contamination during specimen transport

  2. Contamination during processing

    a. Media or solutions

    b. Equipment

  3. Use of inadequate method or technique

C. Related to case-finding

  1. Increased surveillance efficiency

  2. Improved laboratory techniques for identification

D. Related to chance clustering

Adapted in part from the following: McGowan JE Jr., Metchock BG. Infection control epidemiology and clinical microbiology. In: Murray PR, Baron EJ, Pfaller MA, Tenover FC, Yolken RH, eds. Manual of Clinical Microbiology. *6th ed. Washington, DC: American Society for Microbiology; 1995:182-189. McGowan JE Jr. Laboratory approach to an outbreak of nosocomial infection: systems and techniques for investigation. In: Cundy KR, Kleger B, Hinks E, Miller LA, eds.* Infection Control: Dilemmas and Practical Solutions. *New York, NY: Plenum Press; 1990:21-31. McGowan JE Jr., Weinstein RA. The role of the laboratory in control of nosocomial infection. In: Bennett JV, Brachman PS, eds.* Hospital Infections. *3rd ed. Boston, Mass: Little Brown and Co; 1992:187-220.*

problem.[22] Pseudobacteremia results when needle sterilizers on automated bacteremia detection instruments malfunction, allowing the needle to contaminate blood culture vials tested after a true positive vial.[23] Reagents used in such instruments can also be contaminated. For example, 46 specimens were falsely positive for *Mycobacterium gordonae* because an antimicrobial solution (Bactec Panta Plus), which was added to the culture medium, was ineffectively sterilized by the manufacturer.[24] In addition, laboratory personnel may contam-

inate reagents when they reconstitute or activate reagents. For example, contaminated deionized water has caused false-positive Gram-stains.[25] These reagents may also cause pseudo-outbreaks. Of course, clinicians can inadvertently contaminate specimens before they arrive in the laboratory. This situation is illustrated by pseudo-outbreaks of *Mycobacterium abscessus* caused by a contaminated endocope washer[26] and a pseudo-outbreak of *Pseudomonas cepacia* bacteremia caused by contaminated povidone iodine.[27]

Pseudo-outbreaks can take a considerable amount of time to identify. On occasion, someone in the laboratory finds a problem that brings the pseudo-outbreak to light. Usually, however, clinicians or the epidemiologist recognize the problem by noting a great disparity between the laboratory results and the patients' clinical status or the episode's epidemiologic features.[23,25]

Inadequate Quality Control

Because organisms associated with outbreaks usually are isolated at different times, the laboratory characterizes them at different times. The results of many laboratory tests (eg, identification systems, susceptibility testing, and typing procedures) are particularly susceptible to day-to-day and batch-to-batch variation. Therefore, the laboratory must maintain excellent quality control when making media and other reagents. In some cases, the laboratory may need to reevaluate simultaneously isolates recovered at different times to eliminate variability introduced by the testing process.

Overuse of the Laboratory's Resources

To preserve resources, the laboratory should avoid processing too many cultures from personnel or the environment. The laboratory should also judiciously process the organisms obtained from cultures obtained for epidemiologic purposes. For example, if the laboratory uses 20 different antibiotics to determine susceptibility patterns, most epidemiologically linked organisms will be considered different or unrelated.[1]

Typing procedures have substantially improved the epidemiologist's ability to characterize an outbreak. However, typing is still an inexact science. Investigators continue to develop new typing methods and have just begun to standardize criteria for interpreting typing results.[28] In addition, different typing systems may give different results for the same group of organisms.[28,29] Thus, if there is no clinical or epidemiologic "gold standard" that could determine which typing system is correct, several investigators could draw different conclusions from similar typing data. The epidemiologist must consider all these factors when deciding to use typing data.

One must use typing systems selectively, even during outbreaks. Basic infection control measures can resolve some outbreaks without additional microbiologic data or epidemiologic investigation. In other situations, simple typing methods such as biotyping and antibiotic susceptibility testing provide sufficient information and obviate the need for further testing.[30] Wise epidemiologists and microbiologists use more complicated and/or less readily available typing systems only for selected situations in which control measures have failed or those being studied for academic reasons.

Conclusion

Epidemiologic investigations often make exceptional demands on the laboratory service throughout the period of study. The epidemiologist and the microbiologist must investigate the outbreak rapidly and effectively, yet they also must be efficient and cost-effective. The microbiologist who understands epidemiologic methods will support hospital infection control activities more effectively. Likewise, an epidemiologist who is familiar with the laboratory's resources and procedures will achieve better results. To succeed, the epidemiologist and the microbiologist each must prepare in advance for various diagnostic tasks, whether performed on site or by referral to other laboratories. Together, they must make contingency plans that would effectively solve outbreaks caused by the institution's most common nosocomial pathogens. During the past decade, epidemiologic methods and laboratory procedures have improved, benefiting infection control efforts. Despite these advances, regular and frequent communication between the epidemiologist and the microbiologist is still the key to successful investigations.

References

1. McGowan JE Jr. New laboratory techniques for hospital infection control. *Am J Med.* 1991;91(suppl 3B):245S-251S.

2. Arbeit R. Laboratory procedures for the epidemiologic analysis of microorganisms. In: Murray PR, Baron EJ, Pfaller MA, Tenover FC, Yolken RH, eds. *Manual of Clinical Microbiology.* 6th ed. Washington, DC: American Society for Microbiology; 1995:190-208.

3. McGowan JE Jr., Metchock BG. Infection control epidemiology and clinical microbiology. In: Murray PR, Baron EJ, Pfaller MA, Tenover FC, Yolken RH, eds. *Manual of Clinical Microbiology.* 6th ed. Washington, DC: American Society for Microbiology; 1995:182-189.

4. McGowan JE Jr., Laboratory approach to an outbreak of nosocomial infection: systems and techniques for investigation. In: Cundy KR, Kleger B, Hinks E, Miller LA, eds. *Infection Control: Dilemmas and Practical Solutions.* New York, NY: Plenum Press; 1990:21-31.

5. McGowan JE Jr., Weinstein RA. The role of the laboratory in control of nosocomial infection. In: Bennett JV, Brachman PS, eds. *Hospital Infections.* 3rd ed. Boston, Mass: Little Brown and Co; 1992:187-220.

6. McGowan JE Jr. Communication with hospital staff. In: Balows A, Hausler WJ Jr., Herrmann KL, Isenberg HD, Shadomy HJ, eds. *Manual of Clinical Microbiology.* 5th ed. Washington, DC: American Society for Microbiology; 1991:151-158.

7. Brachman PS. Epidemiology of nosocomial infections. In: Bennett JV, Brachman PS, eds. *Hospital Infections.* 3rd ed. Boston, Mass: Little, Brown & Co; 1992:3-20.

8. Weigelt J, Haley R, Siebert G. Necessity and efficiency of wound infection surveillance after discharge. *Am J Infect Control.* 1987;16:75.

9. Ayliffe GAJ, Mitchell K. Incidence of hospital-acquired

infection. *J Hosp Infect.* 1993;24:77-82.

10. Banerjee SN, Emori TG, Culver DH, et al. Secular trends in nosocomial primary bloodstream infections in the United States, 1980-89. *Am J Med.* 1991;91(suppl 3B):86S-89S.

11. Pfaller MA, Epidemiology and control of fungal infections. *Clin Infect Dis.* 1994;19(1 suppl):S8-S13.

12. Herwaldt LA, Wenzel RP. Dynamics of hospital-acquired infection. In: Murray PR, Baron EJ, Pfaller MA, Tenover FC, Yolken RH, eds. *Manual of Clinical Microbiology.* 6th ed. Washington, DC: American Society for Microbiology; 1995:169-181.

13. Bergogne-Berezine E, Decre D, Joly-Guillou ML. Opportunistic nosocomial multiply resistant bacterial infections—their treatment and prevention. *J Antimicrob Chemother.* 1993; 32:39-47.

14. Jones RN, Kehrberg EN, Erwin ME, Anderson SC. Prevalence of important pathogens and antimicrobial activity of parenteral drugs at numerous medical centers in the United States, I: study on the threat of emerging resistances: real or perceived? Fluoroquinolone Resistance Surveillance Group. *Diagn Microbiol Infect Dis.* 1994;19:203-215.

15. McGowan JE Jr., Metchock BG. Penicillin-resistant pneumococci: an emerging threat to successful therapy. *J Hosp Infect.* 1995;30(suppl):472-482.

16. Relman DA. The identification of uncultured microbial pathogens. *J Infect Dis.* 1993;168:1-8.

17. Dale B, Dragon B. Polymerase chain reaction in infectious disease diagnosis. *Lab Med.* 1994;25:637-641.

18. Dixon RE. Investigation of endemic and epidemic nosocomial infections. In: Bennett JV, Brachman PS, eds. *Hospital Infections.* 3rd ed. Boston, Mass: Little, Brown & Co; 1992:109-133.

19. McGowan JE Jr. Nosocomial tuberculosis: new progress in control and prevention. *Clin Infect Dis.* 1995;21:489-505.

20. Kusek JW. Nosocomial pseudoepidemics and pseudoinfections: an increasing problem. *Am J Infect Control.* 1981;9:70-75.

21. Hoffman PC, Arnow PM, Goldmann DA, Parrott PL, Stamm WE, McGowan JE Jr. False-positive blood cultures—association with nonsterile blood collection tubes. *JAMA.* 1976;236:2073-2075.

22. Laussucq S, Schuster D, Alexander WJ, Thacker WL, Wilkinson HW, Spika JS. False-positive DNA probe test for Legionella species associated with a cluster of respiratory illness. *J Clin Microbiol.* 1988;26:1442-1444.

23. Craven DE, Lichtenberg DA, Browne KF, Coffey DM, Treadwell TL, McCabe WR. Pseudobacteremia traced to cross-contamination by an automated blood culture analyzer. *Infect Control.* 1984;5:75-78.

24. Tokars JI, McNeil MM, Tablan OC, et al. *Mycobacterium gordonae* pseudoinfection associated with a contaminated antimicrobial solution. *J Clin Microbiol.* 1990;28:2765-2769.

25. Medcraft JW, New CW. False-positive Gram-stained smears of sterile body fluids due to contamination of laboratory deionized water. *J Hosp Infect.* 1990;16:75-80.

26. Maloney S, Welbel S, Daves B, et al. *Mycobacterium abscessus* pseudoinfection traced to an automated endoscope washer: utility of epidemiologic and laboratory investigation. *J Infect Dis.* 1994;169:1166-1169.

27. Berkelman RL, Lewin S, Allen JR, et al. Pseudobacteremia attributed to contamination of povidone-iodine with *Pseudomonas cepacia. Ann Intern Med.* 1981;95:32-36.

28. Tenover FC, Arbett RD, Goering RV, et al. Interpreting chromosomal DNA restriction patterns produced by pulsed-field gel electrophoresis: criteria for bacterial strain typing. *J Clin Microbiol.* 1995;33:2233-2239.

29. Allen-Bridson K, Dietrich S, Olmsted RN, et al. Dissimilarities in results of phage typing of Staphylococcus aureus when compared to pulsed-field gel electrophoresis. *Am J Infect Control.* 1995;23:117. Abstract.

30. Prevost G, Jaulhac B, Piemont Y. DNA fingerprinting by pulsed-field gel electrophoresis is more effective than ribotyping in distinguishing among methicillin-resistant *Staphylococcus aureus* isolates. *J Clin Microbiol.* 1992;30:967-973.

CHAPTER 22

Epidemiologic Typing Systems

Joel Maslow, MD, PhD, Maury Ellis Mulligan, MD

Abstract

Microbial strain typing is a useful adjunct to clinical epidemiology. Phenotypic typing systems examine expressed characteristics while genotypic systems, including recent PCR-based systems, examine chromosomal or plasmid DNA. Typing systems have successfully evaluated bacteria, fungi, and viruses. The criteria used to assess the use of each system include typeability, reproducibility, and discriminatory power.

Introduction

The hospital epidemiologist must, in addition to many other things, become conversant about various aspects of molecular biology to understand the rapidly expanding field of epidemiologic typing. One must, of course, decide when and how to use typing methods for an epidemiologic investigation. However, one must also be able to evaluate a literature report of "new improved" methods and to converse comfortably with colleagues who seem to speak very rapidly when they discuss the merits of MLEE ETs or IS*6110* RFLPs. (Don't worry, by the end of this chapter you'll be fluent with these abbreviations.)

Epidemiologic typing is a powerful tool that epidemiologists can use to determine whether a small cluster of cases represents an outbreak in the nursing home, to determine if Mr. Jones who has recurrent bacteremia and a long-term intravascular catheter has a new infection or a relapse of his previous infection, and to decide if an outbreak due to highly resistant *Enterobacter* species is the result of selective antimicrobial pressure on the microbial flora of individual patients or due to horizontal spread of a hospital strain. As with any tool, however, epidemiologic typing is only good when used wisely. As a rule, the epidemiologist or investigator should use typing in conjunction with clinical and epidemiologic data and should consider all data before coming to a conclusion.

When selecting a typing method and evaluating the results, one must consider the purpose for using epidemiologic typing. Independent of the organisms in question, different typing systems may give different results. Typing can simplify an epidemiologic investigation, but the hospital epidemiologist must still obtain other necessary data and formulate the specific question that the typing method should answer. In other words, elegant typing methods do not substitute for the epidemiologist any more than the most sophisticated laboratory tests can obviate the need for a doctor.

Practical factors that influence when and how the epidemiologist uses various typing methods include hospital size, budgets for clinical and research laboratories, and the availability of an individual with interest and expertise in typing. When typing methods beyond species and susceptibility determinations are indicated, the epidemiologist can learn about appropriate methods by performing a literature search, evaluating review articles, contacting investigators who do epidemiologic typing, or consulting local, state, or national laboratories.

Epidemiologic typing uses laboratory methods to identify different strains within a species. Typing methods can be classified as phenotypic or genotypic. Phenotypic techniques detect characteristics expressed by the organism (Table 22-1). Genotypic techniques examine the organism's genetic content directly (Table 22-2). Isolates of the same species that give the same results on a test are generally considered to represent the same strain. Isolates that give different test results are considered to represent different strains.

Investigators who use epidemiologic typing have identified several basic criteria for evaluating typing systems. Typeability refers to the ability of the system to give an unambiguous positive result for each isolate. Reproducibility refers both to the method's ability to give the same result when one tests the same isolate repeatedly and also to the typed attribute's stability over time. Discriminatory power refers to the test's ability to differentiate epidemiologically unrelated strains. As a corollary, the criteria used to determine whether isolates are the same or different must be clearly defined. The epidemiologist or investigator should make certain that the typing is performed with appropriate control strains and that repeated testing is done as needed to ensure that the results are accurate. The epidemiolo-gist must also consider other important characteristics of the method including availability, cost, technical requirements (eg, type of equipment, personnel, and difficulty of interpreting results) and speed.

This chapter reviews basic concepts, applications, and relative merits of most typing methods that are presently available. The chapter will emphasize methods presently in use and their use for studies of common nosocomial pathogens. For detailed information about each technique and descriptions of their strengths and weaknesses, we refer the reader to several excellent reviews.[1-3] We have also listed numerous references to give the reader a "portal" into the relevant typing literature (Table 22-3).

The basic information that we present will be current for some time, but the specific applications certainly will be out of date before long, because new typing tools identify new areas for study. For example, the polymerase chain reaction (PCR) has increased our ability to study fastidious and even noncultivable pathogens, and, thus, has allowed investigators to study the epidemiology of such infectious agents.

Thoughts and Caveats

- Organisms cannot be tested unless they are available. The laboratory can easily throw out saved isolates but cannot recover isolates from the autoclave.

- Epidemiologists should determine whether the techniques that are readily available and inexpensive are adequate before using more sophisticated tests.

- Often the best method is one that works, even if the test has theoretical or actual limitations when used for other purposes. This is especially true if a friend knows the technique and will give you advice and help.

- Typing results frequently represent someone's judgment about sameness or relatedness, not a numerical value or a positive versus negative test result.

TABLE 22-1
PHENOTYPIC TYPING METHODS

Typing Method	Typeability	Reproducibility	Discriminatory Power	Ease of Performance	Ease of Interpretation	Availability	Cost
Antimicrobial susceptibility	Excellent	Good	Poor	Excellent	Excellent	Excellent	Low
Biotyping	Excellent	Poor	Poor	Excellent	Excellent	Excellent	Low
Serotyping	Variable	Good	Variable	Good	Good	Variable	Medium
Bacteriophage typing	Variable	Fair	Variable	Poor	Poor	Excellent	Medium
PAGE	Excellent	Good	Unknown	Excellent	Unknown	Good	Medium
Immunoblotting	Excellent	Good	Good	Good	Good	Variable	Medium
MLEE	Excellent	Excellent	Good	Good	Excellent	Variable	High

PAGE = polyacrylamide gel electrophoresis; MLEE = multilocus enzyme electrophoresis.
The subjective rankings are based on the results from bacterial typing; many techniques are not applicable for viruses and fungi.

- Results obtained with different typing systems do not always correlate completely because different systems evaluate different traits. That's not bad; that's life.

- One system may be inadequate because it cannot discriminate one strain from another. Another system may be too discriminatory such that related isolates all appear different.

- Bacteria multiply rapidly and can be promiscuous; like other living entities they also react to outside pressures. As a result, some of their genetic properties (eg, expression of different genes and plasmid content) may be unstable. Consequently, when evaluating typing systems one must consider the stability of the bacterial trait that the tests assess.

- In general, if a method has worked for one organism (eg, *Escherichia coli*), it is likely to work for a related test organism (eg, other *Enterobacteriaceae*).

- There is not always one best method. Different methods may be best for different organisms, different epidemiologic questions, and different research projects.

- Keep an open mind. Despite the strong clinical suspicion that isolates are epidemiologically related, if they are different by one or more typing systems, they are unlikely to represent the same strain. Conversely, strain typing may detect outbreaks that you previously missed.

- One needs some basic knowledge of the population genetics of the organism in question. For organisms with limited genetic diversity (eg, methicillin-resistant *Staphylococcus aureus*), epidemiologically unrelated organisms may appear the same regardless of the typing system and the typing results may be misinterpreted to represent an outbreak.

- Even the experts have a lot more to learn. Many methods have not been compared with others and many have not been evaluated in specific clinical or epidemiologic settings.

- Some laboratories will type organisms for a fee. Some researchers like to collaborate and will help you investigate an outbreak, especially if the project has scientific merit. However, you may need to contribute some money to offset the cost of evaluating the

TABLE 22-2
GENOTYPIC METHODS

Typing Method	Typeability	Reproducibility	Discriminatory Power	Ease of Performance	Ease of Interpretation	Availability	Cost
Plasmid profiles	Variable	Fair	Variable	Fair	Good	Excellent	Medium
Plasmid REA	Variable	Excellent	Good	Excellent	Excellent	Excellent	Medium
Chromosomal REA	Excellent	Variable	Variable	Good	Fair	Variable	Medium
Ribotyping	Excellent	Excellent	Good	Good	Good	Variable	High
PFGE	Excellent	Excellent	Excellent	Good	Good	Variable	High
PCR	Excellent	Excellent	Unknown	Good	Fair	Variable	High

REA = restriction endonuclease analysis; PFGE = pulsed field gel electrophoresis; PCR = polymerase chain reaction.
The subjective rankings are based on the results from bacterial typing; many techniques are not applicable for viruses and fungi.

organisms. You can always call an expert who can always say no.

Phenotypic Methods

Biotyping

Biotyping, which employs a panel of biochemical reactions to produce a numeric code, is used primarily by the clinical laboratory to identify organisms to the genus and species level. The epidemiologist can best use biotyping to evaluate situations in which a particular species is identified with increased frequency or associated with particular factors such as a specific hospital location. Occasionally, a cluster of organisms with an unusual biotype will direct the epidemiolgist's attention to events of epidemiologic import. However, relative to other methods, biotyping has very poor discriminatory power; this method is, therefore, rarely useful for detailed epidemiologic investigations.

Antimicrobial Susceptibility Patterns

The microbiology laboratory routinely performs susceptibility testing for most bacteria. This information may help the epidemiologist recognize different strains. For example, contemporaneous isolates of any species that are initially thought to come from a common source may have such marked differences in susceptibilities that the epidemiologist need not investigate further. Alternatively, if one finds numerous isolates with the same distinctive susceptibility pattern, one may need to determine whether the isolates come from an outbreak.

In many cases, susceptibility patterns are relatively stable and correlate well with the results of other typing systems. However, selective pressure within hospitals may cause organisms to rapidly gain or lose resistance determinants. In that circumstance, antimicrobial susceptibility is an unstable characteristic, and, therefore, it is not a suitable typing method.

Serotyping

Serotyping, one of the oldest typing methods, detects antigenic determinants expressed on the surface of microorganisms. This method can produce rapid and reproducible results. In some cases, particular serotype results have been correlated with virulence or with clinical syndromes (eg, *E coli* O157:H7 as a cause of diarrhea and the hemolytic uremic syndrome). However, this method has limited discriminatory power for isolates within a serogroup. Organisms routinely tested by serotyping include *Streptococcus pneumoniae*, *Legionella pneumophila*, *Salmonella* species, *Shigella* species, *Haemophilus influenzae*, and *Neisseria meningitidis*. Serologic reagents for typing some species are widely available. However standardized reagents are lacking for most species. Furthermore, many isolates of some species, including *H influenzae*, are not typeable. Other organisms, such as *S aureus*, do not have sufficient antigenic heterogeneity to give adequate discriminatory power for most investigations.

Bacteriophage and Bacteriocin Typing

These methods depend on the susceptibility of the test organism to bacteriophages (viruses that lyse bacterial cells) or to bacteriocins (products produced by other bacteria that inhibit the growth of the test organism). Bacteriophage typing was traditionally the standard method used for typing *S aureus*. A combination of bacteriophage and bacteriocin typing was one of the first methods used to evaluate *Clostridium difficile*. Most reference laboratories in the United States no longer keep bacteriophage stocks. Neither of these typing methods is generally available.

Polyacrylamide Gel Electrophoresis (PAGE)

PAGE separates cellular or membrane bacterial proteins according to their respective molecular weights. A stain for proteins detects the bands of different molecular weights. If the isolate is radiolabeled (eg, grown in media containing ^{35}S-methionine before electrophoresis), the pattern of radioactive bands can be detected by autoradiography.[4] PAGE has helped to identify the species of some organisms that are difficult to evaluate by routine laboratory methods and can detect different strains within a species.[5] However, PAGE patterns are often complex and difficult to interpret.

Immunoblotting

An immunoblot is prepared by transferring bacterial cellular materials to nitrocellulose paper after they have been electrophoretically separated by PAGE (Western blot). The nitrocellulose membrane is then reacted with antibodies (either antisera obtained from immunized animals or pooled human sera), an enzyme-labeled antiserum (commercially available), and a substrate to produce a color change. Investigators have used this method to study *C difficile* and *S aureus*. Immunoblotting is inexpensive and relatively rapid. However, one needs some experience to interpret the results and only a few laboratories have evaluated this technique.

Multilocus Enzyme Electrophoresis (MLEE)

This method differentiates bacteria by analyzing the mobilities of numerous metabolic enzymes within starch gels. The location of each enzyme is detected by exposing the gel to a substrate that produces a color reaction with that specific enzyme. Enzyme mobilities reflect variations in numerous genetic loci; the panel of mobilities yields an electrophoretic type (ET) for each isolate. One can use mathematical analysis to quantify the difference between two isolates with different ETs. The method has enabled investigators to analyze rigorously genetic variations within a species. However, for some species, MLEE may have less discriminatory power than other methods that are technically easier.

Genotypic Methods

Plasmid Profile Analysis

Plasmids are extrachromosomal DNA that can be extracted from bacteria and then separated by

TABLE 22-3
TYPING SYSTEMS IN RELATION TO SPECIFIC ORGANISMS

Organism	Serotyping	Phage Typing	PAGE & Immuno-blot	MLEE	PPA	REA	Southern Blot	Ribotyping	PFGE	PCR
						Utility of Typing System for Particular Organism*				
Bacteria										
Acinetobacter	++	++[7]	ND	ND	++[8]	++	++	+++[9]	++++[7,8]	+++[9]
Bacteroides	ND	ND	+++[10]	ND	+[11]	ND	++[12]	+++[12]	+++[11]	+++[12]
Bartonella (rochalimea)	ND	ND	ND	ND	ND	ND	ND	ND	ND	+++[13]
Chlamydia	+/++[14,15]	ND	+[14,16]	ND	ND	+++[14,17]	+++[17,18]	++[18]	ND	++[18]
C difficile, C perfringens	+[19]	+/++[20]	+++[4,19]	ND	+/++[19]	+++[21]	ND	++/+++[21]	+++[21]	++[22]
Enterobacter	++[23]	++[23]	+++[24]	+++	++[25]	++[26]	+++	+++[23]	+++[26]	+++[27,28]
Enterococci	ND	+/++[29]	ND	ND	++[30]	++[31]	+++[30]	+++[31]	++++[32]	+++[28]
E coli	+++[33,34]	++	+	+++[34]	++	++/+++[33]	+++[33]	+++[33,34]	++++[35]	+++[28,36]
Haemophilus	++[37]	ND	+/++[38]	+++[37,39]	+/++[38]	++[39]	++[37]	+++[38,39]	+++[39]	+++[40]
Helicobacter, Campylobacter	++[41,42]	+[41]	+[41]	+++[41]	+	++/+++[41]	++	+++[41,42]	++++[42]	+++[42]
Klebsiella	++	ND	ND	+++	++	++	++[43]	+++[43]	+++[43]	ND
Legionella	++[44]	ND	+++[44,45]	+++[46]	+++[45]	+++[46]	++[47]	+++[47,48]	++++[46,48]	+++[46]
M avium	++[49]	ND	ND	+++[50]	+/++[51]	++	+++/++++[52]	+++[49]	+++[49]	+++[36]
M tuberculosis	++	++[53]	ND	ND	ND	++[54]	+++/++++[55,56]	+	+++[57]	++++[58]
Mycobacterium, other	++[59]	ND	ND	ND	+[60]	++	++	++	+++[61]	++[62]
N meningitidis, gonorrhea	++[63,64]	ND	+[63]	+++[63]	++[64]	+++	+++	++	+++[64]	ND

Organism									
Proteus	++	++[65]	++[66]	+++	+++[66]	ND	++[67]	+++	+++[67]
Pseudomonas, Burkholderia, Stenotrophomonas	++[68,69]	+++/+++	ND	+++[70]	++	+++[71]	+++[68,71]	++++[72]	++++[68]
Rickettsia	ND	ND	++[73]	ND	++/+++[74]	ND	ND	+++[75]	++[76]
Salmonella	++[77]	++[78,79]	ND	+++[77]	++[78]	++/+++[79]	+++[78,80]	++++[80]	ND
Serratia	++[81]	+[81]	+[81]	ND	+[81]	+[81]	ND	+++[82]	ND
Shigella	++[83,84]	ND	ND	+++[85]	++[84]	+++[84]	++/+++[86]	+++[83]	ND
S aureus, MRSA	++[87]	+++[87,88]	+++[88]	+++[88]	++/+++	+++[6,88]	+++[88]	+++[6,88]	+++[28,88]
S epidermidis	++[89]	++[89]	ND	ND	+++[90]	+++[89,90]	+[91]	+++[91,92]	ND
Streptococci	++[93]	+/++[94]	++[93]	+++	ND	+++[93,95]	+++[96]	+++[97]	+++[36]
Fungi									
Aspergillus	ND	ND	+[98]	+++[99]	ND	+++[100]	+++[99,100]	ND	+++[100]
Candida	ND	ND	+[101]	+++[102]	ND	+++[102,103]	+++[103]	+++[102,103]	+++[104]
Cryptococcus	++[105]	ND	ND	ND	ND	ND	ND	+++[105,106]	++
Histoplasma	ND	ND	ND	ND	ND	++++[107,108]	++++[108]	ND	+++[109]
Viruses									
Cytomegalovirus	ND	n/a	n/a	n/a	n/a	+++[110]	n/a	n/a	+++[111,112]
Hepatitis B & C	n/a	n/a	n/a	n/a	n/a	ND	n/a	n/a	+++[113,114]

TABLE 22-3 (continued)
Typing Systems in Relation to Specific Organisms

Organism	Serotyping	Phage Typing	PAGE & Immuno-blot	MLEE	PPA	REA	Southern Blot	Ribotyping	PFGE	PCR
						Utility of Typing System for Particular Organism*				
Herpes simplex, zoster	+	n/a	n/a	n/a	n/a	ND	n/a	n/a	n/a	+++[115]
HIV	n/a	n/a	n/a	n/a	n/a	ND	n/a	n/a	n/a	++++[116]
Rabies	+/++[117]	n/a	n/a	n/a	n/a	ND	n/a	n/a	n/a	++/+++[117]
Rotavirus	++[118]	n/a	n/a	n/a	n/a	+++[119]	n/a	n/a	n/a	+++[118]

PAGE = polyacrylamide gel electrophoresis; MLEE = multilocus enzyme electrophoresis; PPA = plasmid profile analysis; REA = restriction endonuclease analysis; PFGE = pulsed field gel electrophoresis; PCR = polymerase chain reaction.
*The grading system is as follows: ++++ = considered the best method for the organism with a high degree of discriminatory power and typeability; +++ = methodology demonstrates a high degree of discriminatory power and typeability; ++ = fair to moderate discriminatory power or typeability; + = typing method used but low discriminatory power; ND, insufficient data to determine use. Illustrative references are given with the particular techniques. Techniques that are not applicable to the organisms in question are reported as n/a.

agarose gel electrophoresis. Plasmid DNA is detected by staining the gel with ethidium bromide and then exposing the gel to UV light. The plasmid profile is determined by the number and size of plasmids present. Plasmid profile analysis was one of the first DNA-based techniques to be used for epidemiologic studies. This method discriminates poorly among isolates with few or no plasmids. Reproducibility can be poor because supercoiled or circular plasmids can exist in molecular forms that migrate differently during electrophoresis. Thus, one plasmid may produce different numbers of bands in different test runs. Also, plasmids may be lost or gained over time in vivo.

Restriction Endonuclease Analysis of the Plasmids (REAP)

Plasmid DNA can be cut at specific nucleotide sequences by enzymes called restriction endonucleases. This additional step eliminates the problems in profile interpretation caused by supercoiled or circular plasmid DNA and produces consistent patterns by gel electrophoresis. REAP gives better discrimination and reproducibility and is the method of plasmid analysis used most widely at present. Compared with many other methods, REAP is technically simple, inexpensive, and rapid. It has been very useful for studies of many organisms such as staphylococci.

Restriction Endonuclease Analysis of Chromosomal DNA

The same methods are used for chromosomal REA as those described above for plasmid REA except that the entire chromosome is studied. An obvious advantage is that all isolates are typeable, including those lacking plasmids. One technical problem is that the method does not completely remove plasmid DNA. Thus, isolates that have genetically identical chromosomal DNA may have different REA patterns caused by the presence or absence of plasmids. Chromosomal REA patterns,

unlike those obtained with plasmid REA, typically consist of hundreds of bands. Consequently, these patterns are very difficult and time-consuming to interpret and their evaluation requires experience. For these reasons, the method is not commonly used, but it has facilitated epidemiologic studies of organisms such as *C difficile*.

Southern Blot Analysis of Chromosomal DNA

After restriction fragments of DNA are separated by agarose gel electrophoresis (as described above), they can be transferred to nitrocellulose or nylon membranes, producing a blot named after Southern, who described the technique. The Southern blot is then probed with labeled DNA that binds to homologous chromosomal or plasmid DNA fragments. When the membrane exposes radiographic film, fragments of different sizes are visible as black bands called restriction fragment length polymorphisms (RFLPs). Probes can be labeled with radioisotopes or nonradioactive, chemiluminescent compounds. The technique is laborious and time-consuming compared with other methods available for typing most hospital pathogens.

Insertion sequences (IS) and transposons are genetic elements within the chromosome that can also be used as probes. Southern blot analysis using IS*6110* as the probe is now the method of choice for typing *M tuberculosis*. RFLP analysis of *mec* (the gene encoding for methicillin resistance) and Tn*554* (which carries the gene that encodes for erythromycin resistance) has been used to type *S aureus*.[6]

Ribotyping and Other Methods Using Probes

Ribotyping uses Southern blot analysis to detect RFLPs (described above) that are associated with the ribosomal operon. The *E coli* ribosomal operon (DNA or rDNA) is typically used as a probe because the ribosomal genes are highly conserved for all bacteria. The method has been used extensively for epidemiologic studies of *E coli*, *S aureus*, and other hospital pathogens. The discriminatory power is directly proportional to the number of ribosomes (seven for *E coli*, five for *S aureus*, one for *M tuberculosis*) and the genetic diversity of the organism studied (extensive for *E coli*, limited for MRSA).

Pulsed Field Gel Electrophoresis (PFGE) of Chromosomal DNA

PFGE, developed in 1984 by Schwartz and Canter, is a variation of agarose gel electrophoresis. This method is a powerful tool for typing numerous organisms. The orientation of the electric field is changed (or pulsed) periodically. Consequently, PFGE can separate large DNA fragments that conventional agarose gel electrophoresis, which uses a constant electric field, cannot adequately separate. Test organisms are embedded in agarose plugs and the DNA is released in situ, thereby minimizing shearing of the DNA before it is digested with restriction enzymes. PFGE is highly discriminatory and reproducible. PFGE is capable in theory of typing all bacterial isolates. Numerous laboratories have evaluated PFGE and found it to be an excellent method for typing most common bacterial pathogens and also *Mycobacterium avium*. The method, however, is not rapid and it requires relatively expensive equipment. Complete kits are commercially available that include pre-made solutions. The kits and reagents are expensive and do not appear to be more reliable than self-made solutions.

Typing Systems Using the Polymerase Chain Reaction (PCR)

PCR allows the laboratory to use DNA polymerase and two primers (oligonucleotides that correspond to the ends of the template) to replicate (or amplify) a DNA sequence or template rapidly and exponentially. PCR primers represent either known chromosomal DNA sequences that are specific for the species to be tested or unrelated sequences selected "arbitrarily" or "randomly." The procedure can generate substantial amounts of product from minute quantities of template. The product DNA can be digested with restriction enzymes and subjected to electrophoresis. The investigator can then analyze the restriction fragments.

One of the most valuable attributes of PCR is its ability to detect DNA from organisms that cannot be cultivated. A major problem with PCR-based techniques is that they may also amplify minute amounts of contaminating DNA, thus producing erroneous results. Investigators have used PCR to study numerous bacteria and fungi. In addition, researchers are currently comparing PCR with other typing methods and evaluating its use as an epidemiologic typing method. However, problems with reproducibility may limit the usefulness of PCR for epidemiologic studies.

References

1. Maslow JN, Mulligan ME, Arbeit RD. Molecular epidemiology: the application of contemporary techniques to typing bacteria. *Clin Infect Dis.* 1993;17:153-164.

2. Sader HS, Hollis RJ, Pfaller MA. The use of molecular techniques in the epidemiology and control of infectious diseases. *Clin Lab Med.* 1995;15:407-431.

3. Arbeit RD. Laboratory procedures for the epidemiologic analysis of microorganisms. In: Murray PR, Baron EJ, Pfaller MA, Tenover FC, Yolken RH, eds. *Manual of Clinical Microbiology.* 6th ed. Washington, DC: American Society for Microbiology; 1994:190-208.

4. Tabaqchali S. Epidemiologic markers of *Clostridium difficile. Rev Infect Dis.* 1990;12:S192-S199.

5. Tanner AR. Characterization of *Wolinella* spp., *Campylobacter concisus, Bacteroides gracilis*, and *Eikenella corrodens* by polyacrylamide gel electrophoresis. *J Clin Microbiol.* 1986;24:562-565.

6. Kreiswirth B, Kornblum J, Arbeit RD, et al. Evidence for a clonal origin of methicillin resistance in *Staphylococcus aureus. Science.* 1993;259:227-230.

7. Gouby A, Carles-Nurit M-J, Bouziges N, et al. Use of pulsed-field gel electrophoresis for investigation of hospital outbreaks of *Acinetobacter baumannii. J Clin Microbiol.* 1992;30:1588-1591.

8. Seifert H, Schulze A, Baginski R, Pulverer G. Comparison of four different methods for epidemiologic typing of *Acinetobacter baumannii. J Clin Microbiol.* 1994;32:1816-1819.

9. Vila J, Marcos A, Llovet T, Coll P, Jimenez De Anta T. A comparative study of ribotyping and arbitrarily primed polymerase chain reaction for investigation of hospital outbreaks of *Acinetobacter baumannii* infection. *J Med Microbiol.* 1994;41:244-249.

10. Mulligan ME, Kwok RYY, Molitoris D, et al. Immunoblot typing of *Bacteroides gracilis. Clin Infect Dis.* 1995;20:S130-S131.

11. Bedzyk LA, Shoemaker NB, Young KE, Salyers AA. Insertion and excision of *Bacteriodes* conjugative chromosomal elements. *J Bacteriol.* 1992;174:166-172.

12. Podglajen I, Breuil J, Casin I, Collatz E. Genotypic identification of two groups within the species *Bacteroides fragilis* by ribotyping and by analysis of PCR-generated fragment patterns and insertion sequence content. *J Bacteriol.* 1995;177:5270-5275.

13. Matar GM, Swaminathan B, Hunter SB, Slater LN, Welch DF. Polymerase chain reaction-based restriction fragment length polymorphism analysis of a fragment of the ribosomal operon from *Rochalimaea* species for subtyping. *J Clin Microbiol.* 1993;31:1730-1734.

14. Mills SD, Kurjanczyk LA, Shames B, Hennessy JN, Penner JL. Antigenic shifts in serotype determinants of *Campylobacter coli* are accompanied by changes in the chromosomal DNA restriction endonuclease digestion pattern. *J Med Microbiol.* 1991;35:168-173.

15. Vanrompay D, Andersen AA, Ducatelle R, Haesebrouck F. Serotyping of European isolates of *Chlamydia psittaci* from poultry and other birds. *J Clin Microbiol.* 1993;31:134-137.

16. Black CM, Johnson JE, Farshy CE, Brown TM, Berdal BP. Antigen variation among strains of *Chlamydia pneumoniae. J Clin Microbiol.* 1991;29:1312-1316.

17. Timms P, Eaves FW, Girjes AA, Lavin MF. Comparison of *Chlamydia psittaci* isolates by restriction endonuclease and DNA probe analyses. *Infect Immun.* 1988;56:287-290.

18. Scieux C, Grimont F, Regnault B, Grimont PAD. DNA fingerprinting of *Chlamydia trachomatis* by use of ribosomal RNA, oligonucleotide and randomly cloned DNA probes. *Res Microbiol.* 1992;143:755-765.

19. Mulligan ME, Peterson LR, Kwok RYY, Clabots CR, Gerding DN. Immunoblots and plasmid fingerprints compared with serotyping and polyacrylamide gel electrophoresis for typing *Clostridium difficile. J Clin Microbiol.* 1988;26:41-46.

20. Sell TL, Schaberg DR, Fekety FR. Bacteriophage and bacteriocin typing scheme for *Clostridium difficile. J Clin Microbiol.* 1983;17:1148-1152.

21. Kristjánsson M, Samore MH, Gerding DN, et al. Comparison of restriction endonuclease analysis, ribotyping, and pulsed field gel electrophoresis for molecular differentiation of *Clostridium difficile* strains. *J Clin Microbiol.* 1994;32:1963-1969.

22. Silva J, Tang YJ, Gumerlock PH. Genotyping of *Clostridium difficile* isolates. *J Infect Dis.* 1994;169:661-664.

23. Garaizar J, Kaufman ME, Pitt TL. Comparison of ribotyping with conventional methods for the type identification of *Enterobacter cloacae. J Clin Microbiol.* 1991;29:1303-1307.

24. Mulligan ME, Shimoda K, Orakcilar G, et al. *Immunoblot typing of* Enterobacter *spp used to examine epidemiology and development of resistance.* New Orleans, La: American Society of Microbiology; 1992.

25. Markowitz N, Quinn EL, Saravolatz LD. Trimethoprim-sulfamethoxazole compared with vancomycin for the treatment of *Staphylococcus aureus* infection. *Ann Intern Med.* 1992;117:390-398.

26. Haertl R, Bandlow G. Epidemiological fingerprinting of *Enterobacter cloacae* by small-fragment restriction endonuclease analysis and pulsed-field gel electrophoresis of genomic restriction fragments. *J Clin Microbiol.* 1993;31:128-133.

27. Bingen E, Denamur E, Lambert-Zechovsky N, et al. Rapid genotyping shows the absence of cross-contamination in *Enterobacter cloacae* nosocomial infections. *J Hosp Infect.* 1992;21:95-101.

28. Kostman JR, Alden MB, Mair M, et al. A universal approach to bacterial molecular epidemiology by polymerase chain reaction ribotyping. *J Infect Dis.* 1995;171:204-208.

29. Kühnen E, Richter F, Richter K, Andries L. Establishment of a typing system for group D streptococci. *Zbl Bakt Hyg.* 1988;A267:322-330.

30. Patterson JE, Wanger A, Zscheck KK, Zervos MJ, Murray BE. Molecular epidemiology of β-lactamase-producing enterococci. *Antimicrob Agents Chemother.* 1990;34:302-305.

31. Hall LMC, Duke B, Guiney M, Williams R. Typing of *Enterococcus* species by DNA restriction fragment analysis. *J Clin Microbiol.* 1992;30:915-919.

32. Murray BE, Singh KV, Heath JD, Sharma BR, Weinstock GM. Comparison of genomic DNAs of different enterococcal isolates using restriction endonucleases with infrequent recognition sites. *J Clin Microbiol.* 1990;28:2059-

2063.

33. Arthur M, Arbeit RD, Kim C, et al. Restriction fragment length polymorphisms among uropathogenic *Escherichia coli* isolates: *pap*-related sequences compared with *rrn* operons. *Infect Immunol.* 1990;58:471-479.

34. Maslow JN, Whittam T, Wilson RA, et al. Clonal relationship among bloodstream isolates of *Escherichia coli*. *Infect Immunol.* 1995;63:2409-2417.

35. Arbeit RD, Arthur M, Dunn RD, et al. Resolution of recent evolutionary divergence among *Escherichia coli* from related lineages: the application of pulsed field electrophoresis to molecular epidemiology. *J Infect Dis.* 1990;161:230-235.

36. Versalovic J, Kapur V, Koeuth T, et al. DNA fingerprinting of pathogenic bacteria by fluorophore-enhanced repetitive sequence-based polymerase chain reaction. *Arch Pathol Lab Med.* 1995;119:23-29.

37. Musser JM, Kroll JS, Moxon ER, Selander RK. Evolutionary genetics of the encapsulated strains of *Haemophilus influenzae*. *Proc Natl Acad Sci.* 1988;85:7758-7762.

38. Brenner DJ, Mayer LW, Carlone GM, et al. Biochemical, genetic, and epidemiologic characteristics of *Haemophilus influenzae* biogroup aegyptius (*Haemophilus aegyptius*) strains associated with Brazilian purpuric fever. *J Clin Microbiol.* 1988;26:1524-1534.

39. Arbeit RD, Dunn R, Maslow JN, Goldstein R, Musser JM. Resolution of evolutionary divergence and epidemiologic relatedness among *H. influenzae* type b (HIB) by pulsed field gel electrophoresis (PFGE). 30th Intersci Conf Antimicrob Agents Chemother. Atlanta, Ga; 1990.

40. Myers LE, Silva SVPS, Procunier JD, Little PB. Genomic fingerprinting of "*Haemophilus somnus*" isolates by using a random-amplified polymorphic DNA assay. *J Clin Microbiol.* 1993;31:512-517.

41. Patton CM, Wachsmuth IK, Evins GM, et al. Evaluation of 10 methods to distinguish epidemic-associated *Campylobacter* strains. *J Clin Microbiol.* 1991;29:680-688.

42. Stanley J, Linton D, Sutherland K, Jones C, Owen RJ. High-resolution genotyping of *Campylobacter coli* identifies clones of epidemiologic and evolutionary sequence. *J Infect Dis.* 1995;172:1130-1134.

43. Maslow JN, Brecher S, Adams KS, et al. Relationship between indole production and the differentiation of *Klebsiella* species: indole-positive and negative isolates of *Klebsiella* determined to be clonal. *J Clin Microbiol.* 1993;31:2000-2003.

44. Lema M, Brown A. Electrophoretic characterization of soluble protein extracts of *Legionella pneumophila* and other members of the family *Legionellaceae*. *J Clin Microbiol.* 1983;17:1132-1140.

45. Pfaller M, Hollis R, Johnson W, et al. The application of molecular and immunologic techniques to study the epidemiology of *Legionella pneumophila* serogroup 1. *Diagn Microbiol.* 1989;12:295-302.

46. van Belkum A, Struelens M, Quint W. Typing of *Legionella pneumophila* strains by polymerase chain reaction-mediated DNA fingerprinting. *J Clin Microbiol.* 1993;31:2198-2200.

47. Saunders NA, Harrison TG, Haththotuwa A, Taylor AG. A comparison of probes for restriction fragment length polymorphism (RFLP) typing of *Legionella pneumophila* serogroup 1 strains. *J Med Microbiol.* 1994;41:152-158.

48. Schoonmaker D, Heimberger T, Birkhead G. Comparison of ribotyping and restriction enzyme analysis using pulsed-field gel electrophoresis for distinguishing *Legionella pneumophila* isolates obtained during a nosocomial outbreak. *J Clin Microbiol.* 1992;30:1491-1498.

49. Arbeit RD, Slutsky A, Barber TW, et al. Genetic diversity among strains of *Mycobacterium avium* causing monoclonal and polyclonal bacteremia in patients with AIDS. *J Infect Dis.* 1993;167:1384-1390.

50. Yakrus MA, Reeves MW, Hunter SB. Characterization of isolates of *Mycobacterium avium* serotypes 4 and 8 from patients with AIDS by multilocus enzyme electrophoresis. *J Clin Microbiol.* 1992;30:1474-1478.

51. Jensen AG, Bennedsen J, Rosdahl VT. Plasmid profiles of *Mycobacterium avium/intracellulare* isolated from patients with AIDS or cervical lymphadenitis and from environmental samples. *Scand J Infect Dis.* 1989;21:645-649.

52. Guerrero C, Bernasconi C, Burki D, Bodmer T, Telenti A. A novel insertion element from *Mycobacterium avium*, IS*1245*, is a specific target for analysis of strain relatedness. *J Clin Microbiol.* 1995;33:304-307.

53. Snider DE, Jones WD, Good RC. The usefulness of phage typing *Mycobacterium tuberculosis* isolates. *Am Rev Respir Dis.* 1984;130:1095-1099.

54. Collins DM, De Lisle GW. DNA restriction endonuclease analysis of *Mycobacterium tuberculosis* and *Mycobacterium bovis* BCG. *J Gen Microbiol.* 1984;130:1019-1021.

55. Edlin BR, Tokars JI, Grieco MH, et al. An outbreak of multidrug-resistant tuberculosis among hospitalized patients with the acquired immunodeficiency syndrome. *N Engl J Med.* 1992;326:1514-1521.

56. van Soolingen D, Hermans PWM, de Haas PEW, Soll DR, van Embden JDA. Occurrence and stability of inser-

tion sequences in *Mycobacterium tuberculosis* complex strains: evaluation of an insertion sequence-dependent DNA polymorphism as a tool in the epidemiology of tuberculosis. *J Clin Microbiol.* 1991;29:2578-2586.

57. Zhang Y, Mazurek GH, Cave MD, et al. DNA polymorphisms in strains of *Mycobacterium tuberculosis* analyzed by pulsed-field gel electrophoresis: a tool for epidemiology. *J Clin Microbiol.* 1992;30:1551-1556.

58. Haas WH, Butler WR, Woodley CL, Crawford JT. Mixed-linker polymerase chain reaction: a new method for rapid fingerprinting of isolates of the *Mycobacterium tuberculosis* complex. *J Clin Microbiol.* 1993;31:1293-1298.

59. Tsang AY, Denner JC, Brennan PJ, McClatchy JK. Clinical and epidemiological importance of typing of *Mycobacterium avium* complex isolates. *J Clin Microbiol.* 1992;30:479-484.

60. Labidi A, Dauguet C, Goh KS, David HL. Plasmid profiles of *Mycobacterium fortuitum* complex isolates. *Curr Microbiol.* 1984;11:235-240.

61. Burns DN, Wallace RJ, Jr, Schultz ME, et al. Nosocomial outbreak of respiratory tract colonization with *Mycobacterium fortuitum*: demonstration of the usefulness of pulsed-field gel electrophoresis in an epidemiologic investigation. *Am Rev Respir Dis.* 1991;144:1153-1159.

62. Kauppinen J, Mäntyjärvi R, Katila M-L. Random amplified polymorphic DNA genotyping of *Mycobacterium malmoense*. *J Clin Microbiol.* 1994;32:1827-1829.

63. Wedege E, Caugant DA, Frøholm LO, Zollinger WD. Characterization of serogroup A and B strains of *Neisseria meningitidis* with serotype 4 and 21 monoclonal antibodies and by multilocus enzyme electrophoresis. *J Clin Microbiol.* 1991;29:1486-1492.

64. Ng L-K, Carballo M, Dillon J-AR. Differentiation of *Neisseria gonorrhoeae* isolates requiring proline, citrulline, and uracil by plasmid content, serotyping and pulsed-field gel electrophoresis. *J Clin Microbiol.* 1995;33:1039-1041.

65. Schmidt WC, Jeffries CD. Bacteriophage typing of *Proteus mirabilis*, *Proteus vulgaris*, and *Proteus morganii*. *Appl Microbiol.* 1974;27:47-53.

66. Kappos T, John MA, Hussain Z, Valvano MA. Outer membrane protein profiles and multilocus enzyme electrophoresis analysis for differentiation of clinical isolates of *Proteus mirabilis* and *Proteus vulgaris*. *J Clin Microbiol.* 1992;30:2632-2637.

67. Bingen E, Boissinot C, Desjardins P, et al. Arbitrarily primed polymerase chain reaction provides rapid differentiation of *Proteus mirabilis* isolates from a pediatric hospital. *J Clin Microbiol.* 1993;31:1055-1059.

68. Pasloske BL, Joffe AM, Sun Q, et al. Serial isolates of *Pseudomonas aeruginosa* from a cystic fibrosis patient have identical pilin sequences. *Infect Immunol.* 1988;56:665-672.

69. Rabkin CS, Jarvis WR, Anderson RL, et al. *Pseudomonas cepacia* typing systems: collaborative study to assess their potential in epidemiologic investigations. *Rev Infect Dis.* 1989;11:600-607.

70. Boukadida J, de Montalembert M, Gaillard J-L, et al. Outbreak of gut colonization by *Pseudomonas aeruginosa* in immunocompromised children undergoing total digestive decontamination: analysis by pulsed-field electrophoresis. *J Clin Microbiol.* 1991;29:2068-2071.

71. Ogle JW, Janda JM, Woods DE, Vasil ML. Characterization and use of a DNA probe as an epidemiological marker for *Pseudomonas aeruginosa*. *J Infect Dis.* 1987;155:119-126.

72. Anderson DJ, Kuhns JS, Vasil ML, Gerding DN, Janoff EN. DNA fingerprinting by pulsed field gel electrophoresis and ribotyping to distinguish *Pseudomonas cepacia* isolates from a nosocomial outbreak. *J Clin Microbiol.* 1991;29:648-649.

73. Dasch GA, Samms JR, Weiss E. Biochemical characteristics of typhus group *Rickettsiae* with special attention to the *Rickettsia prowazekii* strains isolated from flying squirrels. *Infect Immunol.* 1978;19:676-685.

74. Regnery RL, Tzianabos T, Esposito JJ, McDade JE. Strain differentiation of epidemic typhus Rickettsiae (*Rickettsia prowazekii*) by DNA restriction endonuclease analysis. *Curr Microbiol.* 1983;8:355-358.

75. Roux V, Drancourt M, Raoult D. Determination of genome sizes of *Rickettsia* spp. within the spotted fever group, using pulsed-field gel electrophoresis. *J Bacteriol.* 1992;174:7455-7457.

76. Manor E, Ighbarieh J, Sarov B, Kassis I, Regnery R. Human and tick spotted fever group rickettsia isolates from Israel: a genotypic analysis. *J Clin Microbiol.* 1992;30:2653-2656.

77. Beltran P, Musser JM, Helmuth R, et al. Toward a population genetic analysis of *Salmonella*: genetic diversity and relationships among strains of serotypes *S choleraesuis, S derby, S dublin, S enteritidis, S heidelberg, S infantis, S newport, S typhimurium. Proc Natl Acad Sci.* 1988;85:7753-7757.

78. Altwegg M, Hickman-Brenner FW, Farmer JJ III. Ribosomal RNA gene restriction patterns provide increased sensitivity for typing *Salmonella typhi* strains. *J Infect Dis.* 1989;160:145-149.

79. Rodrigue DC, Cameron DN, Puhr ND, et al. Comparison of plasmid profiles, phage types, and antimicrobial resis-

tance patterns of *Salmonella enteritidis* isolates in the United States. *J Clin Microbiol.* 1992;30:854-857.

80. Baquar N, Burnens A, Stanley J. Comparative evaluation of molecular typing strains from a national epidemic due to *Salmonella brandenburg* by rRNA gene and IS*200* probes and pulsed-field gel electrophoresis. *J Clin Microbiol.* 1994;32:1876-1880.

81. McGeer A, Low DE, Penner J, et al. Use of molecular typing to study the epidemiology of *Serratia marcescens*. *J Clin Microbiol.* 1990;28:55-58.

82. Sader HS, Perl TM, Hollis RJ, et al. Nosocomial transmission of *Serratia odorifera* biogroup 2: case report demonstration by macrorestriction analysis of chromosomal DNA using pulsed-field gel electrophoresis. *Infect Control Hosp Epidemiol.* 1994;15:390-393.

83. Kristjánsson M, Viner B, Maslow JN. Polymicrobial and recurrent bacteremia with *Shigella* in a patient with AIDS. *Scand J Infect Dis.* 1994;26:411-416.

84. Litwin CM, Storm AL, Chipowsky S, Ryan KJ. Molecular epidemiology of *Shigella* infections: plasmid profiles, serotype correlation, and restriction endonuclease analysis. *J Clin Microbiol.* 1991;29:104-108.

85. Selander RK, Caugant DA, Ochman H, et al. Methods of multilocus enzyme electrophoresis for bacterial population genetics and systematics. *Appl Environ Microbiol.* 1986;51:873-884.

86. Strockbine NA, Parsonnet J, Greene K, Kiehlbauch JA, Wachsmuth IK. Molecular epidemiologic techniques in analysis of epidemic and endemic *Shigella dysenteriae* type 1 strains. *J Infect Dis.* 1991;163:406-409.

87. Arbeit RD, Karakawa WW, Vann WF, Robbins JB. Predominance of two newly described capsular polysaccharide types among clinical isolates of *Staphylococcus aureus*. *Diagn Microbiol Infect Dis.* 1984;2:85-91.

88. Tenover FC, Arbeit RD, Archer G, et al. Comparison of traditional and molecular methods of typing isolates of *Staphylococcus aureus*. *J Clin Microbiol.* 1994;32:407-415.

89. Parisi JT, Lampson BC, Hoover DW, Khan JA. Comparison of epidemiologic markers for *Staphylococcus epidermidis*. *J Clin Microbiol.* 1986;24:56-60.

90. Bialkowska-Hobrazanska H, Jaskot D, Hammerberg O. Evaluation of restriction endonuclease fingerprinting of chromosomal DNA and plasmid profile analysis for characterization of multiresistant coagulase-negative staphylococci in bacteremic neonates. *J Clin Microbiol.* 1990;28: 269-275.

91. Goering RV, Duensing TD. Rapid field inversion gel electrophoresis in combination with an rRNA gene probe in the epidemiological evaluation of staphylococci. *J Clin Microbiol.* 1990;28:426-429.

92. Hüebner J, Pier GB, Maslow JN, et al. Endemic nosocomial transmission of *Staphylococcus epidermidis* bacteremia strains in a neonatal ICU over a 10-year period. *J Infect Dis.* 1994;169:526-531.

93. Denning DW, Baker CJ, Troup NJ, Tompkins LS. Restriction endonuclease analysis of human and bovine group B streptococci for epidemiologic study. *J Clin Microbiol.* 1989;27:1352-1356.

94. Skjold SA, Wannamaker LW. Method for phage typing group A type 49 *Streptococci*. *J Clin Microbiol.* 1976;4:232-238.

95. Cleary PP, Kaplan EL, Livdahl C, Skjold S. DNA fingerprints of *Streptococcus pyogenes* are M type specific. *J Infect Dis.* 1988;158:1317-1323.

96. Kell CM, Jordens JZ, Daniels M, et al. Molecular epidemiology of penicillin-resistant pneumococci isolated in Nairobi, Kenya. *Infect Immunol.* 1993;61:4382-4391.

97. Roussel Y, Pebay M, Guedon G, Simonet J-M, Decaris B. Physical and genetic map of *Streptococcus thermophilus* A054. *J Bacteriol.* 1994;176:7413-7422.

98. Burnie JP, Matthews RC, Clark I, Milne LJR. Immunoblot fingerprinting *Aspergillus fumigatus*. *J Immunol Meth.* 1989;118:179-186.

99. Varga J, Croft JH. Assignment of RFLP, RAPD and isoenzyme markers to *Aspergillus nidulans* chromosomes, using chromosome-substituted segregants of a hybrid of *A. nidulans* and *A. quadrilineatus*. *Curr Genet.* 1994;25:311-317.

100. Varga J, Kevei F, Vriesema A, et al. Mitochondrial DNA restriction fragment length polymorphisms in field isolates of the *Aspergillus niger* aggregate. *Can J Microbiol.* 1994;40:612-621.

101. Lee W, Burnie J, Matthews R. Fingerprinting *Candida albicans*. *J Immunol Meth.* 1986;93:177-182.

102. Doebbeling BN, Lehmann PF, Hollis RJ, et al. Comparison of pulsed-field gel electrophoresis with isoenzyme profiles as a typing system for *Candida tropicalis*. *Clin Infect Dis.* 1993;16:377-383.

103. Magee PT, Bowdin L, Staudinger J. Comparison of molecular typing methods for *Candida albicans*. *J Clin Microbiol.* 1992;30:2674-2679.

104. Schönian G, Meusel O, Tietz H-J, et al. Identification of clinical strains of *Candida albicans* by DNA fingerprinting with the polymerase chain reaction. *Mycoses.* 1993;36:171-179.

105. Perfect JR, Magee BB, Magee PT. Separation of chromosomes of *Cryptococcus neoformans* by pulsed field gel

electrophoresis. *Infect Immunol.* 1989;57:2624-2627.

106. Spitzer ED, Spitzer SG, Freundlich LF, Casadevall A. Persistence of initial infection in recurrent *Cryptococcus neoformans* meningitis. *Lancet.* 1993;341:595-596.

107. Keath EJ, Kobayashi GS, Medoff G. Typing of *Histoplasma capsulatum* by restriction fragment length polymorphisms in a nuclear gene. *J Clin Microbiol.* 1992;30:2104-2107.

108. Spitzer ED, Lasker BA, Travis SJ, Kobayashi GS, Medoff G. Use of mitochondrial and ribosomal DNA polymorphisms to classify clinical and soil isolates of *Histoplasma capsulatum. Infect Immunol.* 1989;57:1409-1412.

109. Kersulyte D, Woods JP, Keath EJ, Goldman WE, Berg DE. Diversity among clinical isolates of *Histoplasma capsulatum* detected by polymerase chain reaction with arbitrary primers. *J Bacteriol.* 1992;174:7075-7079.

110. Grillner L, Strangert K. A prospective molecular epidemiological study of cytomegalovirus infection in two day care centers in Sweden: No evidence for horizontal transmission within the center. *J Infect Dis.* 1988;157:1080-1083.

111. Sokol DM, Demmler GJ, Buffone GJ. Rapid epidemiologic analysis of cytomegalovirus by using polymerase chain reaction amplification of the L-S junction region. *J Clin Microbiol.* 1992;30:839-844.

112. Watanabe S, Shinkai M, Hitomi S, et al. A polymorphic region of the human cytomegalovirus genome encoding putative glycoproteins. *Arch Virol.* 1994;137:117-121.

113. Zuckerman MA, Hawkins AE, Briggs M, et al. Investigation of hepatitis B virus transmission in a health care setting: Application of direct sequence analysis. *J Infect Dis.* 1995;172:1080-1083.

114. Allander T, Gruber A, Naghavi M, et al. Frequent patient-to-patient transmission of hepatitis C virus in a haematology ward. *Lancet.* 1995;345:603-607.

115. Haugen TH, Alden B, Matthey S, Nicholson D. Restriction enzyme fragment length polymorphisms of amplified Herpes simplex virus type-1 DNA provide epidemiologic information. *Diagn Microbiol Infect Dis.* 1993;17:129-133.

116. Ou C-Y, Ciesielski CA, Myers G, et al. Molecular epidemiology of HIV transmission in a dental practice. *Science.* 1992;256:1165-1171.

117. Bourhy H, Kissi B, Lafon M, Sacramento D, Tordo N. Antigen and molecular characterization of bat rabies virus in Europe. *J Clin Microbiol.* 1992;30:2419-2426.

118. Das BK, Gentsch JR, Cicirello HG, et al. Characterization of rotavirus strains from newborns in New Delhi, India. *J Clin Microbiol.* 1994;32:1820-1822.

119. Gaggero A, Avendaño L, Fernandez J, Spencer E. Nosocomial transmission of rotavirus from patients admitted with diarrhea. *J Clin Microbiol.* 1992;30:3294-3297.

SPECIAL TOPICS

CHAPTER 23

Epidemiologic Approaches to Quality Assessment

Bryan P. Simmons, MD, Stephen B. Kritchevsky, PhD

Abstract

Hospital epidemiologists have an opportunity to apply their skills to hospital quality problems other than infections. Soon, hospitals will be required to collect and report numerous quality indicators and the results will need epidemiologic interpretation. Hospital epidemiologists who choose to make the transition into quality management must carefully assess the needs of their healthcare facility and plan wisely in order to succeed.

Introduction: The Opportunity

Infection is only one of many adverse events that may occur to hospitalized patients. The majority of adverse events are not related to infection (Table 23-1), but nonetheless are amenable to study by the same epidemiologic techniques used for infection control. In fact, due in part to the success of nosocomial infection control, study of other adverse events has assumed greater importance than infection control in recent debates about healthcare quality. It is clear that before the end of the 1990s someone in each health institution will be performing epidemiologic assessments of many noninfection adverse events. The crucial question is whether those with skills in infection control epidemiology will expand into these new areas of hospital epidemiology, or instead will work for someone who does.

In order to study any event epidemiologically, one needs to develop case definitions and perform surveillance.[1,2] Most infection control professionals feel very comfortable defining nosocomial infection events. Developing such definitions for other adverse events may be quite difficult, especially if one wants to account properly for associated risk factors. For example, what risk factors need to be collected to compare fairly rates of falls among providers and hospitals? Fortunately, expert panels at the Joint Commission on Accreditation of Healthcare Organizations (JCAHO) are developing quality indicators using a rigorous scientific process.[3] These indicators are intended to track precisely defined events that provide clues to patient care quality. More than 50 such indicators are under study by JCAHO. By 1999, it is expected that all hospitals seeking JCAHO accreditation will be required to collect and report either the JCAHO

TABLE 23-1
EXAMPLES OF ADVERSE EVENTS OF HOSPITALIZATION

- Nosocomial infections
- Deaths
- Accidents, such as falls
- Medication errors/reactions
- Strokes
- Pulmonary aspirations
- Pulmonary emboli
- Pain
- Avoidable costs
- Avoidable procedures
- Missed diagnoses
- Decubitus ulcers
- Bleeding
- Organ failure

indicators or a comparable JCAHO-approved set of indicators; soon thereafter, results will be returned to your hospital. Who in your institution will be asked to review these results and, perhaps, to explain why rates of some adverse events are elevated? Certainly, such persons will need epidemiologic skills if they are to perform an accurate, fair investigation. Accreditation of the institution or credentialing of practitioners may depend on the results of an investigation. Because JCAHO expects indicator results to be public information, your institution and practitioners may find themselves compared with other institutions and practitioners in the local paper. The pressure to "look good" on these reports will be substantial. Thus, those who possess epidemiologic skills, who can perform a valid clinical study and produce reliable results, should be in great demand.

JCAHO will not be the only source of quality management surveillance data. The Health Care Financing Administration (HCFA) is beginning an initiative through its peer review organizations (PROs) to "help providers identify problems and

their solutions by monitoring patterns of care and outcomes and allowing providers to conduct the more intrusive and detailed study of who, when, and why."[4] Other initiatives may develop; for example, original plans for national healthcare reform called for a national health board to monitor a number of indicators. Furthermore, institutions may elect to develop their own homegrown indicators to follow special concerns within the institution, possibly using clinical practice guidelines as a starting point. Given the difficulty of developing and interpreting indicators and surveillance data, those who have experience in these processes likely will have opportunities to participate. These opportunities should not be dismissed quickly or without much thought.[5] At the very least, hospital epidemiologists should ensure that they are aware of mandated infection control indicators and closely track their results.

Transition into Quality Assessment

Making the transition into quality assessment may be difficult for many infection control personnel, despite their epidemiologic skills. Many hospital epidemiologists come from a background of infectious diseases training, or at least have become comfortable with infection control. Given the desire to do so, how can a hospital epidemiologist move into quality assessment? Your transition should include self-education, an institution-specific assessment of quality assessment needs, and then development of a plan.

Education should begin with reading but also should include some educational courses (Table 23-2). Perhaps the dominant quality management initiative in use in healthcare institutions today is total quality management (TQM) or continuous quality improvement (CQI).[6,7] JCAHO has encouraged healthcare institutions to adopt CQI. CQI is based on several underlying assumptions that are very compatible with hospital epidemiology. First, in CQI most problems are assumed to be due to inherent weaknesses in the system for getting things done rather than to the failures of individual workers. For example, most medication errors are believed to result from error-prone systems to deliver and administer medications; improving these systems, perhaps by bar-coding medications and tracking them by computer, probably would have a greater impact on drug errors than disciplinary action against those involved in errors.[8] Second, CQI is customer-focused. That is, efforts at improvement are geared to the desires of the customer rather than the institution. Thus, unbridled efforts to limit costs are not supported by CQI theory. Costs are controlled by improving quality and lessening the cost of complications and errors. Third, CQI is data-driven.[7] Processes must be measured in order to be improved. Thus, there has been tremendous emphasis by JCAHO and others on developing indicators to monitor both processes of care and patient outcomes. In order for data to drive clinical process improvements, someone must be capable of correctly interpreting clinical epidemiologic data. Administrators who are comfortable applying CQI to nonclinical processes, such as admissions and meal delivery, probably will shy away from interpreting clinical data that reflect on physician care.

Of the many tools used by CQI,[9] perhaps the most important for the epidemiologist to understand is the control chart.[10,11] A control chart displays data trends (eg, indicator results) graphically over time. Upper and lower boundaries (control limits) are determined statistically such that, when an indicator value falls outside these boundaries, there is statistical evidence that something new has been introduced into the process under study. Each such statistical event (often called a "special cause" by industrial quality managers) requires a special investigation. If the indicator is monitoring an outcome rather than a process, then a change in patient demographics (eg, severity of illness) may be responsible for this statistical event. An epidemiological investigation is needed to determine the sig-

TABLE 23-2
EDUCATIONAL RESOURCES

Society for Healthcare Epidemiology of America (SHEA)
19 Mantua Rd
Mt Royal, NJ 08061
Telephone: 609-423-0087 Fax: 609-432-3420
Offers: courses, annual meeting, journals (*Infection Control and Hospital Epidemiology, Clinical Performance and Quality Health Care*)

Institute for Healthcare Improvement
135 Francis St
Boston, MA 02115
Telephone: 617-754-4800 Fax: 617-754-4848
Offers: courses, annual meeting (The National Forum on Quality Improvement in Health Care), newsletter (*Quality Connection*)

Joint Commission on Accreditation of Healthcare Organizations
One Renaissance Blvd
Oakbrook Terrace, IL 60181
Telephone: 630-916-5600, Fax: 630-792-5005
Offers: courses, publications, annual meeting (National Forum on Health Care Quality)

Agency for Health Care Policy and Research
Executive Office Center
2101 E Jefferson St
Rockville, MD 20852
Telephone: 301-594-6662
Offers: publications, research grants, clinical practice guidelines

nificance of an indicator exceeding its control limits adversely. Thus, control charts can replace the traditional repeated hypothesis testing that is used to monitor infection control indicators for significant changes. Anyone interested in quality assessment should become familiar with the control chart. However, the epidemiologist should keep in mind that the greatest opportunities for quality improvement lie not with addressing special causes but with addressing common causes of quality problems[7] (ie, the characteristics of the process).

Once you understand the major forces of quality assessment that will affect your institution, you should take inventory of your institution's capabilities to address these forces. You must ask and answer several questions. First, is your hospital quality management department still primarily reporting quality events (numerator data) rather than rates? There is an important role for reporting single "sentinel events" (a serious, undesirable, low-frequency event), for example, maternal death, but most improvement efforts should be based on rates. Second, is the medical staff still absorbed in traditional review based on the opinion of peers?[12] If so, they should become aware of the increasing body of evidence that suggests that such implicit review is unreliable, even in the best of hands.[12-14] The medical staff needs to prepare itself to interpret the rate-based data that soon will be required by JCAHO and others. Third, is the quality management department directed by someone capable of doing the job and eager to do it? If not, that person may welcome advice and consultation from the hospital epidemiologist. If the director is well qualified to interpret most clinical data, then this person still may welcome input from the hospital epidemiologist or infection control professional. Certainly, many quality assessment projects have a major overlap with infection control. Such projects include, for example, assessing the timing of antibiotic prophylaxis[15]; assessing the appropriate use of antibiotics, including the duration of intravenous therapy[16,17]; interpreting tuberculosis skin-test conversion data; assessing the success of institutional vaccination programs; and assessing employee sharps injuries. These projects that overlap traditional quality assessment and infection control are ideal projects in which to participate if you want to move into quality assessment slowly, staying close to your home base of infection control.

New leadership in your institution's quality management department might be needed if the current leader is unwilling to address patterns of care, emphasizes punishment rather than education for quality problems, has poor rapport with physicians, manages data poorly, or is a poor adminis-

trator. If you believe the quality management department needs new direction and leadership, then you may need to talk directly to the hospital administrator. When considering this option, you should have a definite plan, including a plan for your participation. If you can negotiate a plan for your involvement in quality management, then you can determine an appropriate amount of reimbursement based on your practice setting (eg, university versus private practice) and additional duties.

If you are assigned the role of quality management epidemiologist, once again you should take an inventory of your resources. Does your department need new computer capabilities to manage data?[18,19] Our institution uses portable notebook computers for data entry at nursing stations and throughout the hospital. Data then are downloaded into a central computer for analysis, eliminating paper forms and the attendant problems of additional data entry. You also should determine what data already are being collected. Your computer billing data sometimes can be used as the starting point for a quality assessment project. We were able to review primary cesarean section rates, by surgeon, from such data. Mortality after coronary artery bypass surgery also was obtained easily. Although interpretation of mortality data is difficult, we could generate these data rapidly and easily to screen for potential problems that may require more in-depth study. Data that are easy to obtain and essentially free should not be overlooked as a quality screening tool, especially given the resources that are invested in implicit peer review with such little return and so few questions asked.

Once you get on your feet and are comfortable with your role in quality assessment, you should give serious thought to long-range planning. Where do you want your institution's quality assessment program to be in 10 years? What initiatives do you need to start now to get it there? Part of this assessment should include consideration of "damage control." Because the JCAHO and federal government have plans to make quality data public, you should look closely at those areas in your hospital most in need of quality improvement. Is your institution at risk for appearing on the front page of the newspaper showing a 40% cesarean section rate? Are there other areas of your hospital that might look poor when measured by JCAHO's planned indicators? If so, you should consider giving priority to quality assessment and improvement in these areas. Otherwise, the priorities for assessment and improvement should be determined by identifying clinical programs that are high volume, high risk, or problem prone. This assessment should lead to projects that will keep you busy for quite a while.

In summary, several organizations, including JCAHO and the federal government, plan to monitor a number of quality assessment indicators for each healthcare institution. Results of these indicators will require epidemiologic interpretation and will create unprecedented opportunities for the hospital epidemiologist. To take full advantage of these opportunities, the hospital epidemiologist must become familiar with new developments in quality assessment including the methods and tools of continuous quality improvement, assess the current status of his or her institution's quality assessment program, and make concrete plans for future personal involvement in the program.

References

1. McGeer A, Credé W, Hierholzer WJ Jr. Surveillance for quality assessment, II: surveillance for noninfectious processes: back to basics. *Infect Control Hosp Epidemiol.* 1990;11:36-41.

2. Credé WB, Hierholzer WJ Jr. Surveillance for quality assessment, III: the critical assessment of quality indicators. *Infect Control Hosp Epidemiol.* 1990;11:197-201.

3. Joint Commission on Accreditation of Healthcare Organizations. *Primer on Clinical Indicator Development and Application.* Oakbrook Terrace, Ill: Joint Commission on Accreditation of Healthcare Organizations; 1990.

4. Jencks SF, Wilensky GR. The health care quality improvement initiative. *JAMA.* 1992;268:900-903.

5. Wenzel RP. Instituting health care reform and preserving quality: role of the hospital epidemiologist. *Clin Infect Dis.* 1993;17:831-836.

6. Decker MD. Continuous quality improvement. *Infect Control Hosp Epidemiol.* 1992;13:165-169.

7. Kritchevsky SB, Simmons BP. Continuous quality improvement: concepts and applications for physician care. *JAMA.* 1991;266:1817-1823.

8. Berwick DM. Continuous improvement as an ideal in health care. *N Engl J Med.* 1989;320:53-56.

9. Plsek PE. Resource B: a primer on quality improvement tools. In: Berwick DM, Godfrey AB, Roessner J. *Curing Health Care: New Strategies for Quality Improvement.* San Francisco, Calif: Jossey-Bass Inc; 1990.

10. Sellick JA. The use of statistical process control charts in hospital epidemiology. *Infect Control Hosp Epidemiol.* 1993;14:649-656.

11. Blumenthal D. Total quality management and physicians' clinical decisions. *JAMA.* 1993;269:2775-2778.

12. Haywood RA, McMahon LF, Bernard AM. Evaluating the care of general medicine inpatients: how good is implicit review? *Ann Intern Med.* 1993;118:550-556.

13. Goldman RL. The reliability of peer assessments of quality of care. *JAMA.* 1992;267:958-960.

14. Rubin HR, Rogers WH, Kahn KL, Rubenstein LV, Brook RH. Watching the doctor-watchers: how well do peer review organization methods detect hospital care quality problems? *JAMA.* 1992;267:2349-2354.

15. Classen DC, Evans RS, Pestotnik SL, Horn SD, Menlove RL, Burke JP. The timing of prophylactic administration of antibiotics and the risk of surgical-wound infection. *N Engl J Med.* 1992;326:281-286.

16. Evans RS, Larsen RA, Burke JP, et al. Computer surveillance of hospital-acquired infections and antibiotic use. *JAMA.* 1986;256:1007-1011.

17. Ehrenkranz NJ, Nerenberg DE, Slater KC, Schultz JM. Interventions to discontinue parenteral antimicrobial therapy in hospitalized patients with urinary tract infection, skin and soft tissue infection, or no evident infection. *Infect Control Hosp Epidemiol.* 1993;14:517-522.

18. Classen DC, Burke JP, Pestotnik SL, Evans S, Stevens LE. Surveillance for quality assessment, IV: surveillance using a hospital information system. *Infect Control Hosp Epidemiol.* 1991;12:239-244.

19. Beyt Jr EE. Computer monitoring—the next step in surveillance. *JAMA.* 1986;256:1042.

CHAPTER 24

Disinfection and Sterilization of Patient Care Items

William A. Rutala, PhD, MPH

Abstract

This chapter provides recommendations on the preferred method for disinfection and sterilization of patient care items based on the intended use of the item (ie, critical, semicritical, and noncritical items). The chemical disinfectants recommended for patient care items and instruments include: glutaraldehyde; hydrogen peroxide; peracetic acid; sodium hypochlorite; alcohol; iodophors; phenolics and quaternary ammonium compounds. The choice of disinfectant, concentration, and exposure time is based on the risk of infection associated with the use of the item. The sterilization methods briefly discussed include: steam sterilization, ethylene oxide, dry heat, and the new low temperature sterilization technologies. When properly used, these disinfection and sterilization processes can ensure the safe use of invasive and noninvasive medical devices. However, this requires strict adherence to current cleaning, disinfection, and sterilization guidelines.

Introduction

Numerous articles that document infections after improper decontamination of patient care items have emphasized the necessity for appropriate disinfection and sterilization procedures. Because it is unnecessary to sterilize all patient care items, hospital policies must identify whether cleaning, disinfection, or sterilization is indicated. The hospital epidemiologist should make these decisions based primarily on the intended use of each item but should also consider other factors including cost. In this chapter, a pragmatic approach is presented to the judicious selection and proper use of disinfection and sterilization processes.

Definition of Terms

The precise use of scientific terms is crucial to an informed discussion of disinfection and sterilization practices. For this reason, a brief review of relevant terms follows. Sterilization is the complete elimination or destruction of all forms of microbial life and is accomplished in the hospital by either physical or chemical processes. Steam under pressure, dry heat, ethylene oxide gas, new low temperature sterilization technologies and liquid chemicals are the principal sterilizing agents used in the hospital. Sterilization is intended to convey an absolute meaning, not a relative one. When chemicals are used for the purpose of destroying all forms of microbiological life, including fungal and bacterial spores, they may be called chemical sterilants. These same germicides used for shorter exposure periods may also be part of the disinfection process.

Disinfection describes a process that eliminates from inanimate objects many or all pathogenic microorganisms with the exception of bacterial endospores. In healthcare settings, disinfection is usually accomplished by soaking equipment in liquid chemicals or by wet pasteurization. A number of factors may nullify or limit the efficacy of disinfection, including whether the object has been cleaned; the organic load present; the type and level of microbial contamination; the concentration of the germicide; the exposure time to the germicide; the nature of the object (eg, crevices, hinges, lumens); and the temperature and pH of the disinfection process.

Cleaning, a process that removes all foreign material (eg, soil, organic material) from objects, is normally accomplished using water with detergents or enzymatic products. Cleaning must precede disinfection and sterilization procedures. Decontamination is a procedure that removes pathogenic microorganisms from objects so they are safe to handle.

Disinfection, unlike sterilization, by definition, does not kill spores. However, a few products called disinfectants will kill spores if the exposure time is long enough (6 to 10 hours). Under these conditions, these products are called chemical sterilants. At similar concentrations but with shorter exposure periods (45 minutes or less), these same disinfectants kill all microorganisms except high numbers of bacterial spores. Under these conditions, the products are called high-level disinfectants. Other disinfectants (low-level) kill most vegetative bacteria, some fungi, and some viruses in a practical period of time (10 minutes or less), whereas others (intermediate-level) may kill tubercle bacilli, vegetative bacteria, most viruses, and most fungi but do not necessarily kill bacterial spores. A germicide is an agent that destroys microorganisms, particularly pathogenic organisms ("germs"). The term germicide applies to compounds used on both living tissue and inanimate objects, whereas, the term disinfectant applies only to compounds used on inanimate objects. Products with the suffix "cide" (eg, virucide, fungicide, bactericide, sporicide, tuberculocide) in their name destroy the microorganism identified by the prefix. For example, a bactericide is an agent that kills bacteria.[1-5] Thus, the antimicrobial spectrum and rapidity of action differs markedly among disinfectants and germicides (Table 24-1).

A Rational Approach to Disinfection and Sterilization

Nearly 30 years ago, Earle H. Spaulding developed a rational approach to disinfection and sterilization of patient care items or equipment.[2] This classification scheme is so clear and logical that it has been retained, refined, and successfully used by infection control professionals and others when planning methods for disinfection or sterilization.[1,3,6] Spaulding believed that the nature of disinfection could be understood more readily if instruments and items for patient care were divided into three categories based on the risk of infection involved in the use of the items. The three categories he described were critical, semicritical, and noncritical. The Centers for Disease Control and Prevention (CDC) employed this terminology in the following publications: "Guideline for Handwashing and Hospital Environmental Control"[6] and the "Guideline for the Prevention of Transmission of Human Immunodeficiency Virus (HIV) and Hepatitis B Virus (HBV) to Health-Care and Public-Safety Workers."[7]

Critical Items

Critical items are so called because of the high risk of infection if such an item is contaminated

TABLE 24-1

METHODS OF STERILIZATION AND DISINFECTION

Object	Sterilization — Critical Items (Will Enter Tissue or Vascular System or Blood Will Flow Through Them) Procedure	Sterilization Exposure Time (Hr)	Disinfection — High-Level (Semicritical Items; [Except Dental]* Will Come in Contact With Mucous Membrane or Nonintact Skin) Procedure (Exposure Time ≥20 Min)[b,c]	Disinfection — Intermediate Level (Some Semicritical Items[a] and Noncritical Items) Procedure (Exposure Time ≤10 Min)	Disinfection — Low Level (Noncritical Items; Will Come in Contact With Intact Skin) Procedure (Exposure Time ≤10 Min)
Smooth, hard surface[a]	A	MR	C	I	I
	B	MR	D	K	J
	C	MR	E	L	K
	D	6	F		L
	E	6	G[d]		M
	F	MR	H		
Rubber tubing and catheters[c]	A	MR	C		
	B	MR	D		
	C	MR	E		
	D	6	F		
	E	6	G[d]		
	F	MR			
Polyethylene tubing and catheters[c,e]	A	MR	C		
	B	MR	D		
	C	MR	E		
	D	6	F		
	E	6	G[d]		
	F	MR			
Lensed instruments	B	MR	C		
	C	MR	D		
	D	6	E		
	E	6	F		
	F	MR			
Thermometers (oral and rectal)[f] Hinged instruments	A	MR	C	I[f]	
	B	MR	D		
	C	MR	E		
	D	6	F		
	E	6			
	F	MR			

A = Heat sterilization, including steam or hot air (see manufacturer's recommendations).

B = Ethylene oxide gas (see manufacturer's recommendations).

C = Glutaraldehyde-based formulations (≥2%). (Caution should be exercised with all glutaraldehyde formulations when further in-use dilution is anticipated.)

D = Demand-release chlorine dioxide (will corrode aluminum, copper, brass, series 400 stainless steel and chrome with prolonged exposure).

E = Stabilized hydrogen peroxide 6% (will corrode copper, zinc, and brass).

F = Peracetic acid, concentration variable but ≤1% is sporicidal.

G = Wet pasteurization at 70°C for 30 minutes after detergent cleaning.

H = Sodium hypochlorite (1000 ppm available chlorine; will corrode metal instruments).

I = Ethyl or isopropyl alcohol (70% to 90%).

J = Sodium hypochlorite (100 ppm available chlorine).

K = Phenolic germicidal detergent solution (follow product label for use-dilution).

L = Iodophor germicidal detergent solution (follow product label for use-dilution).

M = Quaternary ammonium germicidal detergent solution (follow product label for use-dilution).

MR = Manufacturer's recommendations.

Modified from Simmons BP. Am J Infect Control. 1983;11:96-115 and Rutala WA. Am J Infect Control. 1990;58:99-117.

*Semicritical dental items (eg, handpieces, amalgam, condensers) should be heat sterilized.

[a]See text for discussion of hydrotherapy.

[b]The longer the exposure to a disinfectant, the more likely it is that all microorganisms will be eliminated. Ten-minute exposure is not adequate to disinfect many objects, especially those that are difficult to clean because they have narrow channels or other areas that can harbor organic material and bacteria. Twenty-minute exposure at 20°C is the minimum time needed to reliably kill M tuberculosis and nontuberculous Mycobacteria with glutaraldehyde.

[c]Tubing must be completely filled for disinfection; care must be taken to avoid trapping air bubbles when the item is immersed.

[d]Pasteurization (washer disinfector) of respiratory therapy and anesthesia equipment is a recognized alternative to high-level disinfection. Some data challenge the efficacy of some pasteurization units.

[e]Thermostability should be investigated when appropriate.

[f]Do not mix rectal and oral thermometers at any stage of handling or processing.

with any microorganism, including bacterial spores. Thus, it is critical that objects that enter sterile tissue or the vascular system be sterile. This category includes surgical instruments, implants, needles, and cardiac and urinary catheters. Most of the items in this category should be purchased as sterile or be sterilized by autoclaving if possible. If heat-labile, the object may be treated with ethylene oxide or new low temperature sterilization technology. Critical items may rarely be treated with chemical sterilants if other methods are unsuitable. Table 24-1 shows several germicides categorized as chemical sterilants. These include 2% glutaraldehyde-based formulations, 6% stabilized hydrogen peroxide, peracetic acid, and demand-release chlorine dioxide. Demand-release chlorine dioxide sterilizes only if the equipment is thoroughly cleaned and if the guidelines for organic load, contact time, temperature, and pH are followed carefully.

Semicritical Items

Semicritical objects contact mucous membranes or nonintact skin. These items must be free of all microorganisms except high numbers of bacterial spores. Intact mucous membranes are generally resistant to infection by common bacterial spores but are susceptible to other organisms such as tubercle bacilli and viruses. Endoscopes, thermometers, and respiratory therapy and anesthesia equipment are included in this category. Most semicritical items require at least wet pasteurization or high-level disinfection using chemical disinfectants such as glutaraldehyde, stabilized hydrogen peroxide, peracetic acid, chlorine, and chlorine compounds (see Table 24-1). However, some semicritical items such as thermometers or hydrotherapy tanks used for patients whose skin is not intact, may be effectively disinfected with high-level disinfectants (ie, chlorine) or intermediate-level disinfectants (ie, phenolic, iodophor, alcohol).

When selecting a disinfectant for use, one must consider whether the chemical will be safe for certain patient care items after they have been exposed to numerous disinfection cycles. For example, chlorine and chlorine-releasing compounds are high-level disinfectants. However, they corrode many semicritical items, and, thus, are not usually used to disinfect these items.

Laparoscopes and arthroscopes enter sterile tissue and ideally should be sterilized between patients. However, in the United States, they commonly undergo only high-level disinfection between patients. Although limited data are available, there is no evidence to demonstrate that high-level disinfection of these scopes increases the risk of infection.[8]

In general, one should rinse semicritical items with sterile water to prevent organisms that may be in tapwater (eg, nontuberculous mycobacteria and Legionella species) from contaminating the instruments.[6,8-10] If one cannot rinse items with sterile water, one should rinse the items first with tap water and then with alcohol. One should then dry the items with forced air[8,10] and store them (eg, packaged) in a manner that does not recontaminate the item.

Noncritical Items

These items come in contact with intact skin but not with mucous membranes. Intact skin is an effective barrier to most microorganisms. Thus, items that contact the skin do not need to be sterile and are considered to be "not critical." Examples of noncritical items include bedpans, blood pressure cuffs, crutches, bedrails, linens, some food utensils, bedside tables, furniture, and floors. In contrast to critical and some semicritical items, most noncritical reusable items may be cleaned where they are used and do not need to be transported to a central processing area. There is little risk of transmitting infectious agents to patients via noncritical items.[11] However, these items could contribute to secondary transmission by contaminating the hands of healthcare workers or medical equipment that will subsequently be used for other patients.[1,12] The low-level disinfectants may be used to process noncritical items (see Table 24-1).

Problems with Disinfection and Sterilization of Hospital Equipment

One problem associated with the aforementioned scheme is that it oversimplifies these processes. For example, the scheme does not address problems with processing complicated medical equipment that is often heat-labile or problems of inactivating certain microorganisms. Thus, after considering the categories of risk to patients, the hospital epidemiologist will still have difficulty choosing a method of disinfection in some situations. This is especially true for a few medical devices (eg, arthroscopes, laparoscopes) in the critical category because experts dispute whether one should sterilize or high-level disinfect these patient care items. Sterilizing this equipment would not be problematic if these items could be steam sterilized. However, most of these items are heat-labile. They can be sterilized by ethylene oxide, but this process may be too time-consuming to use between patients. The value of sterilizing these items at first seems obvious; however, evidence that sterilization of these items improves patient care by reducing the infection risk is lacking. Many hospitals have used these reasons as the basis for their decision to process arthroscopes and laparoscopes by high-level disinfection not sterilization.[8]

Physicians frequently use endoscopes to diagnose and treat numerous medical disorders. To prevent spread of nosocomial infection, all endoscopes should be cleaned and high-level disinfected following each use. The Food and Drug Administration (FDA) has approved a package label for one 2.4% glutaraldehyde that requires a 45-minute immersion at 25°C to achieve high-level disinfection (ie, 100% kill of *Mycobacterium tuberculosis*). Scientific data suggest that one can reduce *M tuberculosis* contamination at least 8 logs with cleaning (4 logs) followed by chemical disinfection for 20 minutes at 20°C (4

to 6 logs).[13] On the basis of these data, the Association for Professionals in Infection Control and Epidemiology (APIC) recommend that equipment be immersed in a 2% glutaraldehyde at 20°C for at least 20 minutes for high-level disinfection.[14]

Endoscopes are particularly difficult to disinfect because of their intricate design. Reports in the literature indicate that gastrointestinal endoscopes transmitted 281 infections and bronchoscopes transmitted 96 infections. The clinical spectrum of these infections ranged from asymptomatic colonization to death. Gastrointestinal endoscopes have most often transmitted *Salmonella* species and *Pseudomonas aeruginosa*, and bronchoscopes have most often transmitted *M tuberculosis*, nontuberculosus mycobacteria, and *P aeruginosa*. In general, the implicated equipment was not handled properly. For example, the equipment was improperly cleaned, the equipment was treated with the wrong disinfectant, and recommended cleaning and disinfection procedures were ignored.[15]

The hospital epidemiologist may be asked whether semicritical medical devices contaminated with blood from patients infected with the human immunodeficiency virus (HIV) or Hepatitis B virus or respiratory secretions from patients with pulmonary tuberculosis should be sterilized or high-level disinfected. The CDC recommends that such equipment be treated with high-level disinfection because experiments have shown that high-level disinfectants inactivate HIV, HBV, and *M tuberculosis*.[5,13,16] Nonetheless, more than half of the hospitals in one state modified their disinfection procedures when endoscopes had been used on patients known or suspected to be infected with HIV, HBV, or *M tuberculosis*.[8] This procedure is inconsistent with the concept of universal precautions (now included in standard precautions), which presumes that all patients are potentially infected with bloodborne pathogens.[16] Several studies have highlighted that clinicians cannot distinguish patients infected with HIV or HBV from noninfected patients.[17,18] Similarly, clinicians may not be able to identify immediately many patients with mycobacterial infection. In most cases, hospitals gas sterilized the endoscopic instruments because they believed this practice reduced the risk of infection.[8]

The Creutzfeldt-Jakob prion is the only infectious agent that requires unique decontamination procedure. A subpopulation of prions is extremely resistant and the agent is protected by its association with tissue. The preferred method for the treatment of contaminated instruments is steam sterilization for at least 30 minutes at a temperature of 132°C. Alternatively, critical and semicritical items can be immersed in 1 N sodium hydroxide (which is caustic) for 1 hour at room temperature and then steam sterilized at 121°C for 30 minutes. Because noncritical patient care items or surfaces (eg, autopsy tables, floors) have not transmitted this disease, these surfaces may be disinfected with either bleach (undiluted, or up to 1:10 dilution) or 1 N sodium hydroxide at room temperature for 15 minutes or less. Formalin-formic acid treatment is required to inactivate the virus in tissue samples from patients with Creutzfeldt-Jakob disease.[5,19] We refer the reader to several texts and comprehensive chapters for a more detailed discussion of disinfection issues.[1,4,5,9,20]

Sterilization

Sterilization removes or destroys all microorganisms on the surface of an article or in a fluid. However, this oversimplifies the concept of sterility, which is measured as a probability of sterility for each item. This probability is commonly referred to as the sterility assurance level of the product and is defined as the $\log_{10}$ of the probability that an organism would survive on a single item. For example, if the probability of a spore surviving is one in one million, the sterility assurance level would be 6.[1] The following items must be sterilized: items that enter tissue or the vascular system and equipment (eg, extracorporeal circulator, hemodialysis coil) through which blood or sterile fluids circulate. Several detailed reviews, which delineate the principles of ethylene oxide and steam sterilization, were used as references for this section.[20-26]

Steam Sterilization

Of all the methods available for sterilization, moist heat in the form of saturated steam under pressure is the most widely used and the most dependable. Steam sterilization is nontoxic, inexpensive, and sporicidal. It rapidly heats and penetrates fabrics. For these reasons, steam sterilization should be used whenever possible for all items that are not heat and moisture sensitive (eg, steam-sterilizable respiratory therapy and anesthesia equipment), even when not essential to prevent disease transmission.

The basic principle of steam sterilization, as accomplished in an autoclave, is to treat each item with steam at the required temperature and pressure for the specified time to destroy the organism by irreversibly coagulating and denaturing enzymes and structural proteins. Thus, there are four parameters for steam sterilization—steam, pressure, temperature, and time. The ideal steam for sterilization is 100% dry saturated steam, no saturated water in the form of a fine mist. Pressure produces the high temperatures necessary to kill microorganisms quickly. A specific temperature must be obtained to ensure microbiocidal activity. The two common steam sterilizing temperatures are 121°C (250°F) and 132°C (270°F). These temperatures must be maintained for a minimum time to kill microorganisms. *Bacillus stearothermophilus* spores are used to monitor the efficacy of steam sterilization. In general, the exposure periods required to sterilize wrapped hospital supplies are 30 minutes at 121°C in a gravity displacement sterilizer or 4 minutes at 132°C in a prevacuum sterilizer. However, at constant temperatures, sterilization times vary depending on the size and type of items as well as the sterilizer type.

The two basic types of steam sterilizers are the gravity displacement autoclave and the high-speed prevacuum sterilizer. In the former, steam is admitted at the top of the sterilizing chamber. Because steam is lighter than air, it forces air out the bottom of the chamber through the drain vent. Gravity displacement autoclaves are primarily used to process laboratory media, water, pharmaceutical products, infectious waste, and nonporous articles. However, the penetration time is prolonged by incomplete air elimination. High-speed prevacuum sterilizers are similar to the gravity displacement sterilizers except they are fitted with a vacuum pump to ensure that air is removed from the sterilizing chamber and the load before the steam is admitted. The advantage of this process is that the steam can penetrate almost instantaneously even into porous loads.

Ethylene Oxide Sterilization

In the United States, ethylene oxide (ETO) is commonly used to sterilize medical products that cannot be steam sterilized. ETO is a colorless, flammable, and explosive gas. Mixtures of ETO (10% to 12%) with carbon dioxide or chlorofluorocarbon (CFC) reduces the fire and explosion hazards. Because CFC could adversely affect the ozone layer, CFC cannot be produced for general use as of December 31, 1995. Hospitals will have three alternatives to ETO-CFC: 8.5% ETO and 91.5% carbon dioxide; ETO mixed with hydrochloroflurocarbons; and 100% ETO.[27]

The microbiocidal activity of ETO is considered to be the result of alkylation of protein, DNA, and RNA. Alkylation, or the replacement of a hydrogen atom with an alkyl group, within cells prevents normal cellular metabolism and replication. The effectiveness of ETO sterilization is influenced by four essential elements: gas concentration, temperature, humidity, and exposure time. The operational ranges for each of these four parameters are 450–1200 mg/L, 29°–65°C, 45%–85%, and 2–5 hours, respectively. Within certain limitations, increasing the gas concentration and temperature may shorten the time necessary to sterilize medical equipment. ETO inactivates all microorganisms although bacterial spores (especially *Bacillus subtilis*) are more resistant than other microorganisms. Thus, *B subtilis* is used as a biological indicator.

The primary advantage of ETO is that it can sterilize heat or moisture-sensitive medical equipment without deleterious results, whereas the main disadvantages of ETO are the lengthy cycle time, the high cost, and its potential hazards to patients and staff. The basic ETO sterilization cycle consists of five stages (ie, preconditioning and humidification, gas introduction, exposure, evacuation, and air washes) that require approximately 2.5 hours excluding aeration time. Mechanical aeration for 8 to 12 hours at 50° to 60°C removes the toxic ETO residual contained in exposed absorbent materials. Ambient room aeration desorbs the toxic ETO but requires 7 days at 20°C.

In recent years, various groups have become increasingly concerned about the toxicity of ETO to employees. Thus, on June 22, 1984, Occupational Safety and Health Administration (OSHA) reduced the permissible exposure limit for ETO to a time-weighted average of 1 ppm.

Other Sterilization Methods

Dry Heat Sterilizers

Dry heat sterilizers kill microorganisms by oxidizing cell constituents. This method should be used only for materials (eg, powders, petroleum products, sharp instruments) that might be damaged by moist heat or for materials that are impenetrable to moist heat. The advantages are that dry heat penetrates well and it does not corrode metal and sharp instruments. The disadvantage is that dry heat penetrates slowly and kills microorganisms slowly. The most common time-temperature relationship for sterilization with hot air sterilizers are: 170°C (340°F) for 60 minutes, 160°C (320°F) for 120 minutes, and 150°C

TABLE 24-2
SUMMARY OF ADVANTAGES AND DISADVANTAGES FOR NEW LOW-TEMPERATURE STERILIZATION TECHNOLOGIES

Sterilization Method	Advantages	Disadvantages
Liquid peracetic acid (Steris®)	Rapid cycle time (30-45 min) Environmental friendly by-products (acetic acid, O_2, H_2O) Fully automated No adverse health effects to operators Compatible with wide variety of materials and instruments	Potential material incompatibility (ie, aluminum anodized coating become dull) Used for immersible instruments only Biological indicator may not be suitable for routine monitoring One scope or a small number of instruments can be processed in a cycle
Hydrogen peroxide plasma sterilization (Sterrad®)	Safe for the environment and healthcare worker It leaves no toxic residuals Rapid cycle time (75 min); no aeration necessary Ideal for heat and moisture sensitive items since processing temperature is 50°C Simple to operate, install (208 V outlet), and monitor	Cellulose (paper), linens and liquids cannot be processed Sterilization chamber is small, about 3.5 ft³ Endoscopes or medical devices with lumen lengths or channels >12" (31 cm) or a diameter of <1/4" (6 mm) cannot be processed at this time
Plasma Sterilization (Plazlyte®)	Safe for the environment and healthcare workers Cycle time depends on load and varies from 4 h to 6 h; no aeration necessary Ideal for heat sensitive items No corrosive effects and no harmful residues	Sterilization chamber is small, 5.5 ft³ Liquids or products that are harmed by vacuum cannot be processed Effectiveness has not been verified in peer-reviewed literature Limited to stainless steel surgical instruments (excludes devices with lumens or hinges) at this time

(300°F) for 150 minutes. *B subtilis* spores should be used to monitor the sterilization process for dry heat because these spores are more resistant to dry heat than *B stearothermophilus*.

New Low-Temperature Sterilization Technology

Reprocessing heat-labile medical devices is a major problem in hospitals. ETO has been the sterilant of choice for sterilizing heat-labile medical devices. Despite its excellent properties, ETO is toxic and mutagenic and it is suspected to be carcinogenic. For this reason, alternative, low-temperature sterilization technologies are being investigated as replacements for ETO. The FDA has cleared the following for marketing: liquid peracetic acid

sterilization, hydrogen peroxide gas plasma sterilization, and a plasma sterilization system that uses two alternating gases. Infection control personnel must realize that newly introduced technologies will have limited applications (eg, may not be appropriate for instruments with lumens or instruments) when they first enter the marketplace. Furthermore, no single method will work for all hospitals. Table 24-2 provides a summary of the advantages and disadvantages of the new low temperature sterilization alternatives.

Joint Commission on Accreditation of Healthcare Organizations

The goal of disinfection and sterilization is to reduce the risk of endemic and epidemic nosocomial infections in patients. The Joint Commission on Accreditation of Healthcare Organizations (JCAHO) monitors compliance with the above principles.[28] First, the JCAHO will want to know how infection control personnel are involved in performance testing and inspecting sterilizers in your facility. When monitoring sterilizers, one should always record the temperature of each steam sterilization load, use chemical indicators with each item sterilized, and use biological indicators at least weekly and for every load containing implantable items. Data generated by monitoring sterilizers should be presented to the hospital's Infection Control Committee on a regular basis (eg, quarterly). Second, the JCAHO will want to know whether the recommendations for disinfection or sterilization of endoscopes and endoscopic accessories are incorporated into hospital policies and are strictly enforced. To ensure compliance with institutional policies and procedures, infection control personnel should make rounds in areas where endoscopes are used commonly such as the bronchoscopy suite, the gastroenterology clinic, and the operating room. Components of the disinfection procedures that should be implemented include appropriate cleaning, disinfection, and rinse procedures; the use of a chemical sterilant with adequate immersion time and temperature; and proper storage. Third, the JCAHO will want to know whether there are mechanisms for handling (eg, recalling, disposing, reprocessing) outdated sterile supplies if a time-related shelf life designation is used. The JCAHO will also evaluate whether continued sterility of hospital-sterilized and commercially prepared items are ensured through appropriate packaging and storage. Infection control personnel should conduct rounds in the Central Sterile Service area to monitor the following: methods for decontamination of reusable items, use of biological indicators, response to a positive biological indicator (which should include recall of equipment), storage of sterile supplies, and housekeeping practices. Fourth, the JCAHO will

want to know whether the organization's disinfection and sterilization practices are consistent in intent and application throughout the institution and among patients. For example, semicritical equipment should be high-level disinfected between patients. However, some institutions choose to sterilize semicritical equipment after it is used on patients with certain infectious diseases. This practice may lead to a "double standard" after equipment used on patients with known infectious diseases (eg, tuberculosis, HIV infection) is sterilized but the same equipment is only high-level disinfected after it was used for other patients. Under these circumstances, sterilization should not be performed in the belief that it is providing a greater margin of safety.

Note

This chapter has been extensively adapted and updated with permission Rutala WA. Disinfection, sterilization and waste disposal. In: Wenzel RP, ed. *Prevention and Control of Nosocomial Infections.* 2nd ed. Baltimore, Md: Williams & Wilkins; 1993:460-495.

References

1. Favero MS, Bond WW. Chemical disinfection of medical and surgical materials. In: Block SS, ed. *Disinfection, Sterilization and Preservation.* 4th ed. Philadelphia, Pa: Lea & Febiger; 1991:617-641.

2. Spaulding EH. Chemical disinfection of medical and surgical materials. In: Lawrence CA, Block SS, eds. *Disinfection, Sterilization and Preservation.* Philadelphia, Pa: Lea & Febiger; 1968:517-531.

3. Simmons BP. Guideline for hospital environmental control. *Am J Infect Control.* 1983;11:97-115.

4. Block SS. Definition of terms. In: Block SS, ed. *Disinfection, Sterilization and Preservation.* 4th ed. Philadelphia, Pa: Lea & Febiger; 1991:18-25.

5. Rutala WA. Disinfection, sterilization and waste disposal. In: Wenzel RP, ed. *Prevention and Control of Nosocomial Infections.* 2nd ed. Baltimore, Md: Williams & Wilkins; 1993:460-495.

6. Garner JS, Favero MS. Guidelines for handwashing and hospital environmental control, 1985. *Am J Infect Control.* 1986;14:110-126.

7. Centers for Disease Control. Guidelines for prevention of transmission of human immunodeficiency virus and hepatitis B virus to health-care and public-safety workers. *MMWR*. 1989;38(S-6):1-37.

8. Rutala WA, Clontz EP, Weber DJ, Hoffmann KK. Disinfection practices for endoscopes and other semicritical items. *Infect Control Hosp Epidemiol*. 1991;12:282-288.

9. Rutala WA. APIC guideline for selection and use of disinfectants. *Am J Infect Control*. 1990;58:99-117.

10. *Recommended Guidelines for Infection Control in Endoscopy Settings*. Rochester, NY: Society of Gastroenterology Nurses and Associates; 1990.

11. Rutala WA, Weber DJ. Environmental issues and nosocomial infections. In: Farber BF, ed. *Infection Control in Intensive Care*. New York, NY: Churchill Livingstone; 1987:131-171.

12. Sattar SA, Lloyd-Evans N, Springthorpe VS. Institutional outbreaks of rotavirus diarrhea: potential role of fomites and environmental surfaces as vehicles for virus transmission. *J Hyg*. 1986;96:277-289.

13. Rutala WA, Weber DJ. FDA labeling requirements for disinfection of endoscopes: a counterpoint. *Infect Control Hosp Epidemiol*. 1995;16:231-235.

14. Rutala WA, 1994, 1995, and 1996 APIC Guidelines Committee. APIC guideline for selection and use of disinfectants. *Am J Infect Control*. 1996;24:312-342.

15. Spach DH, Silverstein FE, Stamm WE. Transmission of infection by gastrointestinal endoscopy and bronchoscopy. *Ann Intern Med*. 1993;118:117-128.

16. Centers for Disease Control. Recommendations for prevention of HIV transmission in health-care settings. *MMWR*. 1987;36(suppl);S3-S18.

17. Handsfield HH, Cummings MJ, Swenson PD. Prevalence of antibody to human immunodeficiency virus and hepatitis B surface antigen in blood samples submitted to a hospital laboratory: implications for handling specimens. *JAMA*. 1987;258:3395-3397.

18. Kelen GD, Fritz S, Qaqish B, et al. Unrecognized human immunodeficiency virus infection in emergency department patients. *N Engl J Med*. 1988;318:1645-1650.

19. Taguchi F, Tamai Y, Uchida K, et. al. Proposal for a procedure for complete inactivation of the Creutzfeldt-Jakob disease agent. *Arch Virol*. 1991:297-301.

20. Russell AD, Hugo WB, Ayliffe GAJ. *Principles and Practice of Disinfection, Preservation and Sterilisation*. Oxford: Blackwell Scientific Publications; 1992.

21. Perkins JJ. *Principles and Methods of Sterilization in Health Sciences*. 2nd ed. Springfield, Ill: Charles C. Thomas; 1969.

22. American Society for Hospital Central Service Personnel. *Ethylene Oxide Use in Hospitals*. Chicago, Ill: American Hospital Association; 1982.

23. Association of Operation Room Nurses. Proposed recommended practices: sterilization. *AORN J*. 1991;54:82-96.

24. Joslyn L. Sterilization by heat. In: Block SS, ed. *Disinfection, Sterilization and Preservation*. 4th ed. Philadelphia, Pa: Lea & Febiger, 1991:495-526.

25. Caputo RA, Odlaug TE. Sterilization with ethylene oxide and other gases. In: Block SS, ed. *Disinfection, Sterilization and Preservation*. 3rd ed. Philadelphia, Pa: Lea & Febiger; 1983:47-64.

26. Mallison GF. Decontamination, disinfection and sterilization. *Nurs Clin North Am*. 1980;15:757-767.

27. Anonymous. Ethylene oxide sterilization: how hospitals can adapt to the changes. *Health Devices*. 1994;23:485-492.

28. Joint Commission on Accreditation of Healthcare Organizations. *Accreditation Manual for Hospitals*. Oakbrook Terrace, Ill: Joint Commission on Accreditation of Healthcare Organizations; 1994.

CHAPTER 25

Controlling Use of Antimicrobial Agents

Robert A. Duncan, MD, MPH

Abstract

Physicians and hospitals must curtail the excessive use of antimicrobial agents to limit the emergence and spread of multiply resistant organisms. This chapter describes how to organize an antimicrobial control program and provides options for hospitals working with a range of resources.

Introduction

Antimicrobial agents comprise the second most commonly used class of drugs in hospital formularies. They are unique among pharmaceuticals in that they affect not only individual patients but the larger microbiological environment as well. Nearly all practicing physicians readily prescribe antimicrobial agents, with varying levels of competence. It is estimated that 40% to 50% of antimicrobial use in hospitals is inappropriate, and hospitals are often where patterns are set for outpatient practice. Physicians usually focus their attention on the individual patient and are rarely aware of the ecologic effects of antimicrobial agents on the patient, the hospital, long-term care facilities, the community, or the world at large.[1]

Excessive use of antimicrobial agents is linked not only to the emergence and spread of resistance[2] but also to adverse drug reactions and added cost. As a result, both clinicians and the pharmaceutical industry increasingly have been concerned about antimicrobial resistance.[3,4] In response, a joint committee of the Society for Healthcare Epidemiology of America and the Infectious Diseases Society of America has prepared *Guidelines for the Prevention of Antimicrobial Resistance in Hospitals.*[5] Hospital administrators and insurers also have begun to appreciate the financial benefits of controlling the use of antimicrobials and preventing the spread of resistant organisms. This economic incentive may force physicians to implement necessary clinical and ecological reforms that hitherto concerned only infectious disease specialists and hospital epidemiologists.

Organization and Personnel

An effective program for antimicrobial reform requires a team approach. As a first step, the hospital should form an antimicrobial utilization committee, chaired by a member of the infectious dis-

TABLE 25-1

COMPOSITION OF AN ANTIMICROBIAL UTILIZATION
COMMITTEE

- Infectious disease staff (chair)
- Pharmacy director
- Infectious disease pharmacist
- Microbiology director
- Infection control professional(s)
- Surgeon
- General internist
- Pediatrician
- Intensivist
- Emergency room staff
- Residency staff
- Ward nurse
- Quality assurance reviewer
- Administrator
- Data manager

ease staff or someone with sophisticated knowledge of infectious diseases and their treatment. Staff from the pharmacy, the microbiology laboratory, and infection control should participate on the committee. Depending on the size and structure of the hospital, individuals from several other departments (Table 25-1) may provide important clinical perspective and facilitate change. In training hospitals, residents should be included, because they typically prescribe most (or all) antimicrobial agents. A key administrator also should be a member of the committee, because this individual can act as a liaison to higher levels of the hospital administration and support reform efforts among the medical staff.[6] The antimicrobial utilization committee may want to coordinate its activities with those of the quality assurance staff.

Data Collection

The quality of primary data sources for studies of antimicrobial utilization varies substantially. Possible sources range from the pharmacy's purchasing records or individual patient records to computerized databases developed by the pharmacy. Purchase data are influenced by fiscal policies that can produce spurious variations in drug utiliza-

tion. Medical record review yields actual dispensed doses, but is extremely laborious. Computerized systems provide the time, date, location, prescriber, and dose of the administered drug. These data allow appropriate individuals to calculate defined drug densities and to measure the intensity of drug utilization in a given geographic area (eg, vancomycin use per patient-day in an intensive care unit). The antimicrobial utilization committee subsequently can pinpoint areas of misuse. Finally, summary data from health maintenance organizations (HMOs) and Medicare allow researchers to analyze utilization of antimicrobial agents on a broader scale. However, nationwide data on utilization of antimicrobial agents currently are both inadequate and difficult to obtain.

Drug utilization evaluations (DUEs) identify usage patterns and trends, according to service or hospital unit.[7] These projects focus on use of a particular drug or class of drugs, or may expand to include invasive procedures (eg, appropriate use of endoscopy) and strategies for managing specific diseases (eg, appropriate management of congestive heart failure). A DUE should examine a few questions, rather than attempt a comprehensive review. The DUEs provide baseline data that the committee needs to identify problems, design interventions, and monitor the efficacy of the interventions. The DUEs also can identify variability in practice. Follow-up DUEs give essential feedback to clinicians and document whether or not the reforms were effective. Initial projects usually reflect the concerns of clinicians, microbiologists, and pharmacists. Such concerns might include emergence of resistant pathogens (eg, vancomycin-resistant enterococci or imipenem-resistant Gram-negative bacilli), overutilization of antimicrobial agents, dosing regimens that are ineffective or toxic, or specific clinical practices. A list of the pharmacy's "Top 100" expenditures reveals crude patterns of drug use and helps the hospital to identify targets that could decrease costs substantially.

The list could include 200 to 300 items in larger hospitals with broader agendas for change. The antimicrobial utilization committee also can select and assess potential interventions.

The microbiology laboratory must provide the committee with data about the frequency of various resistant pathogens. The laboratory also must inform the committee about emerging problems with resistant organisms and document changes in susceptibility patterns that are attributable to changes in use of antimicrobial agents. Unfortunately, the latter has been difficult to prove in individual institutions.[8] Multicenter collaborative studies may be necessary to achieve this goal.

Interventions

Choosing Interventions

When designing interventions, the committee should consider several factors: hospital size, special patient populations (eg, solid organ or bone marrow transplants, trauma, burns, human immunodeficiency virus, pediatrics), local resistance problems, referral sources (eg, chronic-care facilities), financial resources, and politics.

In the early stages of an antimicrobial control program, the committee should limit the scope of its projects. Projects should be of significant concern to the hospital staff, have potential for improving clinical care and decreasing costs, and have a high probability of success. As the program matures, active surveillance of antimicrobial resistance, drug utilization, and clinical practice will be needed to identify less obvious problems. The committee subsequently may choose to evaluate other types of drugs or may focus on efforts to improve clinical practice, applying the same epidemiologic methods used for reforming antimicrobial use.

Kunin[1] and Bryan[9] have reviewed many reform efforts reported by others (Table 25-2). I will discuss some of these reforms in the following sections and will present some precautions in Table 25-3.

Revising the Formulary

The most effective and easily implemented means of controlling antimicrobial use may be formulary revision. This method eliminates agents that are used rarely and limits the number of drugs within a therapeutic class to one or a few drugs with the best efficacy, safety, side-effect profile, patient compliance, and, finally, cost. Once cost has become the determining factor, the hospital may be able to save substantial amounts of money by negotiating with competing pharmaceutical suppliers. Hospitals that belong to large purchasing alliances may be able to save even more.

When making decisions about the hospital's formulary, the committee should consider characteristics of the hospital and the patient population, antimicrobial susceptibility patterns, availability of new agents, and the price of older (ie, off-patent) drugs. Hospitals also may need to consider the formularies of referring HMOs and managed care plans. However, hospitals and HMOs may choose different agents to suit their circumstances and budgets. Ultimately, the committee must choose drugs on the basis of which agents are the most advantageous for the home institution at a given time. The committee may need to revise the formulary periodically.

Reporting Laboratory Data

The microbiology laboratory should report microbial susceptibility only for agents available on formulary. In addition, the laboratory, using a graduated system, should report the susceptibility to more aggressive agents only for organisms that are resistant to first-line drugs.

General Education

To help physicians choose appropriate antimicrobials, the committee can summarize hospital-wide susceptibility patterns in a pocket-sized guide that is distributed to house staff and attending physicians. Ideally, this guide also would identify restrict-

TABLE 25-2

COMPONENTS OF ANTIMICROBIAL CONTROL AND COST-CONTAINMENT PROGRAMS

Data Collection and Target Identification

- Routine monitoring of pharmacy purchasing volume and costs

- Focused, problem-oriented DUEs of individual drugs or practices

- Review of "top 100" high-cost formulary agents

- Comprehensive review of patterns of antimicrobial usage, with feedback by infectious diseases physicians or pharmacists

- Computerized DUEs that integrate pharmacy data with data from the departments of microbiology, chemistry, and radiology

Formulary Revision

- Expert committee selects formulary and limits pharmacy stocks to one or a few optimal drugs within a therapeutic class (decision analysis may be helpful)

- Generic substitution of proprietary agents

- Competitive contract bidding for similar drugs with equivalent efficacy

- Cyclic rotation of formulary agents within a class (eg, aminoglycosides)

Microbiology Testing and Reporting

- Routine susceptibility testing done only for formulary agents

- Graded susceptibility reporting, based on level of resistance and cost-effectiveness

- Regular reporting of susceptibility patterns and empiric drugs of choice, according to ICU, ward, or outpatient isolates. May include level of restriction, usual dosing regimens, renal dose adjustments, and costs

Education

- Direct education by physicians or pharmacists of health-care providers, one-on-one or by group

- Use of clinical pathways or guidelines

- Counter-detailing of drug information

- Concurrent review and advice provided by infectious disease physicians or pharmacists

- Computerized decision support of prescribing choices

- Feedback to providers

- Educate and recruit senior department heads and opinion leaders

Restriction Policies

- Open formulary ◗ unrestricted but closed ◗ monitored ◗ infectious disease telephone approval required ◗ infectious disease consult required

- Limit drugs to clinical scenarios (eg, diabetic foot infections), locations (eg, ICUs), or services

- Remove or restrict specific problem agents (eg, habitual antimicrobial agent choices)

Ordering Policies

- Antimicrobial agent order forms, including common dosing parameters and educational information

- Specified duration of therapy and prophylaxis

- Surgical prophylaxis protocols with specified doses and duration

- Automatic-stop orders for prophylaxis, empiric therapy, and specific therapy

- Computerized orders incorporating decision-support tools or barriers to use of second-line drugs

Drug Administration

- Infectious disease pharmacist clinical intervention program

- Pharmacokinetic consultation

- Revision of standard dosing regimens, based on new pharmacokinetic data

- Antimicrobial agent streamlining of broad-spectrum or multiple-drug regimens

- Once-daily aminoglycoside dosing

- IV-to-PO or step-down conversion

- Home IV therapy

Limiting Contact With Pharmaceutical Representatives

- Restrict the access of pharmaceutical company representatives to clinical care areas

- Review detailing information and coordinate with representatives

- Therapeutic partnering with pharmaceutical firms to coordinate education, clinical pathways, and drug selection according to institutionally selected criteria

---

DUEs = drug utilization evaluations; ICU = intensive care unit; IV-to-PO = intravenous to oral; IV = intravenous.

---

ed or monitored drugs, suggest optimal dosing regimens with adjustments for impaired renal function, and list the cost for each agent. The committee also

might want to develop formalized treatment guidelines for commonly encountered infectious diseases. Departmental and house staff conferences, grand rounds, and memoranda to staff are commonly accepted methods of educating clinicians, yet many of these efforts have not had a lasting effect on practice. Because the membership of the attending and resident physician staffs may change rapidly and the number of pharmaceuticals is increasing, staff must be educated continually, and the content must be updated frequently. If an explanation of changes in the formulary is included, the clinicians may be more likely to support the changes. Lengthy memoranda usually are ineffective, because staff rarely read them. One-on-one or small-group education has been most effective; "counter-detailing" occasionally may be necessary to neutralize promotions by pharmaceutical representatives.

Restricting Agents

Hospitals vary in the extent to which they restrict microbial use. Some hospitals have unrestricted formularies that allow physicians to prescribe any available pharmaceutical. In contrast, other hospitals have heavily restricted formularies and require physicians to consult with the infectious disease service before they can prescribe certain antimicrobial agents. Options are delineated below, in order of increasing restriction.

- Open formulary. Physicians may prescribe any available pharmaceutical agent, without restriction.
- Unrestricted but closed formulary. The formulary is limited to agents approved by the hospital's pharmacy and therapeutics committee, but physicians may prescribe any drug in the formulary without restriction.
- Monitored drugs. The pharmacy monitors use of particular agents and assesses the appropriateness of use. The pharmacy may ask a pharmacist specializing in infectious diseases or the infectious disease service to review cases in which an antimicrobial agent is used inappropriately.
- Limited drugs. Use of some antimicrobial

TABLE 25-3
CAVEATS

- Avoid formulary changes for only short-term gain
- Financial concerns should not be more important than clinical efficacy
- Substitution may alienate devoted users of a specific agent
- Excessive negotiations may poison established relations with pharmaceutical companies
- Formulary changes may necessitate changes in automated susceptibility testing
- Don't add to clinicians' paperwork or burden them with collecting your data
- Provide antimicrobial agent stewardship; don't become a policeman or zealot

agents is limited to specific clinical scenarios (eg, diabetic foot infections), locations (eg, intensive care units), or services. Physicians who want to use the drug for another indication must obtain approval from the infectious disease service.
- Approval required from the infectious disease service. Physicians who want to use specific antimicrobial agents must discuss the case with the infectious disease consultant to obtain approval. In general, the primary physicians are allowed a 24-hour grace period before they must obtain approval to use the antimicrobial agent.
- Consult required from infectious disease service. Physicians who want to use the restricted antimicrobial agent must obtain an infectious disease consult before the pharmacy will release the drug. Some hospitals allow the primary physician a grace period; others do not.

Physicians who have access to an unrestricted formulary must make complex choices for which they have neither the time, information, nor expertise. Indeed, Kunin has argued that "use of high-cost, specialized antimicrobial agents should be a privilege of infectious disease consultants and others trained in their use, just as performance of invasive procedures is limited to those who are qualified."[10] However, excessive restriction of antimicrobial agents fosters an adversarial relationship between infectious disease consultants, house staff, and the medical and surgical services, and can interfere with timely administration of antimicrobial agents. Thus, most hospitals maintain graduated levels of monitoring and restriction, depending on the severity of problems with prescribing and resistance, potential toxicity, and cost. Closely restricted formularies rarely are employed outside of large teaching hospitals, where numerous high-risk patient populations engender major resistance problems. Narrowing, rather than restricting, options may achieve many of the same goals while maintaining collegial relationships with other staff. Supplementary active surveillance then can be used to identify and correct remaining problems with drug utilization.

Antimicrobial Orders

Some institutions use antimicrobial order sheets that incorporate questions about indications for use of antimicrobial agents, suggest dosing regimens, and define the duration of use for prophylactic, empiric, or specific therapy. These forms can facilitate antimicrobial audits, yet the quality of information is dependent on those filling out the forms and thus could be poor. The pharmacy also may use automatic-stop orders for antimicrobials. This technique is most successful for surgical prophylaxis (eg, limit to 24 hours postoperatively). Pharmacies that use automatic-stop orders must institute precautions that prevent inadvertent lapses in continuing therapy.

Surgical Prophylaxis

Surgical prophylaxis accounts for 40% to 50% of all hospital-based use of antimicrobial agents. Furthermore, up to 80% of prophylactic doses are given well after the wound is closed, when antimicrobial agents are least effective. The team that reviews antimicrobial use therefore should deter-

mine which procedures require prophylaxis and then identify optimal agents, timing, dosing interval, and duration of administration. They should simplify the administration protocol whenever possible. The team should include the surgical opinion leaders who will take primary responsibility for developing and instituting the reforms and for educating attending staff and house staff. The committee could encourage staff to undertake such efforts by promoting them as quality-improvement projects (ie, the changes are designed to reduce practice variation and rate of surgical site infections) or as cost-containment projects.

Once-Daily Aminoglycoside Dosing

Mounting evidence suggests that once-daily aminoglycoside dosing regimens yield equal or better efficacy and less toxicity than traditional twice- or thrice-daily regimens.[11,12] The once-daily dosing regimens also are more economical because they require less time and labor by personnel from nursing and pharmacy and less frequent measurements of drug levels. Once-daily dosing may prove more amenable to home infusion therapy than more frequent dosing schedules. Because these drugs can be toxic and their pharmacokinetics are complex, some institutions require physicians to order aminoglycosides "per infectious disease/pharmacy protocol." In other hospitals, an order for aminoglycosides automatically generates a pharmacokinetics consult. An infectious diseases pharmacist easily can monitor and administer such protocols. Further well-controlled trials are needed to validate this method.

Intravenous-to-Oral Conversion Programs

Some antimicrobial agents have good oral bioavailability, such as doxycycline, fluconazole, fluoroquinolones, metronidazole, and trimethoprim-sulfamethoxazole. These agents may be equally effective when given intravenously or orally. Oral agents are easier to give and frequently are 85% to 90% cheaper than equivalent intravenous agents. In addition, patients receiving oral agents do not need intravenous catheters for antimicrobial therapy and may be able to leave the hospital earlier than patients on intravenous therapy. Thus, treatment with oral agents may decrease complications (eg, phlebitis), duration of hospitalization, and costs. For these reasons, it may be appropriate to change from an intravenous preparation to an oral preparation of the same agent or to convert step-down therapy from an intravenous preparation to an oral agent with a similar spectrum of activity. Examples include changing from intravenous ceftriaxone or cefotaxime to oral cefpodoxime or cefuroxime and changing intravenous acyclovir to oral valacyclovir or famciclovir. Controlled trials of step-down conversion are few, but this literature should expand rapidly as additional convenient oral agents appear on the market.

Infectious Disease Pharmacist

Many authors interested in antimicrobial use have reported successful collaborations with pharmacists trained in infectious diseases. After reviewing a patient's medical record, an infectious disease pharmacist will recommend changes in therapy that enhance antimicrobial efficacy, prevent adverse drug reactions or medication errors, and reduce costs. In addition, infectious disease pharmacists can save money by selecting agents that require fewer doses and by streamlining multidrug regimens.[13] A new infectious disease pharmacist in our 300-bed hospital helped us to avert serious adverse drug effects in 2.2 patients per week and to refine use of antimicrobial agents in 18 more patients per week, saving over $47,000 per year.[14] Such savings often exceed the cost of hiring infectious disease pharmacists. While these specialists review the medical records, they can reinforce appropriate antimicrobial use, monitor compliance with guidelines, and identify emerging problems with antimicrobial use and resistance. The infectious disease pharmacist thus may reduce the recidivism that occurs after active reform efforts are completed.

Computerized Decision Support and Analysis

Computerized pharmacy systems, which allow physicians to prescribe antimicrobial agents on-line rather than writing orders in the medical record, can generate drug information screens or computer-assisted decision support automatically.[15] Alternatively, the system may require clinicians to justify their choices of antimicrobial agents or may impose multilayered disincentives designed to decrease use of selected agents. It remains unclear whether educational or restrictive measures will be most effective in this setting. However, the unpopularity of restriction makes it a less attractive avenue. Broadly integrated computer systems may create many opportunities to reform antimicrobial agent use, because they facilitate utilization review and identification of adverse drug reactions. In addition, these computer systems can be coordinated with surveillance for nosocomial infections.[16,17] These systems should become more widely accessible in the near future.

Selling an Antimicrobial Agent Control Program to Administrators

Programs to control the use of antimicrobial agents offer numerous tangible and potential benefits to patients and the institution. These programs benefit patients because they experience fewer adverse events, more efficient antimicrobial therapy, fewer problems with resistant microorganisms, and decreased length of hospital stay. Prescribers gain from simplified therapeutic choices, while the hospital saves pharmacy costs and achieves better outcomes. Third-party payers, contractors, corporations, and hospital administrators particularly are interested in such improvements. However, these benefits often are immeasurable. Proposals to formalize control of antimicrobial agents therefore should focus on both hard and soft benefits, including actual and projected gains. These programs also may attract external funding.

Maintaining and Evaluating the Efficacy of Interventions

There are numerous reports of successful antimicrobial control programs, but most have focused on reducing the use of antimicrobial agents and decreasing costs. Few authors have designed carefully controlled studies or reported endpoints such as improved antimicrobial susceptibility patterns or decreased spread of resistant organisms.[8] In addition, some control measures produce no discernible effects for months or years. Thus, investigators may have difficulty demonstrating these changes in individual institutions. Furthermore, control measures that work in one hospital may not work in another. For example, methicillin-resistant *Staphylococcus aureus* (MRSA) infections in one hospital may result from overuse of β-lactams, whereas in another hospital MRSA may be imported from referring facilities where it is endemic.[18] Draconian controls on the use of antimicrobial agents would have little benefit in the latter situation. All of these factors conspire against our ability to demonstrate whether interventions are efficacious. Thus, coordinated, prospective multicenter trials that consider local patterns and risk factors and that control for confounding factors may help to determine when and where interventions are most effective.

The Intensive Care Antimicrobial Resistance Epidemiology project is a multicenter study designed to correlate use of antimicrobial agents with resistance and to assess the value of various interventions, thus allowing interventions to be tailored to differing circumstances.[19] Studies that combine such computerized databases with multivariate analysis will enhance our ability not only to make fruitful interventions but to demonstrate their value clearly. Until these tools are widely available, we must demonstrate the efficacy of the programs and elicit the hospital's support by showing that we have improved patient care and reduced costs.

The Role of the Hospital Epidemiologist

Infectious disease specialists and hospital epidemiologists are uniquely qualified to lead and organize antimicrobial control programs. Because of the excesses typically encountered in antimicrobial therapy, effective control programs produce better patient care, less resistance to antimicrobial agents, and decreased costs—the proverbial "win-win" situation. Hospitals that benefit from these control efforts will be more likely to survive in an increasingly competitive healthcare environment and, in turn, will be more likely to support individuals who lead such efforts. The hospital epidemiologist, therefore, will find it advantageous to be identified as the driving force behind reforms that benefit the entire hospital. Additionally, although many projects are best handled by the antimicrobial utilization committee as a group, others may be more amenable to a personal approach by the leader. Thus, hospital epidemiologists can use antibiotic control programs as opportunities to reinforce their reputations as innovators and colleagues, rather than policemen and zealots.

References

1. Kunin CM. Problems in antibiotic usage. In: Mandell GL, Douglas RG, Bennett JE, eds. *Principles and Practice of Infectious Diseases*. 3rd ed. New York, NY: Churchill Livingstone; 1990:427-434.

2. McGowan JE Jr. Antimicrobial resistance in hospital organisms and its relation to antibiotic use. *Rev Infect Dis*. 1983;5:1033-1048.

3. Tomasz A. Multiple-antibiotic-resistant pathogenic bacteria: a report on the Rockefeller University Workshop. *N Engl J Med*. 1994;330:1247-1251.

4. Neu HC. The crisis in antibiotic resistance. *Science*. 1992;257:1064-1073.

5. Shlaes DM, Gerding DN, John JR Jr, et al. Society for Healthcare Epidemiology of America and Infectious Diseases Society of America Joint Committee on the Prevention of Antimicrobial Resistance. Guidelines for the prevention of antimicrobial resistance in hospitals: a report from the Society for Healthcare Epidemiology of America and Infectious Diseases Society of America *Infect Control Hosp Epidemiol*. 1997;18:275-291.

6. Goldmann DA, Weinstein RA, Wenzel RP, et al. Strategies to prevent and control the emergence and spread of antimicrobial-resistant microorganisms in hospitals: a challenge to hospital leadership. *JAMA*. 1996; 275:234-240.

7. Marr JJ, Moffet HL, Kunin CM. Guidelines for improving the use of antimicrobial agents in hospitals: a statement by the Infectious Diseases Society of America. *J Infect Dis*. 1988;157:869-876.

8. McGowan JE Jr. Do intensive hospital antibiotic control programs prevent the spread of antibiotic resistance? *Infect Control Hosp Epidemiol*. 1994;15:478-483.

9. Bryan CS. Strategies to improve antibiotic use. *Infect Dis Clin North Am*. 1989;3:723-734.

10. Kunin CM. The responsibility of the infectious disease community for the optimal use of antimicrobial agents. *J Infect Dis*. 1985;3:388-398.

11. Blaser J, Koenig C. Once-daily dosing of aminoglycosides. *European Journal of Microbiology and Infectious Disease*. 1995;14:1029-1038.

12. Gilbert DN. Once-daily aminoglycoside therapy. *Antimicrob Agents Chemother*. 1991;35:399-405.

13. Nightingale CH, Quintiliani R, Nicolau DP. Intelligent dosing of antimicrobials. In: Remington JS, Swartz MN, eds. *Current Clinical Topics in Infectious Diseases*. vol. 14. Boston, Mass: Blackwell; 1994:252-265.

14. Duncan RA, Segarra M, Anderson ER, Chow LS, Needham C, Jacoby GA. A comprehensive approach to reforming therapeutic antibiotic (ABx) use. *Infect Control Hosp Epidemiol*. 1995;16(4, Part 2):37. Abstract.

15. Evans RS, Classen DC, Pestotnik SL, Lundsgaarde HP, Burke JP. Improving empiric antibiotic selection using computer decision support. *Arch Intern Med*. 1994;154:878-884.

16. Pestotnik SL, Evans RS, Burke JP, et al. Therapeutic antibiotic monitoring: surveillance using a computerized expert system. *Am J Med*. 1990;88:43-48.

17. Pestotnik SL, Classen DC, Evans RS, Burke JP. Implementing antibiotic practice guidelines through computer-assisted decision support: clinical and financial outcomes. *Ann Intern Med*. 1996;124:884-890.

18. Monnet D. Relationship between antibiotic resistance and antibiotic use. Proceedings of the 35th Interscience Conference on Antimicrobial Agents and Chemotherapy; San Francisco, Calif; September 17-20, 1995. Abstract.

19. Monnet D, Gaynes R, Tenover F, McGowan J, ICARE pilot hospitals. Ceftazidime-resistant *Pseudomonas aeruginosa* (PA) and ceftazidime (CFZ) usage in NNIS hospitals: preliminary results of project ICARE phase one. *Infect Control Hosp Epidemiol*. 1995;16;4(suppl):19. Abstract.

CHAPTER 26

Employee Health and Infection Control

Daniel J. Diekema, MD, MS, Bradley N. Doebbeling, MD, MS

Abstract

Hospital employees are at risk for exposure to a variety of communicable diseases, which they may transmit to patients and other workers. The employee health service plays a critical role in an effective infection control program. In this chapter, we outline the major responsibilities of the employee health service and summarize key current recommendations for management of exposures.

Introduction

The employee health department provides a crucial link in protecting the health and safety of workers and patients in healthcare facilities. We will outline the various roles of an employee health department in screening workers, providing education and immunoprophylaxis, and participating in the management of employee exposure to infectious agents. The reader is encouraged to review more detailed discussions of these issues that can be found in the Recommended Readings at the end of this chapter.

Serologic Screening and Immunization

At the time of employment, all hospital personnel should be evaluated by the employee health service. The most important aspect of this evaluation is the history, which should, at minimum, elicit immunization status and prior medical conditions, especially those relating to communicable disease susceptibility (eg, varicella-zoster, tuberculosis). Obtaining information about immunocompromising conditions or therapies (eg, steroids, chemotherapy) also is important.

A screening physical examination occasionally may detect undiagnosed illness or provide baseline information for future evaluation of a work-related condition. However, no available data demonstrate that screening physical exams prevent transmission of infectious agents in the hospital.

Laboratory testing generally should be limited to varicella-zoster virus (VZV) serology. Although some institutions with many immunocompromised patients screen all employees with VZV serology, most consider a history of chickenpox to be reliable evidence of immunity. Information about VZV, already important when evaluating employees exposed to cases, may be even more important now that the VZV vaccine is available. Routine serologic screening of potential hepatitis B vaccine recipients is not cost-effective in low prevalence areas such as the United States. Additionally, receipt of the vaccine is not hazardous to persons who already are immune or are chronic carriers. Routine screening for susceptibility to measles, mumps, and rubella also is not necessary. Individuals who cannot document that they were adequately vaccinated or that they had physician-diagnosed infection should receive measles, mumps, and rubella vaccine (MMR), especially given the recent resurgence of these infections among adults. Because a clinical diagnosis of rubella is nonspecific, all healthcare workers should have documentation of positive rubella serology or immunization.

Every employee should receive a Mantoux skin test with purified protein derivative (PPD) of tuberculosis (0.1 mL of 5TU intradermally) during the initial evaluation, unless documentation of a previously positive skin test or completion of therapy for infection (ie, prophylaxis) or active disease is provided. For screening asymptomatic, nonimmunocompromised employees, the use of control skin tests (eg, candida, mumps) is not cost effective and does not alter management decisions. Positive skin tests should be evaluated and managed as described in the current literature. Skin-test-negative individuals should be retested at least annually, and those at higher risk for exposure (eg, house staff, nurses, respiratory therapists, pulmonologists) should be tested more frequently (eg, every 6 months), particularly in high incidence areas.[1]

Many communicable diseases of healthcare workers are vaccine preventable. Appropriate vaccine use (Table 26-1) optimally protects both employees and patients and costs less than managing individual cases and outbreaks of disease. The employee health service therefore should provide a comprehensive immunization program. Recent data on vaccine acceptance by healthcare workers can help employee health personnel design such programs. Notably, vaccine acceptance rates are highest when vaccination is mandatory, free, and readily available (eg, provided at the worksite, on the wards, at department meetings). Reminder letters to return for follow-up vaccine doses may be beneficial.

Education

Education is the cornerstone of preventive care and should be given high priority by any employee health service. Educational activities should be varied and innovative, including the use of printed materials, lectures, workshops, small group discussions, and inservice programs. Important infection control concepts should be emphasized repeatedly. Furthermore, all employees should have ready access to advice and information about infection transmission and other aspects of employee health.

Educational efforts should focus on the use of universal precautions (now included in standard precautions) and handwashing to decrease the risk of transmitting infection. Studies have documented:

- Generally poor compliance with universal precautions and handwashing.
- Improved compliance with universal precautions following educational programs.
- Association of compliance with universal precautions and decreased rates of exposure to blood and body fluids.
- Association of handwashing with decreased rates of nosocomial infection.

Other important educational objectives should include improving vaccine acceptance rates (especially during the annual influenza vaccine campaign), and increasing awareness of illnesses or symptoms that require evaluation by the employee health service, particularly those that might call for possible work or patient care restriction (eg, conjunctivitis, shingles, jaundice, diarrhea).

TABLE 26-1
IMMUNIZATIONS RECOMMENDED FOR HOSPITAL EMPLOYEES

Immunization	Indications	Dose	Contraindications
Hepatitis A	Employees working in high-risk areas (eg, food handlers, cafeteria workers) without serologic evidence of previous HAV infection	1.0 mL IM at 0 and 6–12 months	Known hypersensitivity to any component of the vaccine
Hepatitis B	All employees at risk for occupational exposure to blood or body fluids	1.0 mL IM (deltoid) at 0, 1, and 6 months	None
Influenza	All hospital employees	0.5 mL IM annually	History of anaphylactic reaction to eggs
Measles*	Employees with no history of physician-diagnosed measles or laboratory evidence of immunity	0.5 mL SC of trivalent measles, mumps, and rubella vaccine (MMR)	Pregnancy, history of anaphylactic reaction to eggs or neomycin, severe febrile illness, immunosuppression, recent receipt of IV immunoglobulin
Mumps*	Employees with no history of physician-diagnosed mumps, laboratory evidence of immunity, or proof of vaccination on or after their first birthday	As for measles (above)	As for measles (above)
Pneumococcus	Employees over 65 years of age or with underlying cardiac, pulmonary, liver, renal, or immunocompromising disease	0.5 mL SC or IM; booster dose every 6–10 years	Safety in pregnancy unknown
Rubella	Employees without verification of live vaccine delivery on or after their first birthday or proof of laboratory immunity	As for measles (above)	As for measles (above)
Tetanus	Employees who have not completed their initial series or who have not received a booster dose within 10 years	Initial series: 0.5 mL IM of tetanus-diphtheria toxoid at 0, 1, and 6–12 months booster: 0.5 mL IM	History of neurologic or hypersensitivity reaction following a previous dose; first trimester of pregnancy
Varicella	Employees with patient contact who have no history of chickenpox and negative varicella titer	0.5 mL at 0 and 4–8 weeks	Hypersensitivity to vaccine, gelatin, neomycin; immunosuppression or immunodeficiency; active TB; febrile illness; pregnancy

ICU = intensive care unit; IM = intramuscular; HAV = hepatitis A virus; SC = subcutaneous; IV = intraveneous; TB = tuberculosis.
*Healthcare workers who have never received measles vaccine and have no history of immunity to measles require two doses of MMR, separated by no less than 1 month.

Exposure Management

Hepatitis A Virus

Hepatitis A virus (HAV) is an uncommon nosocomial infection, usually occurring in neonates and children hospitalized for another reason whose hepatitis is inapparent or in the incubation period.

Transmission

HAV is transmitted primarily via the fecal-oral route. Transmission by needlestick or mucous membrane exposure to blood has not been documented, although rare cases of transfusion-associated HAV have occurred. Fecal excretion of HAV (and associated infectivity) is greatest during the 2 weeks before clinical symptoms and jaundice (if jaundice occurs). Although infants can shed virus in their stools for months after infection, most patients are no longer shedding virus by 1 week after they become jaundiced. There is no carrier state.

Criteria for Exposure

Those employees at greatest risk for infection include:

- Hospital employees who are exposed to the stool of infected patients.
- Patrons consuming food not cooked after preparation by an infected kitchen employee.
- Close personal contacts of patients (ie, household, sexual).

Postexposure Prophylaxis

In the absence of an outbreak, the Centers for Disease Control and Prevention (CDC) does not recommend routine postexposure prophylaxis for healthcare workers. However, we support postexposure prophylaxis with immune globulin (0.02 mL/kg intramuscularly) for healthcare workers who are directly exposed to the stools of infected patients (serologic confirmation of the index case should be obtained before contacts receive prophylaxis). If given within 2 weeks of exposure, immune globulin prevents disease or lessens the severity of clinical illness with 80% to 90% efficacy.

Control Measures

Healthcare workers with suspected HAV infection should be relieved of patient care duties. If infection is confirmed, the healthcare worker should not return to patient care duties until 7 days after the onset of jaundice or other clinical symptoms. To prevent HAV transmission, healthcare workers should wash their hands, use gloves, avoid eating or drinking in patient care areas, and comply with general hygienic measures. Prophylaxis of susceptible healthcare workers with hepatitis A vaccine may be beneficial, especially in high-risk areas (eg, dietary and pediatric departments).

Hepatitis B Virus

Occupationally acquired hepatitis B virus (HBV) infection is a serious threat to healthcare workers and other hospital personnel who come in contact with blood and body fluids. Before the HBV vaccine was available, 10% to 25% of healthcare workers had evidence of previous HBV infection (compared to only 6% of blood donors).

Transmission

HBV is transmitted parenterally, with percutaneous exposure to infected blood the most important mode of occupational transmission. HBV also is transmitted sexually and perinatally. Only hepatitis B surface antigen (HBsAg)-positive individuals are infectious, and the risk for transmission from each percutaneous (ie, needlestick) exposure is from 10% to 40%, depending on hepatitis B "e" antigen (HBeAg) status. HBeAg-positive patients are highly infectious; the risk of transmission after parenteral exposure is up to 40%. The transmission risk after mucous membrane or nonintact skin exposure is much lower but not well quantified.

Criteria for Exposure

Any worker who sustains a percutaneous, mucous membrane, or nonintact skin exposure to the blood or body fluid of an HBsAg-positive patient (or a patient with undetermined serology) should be considered exposed. Source patients with unknown serology should be tested as soon as possible after the exposure.

Postexposure Prophylaxis

In the unvaccinated healthcare worker, one intramuscular (IM) dose of hepatitis B immune globulin (HBIG) (0.06 mL/kg) should be administered within 24 hours of the exposure, followed by the HBV vaccine series at 0, 1, and 6 months.

For vaccinated workers, the anti-HBs level should be measured. Workers whose anti-HBs levels are at least 10 mIU/mL need no prophylaxis. Employees who previously have had protective antibody levels but whose levels have fallen below 10 mIU/mL should receive an additional dose of the HBV vaccine. Employees with low levels of protective antibody who were never documented to have responded to vaccine should receive both a single dose of HBIG and a vaccine booster.[2]

Control Measures

Universal vaccination of healthcare workers against HBV should be a primary goal of the employee health service, and education and vaccination campaigns should focus on achieving that goal.

Although iatrogenic transmission of HBV occurs infrequently, at least 400 patients have been infected with HBV after being treated by an infected healthcare worker. Most cases were related to dental or operative procedures, and in almost every case in which HBeAg was measured in the source, it was positive. Standard precautions and glove use should be required for all procedures. Employee health programs may choose to restrict HBeAg-positive workers from performing invasive or "exposure-prone" procedures.[3] Heptonstall et al recently reported transmission of HBV to patients from four infected surgeons who were HBeAg negative, but HBSAg positive. This report raises new concerns about whether all HBSAg positive workers should be restricted from performing "exposure prone" procedures.[4]

Hepatitis C Virus

Hospital personnel are at elevated risk for hepatitis C virus (HCV) infection (seropositivity ranges from 1.4% to 5.5%). Infection is chronic in up to one half of individuals, and many develop end stage liver disease.

Transmission

The relative importance of different modes of HCV transmission is still unknown. Parenteral transmission clearly occurs, and HCV is the leading cause of post-transfusion hepatitis. Transmission due to percutaneous injury has been well documented, with frequency of transmission estimated at 3% to 10% per exposure. Mucosal or nonintact skin exposure represents a theoretical, if not well-quantified, risk for transmission.

Criteria for Exposure

Any worker who sustains a percutaneous, mucous membrane, or nonintact skin exposure to the blood or body fluid of an HCV-positive patient should be considered exposed. If the source of the exposure is unknown, not tested, or at high risk of HCV infection, the worker also should be considered exposed.

Postexposure Prophylaxis

The administration of immune globulin after HCV exposure is unlikely to prevent infection. No neutralizing antibody to HCV has been found. Additionally, it is unlikely that such antibody would be present in current immune globulin preparations, because donors are now screened for hepatitis C antibody. Therefore, the CDC does not recommend postexposure prophylaxis for HCV exposure.

Control Measures

Exposed individuals should be tested for HCV with a second-generation antibody test at baseline and again at least 15 weeks after exposure. The healthcare worker should be advised to seek prompt medical attention for any symptoms suggestive of acute hepatitis.

The risk of HCV transmission from healthcare worker to patient has not been determined but has been demonstrated.[5] Until additional data or better markers for HCV infectivity are available, the decision to restrict HCV-infected personnel from performing invasive procedures will remain extremely difficult.

Human Immunodeficiency Virus

Although the magnitude of risk from each exposure to human immunodeficiency virus (HIV) is much lower than that for many other occupational bloodborne pathogens, healthcare workers are extremely concerned about acquiring this virus through occupational exposure.

Transmission

HIV is transmitted parenterally, sexually, and vertically (transplacentally or via breastfeeding). Occupational transmission has been reported after percutaneous, mucous membrane, and nonintact skin exposure to HIV-infected blood. HIV is present in much lower amounts in other body fluids, including inflammatory exudates, amniotic fluid, saliva, and vaginal secretions.

Many studies now have placed the risk for HIV seroconversion following percutaneous (hollow-bore needlestick) exposure to HIV-infected blood to be 0.3% per exposure. The risk of seroconversion following mucous membrane or nonintact skin exposure is not zero, but is too low to be estimated reliably given the limits of available data. Similarly, some nonbloody body fluids of infected patients theoretically could transmit HIV; however, the risk is difficult to quantify.

Criteria for Exposure

Any employee who sustains percutaneous, mucous membrane, or nonintact skin contact with HIV-infected blood or body fluid should be considered exposed. The risk of each exposure varies based on the mechanism (eg, deep hollow-bore needlestick exposure to blood versus abraded skin exposure to amniotic fluid), as well as on the clini-

cal status of the source patient (late-stage acquired immunodeficiency syndrome [AIDS] versus early asymptomatic disease). However, each exposure represents a finite risk, may cause considerable anxiety for the employee exposed, and thus should be treated very seriously.

Because some personnel are so concerned about HIV exposure in the workplace, they will report apparently minimal exposures (eg, urine splashed on intact skin). In most of these situations, employees should be evaluated as if exposed and counseled regarding the risks involved. However, testing the source patient and postexposure prophylaxis with zidovudine (AZT) is difficult to justify in such instances.

Postexposure

Prophylaxis

The efficacy of zidovudine (AZT) chemoprophylaxis after occupational HIV exposure has not been established in a prospective clinical trial, although its failure in particular cases has been well documented. Unfortunately, the low transmission risk following occupational HIV exposure, combined with the reluctance of personnel to enroll in a placebo-controlled trial after exposure, makes it difficult to demonstrate the efficacy of AZT (or any prophylactic regimen). However, data from a case-control study suggest that AZT prophylaxis may decrease the risk of seroconversion after percutaneous exposure to HIV-infected blood.[6]

The Public Health Service continues to revise recommendations for chemoprophylaxis after occupational HIV exposure, taking into account the development of new potent antiretroviral agents and concerns about increasing AZT resistance. These recommendations must take into account the likelihood of transmission given the mechanism of injury and status of the source patient. Exposed healthcare workers must be evaluated without delay, because early administration is likely to be critical to any protective effect that antiretrovirals may have.

Other Considerations

Counseling and serologic testing of exposed personnel should be performed as soon as possible after exposure. These services should be available 24 hours per day. All personnel involved in postexposure evaluation and counseling, including emergency room workers, must be trained in and familiar with institutional protocols.

Follow-up serologic testing should be performed at 6 weeks, 3 months, and 6 months after the exposure. Healthcare workers who elect to receive prophylaxis should be tested at 1 year. Exposed workers should return for evaluation if they develop symptoms of acute retroviral infection (eg, fever, rash, lymphadenopathy).

Occupational HIV exposure can cause severe psychological reactions, including depression, anxiety, anger, fear, sleep disturbances, conversion symptoms, suicidal ideation, and psychosis. Postexposure counselors should be alert to these possibilities and refer the employee to specialists in crisis intervention and counseling if necessary.

Transmission of HIV from healthcare worker to patient is extremely unlikely but has been documented in a well-known cluster, in which a dentist transmitted the virus to several patients. Additionally, an unpublished investigation suggests that iatrogenic transmission of HIV probably occurred from an orthopedic surgeon to a single patient (unpublished report, French National Public Health Network). Numerous retrospective studies involving surgical and nonsurgical clinicians and thousands of patients have not confirmed transmission in other settings. Therefore, if HIV-positive employees follow usual infection control guidelines, the risk of HIV transmission during routine patient care is negligible. The CDC's guidelines[3] allow institutions some flexibility as they develop policies regarding HIV-positive personnel who perform inva-

sive or "exposure prone" procedures. Beekmann and Henderson discuss in detail the complex issues involved in formulating such policy.[8]

Cytomegalovirus

Cytomegalovirus (CMV) may be transmitted from patients to hospital employees, but the risk appears to be small. Infants and immunosuppressed patients (eg, AIDS, organ transplant) serve as the largest reservoirs for CMV in the hospital.

Transmission

CMV can be transmitted by several routes: direct contact, sexual contact, congenitally, and by transfusion. Healthcare workers most likely become infected by direct inoculation when their hands become contaminated with infected bodily fluid and they touch their noses or mouths. CMV can be found in blood, urine, saliva, respiratory secretions, tears, feces, breast milk, semen, and cervical secretions.

Control Measures

If hospital personnel follow good handwashing and infection control practices, their risk of acquiring CMV is minimal. Available data suggest that staff who work regularly with adult patients who are likely to shed CMV in large amounts (AIDS, oncology, or transplant patients) are no more likely to contract CMV than employees without patient contact. Data regarding the risk of CMV infection from working closely with pediatric patients, who also commonly shed virus, are contradictory.

Screening employees for evidence of previous CMV infection is not practical or cost-effective, especially because no study clearly demonstrates that CMV-negative employees can be protected by transfer to areas without high-risk patients. However, because primary infection with CMV during pregnancy can damage the fetus, some institutions allow CMV-negative pregnant employees the opportunity to transfer to "lower risk" units if they wish, provided that staffing levels are adequate.

Employees with acute CMV-related illness do not need to be relieved of patient care duties. By following careful handwashing and routine infection control practices, they can protect patients adequately from infection transmission.

Varicella-Zoster Virus

Varicella-zoster virus (VZV), the etiologic agent of varicella (chickenpox) and herpes zoster (shingles), is highly communicable and a well-recognized cause of nosocomial outbreaks among patients and employees.

Transmission

VZV is transmitted primarily via direct contact with respiratory secretions or vesicle fluid. Transmission also occurs by the airborne route, through inhalation of small particle aerosols produced by patients with varicella and disseminated zoster infection.

The incubation period of varicella is 11 to 20 days (although varicella-zoster immune globulin [VZIG] may prolong this to 28 days). Viral shedding occurs during late incubation; patients with chickenpox should be considered infectious from 48 hours before lesion onset to the time the lesions crust over. Patients and employees with zoster should be considered infectious from 24 hours prior to the appearance of the first lesion to the time the lesions crust over.

Criteria for Exposure

Any household contact of a person with varicella or disseminated zoster should be considered to be exposed. Any employee who worked either face-to-face, in the same two- to four-bed room, or at an adjacent bed on a larger ward with a varicella or disseminated zoster patient should be considered exposed. With respect to zoster or shingles (nondisseminated), exposure requires direct contact with the lesions (ie, not exposure to a patient whose lesions are covered with a bandage or clothing). Healthcare workers who have prolonged contact with the patient's clothing or bedding, as during a bedchange or bed bath, also should be considered exposed.

Postexposure

Prophylaxis

Varicella-zoster immune globulin is available for prophylaxis of selected exposed individuals. If given within 96 hours of exposure, VZIG (125 units/10 kg up to 625 units) modifies and attenuates disease rather than preventing infection. If the exposed employee does not report a history of chickenpox, serology should be obtained. Exposed employees without measurable antibody should be considered candidates for VZIG. All immunocompromised seronegative contacts, regardless of age, and all nonimmunocompromised susceptible pregnant women should receive VZIG.

Control Measures

Exposed employees should be placed on work restriction or furloughed from day 8 to day 21 postexposure (day 28 if VZIG is given). Work restrictions should include:

- No direct patient contact.
- Working only around other immune individuals.
- No group meetings.
- No cafeteria use.
- Entering and exiting the hospital by the shortest and safest route (ie, not through the lobby).

Potentially susceptible employees should be identified at preemployment evaluation. A history of previous chickenpox is reliable evidence of immunity. All without such history should be tested for serologic evidence of immunity; an effective vaccine is now available. Susceptible healthcare workers are among those for whom the vaccine is recommended. The role of vaccination in postexposure prophylaxis is unclear.

Herpes Simplex Virus

Herpetic whitlow and other localized HSV infections occur after occupational exposure, but serious or disseminated HSV disease from occupational exposure is unlikely in nonimmunocompromised employees. However, hospital employees can transmit herpes simplex virus (HSV) infections to high-risk patients with serious consequences.

Transmission

Transmission of HSV occurs through direct contact with open lesions or body fluids from individuals shedding virus.

Control Measures

Because parents with herpes labialis can transmit the virus to infants, these parents should not kiss infants. Employees also should not work with infants or immunocompromised hosts during a herpes labialis episode. Similarly, employees with herpetic whitlow should not care for patients until the lesion has healed. Although such employees probably do not pose a significant risk to patients if they wear gloves, the risk of transmission in this setting has not been well studied.

Influenza

Both community and nosocomial outbreaks of influenza are common and can cause significant morbidity and mortality, especially in elderly and immunocompromised patients.

Transmission

Influenza is transmitted via small-particle aerosols. Viral shedding begins approximately 24 hours before the onset of symptoms and can continue for up to 10 days. Young children may be infectious even longer. Because one infected patient may transmit the infection to many others, nosocomial outbreaks can be explosive.

Control Measures

Prevention of influenza among hospital employees depends on the success of the annual immunization campaign. Employee health programs should use the concepts outlined earlier to achieve near universal vaccination of hospital employees. Vaccination of high-risk patients prior to influenza season also is essential. Early recognition of influenza combined with droplet isolation precautions for suspected or confirmed cases is critical in the prevention of nosocomial outbreaks.

Once an outbreak occurs, all at-risk individuals should receive amantadine or rimantidine chemoprophylaxis and the influenza vaccine. Chemoprophylaxis should be given for 2 weeks if immunization is performed simultaneously.

Employees with suspected or confirmed influenza should not work until symptom-free and at least 5 to 7 days following initial symptoms.

Adenovirus (Epidemic Keratoconjunctivitis)

Adenovirus accounts for most highly contagious episodes of keratoconjunctivitis. Outbreaks of epidemic keratoconjunctivitis (EKC) are common in hospitals, especially among personnel working in outpatient settings such as an ophthalmology clinic.

Transmission

Adenoviral keratoconjunctivitis is spread by direct contact with infected persons and contaminated inanimate reservoirs (eg, tonometry equipment, ophthalmologic solutions). The incubation period ranges from 4 to 24 days, and the illness lasts up to 4 weeks. The conjunctivitis often (but not always) is accompanied by upper respiratory tract symptoms and other systemic symptoms (eg, fever, diarrhea, myalgia).

Control Measures

Effective control measures include relieving infected healthcare workers of patient care duties (and sending them home), emphasizing strict hand-washing, and eliminating potential environmental reservoirs. Personnel should be educated to report to the employee health service if they develop conjunctivitis.

Parvovirus B19

Human parvovirus B19 causes erythema infectiosum (fifth disease) in children and an illness manifested by fever, rash, and arthropathy in adults. Most parvoviral infections are mild and self-limited (many cases are asymptomatic). Persons at high risk for serious disease include:

- Patients with chronic hemolytic anemia, who may develop aplastic crisis during acute infection.
- Pregnant women, in whom parvovirus can cause hydrops fetalis and fetal demise.
- Immunodeficient patients, including those with AIDS and hematologic malignancies, who may develop chronic anemia.

Transmission

Parvovirus B19 is found in blood and respiratory secretions during days 5 to 15 of illness and is associated with systemic symptoms. Transmission is by direct person-to-person contact, fomites, or droplet nuclei.

Control Measures

Placing patients with known or suspected infection in droplet isolation precautions effectively prevents nosocomial parvovirus transmission. Women in the first half of pregnancy should not work with patients known or suspected to be infected with parvovirus. An exposed pregnant employee should be tested for evidence of prior infection. A positive IgG titer at the time of exposure represents prior infection and immunity.

Susceptible pregnant employees who are exposed should be referred to an obstetrician and followed for an IgM response (representing acute parvovirus B19 infection). Nonpregnant employees who are exposed should be observed for the development of symptoms.

Employees with acute parvovirus B19 infection should not work until several days after symptoms resolve. No employee with suspected parvovirus B19 infection should work directly with patients at risk for serious sequelae from infection.

Respiratory Syncytial Virus

Respiratory syncytial virus (RSV) is the most common cause of lower respiratory infection in infants and young children. Severe and sometimes fatal illness can occur in infants who have cardiopulmonary disease or who are immunocompromised. During the winter, nosocomial outbreaks frequently occur in association with community outbreaks. Because protective antibody responses rarely develop after infection, everyone is susceptible and nosocomial RSV transmission is common.

Transmission

Patients who have RSV infection secrete large numbers of virus, and the virus survives on inanimate objects for hours. Thus, healthcare workers may contaminate their hands and then inoculate their own conjunctivae or nasal mucosa. Alternatively, close contact can result in transmission via large droplet nuclei produced when patients sneeze, cough, or talk.

Control Measures

Control measures include strict handwashing (whether or not gloves are worn) after contact with patients or potentially contaminated articles. Healthcare workers also should wear eye-nose goggles (if available) for all contact with potentially infected patients and wear gowns when soiling is likely. Masks alone do not completely prevent transmission, because they do not adequately protect the conjunctivae from viral inoculation.

RSV-infected employees or those with symptoms of upper respiratory tract infection should not work with infants or young children. Cohorting patients and staff and limiting visitors (especially siblings and others with respiratory symptoms) also are important in preventing RSV transmission.

Measles, Mumps, and Rubella

A resurgence of measles in the United States began in 1989 and has been associated with an increase in measles transmission in hospitals. Likewise, rubella outbreaks continue to occur and have involved nosocomial transmission. Importantly, index cases in many nosocomial rubella outbreaks are employees, rather than patients. Because rubella can devastate the fetus during the first trimester of pregnancy, hospital outbreaks can have major medical and financial sequelae. Mumps incidence has increased since 1987, largely on college campuses, although hospital transmission also occurs.

Transmission

Measles, one of the most communicable of infectious diseases, is transmitted by aerosol over large areas. Viral shedding begins 9 to 10 days after exposure and lasts up to 10 days.

Rubella also is highly communicable, but is spread by direct contact with infectious nasopharyngeal secretions. Infected individuals can shed virus for up to 1 week before they develop the rash. Asymptomatic persons also may shed virus and transmit disease. Adults shed virus for approximately 4 days after rash onset, but infants with congenital rubella syndrome can shed virus for months.

Mumps is spread by droplet nuclei and direct contact with the saliva of infected persons. Viral shedding may occur for up to 9 days before parotitis develops and for an equal period thereafter.

Control Measures

Employees can be protected from measles, mumps, and rubella by appropriate vaccination, as outlined in Table 26-1. Routine serologic screening of employees for immunity to these pathogens is not cost-effective, and no increased risk is involved in giving MMR to immune individuals. Immunocompromised persons who cannot receive live virus vaccines (with the exception of HIV-infected persons, who are candidates for MMR) may be protected from severe measles infection if they receive immunoglobulin within 3 days after a documented exposure.

Pregnant employees who are seronegative for rubella should not work with patients suspected of having rubella infection, and should be relieved from patient care duties during rubella outbreaks. Due to theoretical risk of the rubella vaccine to the fetus, women of childbearing age should not receive the vaccine unless they are not pregnant. Susceptible pregnant employees who are exposed to patients with rubella should be referred to their obstetrician for careful follow-up, including testing for anti-rubella IgM, which indicates acute infection.

Employees with measles, rubella, or mumps infection should not care for patients until 7 days after the rash appears for measles, until 5 days after the rash appears for rubella, or until 9 days after the onset of parotitis for mumps. Susceptible personnel who are exposed to the above pathogens should be relieved from patient care duties from day 5 through 21 after exposure for measles, from day 7 through 21 after exposure for rubella, and from day 5 through 26 after exposure for mumps.

Meningococcal Meningitis and Meningococcemia

Neisseria meningitidis transmission in the hospital setting is uncommon, but the potentially devastating nature of meningococcal disease produces a great deal of concern and anxiety whenever a meningococcal infection is diagnosed.

Transmission

N meningitidis is transmitted by direct contact with respiratory secretions or with cultures of the organism. Risk from casual or brief contact with infected patients is minimal. Transmission within the hospital is rare. Patients are infectious for 24 to 48 hours after appropriate antibiotic therapy is initiated.

Criteria for Exposure

Only employees who have direct contact with infected respiratory secretions (eg, mouth-to-mouth resuscitation) or laboratory employees who handle *N meningitidis* cultures without appropriate protection (gowns and gloves for routine procedures and biologic safety hood for procedures that aerosolize organisms) require chemoprophylaxis. Chemoprophylaxis often is requested by many more employees than are meaningfully exposed.

Postexposure

Prophylaxis

Exposed healthcare workers can be treated with rifampin (600 mg orally bid for 2 days). Ciprofloxacin (500–750 mg orally) or ceftriaxone (250 mg IM or IV) are acceptable single-dose alternatives. Due to its ease of delivery, single-dose ciprofloxacin has replaced rifampin as the prophylactic therapy of choice at many institutions. However, ciprofloxacin should not be administered to children or pregnant women. Laboratory employees who sustain percutaneous exposure to *N meningitidis* require penicillin (not rifampin) prophylaxis. Susceptibility testing should be performed on all isolates to ensure effective chemoprophylaxis. Immunization of hospital personnel offers no further benefit after chemoprophylaxis for sporadic cases of meningococcal disease.

Control Measures

Patients with meningococcal disease should be placed in droplet isolation precautions (a negative pressure room is not required) for the first 24 to 48 hours of antibiotic therapy, despite the low risk of nosocomial transmission. The local health department should be notified to arrange prophylaxis of household and community contacts.

Methicillin-Resistant *Staphylococcus aureus*

Methicillin-resistant *Staphylococcus aureus* (MRSA) infection and carriage have increased dramatically over the past decade. Although hospital employees do not appear to be at risk for acquiring serious staphylococcal disease from patients, patients can develop infection after contact with employees who are MRSA carriers.

Transmission

MRSA is transmitted by direct contact. Healthcare workers who are transient carriers can transmit MRSA between colonized and susceptible patients. Less commonly, healthcare workers who are chronically colonized or infected may transmit MRSA to patients. The anterior nares is the primary reservoir for MRSA, but the axilla, hands, and perineum also can be colonized.

Control Measures

During nosocomial outbreaks, cultures should be obtained of the hands and anterior nares of healthcare workers who are epidemiologically linked to infected patients, and MRSA-colonized employees should be treated. Mupirocin (1 cm length of ointment bid intranasally for 5 days) eliminates carriage in most employees, although many recolonize with time. Employees who have skin conditions and are MRSA carriers should receive dermatologic care.

Group A Streptococci

Semmelweis first demonstrated nosocomial transmission of group A streptococci. While pharyngitis and skin infections are the most common manifestations of group A streptococcal infection, invasive disease is increasing in frequency. Nosocomial group A streptococcal outbreaks have been linked to employees who were infected or colonized.

Transmission

Transmission occurs following direct contact with infected secretions, although airborne spread is also likely, as suggested by outbreaks associated with rectal, vaginal, and scalp carriers.

Control Measures

When a nosocomial case of group A streptococcal disease is identified, an investigation should be instituted to locate carriers. Only employees who are epidemiologically linked to cases should have cultures obtained. Pharyngeal, rectal, vaginal, and skin lesion cultures should be obtained. If culture-positive and epidemiologically linked to transmission, an employee should be removed from patient care until carriage is eliminated. Oral or intramuscular penicillin is the drug of choice; erythromycin is effective for patients with penicillin allergy.

Tuberculosis

The national incidence of tuberculosis (TB) has increased during the AIDS epidemic, and the disease is once again a primary concern for employee health practitioners. Reports of nosocomial transmission of multidrug-resistant (MDR) tuberculosis are even more alarming and require increased vigilance to protect hospital employees.

Transmission

Mycobacterium tuberculosis is transmitted by droplet nuclei produced during the expiratory efforts (coughing, sneezing, talking) of patients with pulmonary or laryngeal TB.

Criteria for Exposure

Any close or even casual (ie, same ward or clinic) contact with an infectious (smear-positive) patient who is not appropriately isolated should be considered an exposure.

Control Measures

The best way to protect employees from work-related TB infection is to engender a high index of suspicion, so that all patients with suspected TB are isolated before people are exposed.

Exposed employees should have Mantoux tuberculin skin testing with PPD at baseline and then 6 weeks after exposure. Skin test converters should be treated according to currently published guidelines. An infectious diseases consultant should help manage those employees who convert their PPD after exposure to a patient with MDR-TB. Because MDR-TB infection usually is rapidly fatal in HIV-positive persons, employees infected with HIV in areas of high MDR-TB prevalence should be advised against working with high-risk patient populations (eg, AIDS and pulmonary patients).

When an employee develops TB, the employee health service, the infection control service, and public health authorities must collaborate to identify contacts and arrange evaluation and management.

Conclusion

For centuries, healthcare workers have risked the development of infections while caring for patients. As our understanding of these infectious agents has deepened, so has our ability to protect the healthcare worker. Indeed, rapid progress in this area continues, and recommendations designed to protect personnel from infections with VZV, HCV, HIV, TB, and other pathogens are likely to evolve substantially over the next few years, requiring revision of the recommendations we have outlined in this chapter. Responsible infection control professionals and hospital epidemiologists therefore should keep abreast of the current medical literature, particularly CDC recommendations as outlined in the *Morbidity and Mortality Weekly Reports*. By protecting the healthcare worker from occupationally acquired infection, we benefit every patient.

Note

The recommendations in Chapters 26 and 15 vary slightly because different sources were used to formulate them. Infection control staff should evaluate the recommendations and apply those that best suit their institution.

References

1. Centers for Disease Control and Prevention. Guidelines for preventing the transmission of *Mycobacterium tuberculosis* in health-care facilities. *MMWR*. 1994;43(No.RR 13):1-132.

2. Centers for Disease Control. Protection against viral hepatitis. Recommendations of the Immunization Practices Advisory Committee (ACIP). *MMWR*. 1990;39(No.RR 2):5-22.

3. Centers for Disease Control. Recommendations for preventing transmission of human immunodeficiency virus and hepatitis B virus to patients during exposure-prone procedures. *MMWR*. 1991;40:1-9.

4. The Incident Investigation Teams et al. Transmission of hepatitis B to patients from four infected surgeons without hepatitis B e antigen. *N Engl J Med*. 1997;336:178-184.

5. Esteban JI, Gomez J, Marlett M, et al. Transmission of hepatitis C virus by a cardiac surgeon. *N Engl J Med*. 1996;334:555-560.

6. Centers for Disease Control and Prevention. Case-control study of HIV seroconversion in health care workers after percutaneous exposure to HIV-infected blood—France, United Kingdom, and United States, January 1988-August 1994. *MMWR*. 1995;44:929-933.

7. Centers for Disease Control and Prevention. Update: provisional public health service recommendations for chemoprophylaxis after occupational exposure to HIV. *MMWR*. 1996;45:468-472.

8. Beekmann SE, Henderson DK. Nosocomial human immunodeficiency virus infection in healthcare workers. In: Mayhall GH, ed. *Hospital Epidemiology and Infection Control*. Baltimore, Md: Williams & Wilkins; 1995.

Recommended Reading

Beekmann SE, Doebbeling BN. Frontiers of occupational health: new vaccines, new prophylactic regimens, and management of the HIV-infected worker. *Infectious Disease Clinics of North America*. 1997;11. In press.

Benenson AS, ed. *Control of Communicable Diseases in Man*. 16th ed. Washington, DC: American Public Health Association; 1995.

Centers for Disease Control. Update: universal precautions for prevention of transmission of human immunodeficiency virus, hepatitis B virus, and other bloodborne pathogens in health-care settings. *MMWR*. 1988;37:377-382, 387-388.

Doebbeling BN. Protecting the healthcare worker from infection and injury. In: Wenzel RP, ed. *Prevention and Control of Nosocomial Infections*. 3rd ed. Baltimore, Md: Williams & Wilkins; 1997:397-435.

Doebbeling BN, Wenzel RP. Nosocomial viral hepatitis and infections transmitted by blood and blood products. In: Mandell GL, Bennett JE, Dolin R, eds. *Principles and Practice of Infectious Diseases*. 4th ed. New York, NY: Churchill Livingstone; 1995:2616-2632.

Gerberding JL, Henderson DK. Management of occupational exposures to bloodborne pathogens: hepatitis B virus, hepatitis C virus, and human immunodeficiency virus. *Clin Infect Dis*. 1992;14:1179-1185.

Lewy R. Organization and conduct of a hospital occupational health service. State of the art reviews. *Occup Med*. 1987;2:617-638.

Polder JA, Tablan OC, Williams WW. Personnel health services. In: Bennett JV, Brachman PS, eds. *Hospital Infections*. 3rd ed. Boston, Mass: Little, Brown and Co; 1992:31-61.

Sepkowitz KA. Occupationally acquired infections in healthcare workers. *Annals Int Med*. 1996;125(pts. 1 and 2):826-834, 917-928.

CHAPTER 27

Tuberculosis Control in Healthcare

Gina Pugliese, RN, MS, Michael L. Tapper, MD

Abstract

This chapter describes the basic framework for developing a tuberculosis (TB) control program. We suggest how to assess the risk of TB in a healthcare delivery setting, how to prioritize control measures based on their effectiveness, and how to meet current regulatory requirements. In addition, we discuss some problematic issues, examples of how other hospitals have confronted these issues, and where to obtain additional information on nosocomial TB.

Introduction

Nosocomial tuberculosis (TB) is of major concern to both healthcare workers and the public. Few other problems have affected hospital epidemiology so profoundly.[1] Recently, multidrug-resistant (MDR) and drug-susceptible strains of *Mycobacterium tuberculosis* have caused dramatic outbreaks in which both patients and healthcare workers were infected.[2-4]

However, nosocomial transmission of TB is not a new issue. It has been known for decades that the risk of TB to healthcare workers is 2 to 10 times greater than the risk to the general public. However,

characteristics of recent outbreaks, including their magnitude and the degree to which they proceeded unchecked, have alarmed many and have raised questions concerning the safety of receiving or providing healthcare.

Several factors have contributed to the recent outbreaks of TB in hospitals. Breaks in basic TB control strategies, such as delays in the suspicion and diagnosis of TB, delays in identification of drug resistance, and delays in initiation of appropriate therapy, have postponed proper isolation and prolonged infectiousness of patients. Second, respiratory isolation often is inadequate. For example, isolation rooms have had positive rather than negative pressure, air recirculated from isolation rooms to other areas, doors to isolation rooms were left open, isolation precautions were discontinued too soon, and healthcare workers did not wear adequate respiratory protection.[2] Appropriate TB control measures have reduced transmission significantly or prevented transmission. However, the effectiveness of specific interventions during outbreaks cannot be determined, because many of the interventions were implemented simultaneously.

TB outbreaks in hospitals and concern for the safety of healthcare workers motivated the Occupational Safety and Health Administration (OSHA) to develop enforcement policies specifying measures to reduce occupational exposure to TB.[5,6] In response to the same concerns, the Centers for Disease Control and Prevention (CDC) produced a 132-page publication *Guidelines for Preventing the Transmission of Mycobacterium tuberculosis in Health-Care Facilities, 1994*.[4]

Infection control personnel face yet another daunting challenge: designing and implementing a comprehensive TB control program that enables hospitals to comply with these enforcement policies and guidelines. Implementing all components may be beyond a hospital's means, and few data support the efficacy or cost-effectiveness of many of the prescribed requirements; yet, infection control personnel still must implement control measures, despite the imperfect state of knowledge.

This chapter is not intended to provide an exhaustive summary of TB control measures; the CDC's 1994 TB guidelines have discussed these measures in detail. Rather, we describe the basic framework for developing a TB control program. We suggest how to assess the risk of TB in a health-care delivery setting, how to prioritize control measures based on their effectiveness, and how to meet current regulatory requirements. In addition, we discuss some problematic issues, examples of how other hospitals have confronted these issues, and where to obtain additional information about nosocomial TB.

Assemble a Task Force

A specific person or group of persons should be responsible for developing the TB control program. Ideally, the designated person or group should have expertise (or access to expertise) in infection control, hospital epidemiology, employee health, and engineering, particularly air handling and ventilation. Because noncompliance with established infection control policies frequently has contributed to nosocomial outbreaks, this person needs the authority to implement and enforce TB control policies. Small healthcare facilities may employ an existing committee, such as the infection control committee, to handle this task. A larger facility might convene a special task force or subcommittee of a standing committee. The composition of the group may change over time as the institution addresses specific aspects of the TB control program.

The task force should be charged with developing a written TB control plan based on a TB risk assessment of the healthcare facility, outlining a time line and mechanism for implementing the plan, identifying the individuals who are responsible for implementing the plan, and developing a method for evaluating the effectiveness of the TB control program and for correcting deficiencies.

Conduct a Risk Assessment

One size does not fit all when it comes to TB control measures. If a healthcare facility is located in an area of the United States that has no reported cases of TB, the program should be very different from one in New York City, where the TB incidence ranks among the highest in the country. Infection control personnel must begin by assessing the risk of TB transmission in their particular setting. The CDC classifies TB risk as minimal, very low, low, intermediate, and high. The CDC suggests that risk classification (for facility, area, or occupational group) be based on the number of patients admitted to the area, the results of purified protein derivative (PPD) skin-test conversions among workers (eg, clusters of conversions or conversion rates higher than rates for areas or groups without occupational exposure), and evidence of person-to-person transmission. Within each risk classification, the CDC guidelines also recommend specific components for the program. These include the frequency for conducting a number of activities, including reassessing the TB risk, skin testing employees, reviewing medical records to evaluate compliance with infection control policies, observing infection control and work practices (eg, keeping isolation room doors closed), and evaluating engineering controls. The basic elements of this risk assessment are summarized in Table 27-1.

Local or state public health departments can help infection control personnel obtain information about their community's TB profile. Other sources of information on TB cases include extended-care facilities, schools, homeless shelters, and prisons. Even if there are no reported cases of TB in a community, epidemiology staff still should determine if patients with TB may have been admitted or treated in the facility. Good sources for this information are the microbiology laboratory's database, infection control records, and medical records databases containing discharge diagnoses, autopsy, and surgical pathology reports.

Infection control personnel should use the CDC's 1994 TB guidelines to classify the facility's TB risk.[4] If TB patients have been admitted or treated in a facility during the past year, epidemiology staff will need to determine the risk classification for the entire facility and for each specific area of the facility (eg, medical wards, human immunodeficiency virus [HIV] or pulmonary clinics, emergency departments, and other areas where TB patients might receive care or where cough-inducing procedures are performed). The staff also must classify the risk for groups of employees who work throughout the facility rather than in a specific area (eg, respiratory therapists, interns, and environmental services).

On the basis of these data and the CDC guidelines, infection control personnel should determine the appropriate risk classification for their entire facility and, if applicable, for specific areas, departments, or worker groups.[4] Epidemiology staff need to develop different program components for specific areas, departments, or occupational groups.

According to the CDC's statistics, 42% of the counties in the United States have not reported any TB cases in the past year, and another 47% have

---

TABLE 27-1

ELEMENTS OF TUBERCULOSIS RISK ASSESSMENT[*]

First:

- Review community TB profile (incidence and prevalence of TB, and drug-susceptibility patterns)

- Review the facility's TB profile (number of TB patients admitted to facility in past year)

If TB Found in Community or Facility:

- Analyze the number of infectious TB patients admitted to each area or ward during past year

- Analyze healthcare workers' PPD skin-test results by area or occupational group to determine if clusters of PPD conversions or person-to-person transmission may have occurred

- Evaluate TB infection control practices by reviewing the medical records of TB patients and by observing practice

- Evaluate whether engineering controls are maintained

TB = tuberculosis; PPD = purified protein derivative.
[*]*Adapted from the Centers for Disease Control and Prevention.[4]*

---

reported fewer than nine cases. Thus, most healthcare facilities are classified as minimal-risk or very-low-risk facilities. This chapter will focus on these institutions.

Minimal Risk Facility

If the TB assessment indicates, for example, that no cases of TB have occurred in the community or healthcare facility within the past year, then there is little risk of exposure to TB, and the facility meets the CDC's criteria for minimal risk. The basic program components of a minimal-risk facility are listed in Table 27-2.

Very-Low-Risk Facility

A very-low-risk healthcare facility is one in which TB patients are not admitted to the facility but may be seen for triage or diagnostic evaluation in a clinic or emergency department. Patients who need inpatient care will be referred to another facility. If

TABLE 27-2

TUBERCULOSIS CONTROL PROGRAM COMPONENTS FOR A MINIMAL-RISK FACILITY*

- Designated person(s) responsible for TB control program

- Baseline risk assessment (including community and facility TB profile) with annual reassessment

- Written TB control plan

- Protocol for identifying patients with active TB

- Triage system for identifying patients with active TB in emergency and ambulatory-care settings

- Protocol for referring patients who may have active TB to a collaborating facility (if TB patients are admitted, a more comprehensive plan is required†)

- Baseline PPD testing of workers‡

- Educate and train workers regarding TB

- Protocol for identifying, evaluating, and managing workers with positive PPD tests or active TB

- Protocol for investigating PPD conversions among workers

- Protocol for investigating possible patient-to-patient transmission

- Protocol for investigating contacts of TB patients who were not diagnosed or isolated

- Mechanism for reporting patients with TB to health department

TB = tuberculosis; PPD = purified protein derivative; CDC = Centers for Disease Control and Prevention.
According to the CDC, a minimal-risk facility does not admit or treat TB patients to inpatient or outpatient areas and is located in a county or community with no reported TB cases in the past year.
†*Consult 1994 CDC guidelines for additional requirements.*
‡*An ongoing PPD skin-testing program is not needed. However, baseline PPD testing is advisable, so that if an unexpected exposure occurs, conversion can be distinguished from positive PPD test results from a previous exposure.*

TB cases were reported in the community, but no patients were seen in the emergency area in the past year and the hospital has a protocol for transferring TB patients to a referral center, according to CDC guidelines, both the facility and the emergency area are designated very-low-risk. Infection control personnel should identify areas in which exposure to patients with active TB might occur (eg, specific clinics or the emergency treatment center) and then assess the specific risk classification.

Very-low-risk facilities need the same basic components in their TB programs as minimal-risk facilities (see Table 27-2). Both referring and receiving facilities must agree to provide proper management and follow-up of patients suspected of having TB. In addition, very-low-risk facilities must establish protocols for outpatient areas (eg, clinic and emergency areas) that specify how to evaluate and treat patients, how to report laboratory results to appropriate individuals (eg, clinicians, hospital epidemiologist, infection control staff, collaborating referring and receiving facilities, and local health department), and how to protect staff (eg, a respiratory protection program).

Patients suspected of having TB should be placed in an area separate from other patients during their medical evaluation and while they wait for transfer to another facility. These patients should wear surgical masks and should be instructed to keep the masks on their faces. Ideally, a TB isolation room that meets the CDC's ventilation requirements for negative pressure—six air exchanges per hour vented to the outside or recirculation through a high-efficiency particulate air (HEPA) filter—should be available. As an alternative or interim measure to disinfect the air in areas where potentially infectious TB patients wait for transfer, some facilities use portable HEPA filtration and disinfection devices or ceiling-mounted or wall-mounted ultraviolet lights.

Prioritize Control Measures

A TB control program should achieve the following goals: early identification of patients with TB, prompt isolation, and effective treatment of persons with active disease. The specific control measures can be prioritized based on their relative effectiveness in reducing risk of transmission. This ranking is referred to as the "hierarchy of controls" and separates the measures into administrative controls, engineering controls, and respiratory protection. This hierarchy, which comes from an industrial hygiene model, is the basis for OSHA's enforcement procedures for control of occupationally related exposures. The CDC recommends components for TB programs based on the risk assessment. However, a healthcare facility cannot implement all of these measures simultaneously. Some facilities may need additional resources before they can institute particular control measures. Thus, prioritizing control measures using this hierarchy is extremely useful.[7]

Administrative Controls

A healthcare facility should implement administrative controls first, as these are the controls that most effectively reduce the risk of nosocomial transmission. Even facilities that do not have the resources to tackle more expensive engineering controls can institute these controls. Administrative controls include developing and implementing effective policies and protocols to assure that persons likely to have TB are identified rapidly, isolated properly, evaluated clinically, and treated appropriately. Educating, training, and counseling employees about TB, and screening them for TB infection and TB disease, are also components of administrative controls. Finally, administrative controls include monitoring the facility for compliance with TB control measures and correcting inadequate performance.

Early Identification and Isolation

Surveillance is the key to controlling nosocomial TB.[8] It requires that healthcare workers carefully evaluate patients upon their initial encounter and promptly isolate any patient who they suspect may have TB until laboratory and clinical evidence eliminates this diagnosis. The protocol for early identification and isolation of patients should be based on the prevalence and demographic profile of TB patients in the community. Hospitals that assess compliance with TB isolation precautions can reduce the number of days that potentially infectious patients are not isolated appropriately.[9,10] Moreover, because patients with HIV infection may present with atypical signs and symptoms, some facilities isolate all patients with HIV infection who have clinical symptoms suggestive of TB (eg, fever, cough, or an abnormal chest radiograph) until appropriate cultures are negative.[9] Hospitals can implement an early identification and isolation protocol more efficiently by authorizing both nurses and physicians to isolate patients with suspect TB and by developing policies that allow staff to isolate automatically certain patients (eg, patients for whom TB is in the differential diagnosis or from whom specimens are ordered for mycobacterium smear or culture).

The protocol for early identification of TB patients and the definition of "suspect case" will determine the number of isolation rooms required. Some patients who do not have TB will be isolated (ie, overisolation) to prevent nosocomial transmission; the degree of overisolation will depend on the institution's policy. Some degree of overisolation may be more cost-effective than underisolation, because TB exposures may be very costly. To increase the number of isolation rooms, healthcare facilities have used several strategies, such as using window exhaust fans to create negative pressure or using portable HEPA filtration units to filter the air.

Laboratory Diagnosis

Laboratory tests are necessary to confirm or exclude the diagnosis of TB and to identify resistant isolates of *M tuberculosis*. If a clinical laboratory cannot perform the most rapid tests, the hospital may need to send specimens to a referral laboratory. The healthcare facility must ensure that arrangements comply with the CDC's guidelines for transporting specimens and reporting results (eg, acid-fast bacilli smear results must be reported within 24 hours of specimen collection).

Treatment

Clinicians must start empirical therapy as soon as they suspect that the patient has TB. The current recommendation is to begin empirical therapy with four drugs (isoniazid, rifampin, pyrazinamide, and ethambutol or streptomycin). In areas where the prevalence of primary resistance to isoniazid is ≤4%, three drugs (isoniazid, rifampin, and pyrazinamide) are acceptable for initial therapy.[10] The American Thoracic Society has published the details of antituberculous therapy.[4,11]

Skin Testing Workers

The standard method for identifying persons infected with *M tuberculosis* is the Mantoux tuberculin skin test, for which PPD is injected intradermally (0.1 mL of 5 tuberculin units).[4,12] When TB cases were declining, many hospitals abandoned routine employee PPD skin testing, because it was costly and apparently provided minimal benefit. With the resurgence of TB, OSHA specified its enforcement procedures, including routine PPD skin testing, to protect healthcare workers from occupationally acquired TB. Particularly in high-prevalence areas of the country, PPD skin testing allows healthcare facilities to detect TB infection and disease early, to provide isoniazid or other chemoprophylaxis to staff whose skin tests convert, and, thus, to prevent nosocomial transmission.

The infection control staff should consider a number of important issues when developing a program for screening healthcare workers. First, who is considered an employee? OSHA's authority is limited to enforcing compliance with policies for employees, that is, persons who are paid or who receive compensation from the employer. With respect to TB control, healthcare facilities should broaden the definition of employee to ensure that all paid and unpaid staff, including students,

agency nurses, residents, volunteers, and others who work in high-risk areas, are screened as part of the skin-testing program. In addition, all newly hired employees assigned to high-risk areas should have PPD skin tests.

Regardless of the prevalence of TB in the community, infection control personnel would be prudent to obtain baseline PPD testing of employees at least once and to calculate a facility-wide rate of PPD skin-test positivity. The frequency of additional PPD testing depends on the risk classification of the facility or of specific areas in the facility. For example, the CDC recommends that high-risk facilities or areas conduct repeat testing every 3 months.

All PPD test results should be recorded in the individual employee's health record and in an aggregate database of all PPD skin-test results. PPD conversion rates should be calculated for the facility as a whole and, if appropriate, for specific areas of the facility and for occupational groups. PPD conversion rates should be calculated by dividing the number of PPD-test conversions among healthcare workers in each area or group (ie, the numerator) by the total number of previously PPD-negative healthcare workers tested in each area or group (ie, the denominator).

The infection control personnel must interpret PPD conversion rates. If the number of workers in a particular area is small, the conversion rate may be high, although the actual risk may not be higher than in other areas. In contrast, statistical analysis may miss significant problems when the number of workers is small. If healthcare workers become PPD positive, epidemiology staff should investigate to determine whether the likely source is in the facility or in the community. Of note, healthcare workers in some facilities are more likely to be exposed to TB in the community than in the hospital.[13] In addition, infection control staff should determine whether the hospital has changed brands of PPD, because different preparations give different results.[14,15]

Two-step baseline PPD testing can help infection control staff identify infections in new personnel who otherwise would be classified as recent conversions. This is true especially in hospitals with large numbers of employees who have received bacille Calmette-Guérin (BCG) vaccination.[8,12,16] CDC guidelines recommend using the two-step baseline PPD testing for employees who may be exposed to TB, including those who have had BCG vaccination.

The most difficult part of the skin-testing program will be to ensure that staff report to employee health for PPD placement and for follow-up assessment. Some facilities have improved compliance by offering PPD testing at the work site, thereby removing the time and distance barriers and increasing peer pressure. Some facilities, particularly in high-prevalence areas, have implemented mandatory PPD skin-testing programs for high-risk workers.[9]

Engineering Controls

Engineering controls remove droplet nuclei from the air. These controls include local exhaust ventilation, general or central ventilation, air filtration with HEPA filters, and air disinfection with ultraviolet germicidal irradiation (UVGI).

Local Exhaust Ventilation

Local exhaust ventilation using a booth, hood, or tent can be an efficient engineering control technique, because it captures a contaminant at its source. Local exhaust ventilation should be used whenever aerosol-generating procedures, including bronchoscopy, are performed. For example, some operating rooms place "smoke evacuators" near the operating site during procedures that perforate infected lung tissue.

General Ventilation

General ventilation includes mechanisms that control the direction of airflow to prevent an infectious source from contaminating the air in nearby areas. These mechanisms include maintaining negative pressure and circulating air to dilute and remove infectious droplet nuclei (eg, room air exchanges). The CDC currently recommends that TB isolation rooms should have negative pressure, to prevent the escape of droplet nuclei, and six air exchanges per hour, to decrease the concentration of infectious particles. However, the CDC recently changed the requirements for airflow in isolation rooms from 6 to ≥12 air exchanges per hour for newly constructed or renovated facilities.[4] The recommendations on air exchanges do not have a scientific basis, but are derived from information about maintaining comfortable, odor-free air. Furthermore, air from TB isolation rooms must be exhausted to the outside without recirculation. When air from a TB isolation room must be recirculated, the CDC recommends that air be passed through a HEPA filter before it is returned to general ventilation.

Portable Air Filtration Units

Recent data suggest that some portable HEPA filtration units can effectively remove airborne particles similar in size to infectious droplet nuclei.[17] These portable units are becoming increasing popular as interim engineering control measures. These units enable hospitals to establish TB isolation rooms in outpatient departments and in patient-care areas when other TB isolation rooms are in use. In addition, facilities that do not have isolation rooms can use these units to convert general patient rooms to TB isolation rooms.

Ultraviolet Germicidal Irradiation

The CDC considers UVGI to be a supplementary measure for TB control and recommends that UVGI not be used as a substitute for negative pressure or HEPA filtration. Other experts disagree strongly with the limitations placed on using UVGI, citing advantages of efficacy, ease of application, and relatively low cost.[18-20] Studies suggest that a 30-W UV fixture provides the equivalent of 20 or more room air exchanges, depending on the air-mixing and flow patterns.[19,20]

There are two systems for UVGI: duct irradiation and upper room irradiation. In duct irradiation, UVGI lamps inside ventilation ducts disinfect the air before it is recirculated. In upper-room air irradiation, UVGI lamps are suspended from the ceiling or mounted on the wall with a shield at the bottom of the lamp to direct the rays upward. As the air circulates, nonirradiated air moves from the lower to the upper part of the room, and irradiated air moves from the upper to the lower part of the room.

Clearly, there is a role for upper-room air UVGI irradiation in areas that are difficult to ventilate, such as waiting rooms, emergency rooms, corridors, and other central areas of a facility where patients with undiagnosed TB could contaminate the air. The CDC allows healthcare facilities to use UVGI in these situations. Details about how to use both types of UVGI, their applications, and limitations can be found in the CDC guidelines, and in other resources.[4,19-21]

Other

A few hospitals have used alternative engineering controls successfully in TB isolation rooms, including creating negative pressure with window fans[9] or with UVGI in ventilation ducts without negative pressure.[18]

In summary, the general ventilation recommendations are among the most costly controls to implement. Further, there are no clinical trials establishing the relative efficacy of any recommended method for cleaning the air. Until OSHA develops a formal TB standard that mandates the use of specific engineering controls, employers still have some discretion regarding the strategies they use to control a workplace hazard, if they have data to support the effectiveness of the control. However, facilities that depart from recommended engineering control methods must collect accurate

data on the frequency of nosocomial transmission of TB (eg, PPD skin-test conversions).

Respiratory Protection

Respiratory protection is the last step in the hierarchy of TB control measures. In the past, regulatory agencies, infectious disease experts, and infection control personnel argued about which respiratory protection device was most appropriate. However, all federal agencies involved in this issue (National Institute for Occupational Safety and Health [NIOSH], OSHA, and the CDC) now agree that the minimal acceptable respiratory protection is a NIOSH-certified N-95 respirator.[22] According to OSHA, the N-95 respirators meet the CDC's performance criteria for a TB-control respirator. When first released in September 1995, the disposable N-95 cost between $1 and $3. OSHA permits a healthcare worker to reuse a respirator as long as it maintains its structural and functional integrity and the filter material is not damaged or soiled. Each facility should develop a protocol that defines when a disposable respirator must be discarded (eg, if it becomes contaminated with blood).

In addition to selecting respirators, each healthcare facility needs a complete respiratory protection program. OSHA's respiratory protection standard of 1972[4,23,24] requires that an institution:

- Assign responsibility for the program to a specific person or group.
- Write procedures for all aspects of the program.
- Screen all employees for medical conditions that prevent them from wearing respirators.
- Train and educate employees about respiratory protocols.
- Fit test the respirators on each employee and have employees check the fit each time they use a respirator.
- Develop policies and procedures that describe how to inspect, maintain, and reuse respirators, and define when respirators are

contaminated and must be discarded.

• Evaluate the program periodically.

OSHA's final TB standard will discuss the requirements for use of TB respirators. Until OSHA issues this standard, the 1972 respiratory protection standard applies to all respirator use.

OSHA requires healthcare facilities to fit test each employee when a respirator is selected, and to document the respirator type, model number, and size. OSHA recommends, but does not require, annual fit testing. Many facilities have implemented protocols that specify when repeat fit testing should occur. For example, fit testing may be indicated if employees gain or lose more than 10 lbs or if the shape of their face changes when they lose teeth or receive dentures.

A qualitative method generally is used for fit testing disposable respirators. This method involves exposing the employee to an irritant smoke or odorous chemical (eg, saccharin). Federal agencies do not agree on which chemical is most appropriate for qualitative fit testing. Irritant smoke and saccharin each have advantages and disadvantages. Results of fit testing with irritant smoke may be less subjective than those obtained with saccharin. If the respirator does not fit, the employee automatically will cough when exposed to irritant smoke; however, the smoke can irritate the respiratory tract. In contrast, the results of fit testing using saccharin depend on an employee's subjective response to its taste. Some individuals are not sensitive to saccharin's taste. In addition, some data suggest that saccharin may be a carcinogenic. Hospitals should follow the manufacturer's instructions and recommendations for fit testing. There are few studies that demonstrate the efficacy of fit testing disposable respirators.

Employees must test the face piece of the respirator to detect leaks each time they don these devices. The manufacturer's recommendations should be followed, because the recommended procedures vary substantially between specific products.

OSHA requires that healthcare facilities screen employees to determine whether they can wear respirators, but OSHA does not specify the screening method. Other than severe cardiac or pulmonary disease, few medical conditions should preclude the use of disposable respirators. Many facilities use a general questionnaire to screen employees for medical conditions and to determine whether an employee should be evaluated further.

OSHA's minimum requirement for respiratory protection is the N95 respirator. However, particular situations may warrant more protective respirators. For example, personnel who perform extremely high-risk procedures, such as bronchoscopy, on patients with known MDR-TB may need additional respiratory protection. One example of a more protective respirator is a powered air-purifying respirator. NIOSH recently published a guide on respirators for TB that describes the type of respirators that are available.[25]

A respiratory protection program, including fit testing, can be very costly. Thus, some facilities have limited the number of employees who care for TB patients. In addition, healthcare facilities must develop policies regarding respiratory protection for bearded employees, because most disposable respirators cannot seal tightly in the presence of facial hair. Some facilities have reassigned bearded workers to low-risk areas; other facilities have required employees to shave their beards. In special cases, facilities have provided more protective respirators (eg, powered air-purifying respirators) to bearded employees, particularly those working in very high-risk settings such as the bronchoscopy or autopsy suites.

Compliance With OSHA's Standards

Until OSHA develops a specific TB standard, it recognizes the CDC's TB guidelines as the accepted standards of practice, and it enforces compliance with the key components of the CDC guidelines. Infection control personnel should contact their state or regional OSHA office for information on the most current OSHA enforcement directive that specifies

TABLE 27-3

UNITED STATES DEPARTMENT OF LABOR OCCUPATIONAL SAFETY AND HEALTH ADMINISTRATION REGIONAL OFFICES

Region I

(Connecticut,* New Hampshire, Maine, Massachusetts,
     Rhode Island, Vermont*)
Boston, MA
617-565-9860

Region II

(New Jersey, New York,* Puerto Rico,* Virgin Islands*)
New York, NY
212-337-2378

Region III

(Delaware, Maryland,* Pennsylvania,
     Virginia,* Washington, DC, West Virginia)
Philadelphia, PA
215-596-1201

Region IV

(Alabama, Florida, Georgia, Kentucky,* Mississippi, North
     Carolina,* South Carolina,* Tennessee*)
Atlanta, GA
404-562-2300

Region V

(Illinois, Indiana,* Michigan,* Minnesota,* Ohio, Wisconsin)
     Chicago, IL
312-353-2220

Region VI

(Arkansas, Louisiana, New Mexico,* Oklahoma, Texas)
Dallas, TX
214-767-4731

Region VII

(Iowa,* Kansas, Missouri, Nebraska)
Kansas City, MO
816-426-5861

Region VIII

(Colorado, Montana, North Dakota, South Dakota, Utah,*
     Wyoming*)
Denver, CO
303-844-1600

Region IX

(American Samoa, Arizona,* California,* Guam, Hawaii,*
     Nevada,* Trust Territories of the Pacific)
San Francisco, CA
415-975-4310

Region X

(Alaska,* Idaho, Oregon,* Washington*)
Seattle, WA
206-553-5930

*These states and territories operate their own Occupational Safety and Health Administration-approved job safety and health programs
(Connecticut and New York plans cover public employees only).

the minimum requirements for a TB control program. Table 27-3 lists OSHA's regional offices. In the 25 states with state-run OSHA programs, infection control personnel should contact that office, because states may impose more stringent requirements than those mandated at the federal level.

Epidemiology staff should familiarize themselves with OSHA's enforcement directive because, although the current requirements are based on the CDC's *Guidelines for Preventing the Transmission of Mycobacterium tuberculosis in Health-Care Facilities, 1994,*[4] these two agencies may interpret and apply these guidelines differently, and they may require different methods for recordkeeping and respiratory protection. Noncompliance with these requirements can result in fines of up to $70,000 for each violation. OSHA is writing a for-

mal TB regulation, that was scheduled to be published in late 1996 but has been delayed. Infection control personnel also must know local or state regulations (eg, from the department of health) that set minimum standards for TB control.

OSHA is inspecting healthcare facilities, correctional institutions, long-term care facilities, homeless shelters, and drug treatment centers for compliance with the TB enforcement directive. These inspections usually are instigated by complaints from employees or reports of fatalities or catastrophes. OSHA also can evaluate compliance with the TB enforcement directive when it conducts routine industrial hygiene inspections in facilities that have employees exposed to TB.

Table 27-4 summarizes OSHA's required elements for control of TB in healthcare facilities.

TABLE 27-4

OCCUPATIONAL SAFETY AND HEALTH ADMINISTRATION'S REQUIREMENTS FOR TUBERCULOSIS CONTROL PROGRAMS*

Criteria for Inspection: A Suspect or Confirmed Case of TB in the Past 6 Months

- Protocol for early identification of patients with active TB, including training staff to identify patients with active TB

- Medical surveillance of healthcare workers

    - Offer TB skin testing at no cost to all potentially exposed workers and all new workers before they begin work

    - Base frequency of repeat TB skin testing on risk assessment

    - Evaluate workers who have had unprotected TB exposure

    - Evaluate workers who develop symptoms of TB

- Case management of infected workers

    - Have protocol for follow-up of recent PPD converters

- When first hired, and annually, employees should be given training on modes of transmission, signs and symptoms, medical surveillance, site-specific protocols for TB control, and protocols for exposure incidents

- Use of engineering controls

    - Place patients with possible or confirmed TB in isolation rooms with negative pressure and air that is exhausted directly outside or through a HEPA filter if recirculation is unavoidable

    - Use special booths, hoods, or isolation rooms that meet above isolation criteria for hazardous procedures (eg, aerosolized medication treatment, autopsies)

    - Monitor negative pressure in isolation rooms with smoke tubes or other indicators

    - Use respirators when entering isolation rooms if hazardous procedures are performed without local source control or local exhaust (ie, booth, hood, tent) until air is purged of droplet nuclei

- Have a complete respiratory protection program in place

    - Use NIOSH-approved respirators (eg, N-95) for TB

    - Develop protocol for reuse of disposable respirators (by the same worker) and circumstances when the respirator must be discarded (eg, loss of structural integrity, damaged filter media, or contamination)

- Keep records of employee exposures to TB, results of TB skin tests, and all medical evaluations and treatment

- Use signs or tags outside TB isolation or treatment rooms that describe the necessary precautions (eg, respirators must be donned before entering)

- Record on the OSHA 200 log all TB skin-test conversions and active cases of TB among workers. Assume all TB skin-test conversions are occupationally acquired, unless clear documentation exists for non-occupational exposure

---

TB = tuberculosis; PPD = purified protein derivative; HEPA = high-efficiency particulate air; NIOSH = National Institute for Occupational Safety and Health; OSHA = Occupational Safety and Health Administration.

Adapted from Occupational Safety and Health Administration.[23]

Healthcare facilities should implement, at the very least, the required control measures to be ready for an OSHA inspection.

Until the TB standard is complete, OSHA's authority to conduct inspections for occupational exposure to TB comes from the general duty clause of the Occupational Safety and Health Act of 1970. Under this clause, a hazard must be present (eg, a case of suspected or confirmed TB) in the worksite for OSHA to conduct an inspection and to cite an employer for not having a TB control program. Thus, infection control personnel must conduct a risk assessment first when developing a TB control program to document whether patients with suspected or confirmed TB are treated in the facility.

References

1. Tapper ML. Where are we in tuberculosis infection control? *Infect Control Hosp Epidemiol*. 1995;16:125-128. Editorial.

2. Jarvis WR. Nosocomial transmission of multidrug-resistant *Mycobacterium tuberculosis*. *Am J Infect Control*. 1995;23:146-151.

3. Centers for Disease Control. Guidelines for preventing the transmission of tuberculosis in health-care settings, with special focus on HIV-related issues. *MMWR*. 1990;39(No. RR-17).

4. Centers for Disease Control and Prevention. Guidelines for preventing the transmission of *Mycobacterium tuberculosis* in health-care settings, 1994. *MMWR*. 1994;43(RR-13):1-132.

5. Occupational Safety and Health Administration. Memorandum: Enforcement Policies and Procedures for Occupational Exposure to tuberculosis. October 8, 1993.

6. Decker MD. OSHA enforcement policy for occupational exposure to tuberculosis. *Infect Control Hosp Epidemiol*. 1993;14:689-693.

7. American Hospital Association Technical Panel on Infections. *Tuberculosis Control in the Hospital—A Special Briefing*. Chicago, Ill: American Hospital Association; 1994.

8. McGowan JE Jr. Nosocomial tuberculosis: new progress in control and prevention. *Clin Infect Dis*. 1995;21:489-505.

9. Blumberg HM, Watkins DL, Berschling JD, et al. Preventing the nosocomial transmission of tuberculosis *Ann Intern Med*. 1995;122:658-663.

10. Fazal BA, Telzak EE, Blum S, et al. Impact of a coordinated tuberculosis team in an inner-city hospital in New York City. *Infect Control Hosp Epidemiol*. 1995;16:340-343.

11. American Thoracic Society. Treatment of tuberculosis and infection in adults and children. *Am J Respir Crit Care Med*. 1994;149:1359-1374.

12. Pugliese G. Screening for tuberculosis: an update. *Am J Infect Control*. 1992;20:37-40.

13. Bailey TC, Fraser VJ, Spitznagel EL, Dunagan WC. Risk factors for a positive tuberculin skin test among employees of an urban, midwestern teaching hospital. *Ann Intern Med*. 1995;122:580-585.

14. Johnson JL, Nyole S, Shepardson L, Mugereva R, Ellner JJ. Simultaneous comparison of two commercial tuberculin skin test reagents in an areas with high prevalence of tuberculosis. *J Infect Dis*. 1995;171:1066-1067. Letter.

15. Shands JW, Boeff D, Fauerbach L, Gutekunst RR. Tuberculin testing in a tertiary hospital: product variability. *Infect Control Hosp Epidemiol*. 1994;15:758-760.

16. Horowitz HW, Luciano BB, Kadel JR, Wormser RP. Tuberculin skin test conversions in hospital employees vaccinated with bacille Calmette-Guérin: recent *Mycobacterium tuberculosis* infection or booster effect? *Infect Control Hosp Epidemiol*. 1995;23:181-187.

17. Rutala WA, Jones SM, Worthington JM, et al. Efficacy of portable filtration units in reducing aerosolized particles in the size range of *Mycobacterium tuberculosis*. *Infect Control Hosp Epidemiol*. 1995;16:391-398.

18. Eisenman MD. A leap of faith: what can we do to curtail intrainstitutional transmission of tuberculosis? *Ann Intern Med*. 1992;117:251-253.

19. Nardell EA. Interrupting transmission from patients with unsuspected tuberculosis: a unique role for upper-room ultraviolet air disinfection. *Am J Infect Control*. 1995;23:156-164.

20. Nardell EA. Fans, filters, or rays? Pros and cons of the current environmental tuberculosis control technologies. *Infect Control Hosp Epidemiol*. 1993;14:681-685.

21. Macher JM. The use of germicidal lamps to control tuberculosis in healthcare facilities. *Infect Control Hosp Epidemiol*. 1993;14:723-729.

22. Jarvis WR, Bolyard EA, Bozzi CJ, et al. Respirators, recommendations, and regulations: the controversy surrounding protection of healthcare workers from tuberculosis. *Ann Intern Med*. 1995;122:142-146.

23. Occupational Safety and Health Administration. *Enforcement Procedures and Scheduling for Occupational Exposure to tuberculosis*. OSHA Instruction (CPL 2.106). February 9, 1996.

24. Occupational Safety and Health Administration. Occupational safety and health standards, personal protective equipment, respiratory protection (29 CFR 1910.134). *Federal Register*. 1972;37:1910-1934.

25. National Institute of Occupational Safety and Health. *Protect Yourself Against tuberculosis—A Respiratory Protection Guide for Healthcare Workers*. December 1995.

CHAPTER 28

Infection Control Issues in Construction and Renovation

Cheryl D. Carter, RN, BSN, Brenda A. Barr, RN, MS, CIC

Abstract

Construction or renovation projects in hospitals pose special challenges. Infection control personnel should be involved in all phases of these projects to ensure that patients, visitors, and staff are protected from unnecessary exposure to infectious agents. Infection control personnel must identify the infection risks posed by each project and plan ways to minimize the risk. Infection control personnel also must ensure that municipal, county, state, and federal infection control guidelines and regulations are met. This chapter will discuss basic infection control issues encountered during construction and renovation, offer practical suggestions for addressing these issues, discuss common questions that infection control personnel must address, and describe outbreaks related to construction and renovation.

Introduction

Hospital construction and renovation projects pose many challenges to infection control personnel. These projects can increase the risk of nosocomial infections. In addition, resources important to good infection control practices may be disrupted or may not be available during the projects.

Moreover, many agencies regulate functions and construction within hospitals. Finally, infection control personnel must assess whether or not the plans comply with infection control guidelines and regulations established by their city, county, and state, by regulatory and accrediting agencies, and by the federal government. To successfully meet these challenges, infection control personnel must collaborate with engineers, nurse managers, administrators, architects, and physicians before, during, and after the construction projects.

The primary goals of infection control personnel are to prevent nosocomial infections and to ensure that patients, visitors, and staff are protected from unnecessary exposure to infectious agents. During hospital construction and renovation, these goals may be harder to achieve. For example, construction will increase the amount of dust and dirt in the hospital. Bacterial or fungal microorganisms in the dust and dirt can contaminate air handling or water systems. The contaminated systems then can transmit these organisms to susceptible persons. The air handling or water systems may be shut down for periods to allow modifications or additions. During the time these systems are nonfunc-

TABLE 28-1

QUESTIONS INFECTION CONTROL PERSONNEL OFTEN ARE ASKED ABOUT CONSTRUCTION

- Do the construction workers have to use dedicated halls, elevators, entrances, and exits?
- Can we use a cheaper product?
- Can we install fewer sinks?
- Where should the sinks be placed?
- What type of controls should the sinks have?
- What kind of flooring, ceiling tiles, and wall coverings can we use?
- Can we store clean and dirty items in the same area?
- Can we put a refrigerator for medications in an outpatient clinic's laboratory area?
- Do we need a pass-through window in an outpatient clinic's laboratory?
- Can we put particular pieces of equipment in this area (eg, an endoscope washer in the dirty utility room of an outpatient clinic)?
- Do we need special ventilation in a room containing endoscope washers?
- Can we install shower curtains or shower doors?
- Do we need an anteroom for the isolation rooms?
- When can we start the project? Do we have to wait until winter?
- Can we do the project during the day, or do we have to work nights and weekends?
- Can we use live plants as decorations?
- Can we install a fish tank?

tional, routine infection control measures, such as handwashing, may be difficult to maintain. Reinstituting these systems also may increase the risk of infections such as Legionnaires' disease. Moreover, routine clinical practice and traffic patterns may need to be modified substantially during construction projects to ensure that basic infection control precautions are maintained.

Infection control personnel should participate in construction projects from the inception, so that they can identify potential infection control problems created by the project and can design solutions prospectively. In addition, infection control personnel also should understand the purpose of the project, so they can assess whether or not the

design will facilitate good infection control practice. The old adage "an ounce of prevention is worth a pound of cure" must have been coined by frustrated infection control personnel who were investigating an outbreak of construction-associated *Aspergillus* infections or who were trying to retrofit a newly constructed room to be a tuberculosis isolation room.

A caveat is necessary. During construction projects, infection control personnel will be asked to judge the value of many designs or products. Often, infection control personnel will be asked to determine how much space is necessary for a certain function, which products (eg, Corian® [DuPont Corian, Wilmington, Del] versus laminate) should be used, and what air handling requirements must be met. Table 28-1 reviews questions that we frequently are asked during construction or renovation projects. The persons asking the questions may genuinely want to know the answers, or they may have hidden agendas that they hope the hospital epidemiology program will endorse. In addition, the epidemiology staff may find themselves mediating between opposing sides, including department directors who want vast amounts of space and the latest innovations, and administrators who want to limit the costs. To avoid costly mistakes and political landmines, infection control personnel must ask many questions to determine what the real issues are; how the product, equipment, room, or clinic will be used; what possible solutions are available; what the budgetary limitations are; and what infection control principles or external regulations apply. In addition, infection control personnel may need to review the medical literature, laws from many levels of government, guidelines from architectural and engineering societies and accrediting agencies, and product descriptions, to determine which product or design best balances the infection control requirements with employee and patient safety and satisfaction, and cost constraints.

As healthcare budgets shrink, the expertise of

TABLE 28-2
CONSTRUCTION-RELATED *ASPERGILLUS* OUTBREAKS IN HOSPITALS

Author	Risk Factors	Cause of Outbreak	Reservoir	No. of Cases	No. of Deaths	Control Measures	Organism	Institution
Opal et al[1] 1986	Hematologic malignancy, High-dose corticosteroid therapy, Carcinoma	Renovation	Construction site	11	11	Copper 8 quinolinolate, Barriers, HEPA filters in patient rooms, Negative pressure in construction area	*Aspergillus flavus*, *Aspergillus fumigatus*, *Aspergillus niger*, *Aspergillus* sp	Army medical center
Arnow et al[15] 1978	Immunosuppression (renal transplant)	Renovation	Spores in dust from false ceiling tiles above transplant unit	3	1	Impermeable plastic barriers, Patients moved to other wards, Horizontal surfaces vacuumed, damp mopped and dusted	*Aspergillus fumigatus*, *Aspergillus* sp	VA hospital
Weems et al[16] 1987	Hematologic malignancies	Major construction Interior renovation	Excessive dust from demolition, modification of HVAC system, relocation of interior walls, construction traffic	5	5	Windows in patient rooms permanently sealed	*Aspergillus* Zygomycetes	Pediatric referral center

TABLE 28-2 (continued)
CONSTRUCTION-RELATED *ASPERGILLUS* OUTBREAKS IN HOSPITALS

Author	Risk Factors	Cause of Outbreak	Reservoir	No. of Cases	No. of Deaths	Control Measures	Organism	Institution
Krasinski et al[17] 1985	Prematurity	Renovation of special care unit	Mold in dust from a false ceiling	2	2	Patients moved from area of construction Additional dampers placed in air ducts Impervious dust barriers erected False ceiling and ventilation ducts vacuumed Replaced HEPA filters Air ducts and environmental surfaces disinfected	*Aspergillus* Zygomycetes *Rhizopus indicus*	Tertiary care center for newborn infants
Sarubbi et al[18] 1982	Lung carcinoma COPD Bacterial pneumonia	Construction	Defective ventilation and air filtration system	22 (21 colonized and 1 infected)	1	Pre-filters and filters in ventilation system replaced	*Aspergillus flavus*	University hospital

HVAC = heating, ventilation, and air conditioning; COPD = chronic obstructive pulmonary disease.

TABLE 28-3

CONSTRUCTION-RELATED *LEGIONELLA* OUTBREAKS IN HOSPITALS

Author	Risk Factors	Cause of Outbreak	Reservoir	No. of Cases	No. of Deaths	Institution
Haley et al[19] 1979; Shands et al[20] 1985	Immuno-suppressed Malignancy Renal transplant Grounds privileges	Major construction	External hospital environment Potable water	49*	15*	VA hospital
Thacker et al[21] 1978	Sleeping by open window Proximity to excavation	Construction Installation of lawn sprinkling system	Soil	81	12	Psychiatric hospital
Mermel et al[22] 1995	Myelodysplasia Neutropenia Steroids	Major construction	Water supply pipe	2	2	University-affiliated hospital

VA = Veterans Administration.
*Number of cases and deaths reported in the article by Haley et al[19]; the number of cases and deaths were not enumerated in the article by Shands et al.[20]

infection control personnel will become more important during construction and renovation projects. Simultaneously, infection control personnel will feel increasing pressure to choose the cheapest products or design. Despite the pressures, infection control personnel must remember their primary goals and recommend the products or design that will achieve these goals most effectively. The appropriate products or designs may be more expensive initially; but, in the long run, they probably will be less costly, as they may prevent outbreaks, or they may last longer and require less maintenance.

Infection control personnel should educate unit staff, architects, engineers, maintenance personnel, and construction workers about infection risks associated with construction and about appropriate methods for minimizing these risks. Education will be a continual process, because different hospital staff will be involved in each project and because many of the other personnel will be contract workers. Infection control personnel could develop a brochure, which discusses basic infection control issues in construction projects,

and a checklist, which itemizes infection control essentials, to answer particular questions and problems that occur with each project (eg, number and location of sinks, type of ceiling tiles, type of floor and wall coverings). Infection control personnel should inspect the worksite to make sure that the construction workers are following the guidelines. In general, hospitals would be wise to include infection control rules and needs in a written contract, so the contractors know what they are expected to do. If the construction team consistently ignores the infection control policies, the hospital should levy a fine.

Infection control personnel often are the only clinical personnel who work on all construction and renovation projects. Thus, they may have to be the watchdogs for the entire project to make sure that the design and the construction meets the appropriate standards.

Many of the above comments are based on common sense. However, our experience and the medical literature testify that common sense answers often are not chosen during construction projects. To sup-

TABLE 28-4
DESIGN AND CONSTRUCTION ERRORS

- Air intakes placed too close to exhausts or other mistakes in the placement of air intakes
- Incorrect number of air exchanges
- Air-handling system functions only during the week or on particular days of the week
- Air vents not reopened after the construction is finished
- No negative-air-pressure rooms built in a large, new inpatient building
- Carpet placed where vinyl should be used
- Wet-vacuum system in the operating suite pulls water up one floor into a holding tank rather than down one floor
- Aerators on faucets
- Sinks located in inaccessible places
- Patient rooms or treatment rooms do not have sinks in which healthcare workers can wash their hands
- Doors too narrow to allow beds and equipment to be moved in and out of rooms

port this contention, we offer Tables 28-2 and 28-3, which review reported outbreaks due to construction or renovation projects, and Table 28-4, which lists design and construction errors that we have encountered in our practice of infection control. We would recommend that infection control personnel inspect the construction site frequently to make sure the workers are following the recommendations. We have included a checklist (Table 28-5) that will facilitate these inspections. Infection control personnel could modify this basic list to suit the specific project.

Minimizing the Risk of Infection During Construction and Renovation

Controlling Dust and Dirt

Construction and renovation projects create tremendous amounts of dust or debris that may carry microorganisms. For example, hospital construction projects can disperse large numbers of *Aspergillus* spores.[1] Infection control personnel must collaborate with other staff to devise ways to prevent the dust and dirt from contaminating clean or sterile patient-care surfaces, supplies, and equipment.

Construction or renovation sites must be separated from patient-care areas and critical areas (eg, pharmacy and central sterile supply) by barriers that keep the dirt and dust inside the worksite, decreasing the risk of nosocomial infections. Plastic sheeting and sheetrock are the two materials that are used most commonly for barriers during construction in hospitals. Plastic sheeting sealed with duct tape can be used for small, short-term projects (24 to 48 hours) if it meets the local fire codes; framed sheetrock sealed with duct tape or spackling compound should be used for major, long-term projects. The latter must contain a closable door through which the workers access the construction site. A sign should be posted by the entrance stating that this is a construction zone and that only authorized persons may enter the area.

Other measures that may limit the spread of dust, dirt, and nosocomial pathogens include the following:

- Schedule major projects during the winter when the risk is lower for *Aspergillus* and other fungal infections (eg, histoplasmosis).
- Clean and vacuum areas under construction and the surrounding areas frequently.
- Have construction workers step on a mat that has been saturated with a disinfectant.
- Wet mop the area just outside the door to the construction site daily, or more often if necessary.
- Use a high-efficiency particulate air (HEPA)-filtered vacuum to clean carpeted areas daily, or more often if necessary.
- Shampoo carpets when the construction project is completed.
- Transport debris in containers with tight-fitting lids, or cover debris with a wet sheet.
- Remove debris as it is created; do not let it accumulate.
- Remove debris through a window when construction occurs above the first floor.
- Do not haul debris through patient-care areas.

TABLE 28-5
DAILY CONSTRUCTION SURVEY

Date: _____	Time: _____		Time: _____	
Barriers				
Construction signs posted for the area	❏ Yes	❏ No	❏ Yes	❏ No
Doors properly closed and sealed	❏ Yes	❏ No	❏ Yes	❏ No
Floor area clean, no dust tracked	❏ Yes	❏ No	❏ Yes	❏ No
Air handling				
All windows closed behind barrier	❏ Yes	❏ No	❏ Yes	❏ No
Negative air at barrier entrance	❏ Yes	❏ No	❏ Yes	❏ No
Negative air machine running	❏ Yes	❏ No	❏ Yes	❏ No
Project area				
Debris removed in covered container daily	❏ Yes	❏ No	❏ Yes	❏ No
Trash in appropriate container	❏ Yes	❏ No	❏ Yes	❏ No
Routine cleaning done on job site	❏ Yes	❏ No	❏ Yes	❏ No
Traffic control				
Restricted to construction workers and necessary staff only	❏ Yes	❏ No	❏ Yes	❏ No
All doors and exits free of debris	❏ Yes	❏ No	❏ Yes	❏ No
Dress code				
Appropriate for the area (OR, CSS, OB, BMTU)	❏ Yes	❏ No	❏ Yes	❏ No
Required to enter	❏ Yes	❏ No	❏ Yes	❏ No
Required to leave	❏ Yes	❏ No	❏ Yes	❏ No

Comments:

Surveyor: _____

_____

OR = operating room; CSS = central sterile supply; OB = obstetric; BMTU = bone marrow transplant unit.

- Remove debris after normal work hours through an exit restricted to the construction crew.
- Designate an entrance, an elevator, and a hallway that the construction workers must use and that are not used by patients, visitors, or healthcare workers.

Traffic Patterns

To reduce the amount of dust and dirt in the hospital and the risk of exposure to infectious agents, patients, visitors, and staff may need to traverse the hospital by alternate routes. Infection control personnel should help identify the appropriate detours before construction begins. Staff should design these routes in a logical manner, so that they do not increase inadvertently the risk of nosocomial infections or of noninfectious hazards such as falls. They also should consider whether housekeeping personnel can maintain the new route, whether the new route interferes with the work done in the area, and whether the route meets minimum aesthetic requirements. If construction is necessary in or near operating suites, surgical personnel must be able to move from place to place without contaminating their surgical scrubs.

The routes by which inanimate items are transported throughout the hospital may need to be altered during construction. In general, all materials including food, linens, medical supplies and equipment, and janitorial supplies and equipment must be handled in a manner that minimizes the risk of contamination.[2] Before the construction project begins, infection control personnel should help staff from the affected units plan the routes by which various supplies and equipment will be transported. Clean or sterile supplies and equipment must be transported to storage areas by a route that minimizes contamination from the construction site and prevents contact with soiled or contaminated trash and linen. To prevent unnecessary contamination with dirt and dust, used supplies and equipment should be moved in enclosed containers from the point of use to the point at which they will be processed.

Traffic patterns in critical areas, such as the operating room, labor and delivery rooms, nurseries, laboratories, and pharmacies, may not be altered easily to meet these infection control requirements. In such cases, the construction crew may need to work during off hours and on weekends. If infection control requirements still cannot be met, some areas may need to relocated or closed temporarily.

Storage Areas

During construction, basic principles of infection control still apply. Thus, clinical areas must maintain appropriate storage areas, which may be difficult, because the allotted space may be small or may lack essential features. Before construction begins, infection control personnel should help the staff identify the locations in which they will store equipment and supplies. Temporary storage areas should allow staff to do the following:

- Easily monitor the supplies (eg, look at expiration dates).
- Store sterile supplies and equipment away from soiled items (ie, separate clean and dirty areas must be maintained).
- Store clean or sterile supplies at an appropriate distance from sinks to prevent the supplies from becoming wet.
- Store contaminated wastes in a designated dirty area outside of direct patient-care areas.
- Move items without placing them on the floor (ie, have adequate work space).

In addition, the temporary storage space should be clean, have adequate temperature and humidity control, and be free of rodents.

An outbreak of four surgical and burn wound infections that occurred when a large tertiary-care hospital renovated its central inventory control area illustrates the importance of storing supplies properly during construction.[3] The investigators identified several *Aspergillus* species on the outside packages of materials from the main floor of Inventory Control; on intravenous bags, the outsides of sterile paper wrappers, and storage bins in the pharmacy, which was adjacent to the area under construction; from the outsides of packages containing burn dressings, elastic adhesive, Elastoplast, gloves, and disposable scissors, which were stored on the burn unit and in the intensive care unit. The investigators postulated that the supply boxes were contaminated during construction. The outside packages became contaminated when the boxes were opened, and the fungus was inoculated directly into the patients' wounds when the packages were torn open during dressing changes.[3]

Major Infection Control Considerations Associated With Construction and Renovation Projects

Air Handling Systems

Generally, air-handling systems do not transmit

nosocomial pathogens. However, at times, these systems can transmit pathogens such as *Mycobacterium tuberculosis, Aspergillus* species, *Legionella pneumophila,* and varicella-zoster virus. Air-handling systems can increase the risk of infection in other ways. For example, if the humidity level is high and the number of air exchanges is inadequate, walls, ceilings, and vents may drip water onto sterile supplies or clean surfaces. Thus, infection control personnel should make sure that the air-handling systems planned for new or renovated buildings will meet basic infection control requirements.

During the planning phase, infection control and engineering personnel should ensure that the air-handling systems can provide adequate air exchanges. For example, the minimum number of air exchanges is two per hour in patient rooms and 15 per hour in an operating room.[4] The Centers for Disease Control and Prevention now requires 12 air exchanges per hour in newly constructed or renovated respiratory isolation rooms and requires that the air is exhausted either directly outside or passed through a HEPA filter before it is recirculated.[5] A number of areas in the hospital have special requirements for air circulation and purity. These requirements are detailed in the American Institute of Architects' publication, *Guidelines for Construction and Equipment of Hospital and Medical Facilities*[4] and in the American Society of Heating, Refrigerating, and Air Conditioning Engineers' publication *ASHRE 1985 Fundamentals.*[6] We have found both of these books to be invaluable resources.

When reviewing the designs for the project, infection control personnel should ensure that the air intakes are placed properly. Air intakes should be placed at least 8 m from exhaust outlets. The bottom of an intake should be at least 2 m above the ground or 1 m above the roof level. Intakes should be located away from cooling towers, trash compactors, loading docks, heliports, exhaust from biological safety hoods,[7] ethylene oxide sterilizers, aerators, and incinerators. Infection control and engineering personnel should evaluate the design and operation of ventilation systems carefully to ensure that potentially contaminated air is discharged safely to prevent airborne disease transmission.[8] Infection control personnel may need to tour the air intake and exhaust sites to make sure that these items are placed properly.

During construction projects, selected air intakes (particularly those near excavation sites) or air ducts in the construction area may need to be shut down to prevent large amounts of dust from entering the air-handling system. In addition, engineering or maintenance personnel should ensure that elevator shafts are not transmitting dust and fumes. These personnel also should check air filters frequently and change them when necessary. Air-handling units in areas that care for immunocompromised patients should contain HEPA filters to decrease the amount of particulate matter and the number of microbes in the air. However, the presence of HEPA filters alone is not adequate; they must be placed properly. One of the authors of this chapter investigated an outbreak of surgical site infections that occurred because a HEPA filter in an operating room was put in backwards.

The air quality must be maintained and monitored carefully in areas caring for immunocompromised patients, including patients receiving treatment for malignancies, patients with bone marrow or solid organ transplants, and premature neonates. We recommend that infection control personnel work with staff in the appropriate departments to develop policies that describe in detail what must be done when any modifications, renovations, demolition, or construction is done in these areas. Activities as seemingly minor as installing computer cables or conduits in the ceiling space or crawling through this area could stir up *Aspergillus*-laden dust that would be hazardous for immunocompromised patients. We would suggest the following precautions:

- Large projects must be enclosed as described above, and a double door should be used, so that the air pressure inside the barriers is negative with respect to the area outside the barrier. The air pressure should be monitored daily.

- Before the ceiling is entered for small projects, a barrier must be erected that reaches from floor to ceiling, surrounds the affected area entirely, and is sealed with duct tape at the ceiling, floor, and sides.
- Existing air ducts and the space above the ceiling tiles must be cleaned with a HEPA-filtered vacuum before undertaking any project that involves opening these areas.
- If workers must traverse patient-care areas, they must remove dust from their bodies and clothes and then put on gowns, shoe covers, and head covers before walking through the unit. In particular areas of the hospital (eg, the operating suite), workers may need to wear protective clothing while working in the construction site.
- For small projects, the tool carts should be cleaned before entering the unit and left at the exit to the barrier. For larger projects, the carts and equipment should go into the barrier and stay there until the project is done. Before removing carts and equipment from inside the barrier, the construction crew should clean the items and cover them with a clean sheet. They should be moved off the unit by the designated route.
- The area inside the barrier must be cleaned and vacuumed before the barrier is removed.
- The area must be vacuumed again after the barrier is removed.

In addition to these precautions, portable HEPA filters may improve the air quality in rooms housing immunocompromised patients. If the air quality cannot be assured near the construction zone, units caring for immunocompromised patients must be moved temporarily to other areas of the hospital; nonemergency admissions of immunocompromised patients may need to be delayed.

Isolation Rooms

Given the resurgence of tuberculosis and the emergence of many different resistant pathogens, infection control personnel must ensure that the number, type, and placement of isolation rooms is adequate. Infection control personnel should evaluate the proposed isolation rooms during the design phase, because retrofitting regular patient rooms to meet the requirements of isolation rooms can be very costly.

Typically, a hospital should have one isolation bed for every 30 acute-care beds.[4] Pediatric areas require more isolation rooms per total beds than other areas of the hospital,[7] because respiratory or enteric infections that require isolation are more frequent in children than in adults.[9] The number of patients needing isolation on pediatric units will vary with patient age and the season.[9]

In general, isolation rooms for nonrespiratory diseases do not require special features. If the isolation room has an anteroom, both the room and the anteroom should have handwashing sinks. Built-in nurse-server cabinets or isolation carts can be used to store necessary supplies such as gowns, masks, and gloves.

Infection control personnel should ensure that the hospital has an adequate number of isolation rooms and that these rooms are placed in appropriate locations. Patients who have tuberculosis, varicella, or meningococcal meningitis often are seen in emergency rooms, recovery rooms, and outpatient clinics. Thus, appropriate isolation rooms will be beneficial in these areas. In addition, rooms in which high-risk procedures, such as bronchoscopy and aerosolized pentamidine treatments, are performed should have negative pressure or should have a flexible ventilation system that allows the pressure to be changed from positive to negative. Some hospitals have chosen to use flexible ventilation systems for their patient-care areas, so that the rooms can be used optimally.

When negative–air-pressure rooms are occupied, the direction of airflow must be checked daily to ensure that the room is indeed under negative air pressure.[5] In addition, the doors of negative-pressure rooms must remain closed to maintain negative pressure.[5,8]

Handwashing Facilities

Each patient-care room, examination room, procedure room, and restroom needs at least one handwashing sink that should be located as close to the room's exit as possible. Sinks should be large enough to prevent splashing. All sinks must have an associated soap dispenser (built-in stainless steel soap dispensers should not be used) and a paper-towel holder that are located at a level that is comfortable for the user. A trash receptacle should be placed near the sink, so paper towels can be discarded properly.

A variety of mechanisms exist to control water-flow. Conventional hand controls are the least expensive, but may not be appropriate for all areas. Foot, knee, or electric eye controls allow staff to wash their hands or scrub without touching the sink (no-touch method). Such sinks would be appropriate in operating suites, isolation rooms, and critical-care units. The electric-eye devices break frequently, and they are more expensive than the foot or knee controls. Infection control personnel should help the unit staff and architects select the best equipment for the location, placement, and purpose.

Water Supply and Plumbing

Not uncommonly, the hospital's water supply will be disrupted intentionally or accidentally during construction projects. Hospitals should have emergency plans that are activated if the water supply to the hospital is disrupted or contaminated. Infection control personnel should help develop this plan, because water is crucial to many infection control practices and because contaminated water can spread pathogenic organisms.

During the summer of 1993, the University of Iowa Hospitals and Clinics, Iowa City, was faced with the possibility of losing its water supply because the Iowa River was flooding. Our contingency plan included water conservation measures such as shutting down drinking fountains and ice machines, replacing showers and full-tub or bed baths with partial baths, using alcohol-based hand cleaners rather than soap and water, and serving meals on disposable dishes. Our alternative water system was a well, which was tested for coliform organisms, nitrates, and iron. Our plant operations department was prepared to adjust the plumbing system in order to use the well water. The well water could be used if the water supply was shut down during hospital or road-construction projects. Hospitals that do not have wells must design alternative plans. If the water supply will be disrupted only for a short time, staff can fill large plastic containers with water to be used while the water system is turned off. If the water supply will be off for a longer period of time, the hospital may need to have a company deliver bottled water. During emergencies, agencies such as the National Guard may be able to provide water. If the water supply will be turned off for more than 4 hours, the contractor should do this work during times of nonpeak water use, such as evenings, nights, or weekends.

Space for Personal Protective Equipment

Each patient room and treatment room should have a container in which personal protective equipment such as gloves are stored. In addition, these rooms must have sharps containers that allow staff to use one hand when discarding the sharp item.[10] Wall-mounted sharps containers should be placed at a height of 57 inches or less, so that all staff, regardless of their height, can discard sharp items safely.[10] Small plexiglas boxes could be installed outside the rooms of patients in airborne precautions, so that healthcare workers can store their masks.

Waste

Infection control personnel should help clinical staff plan how urine and feces will be discarded in patient-care areas, clinics, and laboratories. A variety of bedpan flushing devices are available such as spray hoses, spray arms, or Vernacare® units (Woodbridge, Ontario, Canada). Some of these options create splash hazards, clean poorly, or allow water to pool in hoses or nozzles. Waste disposal units such as Vernacare® units are quite expensive. Soiled utility rooms should contain a clinical sink or a flushing-rim fixture. This room also must contain a separate handwashing sink.[4] Other human waste can be solidified with a commercial product such as the Liquid Treatment System (LTS®, Isolyser Healthcare Co, Norcross, Ga) and then incinerated.

Finishes

General Considerations

During the design and development phase, the infection control personnel should help the clinicians and architects choose the finishes—flooring, wall coverings, ceiling tiles, etc. For example, these individuals must decide which flooring—carpet or vinyl—and which wall covering—paint or vinyl —should be used.[11] Ideal finishes are those that are washable and easy to clean. Porous or textured materials can be difficult to clean and thus may allow bacteria and fungi to grow. The finishes should be durable and able to withstand repeated cleaning with abrasive solutions. In addition, countertops, backsplashes, and floors should have as few joints as possible, so they are easy to clean.

Ceilings

Ceiling tiles should be appropriate for the areas in which they are being placed. Acoustical tiles may be used in hallways, waiting rooms, and patient rooms. If acoustical tiles become wet, they may support fungal and bacterial growth. Thus, metal flat-pan ceiling tiles should be placed in areas where there is a risk of splashing, such as in procedure rooms. Metal flat-pan tiles also should be used to prevent dust particles from falling on patients or sterile supplies in areas such as operating rooms, delivery rooms, critical-care areas, and central sterile supply. Perforated flat-pan ceiling tiles can be used in areas requiring laminar air flow to allow adequate air exchanges.

Flooring

Vinyl flooring is easier to maintain than carpeting and is more durable in high traffic areas. In addition, carpets may be more costly to maintain than vinyl flooring, because carpets are more difficult to clean, and cleaning requires special equipment. Isolation rooms, operating rooms, critical-care units, kitchens, laboratories, autopsy rooms, dialysis units, and other areas where liquids are likely to be spilled or where heavy soiling is likely to occur should have vinyl flooring.

As carpet has become an increasingly popular floor covering in hospitals, a veritable Pandora's box has opened, releasing a bewildering variety of products, innumerable federal regulations, and endless questions about installation, air quality, cleaning, and maintenance.[12] Carpets used in hospitals should have an impermeable moisture barrier and, if necessary, can be treated with an antimicrobial agent to inhibit growth of bacteria and fungi.[13] Some hospitals have been reluctant to install carpets, because various individuals have alleged that flu-like or allergy-like symptoms are caused by exposure to new carpet and the adhesives used to install carpets. However, there is no conclusive evidence that links carpeting and carpet adhesives to illness.[13] Although carpets may harbor microorganisms, there is no evidence that carpeting increases the risk of nosocomial infections.

Walls

Paint and wall coverings should be washable. Wall finishes should be chosen on the basis of wall protection, soil protection, and toxicity, as well as aesthetics.[11] Wall finishes in areas where blood or body fluids could splatter (eg, operating rooms and cardiac catheterization laboratories) should be fluid resistant (eg, vinyl) and easy to clean. Wall finishes around plumbing fixtures should be smooth and water resistant.[4] Wall bases and floors should not have joints or should have joints that are sealed tightly. This is especially important around small pipes and other structural elements, to prevent vermin or insects from infesting the area.[4] Tile in showers should be mounted on cement board or water-resistant sheetrock to prevent growth of mold. Ceramic-tile walls can be treated with a waterproof sealant, which is expensive, but it may be more cost-effective over time. Fiberglass shower stalls could be used instead of tile.

Countertops

Countertops typically are composed of a nonporous solid material, such as Corian, stainless steel, or laminate, with a protective sealant.

Final Check

After the project is completed, infection control personnel should inspect the area to make sure that all requirements have been met. Infection control personnel should verify the following steps have been done:

- Check the location of soap and towel dispensers, the sharps container, and the wastebasket.
- Check all areas to ensure that the appropriate flooring, ceiling tiles, and wall finishes have been installed.
- Check all procedure rooms, kitchens, and utility rooms to ensure that they have the appropriate scrubbable flooring and splash guards on sinks.

- Inspect water faucets to ensure that they do not have aerators.
- Check pressure and drainage in the water system.
- Have personnel from maintenance or housekeeping run all faucets the day before patients occupy the unit to decrease the risk of *Legionella* infection.
- Evaluate the direction of air flow in negative–air-pressure rooms, and ensure that the meters that monitor the air pressure are placed and functioning properly.
- Check the location of air intakes and exhaust vents.
- Inspect the area 1 week after the barriers have been removed (it takes that long for the dust to settle) to make sure it has been cleaned thoroughly.
- Have an exterminator check for insects and rodents.

In areas such as the bone marrow transplant unit or operating room, air sampling can be performed with an air sampling device such as the SAS® compact air sampler (PBI International, Milan, Italy) to check for contaminated air. Alternatively, settle plates can be placed in various areas throughout the room for ½ to 1 hour while ventilation is running and the room is vacant. The door should be closed and taped shut, so that persons do not enter the room while the settle plates are in place. If the ventilation system is running properly, the settle plates should be negative for pathogenic microbial growth.[7] A certified engineer can evaluate the effectiveness of laminar air flow.

Conclusion

Construction and renovation projects pose special challenges for infection control personnel. Although not specifically discussed in this chapter, demolition of buildings near patient-care areas poses many similar challenges. Infection control personnel who must deal with demolition projects should read the article by Streifel et al.[14] In many hospitals, infection control personnel are the only clinical staff who assist in all construction and renovation projects. Therefore, they may find themselves having to ensure that both infection control guidelines and general building codes are met. We would encourage infection control personnel to be involved in all phases of these projects to avert outbreaks and to ensure that newly constructed or renovated areas allow staff to follow good infection control practices. We think that the role of infection control personnel in these projects will increase as the complexity and immunosuppression of hospitalized patients increase, while hospitals are required to decrease their budgets drastically and regulatory and accrediting agencies increase the number of infection control guidelines. Infection control aspects of construction and renovation projects require large amounts of time and hard work. We would argue that the time and energy invested before and during the project will save hours of time, huge sums of money, and the lives of patients and healthcare workers after the project is finished.

References

1. Opal SM, Asp AA, Cannady PB Jr, Morse PL, Burton LJ, Hammer PG II. Efficacy of infection control measures during a nosocomial outbreak of disseminated aspergillosis associated with hospital construction. *J Infect Dis.* 1986;153:634-637.

2. Fitch H. Hospital and industry can benefit by sharing contamination control knowledge. *Clean Rooms.* 1993;7:8-9.

3. Bryce EA, Walker M, Scharf S, et al. An outbreak of cutaneous aspergillosis in a tertiary-care hospital. *Infect Control Hosp Epidemiol.* 1996;17:170-172.

4. The American Institute of Architects Committee on Architecture for Health. *1992-1993 Guidelines for Construction and Equipment of Hospital and Medical Facilities.* Washington, DC: The American Institute of Architects Press; 1992.

5. Centers for Disease Control and Prevention. Guidelines for preventing the transmission of *Mycobacterium tuberculosis* in health care facilities, 1994. *MMWR.* 1994;43:29.

6. American Society of Heating, Refrigerating, and Air Conditioning Engineers, Inc. *ASHRE Handbook 1985 Fundamentals.* Atlanta, Ga: ASHRE; 1985.

7. *The APIC Curriculum for Infection Control Practice, Volume II.* Soule BM, ed. Dubuque, Iowa: Kendall/Hunt Publishing Co; 1983.

8. Neill HM. Isolation-room ventilation critical to control disease. *Health Facil Manage.* 1992;5:30-38.

9. Langley JM, Hanakowski M, Bortolussi R. Demand for isolation beds in a pediatric hospital. *Am J Infect Control.* 1994;22:207-211.

10. Hankin RL. Disposal related sharp object injuries. *Advances in Exposure Prevention.* 1995;1:5,11.

11. Madden C. Environmental considerations in critical care interiors. *Crit Care Nurse Q.* 1991;14:43-49.

12. Wise KO. Carpet choices for healthcare facilities. *Healthcare Material Management.* 1994;12:35-39.

13. Hospitals and indoor carpeting. *Hospital Facilities Management Report.* 1993;1:12-14.

14. Streifel AJ, Lauer JL, Vesley B, Juni B, Rhame FS. *Aspergillus fumigatus* and other thermotolerant fungi generated by hospital building demolition. *Am Soc Microbiol.* 1983;46:375-378.

15. Arnow PM, Anderson RL, Mainous D, Smith EJ. Pulmonary Aspergillosis during hospital renovation. *Am Rev Respir Dis.* 1978;118:49-53.

16. Sarubbi FA Jr, Kopf HB, Wilson MB, McGinnis MR, Rutala WA. Increased recovery of *Aspergillus flavus* from respiratory specimens during hospital construction. *Am Rev Respir Dis.* 1982;125:33-38.

17. Krasinski K, Hilzman RS, Hanna B, et al. Nosocomial fungal infection during hospital renovation. *Infect Control.* 1985;6:278-282.

18. Weems JJ Jr, Davis BJ, Tablan OC, Kaufman L, Martone WJ. Construction activity: an independent risk factor for invasive aspergillosis and zygomycosis in patients with hematologic malignancy. *Infect Control.* 1987;8:71-75.

19. Haley CE, Cohen ML, Halter J, Meyer RD. Nosocomial Legionnaires' disease: a continuing common-source epidemic at Wadsworth Medical Center. *Ann Intern Med.* 1979;90:583-586.

20. Shands KN, Ho JL, Meyer, RD, et al. Potable water as a source of Legionnaire's disease. *JAMA.* 1985;253:1412-1416.

21. Thacker SB, Bennett JV, Tsai TF, et al. An outbreak in 1965 of severe respiratory illness caused by the Legionnaires' disease bacterium. *J Infect Dis.* 1978;138:512-519.

22. Mermel LA, Josephson SL, Giorgio CH, Dempsey J, Parenteau S. Association of Legionnaires' disease with construction: contamination of potable water. *Infect Control Hosp Epidemiol.* 1995;16:76-81.

CHAPTER 29

Hospital Epidemiology in Smaller Hospitals

John M. Boyce, MD

Abstract

In hospitals with 200 to 300 beds, hospital epidemiologists serve primarily as medical and epidemiology consultants to the infection control professionals, as advocates for the infection control programs, and as chairpersons of the infection control committees. Because smaller hospitals often have limited resources for infection control, surveillance and control activities must focus on issues that have caused problems for the facility and on compliance with mandates and recommendations made by healthcare agencies. The clinical microbiology laboratory plays an important role in ongoing surveillance activities and often is responsible for performing cultures obtained during point prevalence culture surveys or outbreak investigations. Because laboratory support often is limited, the indications for obtaining a culture from patients, personnel, or the inanimate environment for infection control purposes must be reviewed and discussed carefully with the clinical laboratory in advance.

Introduction

Many of the best examples of how to investigate and control nosocomial infections have come from large medical centers that have considerable resources devoted to their infection control programs. In addition to several infection control professionals (ICPs), such institutions often have laboratory space and personnel assigned specifically to the program and a hospital epidemiologist who may spend a majority of his or her time addressing infection control issues. Although hospitals with 200 to 300 beds often experience nosocomial infection problems similar to those of large medical centers, smaller hospitals often have only one ICP, no laboratory space or personnel dedicated to the program, and a part-time hospital epidemiologist who has limited time to devote to infection control. Consequently, it often is difficult for infection control programs in smaller hospitals to duplicate the investigations and surveillance activities that are feasible in large hospitals. This chapter discusses a variety of issues that relate to practicing hospital epidemiology in small- or medium-sized hospitals.

The Hospital Epidemiologist Position

Many physicians who are seeking a position as hospital epidemiologist or who find they will be appointed to serve as chairperson of an infection control committee at a small hospital have received little or no specific instruction in the epidemiology and control of nosocomial infections. Such individuals may find it helpful to attend a workshop or short course dealing with healthcare epidemiology before assuming the new position. For instance, the Society for Healthcare Epidemiology of America, in conjunction with the Centers for Disease Control and Prevention (CDC), conducts 3-day workshops that are designed for physicians who have finished their residency or fellowship training and find that they require additional training in hospital epidemiology.

Also, before accepting a position as hospital epidemiologist, the physician should meet with representatives of the hospital administration to discuss issues that relate to the scope of activities and responsibilities of the epidemiologist; the extent to which the epidemiologist will influence the priorities of the infection control program; the time allotted to various activities by infection control program personnel; office space, computer support, and clerical assistance available to the ICP and epidemiologist; and the salary that will be paid to the epidemiologist by the hospital. Whenever possible, any contractual agreement between the physician and the hospital should cover these issues.

To persuade the hospital administrators that hiring a hospital epidemiologist is a good idea, those concerned with infection control may need to provide the administrators with data outlining the costs due to nosocomial infections and demonstrate savings as a result of practicing prevention measures.[1] Also, administrators may need information about the range of salaries paid to hospital epidemiologists at other facilities.

The Role of the Hospital Epidemiologist

The primary function of a hospital epidemiologist in a small hospital is to serve as a medical and epidemiologic consultant to the ICP and as chairperson of the infection control committee. When the institution develops or revises infection control policies, the epidemiologist may need to assist the ICP with critical review of pertinent literature on the topic and should review revised policies before they are presented to the infection control committee. During investigations of endemic or epidemic infections, epidemiologists with training in outbreak investigation and statistical methods may need to design and conduct appropriate case-control studies, perform statistical analysis of data, and prepare formal reports for presentation to the infection control committee or medical staff. Epidemiologists may advise laboratory personnel regarding special typing methods for nosocomial isolates. Physician epidemiologists may assist the ICP with clinical evaluation of patients who may have communicable diseases or conditions (eg, chickenpox, tuberculosis, scabies) that warrant special isolation and barrier precautions. Occasionally, medical staff members question the ICP's advice, yet will comply with the advice if a physician epidemiologist concurs.

Essential Elements of an Infection Control Program

To provide a minimal level of staffing, hospitals of 200 to 300 beds should have at least one full-time ICP. In such facilities, an experienced ICP can effectively conduct routine surveillance of nosocomial infections, implement isolation and barrier precautions, educate healthcare workers, and develop policies and procedures relating to infection control.

Community hospitals can expect to have an average of one outbreak per year.[2] However, one full-time ICP and one part-time hospital epidemiologist may have difficulty investigating epidemic or endemic nosocomial infections in a timely manner. For this reason, smaller hospitals ideally should have 1.5 to 2.0 full-time equivalents (positions) devoted to the infection control program, particularly if the hospital cares for patients with acute illnesses or performs complex invasive procedures.

To be successful, a program must have the support of the hospital administration and the medical staff. The administration should give the infection control program the authority to determine which nosocomial infection problems will receive greatest priority. At our 230-bed facility, we place a high priority on prompt implementation of appropriate isolation and barrier precautions, prospective surveillance for multidrug-resistant pathogens, investigation of epidemic and various endemic infections, and compliance with mandates or recommendations from outside agencies such as the Occupational Safety and Health Administration, the Joint Commission on Accreditation of Healthcare Organizations, and the CDC.

The hospital administration also must provide the infection control program with an adequate budget. To attract and keep a motivated and experienced individual in the ICP position, the hospital must provide the individual with a salary and benefits package that is competitive with other hospitals in the area. An ICP with only limited experience should be sent, at the hospital's expense, to an approved course or workshop designed for new infection control professionals. To maintain the skills of the ICP, the hospital should provide funds for infection control journals (preferably at least two); reference texts; and, whenever possible, funds for travel to local, regional, or national educational meetings conducted by the Society for Healthcare Epidemiology of America or the Association for Professionals in Infection Control and Epidemiology. The budget also should provide funds to purchase video programs or other educational materials used for training healthcare workers.

The administration also must provide the infection control program with adequate office space, equipment, and computers. Whenever possible, the program should have clerical support for correspondence and for revising written policies and procedures. Unless infection control software programs are available on the hospital's mainframe computer, the infection control staff must have a desktop computer with word processing, database, and graphics software. Several commercially available database programs were designed specifically for use by infection control programs. We have extensively used Epi Info, a software program developed by the CDC and the World Health Organization. This program includes word processing, database, and statistics modules and can produce simple graphics. Small- or medium-sized hospitals that do not have database software already for their infection control program seriously should consider using Epi Info. The program and manual are in the public domain (ie, can be copied legally from a current user) and also are available at a nominal fee (USD Incorporated, Stone Mountain, GA 30087). ICPs also should have access to computerized literature searches through the National Library of Medicine (MEDLINE) or CD-ROM reference databases.

The administration also must provide adequate laboratory support for the infection control program. At a minimum, the program budget must cover the costs of cultures and antimicrobial susceptibility tests needed for surveillance purposes or outbreak investigations. In some small- or medium-sized hospitals, it may be cost-effective for the hospital to devote laboratory space and a part-time technician specifically to the infection control program. The laboratory should be able to save isolates of potential epidemiologic importance, especially during outbreak investigations. In most small hospitals, the only readily available method for typing isolates is analysis of antimicrobial susceptibility patterns (antibiograms), which may be sufficient for many investigations. However, for endemic or epidemic problems spanning many months, or for some pathogens that exhibit little variability in their susceptibility patterns, the infection control program may need to do molecular typing. If laboratory equipment and personnel are not available in the hospital for molecular typing of isolates, the program budget should include funds for sending selected isolates to a reference laboratory.

Infection control staff should collaborate closely with the clinical microbiology laboratory, employee health service, medical records department, nursing service, and infectious diseases specialists. Infection control program personnel and members of the pharmacy and therapeutics committee must work together on issues relating to antibiotic use and the prevalence of multidrug-resistant pathogens.

Surveillance

Because infection control staff in small hospitals often have limited time available for surveillance, they often adopt a problem-oriented approach. At our facility, we focus our surveillance primarily on infections that have posed documented problems for our institution, such as bloodstream infections related to central intravascular catheters, infections related to open heart surgery and vascular surgery, *Clostridium difficile*-related diarrhea, and infections caused by multidrug-resistant pathogens such as methicillin-resistant *Staphylococcus aureus* (MRSA) and vancomycin-resistant enterococci (VRE). We have identified such problems initially through several mechanisms including ongoing prospective surveillance, discussions with nursing personnel, reports from infectious diseases consultants, or, occasionally, reports from concerned physicians. We have made it a point not to participate in surveillance activities, including some suggested by hospital administration, that, in our opinion, would not yield useful information for our program.

At our facility, we enter demographic and microbiologic data regarding patients with pathogens of particular concern (eg, MRSA and multidrug-resistant enterococci) into databases using Epi Info software. We maintain routine surveillance data in notebooks using standardized data collection forms.

In many small hospitals, surveillance for nosocomial infections is laboratory based. For this reason, we emphasize the importance of working closely with the clinical microbiology laboratory. Using criteria recommended by the CDC, the ICP should review clinical microbiology laboratory culture results several times per week to identify patients who may have nosocomial infections, and should review selected medical records to establish if the culture results reflect nosocomial infections.

Whenever possible, the clinical laboratory should provide the ICP with quantitative results of antimicrobial susceptibility tests (ie, zones of inhibition measured in millimeters or minimum inhibitory concentrations) rather than qualitative results (ie, resistant, intermediate, susceptible). Quantitative results provide greater discriminatory power when analyzing antibiograms. At our facility, the clinical laboratory routinely reports zone sizes for disk diffusion susceptibility tests. The infection control program or the clinical microbiology laboratory also may consider obtaining WHO-NET 2 software. Drs. John Stelling and Thomas O'Brien at Brigham and Women's Hospital in Boston designed this program to analyze antimicrobial susceptibility patterns. The program may be obtained by contacting Dr. O'Brien.

Most clinical microbiology laboratories in small hospitals cannot process large numbers of cultures for the infection control program. Therefore, if the infection control program needs to obtain cultures from patients, healthcare workers, or the environment, the hospital epidemiologist or the ICP must talk with the laboratory director in advance. Together they can determine which sites to culture, how many specimens to obtain, and whether to use special selective media. We limit culture surveys of patients to investigations of and surveillance for MRSA and VRE on high-risk units (ie, wards where other cases have occurred). We seldom perform culture surveys of personnel, and, when we do, we limit our survey to personnel who have been epidemiologically implicated as possible sources of transmission.

Outbreak Investigation

The same principles used to investigate outbreaks in large medical centers also are appropriate in smaller community hospitals (Figure 29-1). When prospective surveillance uncovers a possible outbreak, the ICP should make a line-listing of cases. The listing usually includes patient name, medical record number, date of onset, ward, service, body site affected, the responsible organism and its antimicrobial susceptibility pattern, and possible risk factors. We have developed a basic case report form that we use to record such information while we are reviewing medical records. We modify the basic form to suit the type of outbreak that we are investigating (Figure 29-2).

If different organisms have caused infections, or if isolates from cases have many different antibiograms, the hospital epidemiologist usually can rule out a common-source outbreak. However, if the number of cases clearly is greater than the baseline level at the facility, then the infection control staff should investigate to determine if poor technique or inadequate sterilization or disinfection have caused an increase in infections. For example, through routine surveillance activities we detected a cluster of saphenous venectomy surgical site infections among patients undergoing coronary artery bypass grafts. Different pathogens caused the infections, so we reviewed the cardiac surgery team's practices. We found that the team recently had changed techniques for cleansing the skin at the operative site and for suturing the wound, and that these changes led to the cluster of infections.

If a single species is responsible for most cases, then infection control staff must establish whether a single strain or multiple strains caused the outbreak.

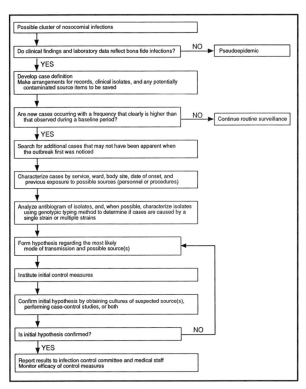

FIGURE 29-1. Steps for investigating possible outbreaks of nosocomial infections.

If a single strain caused most cases, then the hospital epidemiologist or ICP may need to review medical records further to determine if a medication, procedure, piece of equipment, or healthcare worker may have transmitted the epidemic strain. Infection control personnel should try to determine if most cases have some risk factor in common, such as infection involving the same body site (eg, surgical site infection), location on the same service or ward, or exposure to a single team of physicians, or a certain medication or procedure. In some instances, such an analysis will suggest the likely cause of the outbreak. Infection control personnel then could obtain cultures of the suspected source, and institute appropriate control measures.[3] However, infection control personnel may sometimes need to review the medical records of a control group (ie, comparable but unaffected patients) to establish that case patients have been exposed to the putative source significantly more often than control patients.

				─Standard Data─									─Supplementary Data─				
Name	Age	Sex	Ward	Serv	Adm Date	Culture Date	Previous Surgery	Surgeon	NG Tube	Endoscopy	Proximity to a Known Case	Amp/Pip	1st Ceph	2nd Ceph	3rd Ceph	Metro	Imi	Vanc

Adm = admission, NG = nasogastric, Amp/Pip = ampicillin or piperacillin, 1st Ceph = 1st generation cephalosporin, 2nd Ceph = 2nd generation cephalosporin, 3rd Ceph = 3rd generation cephalosporin, Metro = metronidazole, Imi = imipenem, Vanc = vancomycin

FIGURE 29-2. Sample data collection form for use during outbreak investigations. We collect the standard data during all outbreaks and, depending on which risk factors we are considering, we collect different supplementary data.

For example, when results of our ongoing surveillance suggested that we had an outbreak of MRSA cases at our facility, we entered basic information pertinent to the cases into our MRSA database. Using Epi Info software, we sorted the cases by the antibiogram of their organism. We found that isolates with an unusual (epidemic) antibiogram caused the majority of cases, so we hypothesized that this was a common-source outbreak. When we further analyzed cases with the epidemic strain, we found that they had occurred on numerous services and wards. We then focused on previous exposure of case patients to healthcare workers, because personnel may be a source of epidemic *S aureus* infections. We reviewed medical records of affected patients and recorded the names of physicians, nurses, and respiratory therapists who had cared for each case patient between the time the patient was admitted and the time the first culture was positive for the epidemic strain. Three healthcare workers previously had cared for many of the case patients, and when we reviewed the charts of a control group, we found that previous exposure to the three workers had occurred significantly more often among cases than controls. After taking cultures from the three staff members, we identified a respiratory therapist who had chronic sinusitis and persistently carried the epidemic strain in her nares. To confirm that isolates of the epidemic strain recovered from patients and the implicated healthcare worker were the same clone, we sent representative isolates to an outside laboratory for restriction endonuclease analysis of plasmid DNA, which revealed that all isolates carried the same plasmid. By eradicating the epidemic strain from the respiratory therapist, we terminated the outbreak.[4]

If an outbreak investigation implicates a member of an influential practice group, the hospital epidemiologist may need to present a summary of the findings to the chief of service and enlist his or her support before approaching the implicated individual. Infection control personnel always should make every effort to maintain the confidentiality of implicated individuals.

Other Selected Experiences

Bloodstream Infections Associated With Total Parenteral Nutrition

During a 6-month period, 6 (16%) of 37 patients who had received total parenteral nutrition therapy (TPN) developed catheter-related bloodstream infections. We reviewed patient charts and found that physicians who had received little instruction regarding insertion techniques sometimes placed the catheters, that insertion often was performed in the patient's room, and that there was no standardized protocol for aseptic technique.

To address the problem, the infection control program formed a multidisciplinary team that included members of the nutrition committee and nursing service. The team recommended that:

- The central supply service should provide a standardized sterile tray containing all items necessary for TPN catheter insertion.
- Physicians should insert TPN catheters in an operating room or special procedure room.
- The institution should allow physicians to insert TPN catheters only if they have received training in central line placement by a qualified attending physician.

During the next 8 years, we conducted quarterly targeted surveillance of bloodstream infections related to TPN and found that fewer than 3% of patients developed TPN-related bloodstream infections.

Surgical Site Infections Following Open Heart Surgery

Several years ago, a *Staphylococcus epidermidis* strain with an unusual antibiogram caused a case of prosthetic valve endocarditis. The director of the clinical microbiology laboratory reviewed the antimicrobial susceptibility patterns of coagulase-negative staphylococci and found that only patients who had undergone cardiac surgery had isolates with the same antibiogram. We calculated cardiac surgeon-specific infection rates, conducted case-control studies of exposures to personnel, and tested cultures from potential environmental sources and from the cardiac surgery team. Through this epidemiologic investigation, we identified as the source of the outbreak a cardiac surgeon whose hands were colonized with the epi-

demic strain.[5] Dr. Steve Opal performed restriction endonuclease analysis of plasmid DNA from representative isolates, which confirmed that the isolate carried by the surgeon and those recovered from affected patients were the same strain. We presented the findings of the investigation to the chairman of surgery and the implicated surgeon who agreed to comply with recommendations made by the infection control program. By eradicating the epidemic strain from the surgeon's hands, we terminated the outbreak. We continue to perform surveillance for infections related to heart surgery, we adjusted infection rates for patients undergoing coronary artery bypass graft surgery by the National Nosocomial Infections Surveillance System risk index and we report these rates to the chairman of surgery.

Vancomycin-Resistant Enterococci

In early 1991, while prospectively reviewing susceptibility test results from the clinical microbiology laboratory, we found that enterococci with no zone of inhibition around vancomycin disks had been recovered from several patients in the hospital's intensive care unit. To determine if similar cases had gone unnoticed, the director of the clinical microbiology laboratory used WHONET-2 software to review the vancomycin zone diameter results of all enterococcal isolates tested during the preceding 12-month period. In this review, the laboratory director identified several possible isolates of VRE that had zone diameters ranging from 10 mm to 14 mm. These isolates had been classified as susceptible by existing zone-size criteria.

We entered data from patients with VRE into a database using Epi Info software, and an analysis revealed that a majority of cases had been acquired in the ICU.[6] Because cases continued to occur despite body substance isolation precautions, the infection control program required that affected patients be placed in private rooms and that all personnel entering the rooms wear gloves. When these measures failed to control the outbreak, infection control personnel performed cultures of environmental surfaces in the rooms of affected patients and found that VRE often contaminated surfaces near the patients. We became concerned that organisms on surfaces might contaminate the clothing of personnel. Therefore, we required that all personnel entering the rooms of affected patients wear gowns as well as gloves. Through these barrier precautions, periodic point prevalence surveys of patients on affected wards, and continued prospective laboratory-based surveillance we terminated the outbreak.[6] Our experience with the VRE outbreak exemplifies the importance of ongoing communication and cooperation between the clinical microbiology laboratory and the infection control program.

Improving Perioperative Antimicrobial Prophylaxis

To reduce the risks of postoperative surgical site infections, the infection control program audited perioperative antimicrobial prophylaxis. We found that patients frequently received prophylactic antibiotic doses while on call for surgery, sometimes 1 or 2 hours before the procedure began. As a result, we instituted a policy wherein anesthesiologists administer perioperative prophylaxis to patients in the operating room, just before the operation commences. This has led to improved dosing of perioperative prophylaxis.

Improving Empiric and Therapeutic Use of Antibiotics

To promote more appropriate utilization of broad-spectrum antibiotics and of oral vancomycin, our program helped to develop a structured antibiotic order sheet for all inpatient antibiotics. By use of the order sheet, we have reduced the use of broad-spectrum agents such as imipenem and reduced inappropriate dosing of antibiotics among patients with impaired renal function. In addition,

during the first 12 months of the program, the hospital saved an estimated $32,000 on antibiotic acquisition costs.[7]

Other Activities

Over the years, the ICP and the hospital epidemiologist at our facility have investigated nosocomial aspergillosis related to hospital renovation and *Pseudomonas* infections due to inadequately disinfected endoscopes. We also have studied the epidemiology of nosocomial ampicillin-resistant enterococcal infections and the financial impact of selected nosocomial infections under the prospective payment system.[8-10]

Finally, in response to new state regulations that require physicians to obtain continued medical education on universal precautions (now included in standard precautions) and other infection control issues, our infection control program presented several sessions dealing with universal precautions, infection control in the office setting, and the epidemiology and prevention of infections caused by multidrug-resistant nosocomial pathogens.

Acknowledgments

The author wishes to thank Gail Potter-Bynoe, who served as the hospital's infection control coordinator for many years. Her efforts and expertise contributed immensely to the success of the infection control program at this facility. The author also thanks Dr. Antone A. Medeiros, director of the Clinical Microbiology Laboratory, who has assisted the infection control program on many occasions by analyzing antimicrobial susceptibility data from the laboratory and by providing advice on a variety of other important issues.

References

1. Miller PJ, Farr BM, Gwaltney JM Jr. Economic benefits of an effective infection control program: case study and proposal. *Rev Infect Dis.* 1989;11:284-288.
2. Haley RW, Tenney JH, Lindsey JO II, Garner JS, Bennett JV. How frequent are outbreaks of nosocomial infection

in community hospitals? *Infect Control.* 1985;6:233-236.

3. Wenzel RP, Nettleman MD, Jones RN, Pfaller MA. Methicillin-resistant *Staphylococcus aureus*: implications for the 1990s and effective control measures. *Am J Med.* 1991;91(suppl 3B):221s-227s.

4. Boyce JM, Opal SM, Potter-Bynoe G, Medeiros AA. Spread of methicillin-resistant *Staphylococcus aureus* in a hospital after exposure to a health care worker with chronic sinusitis. *Clin Infect Dis.* 1993;17:496-504.

5. Boyce JM, Potter-Bynoe G, Opal SM, Dziobek L, Medeiros AA. A common-source outbreak of *Staphylococcus epidermidis* infections among patients undergoing cardiac surgery. *J Infect Dis.* 1990;161:493-499.

6. Boyce JM, Opal SM, Chow JW, et al. Outbreak of multidrug-resistant *Enterococcus faecium* with transferable vanB class vancomycin resistance. *J Clin Microbiol.* 1994;32:1148-1153.

7. Graham KK, Boyce JM, Medeiros AA, Mahoney GM, Kaufman RL. Improved dosing through use of an antimicrobial order sheet with a table of dosage adjustments for renal function. Presented at the 13th Annual Meeting of the American College of Clinical Pharmacy, Toronto, Ontario, Canada; 1992.

8. Boyce JM, Opal SM, Potter-Bynoe G, et al. Emergence and nosocomial transmission of ampicillin-resistant enterococci. *Antimicrob Agents Chemother.* 1992;36:1032-1039.

9. Boyce JM, Potter-Bynoe G, Dziobek L. Hospital reimbursement patterns among patients with surgical wound infections following open heart surgery. *Infect Control Hosp Epidemiol.* 1990;11:89-93.

10. Boyce JM, Potter-Bynoe G, Dziobek L, Solomon SL. Nosocomial pneumonia in Medicare patients: hospital costs and reimbursement patterns under the prospective payment system. *Arch Intern Med.* 1991;151:1109-1114.

CHAPTER 30

Infection Control in Public Hospitals

Rebecca Wurtz, MD, MPH

Abstract

Public hospitals face challenging infection control problems that differ from those in other hospitals. This chapter reviews some of the unique aspects of infection control in public hospitals—including governance, physical plant, patient mix, communicable diseases, and employee issues—and suggests management strategies.

Introduction

The American Hospital Association's Hospital Directory lists hundreds of "public" hospitals, including federal (such as veterans' hospitals), state (including state university hospitals and state psychiatric facilities), city, county, and local "hospital district" facilities. The number of public hospitals per state ranges from a handful in Connecticut to more than 80 in California. This chapter will focus on hospitals, usually city or county hospitals, that primarily provide medical care for uninsured and indigent patients.

How are public hospitals different? The major determinants of infection control programs—patients, services, employees, facilities, and con-text—differ from other hospitals (Table 30-1). The problems that I will discuss are not necessarily unique to public hospitals, but are exacerbated by the paucity of resources and the high proportion of indigent patients. The Joint Commission on Accreditation of Healthcare Organizations (JCAHO) has recently acknowledged, by writing a guide about public hospitals for its surveyors, that public hospitals have special qualities and problems.[1] Some of the infection control problems facing public hospitals are reviewed here and some management strategies are suggested.

Governance

Public hospitals ultimately are controlled by public (elected) officials whose priorities are sometimes political rather than medical. The direction of the local public healthcare system may change with each election, which changes the administrative leadership. This instability may make sustained infection control program development difficult. Occasionally, elected hospital boards make infection control issues into political issues (eg, whether a human immunodeficiency virus (HIV)-seroposi-

TABLE 30-1

WHAT MAKES INFECTION CONTROL AT A PUBLIC HOSPITAL DIFFERENT?

Facility

Old

Heavy use

Poor maintenance

Patient Mix

High proportion of indigent and foreign-born patients

High census of patients infected with HIV and TB

High number of patients with reportable diseases

Services

Specialized units: jail, burn, trauma, psychiatric

Large outpatient clinics

Employees

Unionized

Represent the community

Large housestaff component

Context

Elected board

Public "fishbowl"

Resources

Limited

Controlled by politicians

TB = tuberculosis.

tive employee may work or how to manage tuberculosis [TB] exposures). The JCAHO standards suggest that hospital boards should be educated about healthcare issues, even if the board is elected annually. Hospital epidemiologists would be wise to take responsibility for educating the board about infection control issues.

Physical Plant/Engineering

Public hospitals range from turn-of-the-century buildings without window screens to modern state-of-the-art facilities. In general, the physical plants of public facilities are older, have more multi-bed rooms, and have fewer sinks than other hospitals. Furthermore, public facilities suffer more wear and tear from the high volume of patients and visitors.

Inadequate capital development and maintenance programs allow the physical plant and equipment to deteriorate further. Engineering systems (including water supply and air handling) may be antiquated, and patchwork repairs may make it difficult to trace the path of ductwork and plumbing. Old plumbing systems that are poorly maintained frequently leak allowing mold and mildew to grow. Recently, the water main supplying all water to Cook County Hospital broke inside the hospital. To repair the pipe, the county turned off the hospital's water supply for 12 hours. Consequently, autoclaves, scrub sinks, ice machines, toilets, sinks, and dishwashers, among other essential equipment for infection control and patient care, were inoperable. Fortunately, the hospital had a water shut-down protocol and had standing contracts with local companies that could supply bottled water in such emergencies.

The hospital epidemiologist must get to know key personnel in the engineering department to learn rudimentary principles of heating, ventilation, and air conditioning (HVAC). Furthermore, the hospital epidemiologist should encourage the engineers to contact the infection control department early if they plan to renovate the physical plant or if disasters, like the one described above, occur.

If the hospital cannot or will not provide additional sinks, the hospital epidemiologist could recommend that the hospital provide soapless handwashing stations. A variety of skin "degermers" are available, and these products can substitute for sinks except in locations where "scrubbing" is necessary. Retrofitting the ventilation for negative air pressure and monitoring the air circulation in isolation rooms can pose significant problems in any hospital, but especially in those that require major structural changes. The hospital may only be able to afford expedient solutions, such as punching exhaust fans through exterior walls. The hospital epidemiologist should ensure that the responsibility and timing for regular review and maintenance of engineering controls are clearly delineated.

Between scheduled reviews, the direction of air flow in negative pressure rooms occupied by tuberculosis patients can be crudely monitored on a daily basis with strips of paper towel or tissue paper held at the door.

If the hospital cannot afford to hire consultants who can evaluate the physical plant, the hospital epidemiologist might be able to enlist faculty or students from industrial hygiene programs at a local university to investigate specific problems as part of a school project.

Surveillance

The patient mix in public hospitals differs from that of other healthcare facilities—public hospitals may not do many transplants or much chemotherapy, but may have a disproportionately high census of patients with HIV and tuberculosis. Public hospitals frequently have specialized intensive care units, such as burn and trauma units, in which nosocomial infection rates are extremely high (see below). Consequently, surveillance for nosocomial infections may have a different emphasis in a public hospital than in a tertiary academic center. Infection control personnel in public hospitals should tailor surveillance to the specific problems and patient population in their hospitals.

Indigent patients may be at greater risk than those from higher socioeconomic strata for some nosocomial infections. For example, indigent status and lack of prenatal care are risk factors for endometritis following delivery. Immigrants and foreign visitors who do not have health insurance also use public hospitals. These patients may come from countries where natural infection for certain diseases, such as measles or varicella, is less common, putting them at higher risk for acquiring disease in crowded waiting areas. Similarly, patients may come from countries where vaccination for diseases, such as tetanus and diphtheria, is inadequate, once again putting them at higher nosocomial risk. A recent study demonstrated that immi-

grants and patients from lower socioeconomic strata have low levels of tetanus antibody. Therefore, infection control personnel must be aware that patients hospitalized following trauma or abdominal catastrophes may develop tetanus. Moreover, people recently arrived from foreign countries can potentially import dangerous communicable pathogens such as Ebola and Lassa viruses.[2]

Infection control personnel in public hospitals may have great difficulty conducting follow-up surveillance for nosocomial problems such as surgical site infections because the patients may go to other hospitals or clinics for subsequent evaluation and treatment. Furthermore, these patients may not speak English, may be homeless, or may not have phones. To complicate post-discharge surveillance and treatment further, patients may be migrant laborers or work for traveling shows and circuses, or may have used an alias during their admission.

The goal of the hospital epidemiologist, who has limited resources, must be to make more of less. The hospital epidemiologist must define the problems that are specific to the institution and design surveillance to detect these infections. It does not make sense to study hospital-acquired *Legionella* or *Aspergillus* infections if *Clostridium difficile* diarrhea and nosocomial TB are more common and more serious. Infection control professionals must identify creative ways to accomplish important tasks. For example, the infection control nurse could enlist clinical nurses who are interested in infection control issues to help collect data. The hospital epidemiologist could recruit eager house staff and medical students to do surveillance as part of research projects. In addition, infection control professional could assemble multidisciplinary groups that conduct surveillance projects, which serve more than one department's needs.

All hospitals face cost cutting, but the impact is greater where there were fewer resources to start. In an era where cost is a major outcome measure and the dollars that support public hospitals are subject to tax-saving maneuvers, the hospital epidemiologist would be wise to calculate the costs and savings attributable to surveillance and prevention of nosocomial infections. The hospital epidemiologist should report these data frequently to the hospital's administrators and the infection control committee, to preserve enough personnel for adequate surveillance.

Isolation and Precautions

Public hospitals care for many patients infected with TB and HIV. Thus, infection control personnel must often cope with inadequate resources for respiratory isolation and must evaluate frequent occupational exposures. Furthermore, drug resistant TB is more common in patient populations seen at public hospitals. Such patients may require prolonged admissions in isolation because their organisms are resistant to antimicrobial agents or because the patients are unlikely to take their medications reliably. Consequently, isolation resources, which are already at a premium, are strained further. Because the patient rooms may contain numerous beds (eg, four-bed rooms or open wards), infection control personnel must maximize resources for isolation by carefully creating cohorts when pathogens such as *C difficile* and vancomycin-resistant enterococcus cause outbreaks. All hospitals must have workable exposure control plans, but public hospitals—because exposures are frequent and the population of employees at risk is large and changes constantly—must have plans for exposures to TB and to bloodborne pathogens that emphasize simple algorithms and automatic mechanisms. Infection control personnel should write protocols in English and Spanish for sharps exposures. The protocols should be easy to understand and should be posted in all clinical areas. Annual education programs are not adequate. Infection control personnel must conduct frequent programs that describe how to prevent exposures and what to do if an employee is exposed to a patient's blood.

Programs that screen patients to identify those with tuberculosis do not cost a lot of money but yield a high return.[3,4] At Cook County Hospital, the point-of-entry triage questionnaire is very simple. The emergency room triage nurse asks all patients whether they have had a cough of more than 3 weeks' duration, or cough of any duration plus hemoptysis, weight loss, or night sweats. The nurse then:

• Gives all patients who answer "yes" to any of those questions a mask and a box of tissues and instructs the patients to cough into them.
• Puts the patients in the emergency room isolation room.
• Sends the patients for expedited CXRs.
• Asks the patients to produce sputum samples.

Another public hospital automatically isolates any patient who has sputum sent for AFB smear and culture.[4] Other hospitals have developed consulting teams that are dedicated to evaluating patients for isolation and to expediting their workup. The consulting teams are labor-intensive, but optimize utilization of isolation resources.[5]

Special Units

Public hospitals have units, including jail wards, that are unique to these facilities. Patients admitted from crowded jails may transfer contagious diseases such as meningococcal and streptococcal infections, varicella, and tuberculosis. Furthermore, detainees must always be accompanied by correctional officers, even into the operating room, which may pose problems for infection control. Wall-mounted needle disposal boxes may not be allowed on jail wards, in which case the infection control program must devise a safe method for sharps disposal. The infection control program should include the correctional officers in annual infection control inservices and infection control screening (eg, tuberculin skin tests). In addition, public hospitals frequently have other units, such as burn and trauma wards, in which nosocomial infections are extremely common.[6] Hospital-acquired infection is the most common cause of death in burn and trauma patients who survive the first few hours after injury.

Emergency Room and Clinics

Infection control personnel justifiably have focused on preventing spread of tuberculosis in outpatient areas. However, other infections, such as measles, varicella, and, potentially, pertussis and diphtheria, can be spread in waiting areas. Many patients in public hospitals have been inadequately vaccinated, and thus may be especially vulnerable to these infections. Infection control personnel should post simple triage procedures in all walk-in areas so that healthcare workers can learn quickly how to evaluate and isolate patients who present with potentially contagious diseases. In addition, the hospital-based infection control program is usually responsible for infection control problems at hospital-associated outlying clinics.

Reporting

The incidence of reportable communicable diseases—such as sexually transmitted diseases, tuberculosis, enteric pathogens, and hepatitis—is disproportionately higher in public hospitals than in other hospitals, and the associated burden of reporting these infections to local departments of health (DOH) is higher. Infection control personnel can decrease this paperwork if the hospital can transfer data electronically to the local DOH. For example, the hospital's diagnostic laboratory could transmit directly to the DOH pertinent results regarding diseases for which extensive demographic information is not required.

Employees and Employee Health

Employees of public hospitals are exposed to a wide range of occupational hazards, from scabies to HIV and multidrug-resistant tuberculosis (MDRTB). It is no wonder that employee morale sometimes suffers, given the difficult, even dangerous, working conditions. The very hospitals in which protective gear and safety needle devices are most indicated—those caring for numerous patients with identified and unidentified airborne and blood-borne infections—can least afford these products.

Public hospitals care for many intravenous drug users, who may be infected with hepatitis B, hepatitis C, and HIV. Thus, healthcare workers in public hospitals are at risk for occupational exposure to those viruses. Hepatitis B vaccination programs should be especially active at public hospitals.

Public hospitals rely heavily on house staff who may know very little about infection control issues and who may not have a personal commitment to the institution. Residents may violate basic infection control practices, and may not report conditions, such as communicable diseases that should be reported to the infection control department. The infection control program should use every opportunity—morning report, conferences, grand rounds, house staff newsletters, paycheck inserts—to educate house staff. Pocket cards summarizing infection control principles and reportable diseases may help infection control personnel educate the house staff.

Employees in public hospitals are often representative of the community in which the hospital is located. These individuals may have higher baseline rates of tuberculin skin test (TST) positivity, and may also be more likely to have community-acquired TST conversions than employees of other hospitals.[7] To establish the baseline community rate of TST positivity, the infection control program should compare TST conversions in employees who care for patients and those who do not. In addition, employees may not be immune to measles, rubella, and varicella, because they have not been exposed or were not vaccinated during childhood. To more easily trace and monitor employees exposed to contagious diseases, infection control and employee health programs should carefully document whether new employees are TST positive and whether they are immune to hepatitis B, rubella, measles, and varicella. Foreign-born staff from countries with tropical climates are less likely to have had chickenpox. Although the Centers for Disease Control and Prevention recommends that antibody-negative healthcare workers receive the new varicella vaccine, the vaccine manufacturers suggest that recipients avoid exposure to immunocompromised people for 6 weeks, which is often not possible for employees with clinical duties. One option is to vaccinate employees immediately before their vacations.

Employee unions are common in public hospitals, and are often extremely sensitive to infection control issues. Unions have powerful voices, and share with the hospital epidemiologist the desire to protect their membership, the hospital employees, from occupational exposure to infectious disease. Thus, union leadership can serve as your allies, even if their approach differs from that of the infection control program. For example, the union leadership may be willing to help you promote vaccination programs, evaluate protective gear, and educate healthcare workers.

Because public hospitals are understaffed, employees may have little time to go to the employee health service for indicated screening. Union rules may preclude the hospital from instituting disciplinary measures, such as holding paychecks, for noncompliance with annual screening. For example, to circumvent these problems, Cook County Hospital instituted a roving employee health service team that goes to the employee's worksite to place PPDs, to obtain baseline and follow-up serology, and to administer hepatitis and influenza vaccine.

Education

The infection control program in public hospitals must use creative strategies to teach infection control principles. This is especially true if a sub-

stantial proportion of employees are functionally illiterate in English (either they can't read or they can't read English). Comic book-style written material, cassette tapes, and videotapes in a variety of languages can convey important infection control messages to employees working during all shifts. In addition, the infection control staff will be more effective if they can speak some of the languages spoken by the employees.

Medical Information Systems

Computerized medical information systems in public hospitals may be less sophisticated and less able to provide aggregate or trend data. Furthermore, the infection control staff may have difficulty locating basic hard copy medical records. Infection control personnel can sometimes arrange to have medical records retrieved expeditiously for quality assurance and infection control purposes.

Inspections

State health departments monitor conditions in local public hospitals. Consequently, state and local politicians may use the hospital as a political football. Infection control problems are easy targets. Some hospital epidemiologists who have worked in both private and public hospitals feel that JCAHO inspections are tougher in the public sector. Perhaps the new JCAHO guide will educate surveyors about the unique characteristics of public hospitals.

The Public Eye

Public hospitals serve the community, and for that reason, are more liable to public scrutiny and controversy. Many infection control issues, such as isolation of tuberculosis patients, management of occupational exposure, and reporting of communicable diseases provoke controversy and, therefore, interest the media. The wise hospital epidemiologist will know the hospital's public information officer and refer questions from the media to that office.

Exciting Directions

Given the diverse populations seen in these institutions, public hospitals may serve as early detectors of new communicable diseases. Antibiotic resistance perhaps is more common in public hospitals because of uncontrolled antibiotic use. A hospital epidemiologist who is curious and energetic will have endless opportunities for research and intervention into hospital infection control and public health issues.

Conclusion

Hospital epidemiologists and infection control professionals will not easily solve the special problems that abound in public hospitals. A daily, steady current of crises sweeps away the time infection control personnel would use to address larger programmatic issues. One could easily surrender to the bureaucratic obstacles that obstruct the practice of infection control. Regardless, the hospital epidemiologist must strive to communicate well with all relevant departments, especially with employee health, engineering, environmental services, quality assurance, the local health department, and local correctional health services. The hospital epidemiologist and infection control professionals will gain great satisfaction when they design creative, cost-effective programs that turn the public hospital's weakness into strengths.

References

1. Joint Commission on Accreditation of Healthcare Organizations. *Joint Commission Surveyor Guide for Surveys of Public Hospitals.* 1995.
2. Holmes GP, McCormick JB, Trock SC, et al. Lassa fever in the United States. *N Engl J Med.* 1990;323:1120-1123.
3. Mathur P, Sacks L, Auten G, Sall R, Levy C, Gordin F. Delayed diagnosis of pulmonary tuberculosis in city hospitals. *Arch Intern Med.* 1994;154:306-310.
4. Blumberg HM, Watkins DL, Bershling JD, et al. Preventing the nosocomial transmission of tuberculosis. *Ann Intern Med.* 1995;122:658-663.
5. Fazal BA, Telzak EE, Blum S, Pollard CL, Bar M, Ernst JA, Trett GS. Impact of a coordinated tuberculosis team in an inner-city hospital in New York City. *Infect Control Hosp Epidemiol.* 1995;16:340-344.
6. Wurtz R, Karajovic M, Dacumos E, Jovanovic B, Hanumadass M. Nosocomial infections in the burn intensive care unit. *Burns.* 1995;21:181-184.
7. Bailey TC, Fraser VJ, Spitznagel EL, Dunagan WC. Risk factors for positive tuberculin skin test among employees of an urban, midwestern teaching hospital. *Ann Intern Med.* 1995;122:580-585.

Infection Control in Long-Term Care Facilities

Lindsay E. Nicolle, MD, Richard A. Garibaldi, MD

Abstract

Although patients in long-term care facilities are at increased risk of infection, little is known about how to practice infection control in this setting. This chapter reviews risk factors for infection, the components of an infection control program, and particular infections that are important in long-term care facilities. In addition, special characteristics of long-term care facilities that challenge the individuals charged with conducting effective infection control programs will be discussed.

Background

Population

Many individuals in developed countries reside for extended periods in long-term care institutions. Many different types of institutions provide a wide variety of services to diverse patient populations. The majority of residents in these facilities, however, are elderly persons who reside in nursing homes. Approximately 43% of Americans who became 65 years old in 1990 will reside in a nursing home for some time before they die.[1] Infection control programs are necessary in these facilities to limit morbidity and mortality from infections and to decrease the cost of care.

Infections in Long-Term Care Facilities

Infections are common in long-term care facilities. Reported rates of infection in nursing homes have varied from 1.8 to 9.4 per 1,000 resident-days (Table 31-1). The prevalence of infection has varied from 1.6% to 14%.[2] This wide variation reflects differences among the patient populations studied and among the definitions of infection and the surveillance methods used.

Common Infections

The most common endemic infections in nursing homes affect the urinary tract, upper and lower respiratory tracts, gastrointestinal tract, conjunctiva, and skin (eg, decubitus ulcers, cellulitis, and vascular ulcers). Surgical site infections, the second most common cause of nosocomial infections in acute-care facilities, are uncommon. Outbreaks of infections occur frequently. The most common etiologic agents of outbreaks are listed in Table 31-2.

TABLE 31-1
REPORTED INCIDENCE AND PREVALENCE OF COMMON INFECTIONS IN NURSING HOMES

	Incidence Per 1,000 Days	Percent of Prevalence
All infections	1.8–9.4	1.6–13.9
Urinary infections		
Symptomatic	0.19–2.2	2.6–3.5
Asymptomatic	1.1	15–50
Respiratory tract		
Lower (pneumonia, bronchitis)	0.3–4.7	0.3–5.8
Sinusitis/otitis	0.003–2.3	1.5
Skin/soft tissue	0.14–1.1	5.6–8.4
Infected pressure ulcers	0.1–0.3	2.6–24
Cellulitis/cutaneous abscesses	0.19–0.23	7.2–8.7
Conjunctivitis	0.17–1.0	5–13
Candida infections	0.28	33–47
Bacteremia	0.2–0.36	—
Gastrointestinal infections	0–2.5	0.5–1.3

Morbidity and Mortality

Residents of long-term care institutions have numerous comorbidities and impaired functional status. In addition, from 10% to 30% of these patients die each year. Consequently, investigators have had difficulty determining the additional morbidity or mortality attributable to infections. Moreover, infections may cause further functional impairment, prolong institutional care, or necessitate transfer to acute-care facilities. Pneumonia, with a reported case-fatality ratio of 6% to 23%, is the only infection that contributes substantially to mortality. Although bacteremia complicates urinary tract infections infrequently, such infections have a case fatality ratio of 10% to 25%.

Costs

At present, little is known about the costs of infections in long-term care facilities. Some factors that may contribute to increased costs include evaluation by nursing and medical staff, laboratory and radiologic tests, antimicrobial therapy, intensified nursing care, infection control efforts, and transfer of residents to acute-care facilities.

Reasons for Increased Risk of Infection

Aging-Associated Changes

As a person ages, the immune and other body systems change, increasing the risk of infection (Table 31-3). The specific contribution of aging-associated immune changes is not clear. Nonimmune aging-associated changes that enhance the patient's susceptibility to infection occur in virtually all body systems.

Comorbidity and Functional Impairment

The institutionalized elderly have numerous comorbidities that substantially increase their risk of infection. For instance, urologic abnormalities, such as prostatic hypertrophy, are associated with urinary tract infections. Chronic obstructive lung disease and congestive heart failure increase a patient's risk of developing pneumonia. Diabetes or vascular insufficiency may lead to more frequent and severe skin infections. Functional impairment, including decreased mobility and incontinence (usually secondary to comorbidities), further increases the risk that a patient will develop an infection.

TABLE 31-2
ETIOLOGIC AGENTS IDENTIFIED AS CAUSES OF OUTBREAKS IN LONG-TERM CARE FACILITIES

	Viral	Bacterial	Other
Respiratory	Common cold viruses	*Streptococcus pneumoniae*	
	Influenza	*Haemophilus influenzae*	
	Respiratory syncytial virus	*Mycobacterium tuberculosis,*	
	Parainfluenza[1,3]	*Bordetella pertussis* (rare)	
		Group A Streptococcus (rare)	
Gastrointestinal	Rotavirus	*Salmonella* sp	*Giardia*
	Norwalk-like viruses	*Escherichia coli* 0157:H7	*lamblia*
	Astroviruses (rare)	*Shigella* sp	(rare)
	Calcivirus (rare)	*Clostridium difficile*	
		Staphylococcus aureus (food poisoning)	
		Clostridium perfringens (food poisoning)	
		Bacillus cereus (food poisoning)	
		Aeromonas hydrophilia (rare)	
		Campylobacter jejuni (rare)	
Skin infections		Group A Streptococcus	Scabies
		Methicillin-resistant *Staphylococcus aureus*	

Interventions

Therapeutic interventions may increase the risk of infection for individual patients. Approximately 5% to 10% of patients in nursing homes will have long-term indwelling urinary catheters, and these subjects always will be bacteriuric.[2] Feeding tubes may allow Gram-negative organisms to colonize the pharynx and the stomach and, possibly, to cause pneumonia. Medications such as antidepressants, with atropine-like side effects, may dry secretions and increase the frequency of pharyngeal colonization. In addition, these drugs inhibit bladder contraction and impede urine flow, which may predispose patients to develop urinary tract infections.

Institutionalization

In institutions, high-risk patients are clustered in one locale, which may facilitate transmission of pathogens among residents. Organisms may be transmitted through the air (eg, tuberculosis,

influenza), on the hands of staff (eg, *Staphylococcus aureus* or uropathogens), and by contaminated items (eg, food).

Special Considerations for Infection Control Programs in Long-Term Care Facilities

There are fundamental differences between long-term care and acute-care facilities. In some cases, these differences require epidemiologists to approach infection control differently in each setting.

Resources

In long-term care facilities, the resources and expertise available for establishing and operating infection control programs are limited. Specific problems include the following:

- In many facilities, individuals responsible for the infection control program are part-time workers. They have numerous other responsibilities that limit the time available

TABLE 31-3

FACTORS THAT MAY PROMOTE INFECTION IN RESIDENTS OF LONG-TERM CARE FACILITIES

Factor	Aging-Associated Changes
Immune system	Thymic involution; decreased antibody production, decreased T cells, decreased mitogen stimulation, decreased fever response, and decreased interleukin-2, and increased autoantibodies
Skin	Epidermal thinning; decreased elasticity, subcutaneous tissue, vascularity, and wound healing
Respiratory tract	Decreased cough reflex, elastic tissue, mucociliary transport, IgA
Gastrointestinal tract	Decreased gastric acidity and motility
Genitourinary tract	Decreased estrogen effect on mucosa, decreased prostatic secretions, and increased prostatic size
Chronic illness	Diabetes, congestive heart failure, vascular insufficiency, COPD, neurologic impairment
Nutritional impairment	Decreased cell-mediated immunity and wound healing
Functional impairment	Immobility, incontinence, impaired mental status
Invasive devices	Indwelling urinary catheter, tracheostomy, feeding tube gastrostomy, central intravenous catheter
Institutionalization	Increased person-to-person transmission

COPD = chronic obstructive pulmonary disease.

for infection control and reduce its priority.

- Some facilities have limited access to personnel with expertise in infectious diseases, microbiology, and standard infection control practices.
- Some facilities have limited or no employee health programs.
- The medical literature provides little data regarding the efficacy of infection control programs in long-term care facilities.

Personnel

Compared with staff in acute-care facilities, staff in long-term care facilities may have less training in infection control and in other patient care practices. Furthermore, staff turnover in long-term care facilities may be higher than that in acute-care facilities, making it difficult to train personnel adequately in infection control practices.

Patient-Related Issues

The clinical approach to the diagnosis and management of patients in long-term care facilities differs from that practiced in the community or in acute-care facilities. The reasons for this include the following:

- Communication may be impaired for many patients in long-term care facilities.
- Access to radiologic and laboratory facilities may be limited, and specimens or patients may need to be transferred off site for testing.
- Clinical diagnostic criteria have been developed for younger populations with fewer comorbidities. Most long-term care residents have chronic symptoms that may make it difficult to identify and evaluate acute changes in clinical status.
- Infectious diseases in the elderly patient may have nonclassical presentations. For instance, impaired elderly patients who have infections may present with confusion, rather than prominent localizing findings. Compared with younger patients, the elderly have a relatively blunted temperature response; therefore, a higher proportion of infected patients may be afebrile.
- Certain microbiologic specimens have limited diagnostic use in this population. For example, Gram-negative organisms frequently colonize the oropharynx of elderly patients who are in institutions. Sputum specimens obtained from these patients may be contaminated by the colonizing organisms. In addi-

tion, 30% to 50% of noncatheterized elderly residents of nursing homes are bacteriuric. Therefore, in these patients, a positive urine culture has a low predictive value for diagnosing invasive urinary infection.[3]

- In general, the use of standard clinical diagnostic tests has not been assessed for patients in long-term care facilities. The optimal use of laboratory tests for management of infection in this population and the appropriate empiric approach to treatment are not established.

Developing an Infection Control Program

Infection control programs should be developed to serve the specific needs of a given institution and its patient population. The fundamental components of such a program include administration, personnel, surveillance, policies, and education.

Administration

An effective reporting structure must be defined. Responsibility and authority should be defined clearly, and the structure developed to ensure a flexible and efficient infection control program.

Personnel

The size and complexity of the institution will determine the number of individuals needed to work on infection control. At least one individual must have responsibility for the infection control program. If an individual is responsible for programs in the institution in addition to infection control, his or her specific commitment to infection control must be defined clearly.

Personnel with responsibility for infection control must have some training in microbiology, infectious diseases, epidemiology, and program management.

Individuals with expertise in areas such as outbreak investigation, infectious diseases, antimicrobial use, and microbiology should be identified and

consulted when needed.

Surveillance for Infections

Surveillance to identify infections and outbreaks is an essential component of the infection control program.[4]

Standard definitions, appropriate for long-term care facilities, should be used to identify infections at each site. Some recommended definitions have been published.[5]

Infection control personnel should use case-finding methods that are appropriate for the available resources and characteristics of the institution. Methods may include walking rounds, nursing-generated reports, chart reviews, kardex reviews, and laboratory or medication record reviews. When an infection control program initially is being developed for a facility, prevalence surveys may be useful. Generally, incidence surveys are more useful for ongoing programs.

Infection control personnel should analyze data, review findings, and report results to the administration and to public health authorities when appropriate. Incidence rates generally should be reported as the number of infections per 1,000 resident days.

The surveillance program should enable personnel to identify quickly outbreaks of influenza, gastrointestinal illness, scabies, and other common problems.

Policies

Policies regarding the identification and control of infections must be developed, reviewed, updated, and monitored to document adherence. Some specific issues to be addressed by institutional policies include the following:

- Handwashing.
- Universal precautions (includes standard precautions).
- Environmental cleaning, laundry, and waste disposal.
- Food preparation, holding, and transport.

- Preadmission screening of residents for infections (eg, tuberculosis).
- Vaccination policies (eg, influenza).
- Management of patients with infections, especially those who may require special infection control precautions.
- Identification and management of residents with antimicrobial-resistant organisms.
- Outbreak identification, investigation, and control.
- Review of antimicrobial use.
- An employee health program that addresses tuberculosis screening, immunizations, and leaves of absence when employees have potentially transmissable infections.

Education

Ongoing education of staff, residents, and visitors is an important component of the infection control program. All individuals working in the facility, including medical staff, should know risk factors for infection and methods for minimizing residents' risk of infection. These programs should be developed with input from the groups of employees for which they are targeted.

Special Infection Problems

Influenza

Influenza outbreaks occur frequently in long-term care facilities,[6] and may be disruptive because many patients and staff become ill within a short time. Outbreaks have been associated with substantial patient mortality. Each facility should develop a specific plan for managing influenza that includes the following:

- Yearly vaccination programs for patients and staff.
- Clinical and epidemiologic definitions of influenza.
- Surveillance for possible outbreaks.
- Criteria defining when and from whom

diagnostic specimens should be collected.
- Response to outbreaks, including isolating residents and restricting visitors.
- Notification of local authorities.
- Recommendations for prophylactic use of amantadine or rimantadine (eg, dose, patient exclusions, triggers for initiating prophylaxis, and criteria for deciding which patients will receive prophylaxis).

Gastrointestinal Illness, Including *Clostridium difficile*

Outbreaks of gastrointestinal illness are common in long-term care facilities.[7] Sporadic episodes of diarrhea frequently are due to *C difficile* or noninfectious causes. Specific components in a program to control gastrointestinal illness include the following:

- Clinical definitions for identification of individual cases and outbreaks.
- Criteria that define when specimens and laboratory tests are obtained.
- A description of infection control practices, including isolation precautions required for patients with sporadic or epidemic gastrointestinal illness.
- A protocol for use of oral rehydration therapy.
- Protocols for antimicrobial therapy (eg, metronidazole for moderate-to-severe *C difficile* colitis) of infected patients and staff.
- Staff education programs.

Clusters of patients with diarrhea may be caused by foodborne pathogens, including those associated with toxins (eg, *Bacillus cereus, Staphylococcus aureus*), as well as bacterial, viral, or parasitic infection. Management of such clusters should include the following:

- Epidemiologic investigation.
- Identification of the source of infection (eg, food item, person, utensil).
- Elimination or treatment of the source.
- Staff education to limit transmission and to

prevent future outbreaks.

- Appropriate management of infected residents and personnel.

Scabies

To manage scabies[8] effectively, personnel in long-term care facilities must understand the disease and follow a systematic approach to identifying and treating affected patients. Issues that must be addressed include clinical and microscopic diagnostic criteria; treatment for infected patients (5% permethrin or 1% lindane); management of exposed patients, staff, or household contacts; handling of contaminated bedding and clothing; and follow-up of treated subjects.

Group A Streptococcal Skin Infections

Long-term care facilities should define how they will identify outbreaks and individual cases of streptococcal disease.[9] They also must define which infection control precautions should be instituted when streptococcal infections are identified.

For severe outbreaks, or in instances when initial control measures are not effective, infection control personnel should consider either performing a culture survey to identify colonized patients and staff or undertaking mass treatment of residents.[9]

Tuberculosis

The most important strategy for preventing spread of tuberculosis is early identification and treatment of possibly infectious cases.[10] Long-term care facilities need to monitor skin-test conversion among residents and staff, identify and evaluate patients with pulmonary symptoms consistent with tuberculosis, isolate patients with potential or proven pulmonary tuberculosis, trace exposed patients and staff, and initiate prophylactic isoniazid therapy.

Bloodborne Pathogens

Policies must be developed for the management of patients with potential bloodborne infec-

tions, including hepatitis B, hepatitis C, and human immunodeficiency virus (HIV) infection. These policies should describe the practice of standard precautions, include guidelines for the use of gloves and other barriers during patient care, and discuss methods to limit needlestick exposures and other percutaneous injury.

Multiply-Resistant Organisms

Patients in nursing homes are at increased risk for acquiring antimicrobial-resistant organisms.[11] Many facilities have been concerned particularly about methicillin-resistant *S aureus*.[12] Institutional programs should define multiply resistant organisms, review and restrict antimicrobial use when appropriate, and provide guidelines for the management of patients who carry or are infected with resistant organisms. Certain patients may require isolation precautions; however, standard infection control practices, such as appropriate handwashing, environmental cleaning, and wound care, usually will be sufficient.

Long-term care facilities should develop policies regarding transferring patients with resistant organisms to other institutions or accepting such patients from other institutions. In general, a resistant organism should not preclude transferring or accepting a patient. However, the institution that transfers the patient always should notify the accepting institution before the patient is transferred so that the staff of the latter can be prepared.[13]

References

1. Kemper P, Murtaugh C. Lifetime use of nursing home care. *N Engl J Med.* 1991;324:595-600.

2. Warren JW. Catheter-associated bacteriuria. *Clin Geriatr Med.* 1992;8:805-819.

3. Nicolle LE. Urinary tract infections in long-term care facilities. *Infect Control Hosp Epidemiol.* 1993;14:220-225.

4. Smith PW. Infection surveillance in long-term care facilities. *Infect Control Hosp Epidemiol.* 1991;12:55-58.

5. McGeer A, Campbell B, Emori TG, et al. Definitions of

infection for surveillance in long-term care facilities. *Am J Infect Control.* 1991;19:1-7.

6. Gravenstein S, Miller BA, Drinka P. Prevention and control of influenza A outbreaks in long-term care facilities. *Infect Control Hosp Epidemiol.* 1992;13:49-54.

7. Bennett RG. Diarrhea among residents of long-term care facilities. *Infect Control Hosp Epidemiol.* 1993;14:397-404.

8. Segelau J. Scabies in long-term care facilities. *Infect Control Hosp Epidemiol.* 1992;13:421-425.

9. Schwartz B, Ussery XT. Group A streptococcal outbreaks in nursing homes. *Infect Control Hosp Epidemiol.* 1992;13:742-747.

10. Centers for Disease Control. Prevention and control of tuberculosis in facilities providing long-term care to the elderly. *MMWR.* 1990;39(No. RR-10):7-13.

11. John JF Jr, Ribner BS. Antibiotic resistance in long-term care facilities. *Infect Control Hosp Epidemiol.* 1991;12:245-250.

12. Kauffman CA, Bradley SF, Terpenning MS. Methicillin-resistant *Staphylococcus aureus* in long-term care facilities. *Infect Control Hosp Epidemiol.* 1990;11:600-603.

13. Boyce JM, Jackson MM, Pugliese G, et al. Methicillin-resistant *Staphylococcus aureus* (MRSA): a briefing for acute care hospitals and nursing facilities. *Infect Control Hosp Epidemiol.* 1994;15:105-115.

Recommended Reading

Smith PW, ed. *Infection Control in Long-Term Care Facilities.* 2nd ed. Albany, NY: Delmar Publishers, Inc; 1994.

Strasbaugh LJ, Joseph C. Epidemiology and prevention of infections in long-term care facilities. In: Mayhall G, ed. *Hospital Epidemiology.* Baltimore, Md: Williams & Wilkins, 1996:1151-1170.

CHAPTER 32

Infection Control in the Outpatient Setting

Loreen A. Herwaldt, MD, Shanon D. Smith, MD,
Cheryl D. Carter, RN, BSN

Abstract

This chapter discusses aspects of ambulatory care that increase the difficulty of practicing infection control in this setting or that require infection control staff to use different methods than they would use in the inpatient setting. The chapter reviews basic infection control precautions that apply to the outpatient setting, in general, and specific precautions that apply to dialysis centers and physical therapy programs. The chapter also describes outbreaks that have occurred in the outpatient setting, defines the deficiencies in infection control practice that caused the outbreaks, and discusses methods to prevent transmission of pathogens in the outpatient setting.

Introduction

Healthcare delivery is undergoing cataclysmic changes. Innovative medical technologies have allowed healthcare workers to do many diagnostic and therapeutic procedures in the outpatient setting. Moreover, third-party payers are insisting that much of medical care be delivered outside of hospitals. Consequently, the proportion of medical care that is given in the outpatient setting is increasing rapidly. Currently, 80% to 90% of all cancer care is delivered in the outpatient setting[1] and 52% of all hospital-based operations are done in ambulatory surgery centers.[1] At the University of Iowa Hospitals and Clinics, the proportion of operations done in the ambulatory surgical center has increased from 5% in fiscal year 1982-1983 to 30% in fiscal year 1991-1992.[2] Some observers predict that, by the year 2000, approximately 80% of operations will be done in the ambulatory setting.[1,3] Concomitantly, the number of inpatient hospital beds in the United States has decreased by 20% in the last 10 years and is expected to decrease by another 20% to 30% in the next 10 years.[1]

Given such statistics, one does not have to be prescient to recognize that hospital epidemiologists and infection control professionals must stop working exclusively in the inpatient setting and begin to develop programs that address infection control issues across the spectrum of care from the acute-care setting to patients' homes. In addition to the clinical and monetary incentives to address infection control issues in the outpatient setting, the

Centers for Disease Control and Prevention (CDC) recommends, and the Occupational Safety and Health Administration (OSHA) mandates, that healthcare workers in the outpatient setting incorporate the Bloodborne Pathogen Standard[4] and tuberculosis guidelines into their practices.[5] Moreover, the Joint Commission on Accreditation of Healthcare Organizations requires that, within a particular healthcare organization, the infection control policies and procedures that are applied in the inpatient setting and in the outpatient setting are consistent in intent and application.[6]

Healthcare workers and infection control personnel traditionally have considered the risk of infection to be low in the ambulatory-care setting. However, few investigators have evaluated systematically the rates of infection in outpatient populations. Investigators who have attempted to conduct surveillance in outpatient populations often have encountered substantial problems that have precluded instituting such programs into the routine practice of infection control.

To date, experts in infection control and agencies such as the CDC have not recommended specific programs or surveillance systems in ambulatory care. Furthermore, there currently are few recommendations or guidelines for infection control in this setting. The standards regarding bloodborne pathogens and tuberculosis must be applied in the outpatient setting, and several subspecialty societies (eg, American Academy of Ophthalmology and the American Society for Gastrointestinal Endoscopy) have published recommendations that can help infection control personnel. However, there are no comprehensive, national guidelines for the practice of infection control in the outpatient setting. Despite the dearth of data and guidelines, infection control staff must develop programs that address the special needs of the ambulatory-care setting, because this is where most medical care will be given in the 21st century.

This chapter will:

- Discuss aspects of ambulatory care that increase the difficulty of practicing infection control in this setting or that require infection control staff to use different methods than they would use in the inpatient setting.
- Review basic infection control precautions that apply to the outpatient setting.
- Describe outbreaks that have occurred in the outpatient setting and the deficiencies in infection control practice that caused the outbreaks.
- Describe methods to prevent transmission of pathogens in the outpatient setting.

In addition, we will discuss basic infection control precautions for dialysis centers and physical therapy programs. However, we will not discuss infection control for ambulatory surgery centers, home healthcare, or dental offices. Readers who need information on those topics are referred to recent reviews.[3,7-9]

Components of Healthcare Delivery in the Outpatient Setting

For the purposes of this chapter, we will define outpatient or ambulatory care as any medical services provided to patients who are not admitted to inpatient hospital units. Infection control in the outpatient or ambulatory setting is a very broad topic, because the scope of medical services provided outside of the traditional inpatient setting and the types of facilities providing these services have expanded exponentially. Even conventional hospitals that specialize in hospital-based care have numerous areas in which persons other than inpatients are waiting, visiting, or undergoing treatment. Examples include the admissions or registration areas, emergency treatment centers, hospital-based clinics, ambulatory surgery centers, and procedure suites (eg, bronchoscopy, gastrointestinal endoscopy, and radiology). In addition, many hospitals have outpatient clinics that are located some distance from the inpatient facility. Although most hospitals have an infection control program, the staff might not have expanded their efforts beyond the inpatient units or might not have been consulted by the persons who planned the new outpatient services.

Numerous outpatient facilities have sprung up that are independent of hospitals, including ambulatory treatment centers, urgent-care centers, outpatient surgical centers, radiology and imaging clinics, dialysis centers, physician-owned clinics, and chemotherapy centers. Third-party payers have encouraged this development and now demand that a large proportion of medical care be given in the outpatient setting and that patients who are admitted to hospitals must be discharged as soon as possible. Consequently, short-term care facilities, such as 23-hour clinics, have been developed to provide subacute and semiurgent care for patients who do not require hospitalization. Staff in such facilities evaluate patients, observe patients for short periods, do some outpatient procedures, and do after-hours telephone triage. Some centers also provide services such as radiation therapy, chemotherapy, and infusion therapy for hydration, parenteral nutrition, or antibiotics.

Many freestanding outpatient medical centers operate for profit. Administrators of such centers may over-emphasize profits and cost-cutting, and might not provide the resources necessary for an effective infection control program, because these programs initially increase costs. The persons who are responsible for infection control in these facilities often have many other pressing duties and might not have appropriate training or experience.

Common Problems Encountered in the Outpatient Setting

Persons who conduct infection control efforts in any outpatient setting will encounter problems that either do not occur in the inpatient setting or are exaggerated in the outpatient setting compared with the inpatient setting. We will discuss some of these problems briefly.

The population of persons in the outpatient setting often is very difficult to define. For example, exposures to communicable diseases such as measles or tuberculosis can occur in clinic waiting areas, hospital registration areas, or in other large open areas in which many people congregate. Infection control personnel may have difficulty identifying which patients, family members, and staff were in the area at a particular time. Similarly, infection control personnel may have difficulty determining the rate of catheter-related bloodstream infections in outpatients, because patients who acquire these infections may be treated elsewhere and because the denominator (ie, the number of persons with catheters) is very difficult to define.

Most surveillance methodologies were developed for use in the inpatient setting and are of limited use in the outpatient setting. The surveillance methods that have been tested in the outpatient setting often are labor-intensive and lack sensitivity and specificity. In addition, few hospitals or freestanding clinics have developed follow-up programs that allow staff to identify infections or other complications that occur after the patient is discharged from the hospital or after outpatient procedures.

Clinic schedules often are very busy and leave little time for formal educational programs. Moreover, unlike hospital-based programs, freestanding facilities might not have on-site continuing-education programs.

Staff in some outpatient facilities turn over rapidly, and, as facilities downsize, they often replace staff with the most education (eg, registered nurses) and experience with persons who have little education (eg, medical assistants) and experience. These changes make it difficult to achieve and maintain an adequate level of infection control knowledge among staff members.

Telephone calls and registration usually are handled by persons with the least medical knowledge. Thus, patients who have contagious diseases might not be identified and triaged appropriately.

Personnel in clinics often care for many patients and do many procedures during a day. Given current budget constraints, the number of staff and the amount of equipment often are limited. Thus, staff might cut corners to meet the demands of the schedule. For example, healthcare workers might not wash their hands when appropriate, or they might not clean, disinfect, or sterilize equipment properly.

Many outpatient medical facilities were not designed with regard for principles of infection control. For example, most outpatient facilities do not have negative-air-pressure rooms, and the air often is recirculated without filtration. In addition, outpatient facilities might have only one entrance and one waiting area, making these clinics ideal places in which airborne pathogens, such as *Mycobacterium tuberculosis*, varicella-zoster virus (VZV), or measles virus can spread. Moreover, many outpatient facilities have inadequate space to allow the staff to maintain separate clean and dirty areas.

Exposures to Bloodborne Pathogens in the Outpatient Setting

The OSHA Bloodborne Pathogen Standard specifies that all healthcare institutions, including outpatient facilities, must implement policies and procedures to protect healthcare workers from exposures to bloodborne pathogens.[4] Infection control personnel must ensure that the inpatient and outpatient facilities within their institution implement the same general policies and procedures (ie, a single standard of practice) to prevent exposures. However, some of the specific policies might be different in the two settings, because the staff provide different services in each setting.

Healthcare workers in the ambulatory setting are at risk for exposure to blood and body fluids.[10 14] Staff in emergency departments may be at the highest risk, because they frequently provide acute care for persons who have traumatic injuries or are criti-

cally ill. Kelen et al demonstrated that 92% of the procedures performed in the emergency department of Johns Hopkins University Hospital, Baltimore, Md, involved exposure to blood or body fluid.[10] In addition, nearly one fourth of the patients seen in their emergency department during 6 consecutive weeks were infected with at least one bloodborne pathogen.[11] Five percent of the samples had hepatitis B surface antigen (HBsAg), 18% had antibody to hepatitis C (HCV), and 6% had antibody to human immunodeficiency virus (HIV).

Despite their exposure to blood and body fluids, healthcare workers in the outpatient setting often do not comply with precautions designed to protect them from bloodborne pathogens.[12-14] For example, Kelen et al found that compliance improved in their emergency room after the hospital mandated use of bloodborne pathogen precautions.[12] However, after the policy was implemented, compliance was only 55% during major procedures and 56% during interventions on patients who were bleeding profusely.[12]

Likewise, staff in medical offices often do not comply with bloodborne pathogen precautions. Thurn et al surveyed 141 physician's offices throughout Minnesota[13] and discovered that personnel in 51% of the offices recapped needles, and 44% of the offices reported at least one needlestick injury in the past year. However, only 38% of the offices had a needlestick protocol. In addition, personnel in some offices discarded needles in cardboard containers or plastic bags. Similar results were obtained from a survey of family practitioners in Ohio.[14] Of 1,409 respondents, only 35% "almost never" or "never" recapped used needles. Thirty-six percent of physicians and 38% of staff had at least one exposure to bloodborne pathogens in the previous year; 2% acknowledged exposures to blood or secretions from patients known to be infected with HIV. Only 80% of the respondents reported that they disposed of sharp instruments in puncture-resistant containers.

Patients also are at risk for acquiring hepatitis B virus (HBV) and HIV through medical care provided in the outpatient setting (Tables 32-1 and 32-2). Several outbreaks of HBV have occurred in alternative healthcare settings,[15-17] but transmission also has occurred in dialysis centers,[18-20] a dermatology practice,[21] a procedure suite in which endomyocardial biopsies were performed,[22] and in oral surgery practices.[23] Contaminated multidose vials and equipment that was cleaned and disinfected improperly were vehicles for transmission of HBV in these settings. HIV has been transmitted in a dental office,[24] a dialysis center,[25] and in a private surgeon's office[26] (see Table 32-2). Specific errors in infection control technique were not identified in two outbreaks.[24,26] In the third outbreak, improperly reprocessed dialysis needles were the likely vehicle for transmission.[25]

Respiratory Infections in the Outpatient Setting

Several outbreaks have illustrated that bacterial and viral pathogens can be transmitted within outpatient facilities by airborne or droplet spread. Particular characteristics of the outpatient setting, such as the following, might enhance the likelihood that these pathogens will be transmitted:

- Many people congregate in waiting rooms.
- Many infectious patients come to outpatient facilities for evaluation and treatment, particularly during endemic or epidemic periods for viral infections.
- Outpatient facilities frequently have inadequate triage systems.
- The number of air exchanges in the building often is low, and the air often is recirculated.

Tuberculosis in the Ambulatory Setting

Several outbreaks illustrate that *M tuberculosis* can be transmitted easily in the outpatient setting (Table 32-3).[27-34] These outbreaks demonstrate that healthcare workers[27-29,34] and patients[30-33] can become infected when exposed to outpatients who

have undiagnosed tuberculosis or to patients with known tuberculosis when the isolation precautions are not optimal. Healthcare workers have transmitted *M tuberculosis* to patients infrequently. For example, Moore et al investigated an outbreak in which a pediatrician transmitted tuberculosis to at least five children.[32]

A few studies have assessed the risk of infection associated with exposure to *M tuberculosis* in the outpatient setting. For example, Couldwell et al[31] observed an attack rate of 3.4% among patients who were exposed while in an HIV clinic, and Haley et al[27] and Griffith et al[34] noted attack rates of 34% and 76%, respectively, among staff exposed in the emergency department. Moreover, Sokolove et al documented that the risk of *M tuberculosis* infection among staff who worked full-time in the emergency department of Harbor-UCLA Medical Center, Torrance, Calif, increased substantially during a time period when tuberculosis controls were less than optimal.[35] After 60 months of full-time work, the risk of tuberculin skin-test conversion was 39.6%. During the study period, emergency department air was exhausted to the outside, and patients and staff wore surgical masks with string ties while in respiratory isolation rooms. However, the emergency department did not have a screening protocol or appropriate engineering controls (ie, negative-pressure rooms, high-efficiency particulate air [HEPA] filters, or ultraviolet irradiation).

The most important element of a tuberculosis control program is early identification and isolation of patients with suspected or confirmed infectious tuberculosis. Triage personnel and staff who perform the initial evaluation in ambulatory-care facilities must know both the signs and symptoms of tuberculosis, including atypical symptoms expressed by immunocompromised patients, and the appropriate isolation precautions for patients who might have tuberculosis.

Healthcare workers in the ambulatory setting

TABLE 32-1
OUTBREAKS CAUSED BY HEPATITIS B VIRUS IN OUTPATIENT HEALTHCARE FACILITIES

Ref	Year*	Duration of Outbreak	Source	No. of Persons Affected	Type of Facility	Infection Control Error	Comments
18	1983 (1981)	>1 mo	Bupivacaine MDV	10	Outpatient dialysis center associated with a general hospital	Contamination of a bupivacaine vial with HBV	MDV may have become contaminated when a patient who carried HBsAg and HBeAg stuck herself with a needle before drawing up bupivacaine Ten of 11 (91%) susceptible patients who subsequently used the MDV were infected The implicated carrier and six cases who had serum available were infected with the Ad subtype
15	1988 (1984)	1 yr	Contaminated acupuncture needles	35	Acupuncture clinic	The acupuncturist did not wear gloves during procedures, did not wash his hands between patients, did not sterilize needles after use, and did not sterilize a device used to apply pressure to bleeding sites	The acupuncturist used solid-metal reusable needles
16	1986 (1980)	4 days during a 3-mo period	Acupuncture needles	6	Chiropractic clinic	Needles were reused after being immersed for 24 hrs in benzalkonium chloride	
17	1990 (1984-1985)	23 mo	Human chorionic gonadotropin injections	60	Weight reduction clinic	Contaminated jet injectors	Persons receiving injections of human chorionic gonadotropin by syringe did not become infected The outbreak stopped when the jet injector was no longer used
21	1993 (1985-1991)	7 yrs	Probably HBsAg-positive patients	Up to 305	Dermatology practice	The dermatologist did not use sterile surgical technique He operated without gloves,	There was serological evidence of HBV infection in 305 unvaccinated patients, 69 of whom had known dates of onset and

No.	Year published (year occurred)	Duration	Setting	No.	Probable source	Comments
			who had procedures in the office		did not wash his hands between patients, reused syringes to obtain medications from MDVs, and reused contaminated electrocautery tips	records available for review; Of the patients with known dates of onset, 72% were operated on by the physician during the incubation period; Spouses of two patients acquired HBV infection
22	1994 (1986-1990)	3.5 yrs	A room in which endomyocardial biopsies were done	67	Patients who carried HBsAg and who underwent endomyocardial biopsy	Patients were at higher risk of becoming infected if they underwent endomyocardial biopsy in the room after a patient who carried HBsAg had the same procedure; Attack rate was 28%; 63 of 67 had the viral subtype Ay; The investigators postulated droplet contamination of instruments or medication vials that were used for subsequent patients
19	1995 (1994)	2-5 mo	Dialysis center	7	Contaminated MDV possibly was the source	Separate rooms and machines were not used for HBsAg carriers and for noncarriers; Staff were not cohorted; Supplies were shared among patients; The attack rate for HBV infection was associated significantly with one shift (RR, 30) and with specific chair locations (RR, 7); Partially used MDVs were returned to a central area, where they were used for other patients
20	1995 (NS)	NS	Community dialysis center	10	Contaminated MDV possibly was the source of one cluster	Two separate transmission events occurred; Many patients were susceptible to HBV and general infection control precautions were suboptimal; One group of patients shared MDVs of medication; A second group was clustered geographically and frequently was cared for by the same technician; No further seroconversions occurred after cohorting was improved and susceptible patients were immunized

MDV = multidose vial; HBV = hepatitis B virus; HBsAg = hepatitis B surface antigen; HBeAg = hepatitis B e antigen; RR = relative risk; NS = not specified.
*The first year is the year the paper was published; the year in parentheses is the year in which the outbreak occurred.

TABLE 32-2
OUTBREAKS OF HIV IN OUTPATIENT HEALTHCARE FACILITIES

Ref	Year*	Duration of Outbreak	Source of the Outbreak	No. of Persons Affected	Type of Facility	Infection Control Error	Comments
24	1992 (1987-1989)	Transmission may have occurred during 20-mo period	A dentist who had AIDS	5	Dentist's office	None identified	Of eight HIV-infected patients, five had no confirmed exposures to HIV other than through an invasive dental procedure done by the dentist after he was diagnosed with AIDS The HIV isolates from the patients and the dentist were related closely
25	1995 (1992)	4 mo	An HIV-positive patient who was dialyzed in the center	9	Dialysis center	Improper reprocessing of patient-care equipment, particularly access needles	The dialysis center reprocessed access needles, dialyzers, and bloodlines Dialyzers were reprocessed separately with 5% formaldehyde and were labeled for use by the same patient Access needles were soaked in a common container with a low-level disinfectant, benzalkonium chloride Four pairs of needles were soaked in one pan, such that needles could become cross-contaminated or could have been used on the wrong patient
26	1993 (1989)	1 day	Probably a patient who had an epidermal cyst removed	4	Private surgeon's office	None identified	The surgeon wore latex gloves, which he changed between patients Scalpel handles were the only reusable items; no MDVs were used Reusable instruments were placed in 1% glutaraldehyde immediately after use and, at the end of session, were scrubbed under running water and then were boiled for 5-10 min

HIV = human immunodeficiency virus; AIDS = acquired immunodeficiency virus; MDVs = multidose vials.
*The first year is the year the paper was published; the year in parentheses is the year in which the outbreak occurred.

should be trained to recognize patients who might have tuberculosis and to initiate isolation precautions and the appropriate clinical evaluation promptly. Patients with risk factors and suspicious symptoms should be given a mask and be instructed to cover their mouth and nose with tissues when coughing or sneezing. These patients should undergo chest radiography immediately. Patients whose signs and symptoms or chest radiographs are suggestive of tuberculosis must not stay in common waiting rooms or in areas where air is recirculated without HEPA filtration but must be placed in airborne precautions immediately. For example, many hospitals in New York City have implemented "rule out tuberculosis" policies.[36] These policies stipulate that patients who are known or suspected to be infected with HIV and who have a fever or cough or any respiratory symptoms but have no obvious nonpulmonary source must be placed in airborne precautions until tuberculosis is ruled out.[36] Such policies may have decreased the spread of tuberculosis within those hospitals.[36]

Moran et al reviewed the records of 55 patients who had culture-proven tuberculosis and were evaluated in an emergency department during 1991 and 1992.[37] Isolation was instituted as follows: 2 (4%) at triage, 26 (47%) in the emergency department, 17 (30%) on admission to the inpatient unit, and 4 (8%) after admission to the unit. Two patients never were isolated.[37] Staff in the emergency department made a presumptive diagnosis of tuberculosis in 39 (71%) of the cases. However, the median time from registration to isolation was 8 hours. Factors that led staff to isolate the patient significantly earlier were a history of exposure to tuberculosis, a chest radiograph that was consistent with tuberculosis, absence of risk factors for HIV infection, current cough, and sputum production. The authors concluded that "tuberculosis is often unsuspected, and isolation measures are often not used."[37]

If staff in outpatient departments or facilities do special procedures such as sputum induction,

bronchoscopy, aerosolized pentamidine treatments, and pulmonary function testing, the units must have adequate facilities (ie, booths or other enclosures meeting ventilation requirements for tuberculosis isolation) to prevent airborne spread of *M tuberculosis*. However, a survey conducted by the CDC in 1992 revealed that patients with tuberculosis often were treated in emergency departments, but few emergency departments were equipped appropriately to care for patients with suspected tuberculosis.[38] Of the 305 emergency departments that responded:

- Fifty-six percent had written policies for their triage area about isolating patients suspected of having tuberculosis.
- Seventy-six percent had written policies for their emergency department proper about isolating patients suspected of having tuberculosis.
- Two percent of triage areas and 20% of emergency departments had tuberculosis isolation rooms that met the CDC's recommendations.
- Seven percent of emergency departments that performed sputum induction did so only in isolation rooms.
- Eighty percent of triage areas and emergency departments recirculated air to some degree.
- Fifteen percent of the triage areas and 17% of the emergency departments used HEPA filters.
- Five percent of the triage areas and 8% of the emergency departments used ultraviolet germicidal light.[38]

Infection control personnel should help staff in the ambulatory-care areas of their healthcare center develop comprehensive protocols for identifying and treating patients with possible tuberculosis. As part of this process, infection control personnel should help create screening tools that staff can use to identify patients who may have tuberculosis. We

TABLE 32-3
Outbreaks Caused by *Mycobacterium Tuberculosis* in Outpatient Healthcare Facilities

Refs	Year*	Type of Infection	Duration of Outbreak	Source of the Outbreak	No. of Persons Affected	Type of Facility	Infection Control Error	Comments
27	1989 (1983)	Active pulmonary TB (6) and TST conversion (11)	1 day	A patient with known cavitary TB who developed severe respiratory distress while riding in an ambulance	17	ED and MICU	Air (60%) was recirculated without filtration in the ED; Most staff wore surgical masks	The patient was intubated and suctioned frequently in the ED; The patient remained in the ED for 4 hrs; The attack rate among staff in the ED was 34%
28, 29	1989 (1988)	TB infection detected by TST conversion	6 mo	Possibilities included a nurse with pulmonary TB, 39 patients with active TB	30, of whom 17 had documented TST conversions	Primary-care health clinic	Air in the clinic was recirculated, and sputum induction and aerosolized pentamidine treatments were done without proper ventilation	The risk of TB infection was increased in persons who worked on the first floor and in those who were present during treatments with aerosolized pentamide; Transmission by face-to-face exposure to TB patients could not be excluded
39	1992 (1989-1990)	MDR TB	Approximately 15 mo	Other HIV-infected patients who had MDR TB	53	Hospital and HIV clinic	Not specified	Multiple logistic regression analysis identified a diagnosis of AIDS and visits to the HIV clinic as independent risk factors; The outbreak was controlled after patients with MDR TB were kept in airborne precautions indefinitely, and all patients and healthcare workers began wearing respirator masks
34	1995 (1992)	TST conversions (10) and pulmonary TB (3)	1 day	A 22-year-old Mexican woman who suffered a cardiopulmonary arrest at home	13	ED and MICU	All healthcare workers wore surgical masks while caring for the patient; The ED did not have an appropriate screening protocol, and neither the ED nor the MICU had	The patient was intubated and resuscitated for 2 hrs in the ED and transferred to the MICU, where she died 10 hrs later; Of 17 HCW with previously negative TST, 10 became TST-positive, and 3 acquired active

						appropriate engineering controls	pulmonary TB (76% attack rate)
31	1996 (1993)	Pulmonary TB	5 wk	A patient from Southeast Asia	3	Outpatient HIV treatment room	The treatment room was ventilated with a recirculating air conditioning system. Seven patients could receive care at one time in the treatment room	Only patients infected with HIV were managed in the treatment room. The attack rate was 3.4%, and the incidence of active TB during the follow-up period was 5.3/100 person years. The secondary cases occurred within 10 wks of exposure to the source patient. The isolates from the source patient and the three secondary cases were identical by chromosomal DNA analysis
33	1997 (1995)	1 TB infection documented by TST conversion, 1 case of active MDR TB, 1 false-positive culture	1 mo	Patient 1	3	Bronchoscopy laboratory	The bronchoscope was cleaned inadequately and never was immersed in disinfectant	Patients 2, 3, and 4 underwent bronchoscopy 1, 12, and 17 days, respectively, after patient 1, who had cavitary TB. Patient 2 had a TST conversion, patient 3 had a false-positive culture, and patient 4 acquired cavitary TB
32	1997 (1995-1996)	TB infection detected by TST conversion	4 mo	A pediatrician with culture-positive TB	At least 5	Pediatrics clinic and an acute-care hospital	The physician practiced while coughing (11/95-2/96)	Only 64% of 1,419 patients seen by the pediatrician during his infectious period presented for evaluation. One US-born child had a documented TST conversion, and four US-born children with TST ≥10 mm had no other known exposure. The four foreign-born children with TST ≥10 mm were from countries with a high prevalence of TB

TB = tuberculosis; TST = tuberculin skin test; ED = emergency department; MICU = medical intensive care unit; MDR TB = multidrug-resistant M tuberculosis; HIV = human immunodeficiency virus.

*The first year is the year the paper was published; the year in parentheses is the year in which the outbreak occurred.

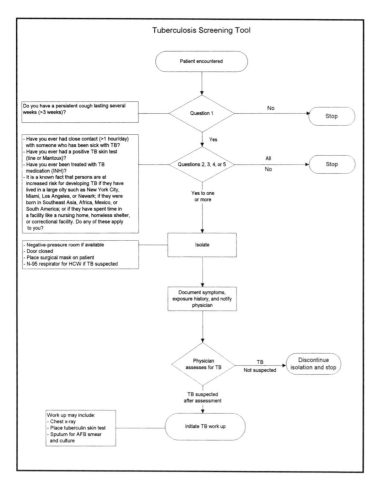

FIGURE 32-1. We incorporated a screening questionnaire into an algorithm to help staff in outpatient clinics and the emergency department identify and isolate patients who may have tuberculosis. Abbreviations: TB = tuberculosis; INH = isoniazid; HCW = healthcare worker; AFB = acid-fast bacilli.

have included a copy of a screening questionnaire and algorithm (Figure 32-1) that we currently use in our emergency department, in our general medicine clinics, and in some subspecialty medicine clinics (ie, the clinics in which most of our patients with tuberculosis are seen).

Measles in Outpatient Healthcare Facilities

The incidence of measles in the United States has decreased substantially since the vaccine was introduced. However, measles continues to be transmitted within healthcare facilities.[39-46] Davis et al reported that 0.7% of measles cases from 1980 to 1982 were acquired in medical settings, and by 1982 that proportion had increased to 2.9%.[39] Istre et al identified 33 cases of measles that occurred in Oklahoma between September 1981 and August 1985,[40] of which 9 (27%) acquired their infection

in a physician's office or waiting room, and 6 secondary cases resulted from exposures to these patients. Thus, 15 (45%) of the patients acquired their infection directly or indirectly from an exposure in a medical office or a waiting room.

Data from several outbreaks confirm that measles virus frequently is transmitted in physicians' offices and emergency departments (Table 32-4). In 1990, 266 measles cases were identified in the state of Washington, which was more cases than had been identified in the previous 10 years.[41] Nearly half of the cases in the epidemic occurred among unvaccinated persons who should have been vaccinated. At least 17% of the infections were acquired through exposures in medical settings, including physicians' offices, hospital wards, and emergency rooms. Serosurveys in two hospitals determined that 7% of the employees lacked immunity to measles.

TABLE 32-4
OUTBREAKS CAUSED BY THE MEASLES VIRUS IN OUTPATIENT HEALTHCARE FACILITIES

Refs	Year*	Source	No. of Persons Affected	Type of Facility	Infection Control Error	Comments
45	1983 (1983)	Not identified	12	Medical clinic and community outbreak in Florida	Not specified	The outbreak occurred within the context of larger outbreak among migrant workers. A vaccination campaign helped terminate the outbreak
43	1984 (1984)	Other children with measles	17	Medical clinics	The office had no plan or procedures for isolating sick children	16 patients who acquired measles visited a physician's office at the same time as a source patient. The visits overlapped 20 to 90 min. One secondary case was seen 45 min after the source patient left the office
42	1985 (1981)	12-year-old boy with measles	8	Pediatric practice	The ventilation system recirculated air. The office had only one entrance/exit	Four patients had transient contact with the source patient when he entered or exited the waiting room, one patient had face-to-face contact with the source patient, and three patients were in the office 1 hr after the source patient left
46	1985 (1982)	7-month-old girl with measles	4	Pediatrician's office	The source patient, who had a febrile exanthem, was in the waiting room for 1 hour. Air was recirculated in the office	Eighty-four persons were exposed in the office on the day the source patient was seen, of whom 19 were <18 years old and had not been vaccinated. Three of four patients who became ill arrived in the clinic 60-75 min after the index case left

*The first year is the year the paper was published; the year in parentheses is the year in which the outbreak occurred.

In a similar outbreak in Hawaii, transmission of measles virus in physicians' offices accounted for 36% of cases in children less than 15 months of age and for 31% of cases in children less than 5 years of age.[43] Interviews with office staff indicated that procedures for isolating sick children from well children were not implemented well. "In many cases parents brought in their children complaining of high fever and rash without appointments and either had to wait in or pass through a common waiting room."[43] Transmission in physicians' offices was terminated after good isolation precautions were implemented.

A study published by Miranda et al documented that the problem of measles transmission in outpatient healthcare facilities also occurred outside of the United States.[44] These investigators noted that children less than 12 years of age who visited an emergency department were 4.1 times more likely to develop measles than were control patients who did not visit an emergency department ($P<.001$). Visits to private physician's offices were not associated significantly with acquisition of measles.[44]

Several infection control precautions can prevent measles transmission in medical settings: proper ventilation, infection control policies stipulating that all staff must be immune,[47] appropriate immunization protocols for patients, and prompt triage of patients who have febrile exanthems. Proper ventilation may be difficult to achieve in many outpatient settings, because buildings are built to be energy efficient, which often means the buildings are airtight, and the ventilation systems recirculate air.[42] In addition, because the incidence of measles is low, few healthcare workers recognize measles. Consequently, patients with measles may be misdiagnosed and may not be isolated appropriately.[41]

Appropriate triage begins with the telephone conversation during which clinic appointments are scheduled. The scheduler should ask the caller for the patient's chief complaint. If the patient has a fever and a rash, the appointment should be scheduled at the end of the day or during times of the day when few patients are present.[43] Patients who must come to the clinic when other patients are present should wear a mask, enter through a separate entrance, and go directly to an examination room. If negative-pressure rooms are not available, a large fan could be put in a window in the examination room to pull air out of the room. This makeshift solution can be used only if examination rooms have windows that can be opened, which may not be the case in many modern medical office buildings. If patients arrive unannounced at clinics or emergency departments, the staff at the registration desk should ask whether the patient has fever and a rash. If the answer to this question is yes, the patient should put on a mask and go to an examining room (preferably one with negative air pressure) immediately.

Rubella in Outpatient Medical Facilities

Outbreaks of rubella continue to occur sporadically in outpatient medical facilities, which are an important site for transmission of this virus. Several outbreaks of rubella have occurred among medical personnel and patients in outpatient clinics.[48-50] Several hundred pregnant women possibly were exposed in each of three outbreaks that we identified.[48] In one outbreak, two patients developed clinical rubella (3.6% attack rate among susceptible patients who had face-to-face contacts with an ill person), and subclinical cases were not detected in women who had follow-up serologic testing.[49] Healthcare workers acquired rubella in all three outbreaks.[48-50]

The most important preventive measure is to ensure that all staff and patients are immune to rubella. Staff members and patients who do not have antibody to rubella or who cannot provide proof that they were vaccinated should be vaccinated against rubella. Other important infection control precautions in the outpatient setting are described in the discussion of measles.

Epidemic Keratoconjunctivitis

Adenovirus, particularly type 8, has caused numerous outbreaks of keratoconjunctivitis in ophthalmology clinics (Table 32-5).[51-63] However, basic infection control precautions could prevent spread of this virus among patients and staff in those clinics. Infection control staff should ensure that their ophthalmology clinic and emergency departments have developed the following appropriate policies and procedures[56,64]:

- Healthcare workers should wash hands before and after examining patients.
- Healthcare workers should wear gloves for possible contact with the conjunctiva.[58,59,62]
- Equipment, including tonometers, should be cleaned and disinfected according to recommendations by the CDC,[59] the American Academy of Ophthalmology,[64] or the manufacturers. (Note that the methods for cleaning and disinfecting tonometers vary with the type of tonometer. Moreover, tonometers must be rinsed appropriately and thoroughly to prevent chemical keratitis).[65]
- If a nosocomial outbreak is identified, all open ophthalmic solutions should be discarded, and the equipment and environment should be cleaned and disinfected thoroughly.
- During an outbreak, unit doses of ophthalmic solutions should be used.[59]
- During outbreaks, patients with conjunctivitis should be examined in a separate room with designated equipment, supplies, and ophthalmic solutions.[59,60]
- During an outbreak, elective procedures such as tonometry should be postponed.
- Healthcare workers who work in any outpatient area and who have adenovirus conjunctivitis should not work until the inflammation has resolved, which may take 14 or more days.[59,62]

Other Transmissible Agents

Bordetella pertussis outbreaks in the community have spread to outpatient settings within hospitals.[66,67] Varicella-zoster virus, influenza virus, and parvovirus B19 all have been transmitted in the inpatient setting, and many exposures to VZV occur in clinics and physicians' offices. However, we did not find published descriptions of outbreaks in the ambulatory setting caused by VZV, influenza virus, or parvovirus B19. Outbreaks may in fact occur, but they might not be recognized, or persons who investigate them might not report them. The general infection control precautions recommended to prevent spread of measles and rubella will help prevent spread of these etiologic agents. Vaccines currently are available for all of these agents except for parvovirus B19.

Infection Control Issues Related to Devices

Infections Related to Bronchoscopic and Gastrointestinal Endoscopic Procedures Done in the Outpatient Setting

Eleven million endoscopic procedures are performed in the United States each year, many of which are done in the outpatient setting. Many inpatient healthcare facilities have bronchoscopy or gastrointestinal endoscopy suites that serve both inpatients and outpatients. Private physicians and physicians in freestanding clinics also do endoscopy in their offices. Moreover, the number and type of procedures performed and the number of patients undergoing these procedures continue to increase.

Given the nature of the procedures and the limitations of surveillance systems, infections associated with endoscopic procedures are very difficult to identify unless they occur in clusters. Despite these limitations, numerous investigators have reported outbreaks of infection related to endoscopic procedures. Most outbreaks could have been prevented if the endoscopy staff had followed basic infection control precautions and had cleaned, dis-

TABLE 32-5
OUTBREAKS OF EPIDEMIC KERATOCONJUNCTIVITIS CAUSED BY ADENOVIRUS IN OUTPATIENT HEALTHCARE FACILITIES

Refs	Year*	Duration of Outbreak	No. of Persons Affected	Type of Facility	Infection Control Error	Comments
51	1950 (1948)	6 wk	24	Ophthalmology office	Not specified	To control the outbreak, the physician and nurse implemented handwashing. Separate syringes and eye droppers were used for patients with conjunctivitis and then sterilized after use. Patients were instructed not to touch things in the office
53	1963 (1961)	Approximately 2 mo	26 patients and 1 physician	Ophthalmology and otolaryngology office	Probably poor compliance by physician with infection control precautions	Zero of 50 ENT patients and 21 of 98 patients who had ophthalmology procedures acquired EKC. No single piece of equipment could account for all cases. All procedures involved manipulation of the eyelid by the physician
54	1981 (1977)	7 wk	86 persons exposed in the office and 106 exposed in the community	Ophthalmology office and community	Not specified. The source case was a nurse who acquired EKC on vacation in Korea. She transmitted the virus to patients and staff in the nursing home in which she worked. These persons were seen by the ophthalmologist in his office. The environment in the office was contaminated with adenovirus type 8	Adenovirus type 8 caused the outbreak. The risk of EKC was increased as the number of invasive ophthalmic procedures increased. Four of seven ophthalmic solutions were contaminated. The outbreak ceased when infection control precautions were improved
55	1983 (1977–1978)	8 mo	83	Ophthalmology office	Not clear, but the environment was contaminated with adenovirus. The outbreak persisted despite improved infection control precautions, including increased handwashing and sterilizing instruments	Adenovirus type 37 caused part of the outbreak. The outbreak occurred in three clusters. Older patients and those who had tonometry were at higher risk of acquiring EKC. Work surfaces, solutions, instruments in the examination room, and mydriatic drops were contaminated
56	1984 (1981)	2 mo	39	Private ophthalmology clinic	Poor handwashing and possible failure to	Of persons seen in clinic, 1.8% acquired EKC. Risk factors were examination by two physicians,

Ref	Year*	No. of cases	Setting	Disinfection	Comments
60	1989 (1985-1986)	110 nosocomial (including 10 ophthalmologists, 3 nurses, 2 support staff; 291 community-acquired	Eye and ear infirmary	Not specified	sterilize ophthalmic equipment tonometry, or foreign body removal. The outbreak was terminated when physicians encouraged staff to wash their hands. The overall attack rate among clinic patients was 4.7 per 1,000 visits. All nosocomial cases were adenovirus type 8; community-acquired cases were caused by adenovirus types 8 and 37. Standard infection control precautions did not interrupt transmission. Stringent measures were required to terminate nosocomial spread
58	1989 (1987-1988)	63 patients, 3 physicians	Ophthalmology clinic in a university medical center	Inadequate handwashing. Staff followed the manufacturer's recommendations to disinfect the pneumotonometer with 70% isopropyl alcohol, which has limited activity against adenovirus 8 and is not a high-level disinfectant	Of patients seen in epidemic period, 17% were affected. Risk factors were exposure to the pneumotonometer and to one healthcare worker. The outbreak was terminated by removing the pneumotonometer from use and increasing compliance with handwashing and glove use
63	1996 (1991)	41	Ophthalmology emergency room	Not specified	Specific infection control measures were developed for patients with viral conjunctivitis. Control measures included designating a room for examination and treatment of patients with conjunctivitis
61	1991 (1986-1987)	At least 132	Eye clinic and the community	Not specified	Of all cases, 85% could be traced to patients who were seen in the eye clinic within 3 to 4 wk of the onset of EKC. Most persons who acquired nosocomial EKC came to the clinic for cataract surgery or for glaucoma follow-up
62	1993 (1986)	126	Outpatient clinic	Inadequate disinfection of instruments, especially pneumotonometers; physicians used inadequate precautions to prevent contamination of their hands	The attack rate was 7%. Risk factors for EKC were pneumotonometry, numerous clinic visits, and contact with an infected physician. Handwashing did not remove adenovirus from hands reliably

ENT = ear, nose, and throat; EKC = epidemic keratoconjunctivitis.
*The first year is the year the paper was published; the year in parentheses is the year in which the outbreak occurred.

infected, and maintained the equipment properly. Thus, infection control personnel should familiarize themselves with the procedures, equipment, current recommendations and guidelines,[68-70] and problems reported in the literature,[71-73] so that they can help endoscopy personnel prevent rather than ameliorate problems.

Fiberoptic endoscopes have allowed physicians to do procedures that are not possible with rigid endoscopes. However, flexible endoscopes present problems not encountered with rigid endoscopes. The most important problem is that flexible endoscopes are very difficult to clean and disinfect because they have several long, narrow internal channels and because they cannot be steam sterilized. Consequently, endoscopes must be reprocessed by persons who understand the internal structure of the devices and who take the time necessary to clean and disinfect these devices meticulously. Although professional societies have published guidelines for reprocessing endoscopes,[68-70] the protocols used for those procedures have not been standardized,[74,75] and different endoscopes must be reprocessed by different methods. Moreover, because endoscopes are very expensive, endoscopy staff may try to save money by using a small number of endoscopes to evaluate and treat a large number of patients. Staff may not be able to process the equipment properly in the time allowed between patients.[76]

The American Society for Gastrointestinal Endoscopy's Technology Assessment Committee estimates that the incidence of infection transmitted by gastrointestinal endoscopic procedures is 1 in 1.8 million procedures.[69] The committee evaluated 28 episodes of transmission that occurred after specific guidelines on cleaning and disinfection of gastrointestinal endoscopes were published. The committee concluded that, in each of the 28 episodes, recommended cleaning or disinfecting procedures had been breached or equipment (eg, endoscopy accessories or an automated endoscope reproces-

sor) was contaminated.[69] In addition, certain procedures, particularly those involving biopsies and those that examine the biliary tree, have higher risks of transmitting infection than do other less-invasive procedures.

Spach et al reviewed articles published in English between 1966 and July 1992, to identify episodes in which infectious agents were transmitted by gastrointestinal endoscopy or by bronchoscopy.[71] These authors identified 281 infections transmitted by gastrointestinal endoscopy and 96 that were transmitted by bronchoscopy.[71] Gastrointestinal endoscopic procedures have transmitted several serotypes of *Salmonella*[71] including *Salmonella typhimurium*[77] and *Salmonella newport*,[78] *Pseudomonas aeruginosa*,[79-82] several species of *Enterobacteriaceae*,[79] *Helicobacter pylori*,[83,84] HBV,[85] *Trichosporon beigelii*,[86] and *Strongyloides stercoralis*.[71] Bronchoscopes have transmitted *M tuberculosis*,[87] multidrug-resistant *M tuberculosis*,[33] *Mycobacterium avium*,[87] *Mycobacterium chelonae*,[88-90] *Mycobacterium gordonae*,[91] other nontuberculous mycobacteria,[71,73] *P aeruginosa*,[92] *Pseudomonas pseudomallei*,[71] *Pseudomonas putida*,[93] *Rhodotorula rubra*,[94] *Sporothrix cyanescens*,[73] and *Blastomyces dermatitidis*.[73] To date, endoscopes have not been documented to transmit HIV.

Tables 32-3, 32-6, and 32-7 describe several outbreaks associated with endoscopy. Readers who want to review tables describing outbreaks associated only with endoscopy should read the review articles by Spach,[71] Ayliffe,[72] and Weber and Rutala.[73] Factors that have allowed flexible endoscopes to transmit pathogenic organisms have included the following:

- Failure to clean and disinfect the blind channel in endoscopes used to examine the biliary tree.[79]
- Failure to disinfect endoscopes and accessory equipment (eg, suction-collection bottles, rubber connection tubing) properly between procedures.[77,82-84]

- Failure to sterilize biopsy forceps.[78,83]
- Failure to dry endoscopes completely before storage.[80]
- Failure to wash endoscopes before disinfecting them.[92]
- Use of contaminated water.[80]
- Use of tap water to rinse endoscopes.[81,89]
- Use of unfiltered tap water in automatic endoscope washers.[95]
- Improper maintenance with subsequent contamination of automatic endoscope washers.[93]
- Use of inadequate disinfectants.[84]
- Use of contaminated suction valves.[87]
- Use of endoscopes with internal defects that prevent adequate cleaning and disinfection.[90]

Despite numerous reports of outbreaks, endoscopy suites often do not reprocess endoscopes properly. Several surveys conducted in different countries document that staff in many endoscopy suites continue to make the same errors that have caused the outbreaks listed above.[75,76,96-100] Many endoscopy staff apparently do not understand standard precautions. The staff often do not employ high-level disinfection to reprocess endoscopes used for patients who were presumed not to have infections,[96] but they employ special cleaning and disinfecting procedures, including sterilization, for endoscopes used for patients known to be infected by agents such as HIV, HBV, or *M tuberculosis*.[97,99]

An observational study conducted by Kaczmarek et al confirmed the results of the mailed surveys.[97] These investigators identified one ambulatory endoscopy center whose staff did not use any disinfecting agent when processing gastrointestinal endoscopes![97] In addition, these authors obtained cultures from reprocessed endoscopes. Twenty-four percent of samples grew 100,000 or more colonies, indicating that the disinfection processes often were not efficacious.[97]

The policies and procedures needed in an endoscopy suite for infection control, cleaning, and disinfection are not more complicated or substantially different from those needed in other healthcare settings. However, the procedures must be followed precisely, because patients undergoing endoscopic procedures may be particularly vulnerable to infections, and because endoscopes are such complex semicritical instruments that they are difficult to clean even when the staff reprocess these devices conscientiously.[101] In addition, infection control staff might be intimidated by the complexity of the endoscopes and the automatic endoscope washers or by the cleaning and disinfection process. To overcome these barriers, infection control staff should read the published recommendations for cleaning and disinfecting endoscopes[68-70] and should understand the basic principles of disinfection and sterilization.[102] Infection control staff also should spend time in the endoscopy suite to learn from the staff and to identify potential infection control problems. Together, staff from both programs should review the policies and procedures to ensure that they are consistent with current recommendations and guidelines and that they are consistent in intent and application throughout the healthcare facility.

Infection control personnel should be aware that new ion plasma, vaporized hydrogen peroxide, and 100% ethylene oxide sterilizers do not reliably kill organisms in narrow lumens when serum and salt are present.[103,104] Thus, these methods may not be adequate for processing flexible endoscopes, especially if they have not been cleaned scrupulously. Infection control personnel should discuss with staff in the endoscopy suite the limitations of these technologies and, at present, probably should discourage their use in this setting.

Endoscopy clinics that are not a part of a larger medical center may not have direct access to infection control personnel or to training in infection control. Regardless of the endoscopy suite's location, staff must be trained to clean and disinfect endoscopes meticulously. The endoscopy staff also

TABLE 32-6
OUTBREAKS CAUSED BY *PSEUDOMONAS* SPECIES IN OUTPATIENT HEALTHCARE FACILITIES

Refs	Year*	Type of Infection	Organism	Duration of Outbreak	Source	No. of Persons Affected	Type of Facility	Infection Control Error	Comments
140	NS (1977)	Septic arthritis	*Pseudomonas cepacia*	Not applicable	Contaminated MDV	1	Medicine clinic	Not determined	Two multidose vials of methylprednisolone were contaminated
141	NP (1991-1992)	Pseudosinusitis	*Pseudomonas pickettii*	6 mo	Contaminated distilled water	4	Otolaryngology clinic	Nonsterile distilled water was used to reconstitute crystalline ephedrine	Use of sterile water to reconstitute the crystalline ephedrine terminated the outbreak
142	1993 (1991)	Bacteremia	*P (Burkholderia) cepacia*	Approximately 2 wk	Contaminated 500-mL intravenous bag of 5% dextrose used to make heparin flush solutions	14	Oncology clinic	One bag of 5% dextrose was used to make the heparin flush solutions between 8/7 and 8/21. The source from which the 5% dextrose solution was contaminated was not identified	The only patients who acquired *P cepacia* bloodstream infections had central venous catheters ($P < .001$). Only clinic visits in which the catheters were flushed were associated with bacteremia ($P < .001$). All 14 patients were hospitalized for treatment of the infections (median 17 days). Ribotyping documented that the isolates from the patients and from the 5% dextrose solution were the same strain
93	1996 (1995)	Pseudo-pneumonia	*Pseudomonas putida*	1 mo	Bronchoscopes and the bronchoscope washer	4	Pulmonary clinic	Improper maintenance of the bronchoscope washer	The enzymatic detergent used in the bronchoscope washer was not discarded every day. The detergent tub remained wet. Glutaraldehyde

No.	Year	Infection	Organism	Duration	Device/Source	Comments 1	Location	No. affected	Comments 2
						treatment for 20 min could not kill the large number of *P putida* contaminating the bronchoscopes			
143	1996 (1995)	Urinary tract infection	*Pseudomonas aeruginosa*	>6 wk	Urodynamic transducers	Urodynamic transducers that were designed for single use were reused. The disinfection process was inadequate	Urodynamic suite	25	Transducers, connecting tubing, and irrigation bags were reused to save money. The disinfection procedure consisted of flushing and soaking the tubing and transducer with Cidex between patients. Reflux of urine from the catheter into the connecting tubing and transducer was noted occasionally during the procedure. A culture from the transducer's connector revealed ciprofloxacin-resistant *P aeruginosa* that was identical by PFGE to the isolates obtained from patients
144	1996 (1992)	Endophthalmitis	*P aeruginosa*, coagulase-negative staphylococci	1 d	Irrigation solutions were contaminated with *P aeruginosa*	The solution was contaminated in the pharmacy, but the mode of contamination was not identified. Common solutions were used for numerous patients	Hospital eye department	13	Intravitreal cultures from four patients grew *P aeruginosa*, from three patients grew coagulase-negative staphylococci, and from three patients were negative

MDV = multidose vials; NP = not published; NS = not specified; PFGE = pulsed-field gel electrophoresis.
*The first year is the year the paper was published; the year in parentheses is the year in which the outbreak occurred.

TABLE 32-7
OUTBREAKS CAUSED BY OTHER AGENTS IN OUTPATIENT HEALTHCARE FACILITIES

Refs	Year*	Type of Infection	Organism	Outbreak Duration	Source	No. of Persons Affected	Type of Facility	Infection Control Error	Comments
145	1976 (1975)	Infectious mononucleosis	EBV	1 mo	Not identified	29	Obstetric and gynecology clinic	Unclear	Close salivary contact was proposed as the most likely route of infection for some patients Airborne dissemination of EBV may have occurred
146	1982 (1978–1980)	Amebic colitis	Entamoeba histolytica	21 mo	Colonic irrigation therapy	36	Chiropractic clinic	The machine had a common tube for inflow of irrigant and outflow of fecal material Consequently, the machine became contaminated with feces The machine and tubing were not cleaned adequately or sterilized between patients	Six patients died
147	1982 (1981)	Soft-tissue abscesses	Group A streptococcus	3 days	Contaminated MDV of DPT vaccine	7	Pediatric clinic	Not identified	Other MDVs in the lot were not contaminated Therefore, the implicated vial must have become contaminated during use
148	1983 (1978)	Pyrogenic reactions	Acinetobacter calcoaceticus	1 wk	Heparin solution contaminated with A calcoaceticus	16	Private dialysis center	Not identified Staff probably used poor aseptic technique when diluting heparin	Diluted heparin solutions were prepared by adding commercially prepared heparin to 0.9% sodium A laboratory experiment suggested the dilute heparin solution was contaminated during the process of withdrawing heparin from the vials and injecting it into the bags of saline Solutions were stored at

149	1985 (1982)	Subcutaneous abscesses	Group A streptococcus	2 days and 14 days, respectively	Contaminated MDV of DTP	12 in one office, 7 in another office	Two private pediatric offices	Not identified	room temperature, which could have allowed the bacteria to multiply The cases were children (12/17 and 7/7) vaccinated consecutively with DTP vaccine
150	1987 (1982)	Wound infection, abscesses, osteomyelitis	*Proteus mirabilis*	1 mo	Three bone drills	6	Private podiatrists' office	The Anprolene gas-bag method used to sterilize the drills was ineffective, possibly because lubricant and other material was present on the drill	All patients had undergone osteotomies Three drills were contaminated with *P mirabilis* and with other Gram-negative organisms The lubricant used for the drills supported the growth of *P mirabilis* The drills served as the reservoir from which *P mirabilis* either was inoculated directly into the wound or was transferred to the hands of the surgeon, who then contaminated the wound The outbreak ended after the drills were thoroughly disinfected and sterilized in ethylene oxide
151	1987 (1981-1982)	Septic arthritis	*Serratia marcescens*	2 days in 12/81 and 5 days in 1/82	MDV and cotton balls soaked in benzalkonium chloride and two partially used MDVs of methylprednisolone	10 patients had definite infections and 1 had a possible infection	Orthopedic office	Cotton balls were soaked in benzalkonium chloride and then used to wipe off the tops of MDVs of lidocaine and methylprednisolone and to prepare the skin at the injection site	The infections were associated with previous joint injections of lidocaine and methylprednisolone The outbreak terminated after the staff stopped soaking cotton balls in benzalkonium chloride
94	1989 (NS)	Pseudo-	*Rhodotorula*	>3 mo	Cleaning	30	Pulmonary clinic	Failure to disinfect	

TABLE 32-7 (continued)
OUTBREAKS CAUSED BY OTHER AGENTS IN OUTPATIENT HEALTHCARE FACILITIES

Refs	Year*	Type of Infection	Organism	Outbreak Duration	Source	No. of Persons Affected	Type of Facility	Infection Control Error	Comments
		pneumonia	rubra		brushes for internal cannula of bronchoscope			contaminated equipment	
152	1990 (1985)	Pneumonia	Legionella pneumophila	>6 mo	Ventilation chiller unit	103	Outpatient department	Design flaws in the ventilation system allowed L pneumophila in the chiller unit to be aerosolized	Twenty-two patients died
153	1990 (1988)	Hypotension	Sodium azide	1 d	The water was contaminated with sodium azide	9	Dialysis unit	Four ultrafilters, which were not rinsed before they were used, were installed in the water treatment system 12 h before the outbreak The ultrafilters were preserved with sodium azide mixed with glycerine High levels of total organic carbons were detected in dialysis water at point-of-use sites at the time of the outbreak, which was consistent with contamination by sodium azide and glycerine	Nine of nine treatments during the epidemic day compared with 0 of 238 treatments between Sep 1 and Nov 2 were associated with hypotension within 30 min after starting dialysis

Ref	Year	Infection	Pathogen	Duration	Source	No.	Setting	Findings	Comments
154	1992 (1988-1990)	Bacteremia	Gram-negative bacteria and *Enterococcus casseliflavus*	2 yr	The blood tubing became contaminated with ultrafiltrate waste when the dialyzer was set up	2	Hemodialysis unit in a military hospital	The venous tubing was attached to the waste container while the membrane was primed	The outbreak was terminated by stopping this practice, emphasizing the need to change gloves and wash hands after contact with ultrafiltrate waste, and decontaminating the ultrafiltrate waste bag daily
118	1992 (1987-1988)	Hepatitis	Hepatitis C	22 mo	Not identified	27	Outpatient dialysis unit associated with a university hospital	A common source and person-to-person spread could not be documented. Numerous errors in infection control technique were identified	The outbreak terminated when the staff implemented infection control precautions designed to prevent the spread of bloodborne pathogens in dialysis units
155	1993 (1988)	Bacteremia	Gram-negative bacteria	9 mo	Dialysis O-rings	11	Outpatient hemodialysis unit associated with a university	The standard automated method of disinfecting Hemoflow F-80 (Fresenius AG Bad Homburg, Germany) dialyzers did not disinfect the O-rings adequately	Cultures of the O-rings grew the organisms causing the outbreak. The outbreak ceased when the dialyzers were disassembled and the O-rings were disinfected completely
156	1993 (1988)	Bacteremia (5) and pyrogenic reactions (9)	Endotoxin and *Pseudomonas (Burkholderia) cepacia*, *Xanthomonas maltophilia*, and *Alcaligenes denitrificans* sp *xylosoxidans*	16 days	Contaminated dialyzers	11	Freestanding hemodialysis center	The technician who prepared the 2.5% Renalin (Minntech, Minneapolis, MN) disinfectant solution did not mix the solution adequately. The levels of disinfectant were low and did not disinfect the dialyzers well. Dialyzers were	The rate of bacteremia or pyrogenic reactions was 4.5 per 100 sessions in which reprocessed dialyzers were used and 0 per 100 sessions in which new dialyzers were used (*P*=.03)

TABLE 32-7 (continued)
OUTBREAKS CAUSED BY OTHER AGENTS IN OUTPATIENT HEALTHCARE FACILITIES

Refs	Year*	Type of Infection	Organism	Outbreak Duration	Source	No. of Persons Affected	Type of Facility	Infection Control Error	Comments
									contaminated with high levels of endotoxin and bacteria (*B cepacia, Pseudomonas paucimobilis, Pseudomonas pickettii,* and *Alcaligenes* sp)
157	1996 (1993)	Endophthalmitis	*Acremonium kiliense*	>1 mo	Ventilation system	4	Ambulatory surgery center	The ventilation system was turned on 5-30 min before procedures began on the first operative day of the week. The air was filtered before it was humidified but not thereafter. Turning the ventilation system on aerosolized a reservoir of *A kiliense*	Compared with control patients, case patients all had surgery on the first operative day of the week or had surgery significantly sooner after the operating room reopened. *A kiliense* that was phenotypically identical to the case patients' isolates was isolated from the humidifier water. One patient required enucleation of the affected eye
158	1997 (1996)	Culture-negative peritonitis in patients treated with CCPD	Endotoxin	5 wk	Dialysate contaminated with high levels of endotoxin	73	Peritoneal dialysis patients in five states	Not specified	The product, which was contaminated with high levels of endotoxin, was distributed to numerous states. Endotoxin levels in dialysate were determined before the solutions were sterilized. This procedure may not reflect the levels after sterilization accurately

EBV = Epstein-Barr virus; DPT = diphtheria-pertussis-tetanus; NS = not specified; CCPD = continuous cyclic peritoneal dialysis.
*The first year is the year the paper was published; the year in parentheses is the year in which the outbreak occurred.

should understand basic principles of infection control, including methods for preventing transmission of routine bacterial pathogens to patients and to staff, methods for preventing spread of bloodborne pathogens, and methods for cleaning and disinfection. One person should be responsible to ensure that staff are educated properly, that they always comply with the specified procedures, and that all equipment is handled and maintained properly.

Disposable Devices

With the increased pressure for cost containment, healthcare workers and administrators are questioning why many devices marketed for single use cannot be reprocessed and reused. This issue is not unique to the outpatient setting, but, in this setting, the pressure to reuse single-use items might be greater, or the infection control oversight might be substantially less than in the inpatient setting. Examples of single-use items that often are reused in the outpatient setting include syringes, plastic vaginal specula, mouthpieces for pulmonary function machines, cardiac catheters, and oral airways. An ambulatory healthcare facility that chooses to reprocess single-use devices must develop a comprehensive quality-assurance program to ensure that the products are cleaned, disinfected, or sterilized adequately and that the items retain their integrity and function.[105] Institutions that reprocess those devices, not the manufacturers, assume the liability. Thus, infection control personnel would be wise to identify which single-use products are being reused and to ensure that the devices are reprocessed and tested for function and integrity appropriately. Readers interested in a more in-depth discussion of this topic should read the recent review by Green.[106]

Flash Sterilization of Surgical Equipment

Steam sterilization of patient-care items for immediate use, or "flash sterilization," was designed to process items that had become contaminated during a sterile procedure but were essential for that procedure. The time required for flash sterilization is very short. Thus, all of the parameters (eg, time, temperature) must be met precisely. The persons doing flash sterilization must keep meticulous records to document that these parameters have been met. In addition, flash sterilization will not work if the device is contaminated with organic matter or if air is trapped in or around the device. The efficacy of flash sterilization also will be impaired if either the sterilizer or the flash pack are not working properly. Moreover, because the devices are used immediately (ie, before the results of biological indicators are known), personnel in ambulatory surgery centers that use flash sterilization must record which devices were used for specific patients, so that they can be followed if the load was not processed properly.

Many institutions have expanded the use of flash sterilization well beyond its intended and approved uses. Some of the changes are reasonable, but some jeopardize the efficacy of sterilization. In particular, staff in ambulatory surgery centers that do numerous procedures in a day and that try to keep their costs low by maintaining a low overhead, including a limited inventory of equipment, may be inadvertently or intentionally stretching the limits of flash sterilization. Infection control professionals whose outpatient facilities use flash sterilization should read two pertinent publications by the Association for the Advancement of Medical Instrumentation (AAMI).[107,108] Infection control professionals then should assess whether their institution is using this process properly.

Other Infection Control Issues in the Outpatient Setting

Multidose Vials

Multidose vials are used frequently in the inpatient and outpatient setting, because they may be more convenient and cheaper than single-dose vials. Studies in the literature indicate that 0% to 27% of used multidose vials are contaminated with bacterial pathogens.[109] However, the studies that reported high rates of contamination were conducted before 1973. Subsequently, the reported contamination rates have been much lower (0.5%-0.6%). In another study, 1 of 69 multidose vials was contaminated with red blood cells.[110]

Although the actual risk of infection associated with multidose vials remains unknown, the risk of infection appears to be low if multidose vials are used properly. However, staff in a busy outpatient clinic might not adhere to appropriate infection control precautions. Indeed, numerous outbreaks in such clinics attest to the fact that multidose vials can be an important reservoir or vehicle for bacterial and viral pathogens (Tables 32-1, 32-5 through 32-8). Although infections and outbreaks of infections occur rarely, the consequences of such infections can be catastrophic.

Vancomycin-Resistant Enterococci

Vancomycin-resistant enterococci (VRE) are spread on the hands of personnel and by contaminated patient-care equipment or environmental surfaces. Consequently, the organisms could be spread in both the inpatient and outpatient settings. Infection control personnel, therefore, must work across the spectrum of healthcare settings (ie, inpatient units, central surgical suites, ambulatory surgical centers, endoscopy suites, hospital-based and freestanding ambulatory clinics, long-term care facilities, and home care) if they want to control the spread of these organisms effectively. In addition, recent media reports about "super bugs" have heightened the public's awareness and concern about these organisms. Hence, infection control personnel probably will have to answer many questions and do much education in the outpatient setting. To help infection control professionals who must answer those questions, we have included a copy of a question-and-answer sheet that we developed for healthcare workers (Table 32-9) and a pamphlet (Figure 32-2) that we use to educate

patients, family members, and staff in external healthcare agencies.

Efforts to control VRE in the outpatient setting will cross disciplines, departments, and organizations. Hence, these efforts may be very difficult to coordinate. Personnel who should be involved in, or at least informed about, these efforts include nurses, schedulers, and triage staff in the various units or institutions, the administrators of each program, office managers, microbiologists, laboratory technologists, phlebotomists, housekeeping staff, staff in the purchasing department, and infection control personnel in other facilities.

Many of the following precautions recommended for inpatient care of patients with VRE are appropriate for outpatient clinics or surgery centers[111]:

- Patients should be placed in contact isolation immediately, which means they should not wait in the waiting room but should be placed in an examination room as soon as they come to the clinic.
- If possible, the floor of the room should be linoleum or vinyl, not carpet, and the furniture should be washable (eg, plastic or vinyl), so it can be decontaminated.
- Reusable equipment (eg, stethoscopes, scissors) must be decontaminated before use on other patients. Alternatively, disposable items (eg, blood pressure cuffs) may be used.
- If the patient spends substantial time in the room or has an infected wound or diarrhea, the room and all permanent equipment in the room must be cleaned thoroughly before another patient may be placed in the room. If the patient is only in the room for a short time and the site of infection or colonization is contained, the items with which the patient had direct contact should be cleaned thoroughly before another patient is placed in the room.
- Ideally, all healthcare workers should wear gowns and gloves when they enter the room and must wash their hands with chlorhexi-

TABLE 32-8

INFECTIONS CAUSED BY NONTUBERCULOUS MYCOBACTERIA IN THE OUTPATIENT SETTING

Refs	Year*	Type of Infection	Organism	Duration of Outbreak	Source of the Outbreak	No. of Persons Affected	Type of Facility	Infection Control Error†	Comments
132	1969 (1966)	Soft-tissue abscesses	*Mycobacterium abscessus*	14 mo	Contaminated histamine solution	12	Outpatient otolaryngology clinic	Actual source was not identified; however, staff put new sterile needles on used disposable syringes to obtain histamine from MDV	Four MDVs from the same lot numbers were found at other clinics Cultures of those MDVs were negative, suggesting that the vaccine was not contaminated intrinsically
133	1973 (1969)	Soft-tissue abscesses	*Mycobacterium chelonae*	7 mo	Contaminated diphtheria, pertussis, tetanus, polio vaccine	50	Health clinic	Syringes and needles were sterilized by boiling A different syringe and needle was used for each child A common needle was used to remove the vaccine from the MDV The needle was left in the stopper of current MDV and transferred to the next vial	
134	1980 (NA)	Subcutaneous abscess	*M chelonae*	NA	Contaminated glass syringe	1	Patient's home	Inactive disinfectant	The patient boiled the glass syringe weekly and stored the syringe in hypochlorite, which she made twice weekly

TABLE 32-8 (continued)
Infections Caused by Nontuberculous Mycobacteria in the Outpatient Setting

Refs	Year*	Type of Infection	Organism	Duration of Outbreak	Source of the Outbreak	No. of Persons Affected	Type of Facility	Infection Control Error	Comments
									She often used boiling water to make the hypochlorite The boiling water would have inactivated the disinfectant by driving off the chlorine
135	1984 (1979)	Keratitis	M chelonae	3 y	No common source identified	3	Ophthalmology clinic	The break in technique was not identified, but possibilities included contamination of ophthalmologic solutions or cocaine anesthetics and inadequate disinfection of instruments	The investigation was conducted 9-17 mo after the exposures Instruments (eg, the needle-knife and forceps) were soaked in benzalkonium chloride, a disinfectant that can support the growth of nontuberculous mycobacteria
136	1988 (1987)	Otitis media	M abscessus that was highly resistant to aminoglycosides	4 mo	Otologic instruments	17	Otolaryngology clinic	Otologic instruments were not treated with high-level disinfection or sterilization but were cleaned with tap water and a liquid detergent The water and detergent were changed weekly	Risk factors were having the ear canal suctioned more than once and undergoing at least five ear examinations M chelonae that was highly resistant to aminoglycosides was identified in tap water

	Year[*]	Infection	Organism	Duration	Source/vehicle	No.	Setting	Findings	Comments
137	1990 (1988)	Subcutaneous abscess	*M abscessus*	4 mo	A gallon jug used to store distilled water	8	Podiatric clinic	The jet injector used to administer lidocaine was not treated with a high-level disinfectant but was held between procedures in a mixture of distilled water and a quaternary ammonium disinfectant	The original source of the *M abscessus* was not identified Tap water specimens did not yield this organism
138	1996 (1995)	Bacteremia and prostatic abscess	Rapidly growing mycobacterium	NS	Prostatic biopsy probe and ultrasound probe	2	Urology office	The biopsy probe tip was covered with a rubber sheath filled with tap water The tap water in the syringe was changed weekly or when cloudy The biopsy forceps were extended through a separate channel, but occasionally the sheaths leaked or ruptured during procedures	Rapidly growing mycobacteria were isolated from water obtained from a syringe used with the biopsy probe and with a separate ultrasound probe The outbreak was terminated when sterile water was used
139	1996 (1996)	Subcutaneous abscess	*M abscessus*	10 mo	Adrenal cortex extract injections	54	Medical clinic	Administration of non–FDA-approved products that were contaminated intrinsically	Patients in several states were treated by a physician to induce weight loss

MDV = multidose vials; NA = not applicable; NS = not specified.
The first year is the year the paper was published; the year in parentheses is the year in which the outbreak occurred.

Vancomycin-resistant enterococci (VRE) are organisms that are carried in the gastrointestinal tract (gut). A stool culture or rectal swab may detect this organism. VRE can cause bloodstream, urinary tract, and wound infections. People who are more prone to carry VRE are those who are immunocompromised, such as a person who has had a transplant, received chemotherapy, or has been on many antibiotics for a long period of time. Other persons at risk include those who have spent long periods of time in the intensive care unit. Because this organism is resistant to certain medications, VRE can be very difficult to treat if an infection occurs.

HOW IS VRE SPREAD?
VRE spread occurs mainly by the hands and on objects that you may touch frequently such as door knobs and tabletops. VRE can live on environmental surfaces for long periods of time.

WHAT CAN I DO TO PREVENT THE SPREAD OF VRE?
Always wear gloves when performing wound care or line care. If you are being cared for at home by family members or a home health nurse, they should wear gloves and gowns when doing these same procedures or for close physical contact. It is very important to wash your hands before and after these procedures. Leisure activities, such as watching TV and eating, do not require these precautions.

ARE THERE SPECIAL SOAPS OR LOTIONS THAT I SHOULD USE?
A special soap with an ingredient called chlorhexidine 4% (such as Hibiclens) or a soap with 60% alcohol (Alcare) is available from your local pharmacist without a prescription. This should be used every time you wash your hands, especially after you use the restroom. You also should use these products before and after performing colostomy care or any dressing changes.

CAN I GO OUTSIDE MY HOME WITH VRE?
Yes, but you should wash your hands **very** well before you leave your home and while you are out if you use the restroom or provide wound or line care.

WHAT SHOULD I USE TO CLEAN MY HOME ENVIRONMENT?
You should use a Lysol-type product to clean surfaces in your home at least twice a week. If you will be sharing a bathroom with other family members, it should be cleaned on a daily basis. Laundry items, such as linens, towels, etc, should be washed in hot soapy water.

CAN I HAVE VISITORS AT HOME?
Yes, but you should suggest to anyone who has had any of the following problems to delay their visit: recent major surgery (such as a transplant, open heart surgery), chemotherapy, or taking antibiotics either currently, in the recent past, or long term. This special group needs to wear a gown and gloves while in your home. They should wash their hands with the special soap before leaving.

HOW LONG WILL I HAVE VRE?
No one knows for sure. Some people can carry VRE in their gut for up to 1 year. When you come back to the hospital for admission or for a clinic visit, let the staff know that you have VRE. A swab will be obtained from stool or your rectal area to determine if you still have the resistant organism.

IF YOU HAVE FURTHER QUESTIONS REGARDING VRE, YOU SHOULD CONTACT YOUR PHYSICIAN.

Prepared by:
C. Carter, RN, Program of Hospital Epidemiology
M. Jensen, RN, Department of Surgery

FIGURE 32-2. We use this pamphlet to educate patients, family members, and staff in external agencies about vancomycin-resistant enterococci.

dine or an alcohol product before leaving the room. If the patient's site of infection or colonization is contained, healthcare workers who will have only minimal contact with the patient may wear gloves but do not need to wear a gown.

• To alert healthcare workers when the patient goes to other clinic visits or is admitted, the patients' paper medical records could be labeled with "resistant organism stickers," and their computerized records could be marked with warnings.

To help infection control personnel who must develop policies for their outpatient settings, we have included a copy of the policy that we use in our clinics (Table 32-10).

Medical Waste in the Outpatient Setting

Like hospitals, healthcare facilities and agencies that operate in the ambulatory setting produce infectious wastes. However, these institutions may not have an expert in waste management on their staff, and they may not have ready access to appropriate processing (eg, autoclaves) and disposal facilities (eg, incinerators). In addition, because these facilities often operate for profit, staff might feel pressured to take shortcuts.

An in-depth discussion of medical waste is beyond the scope of this chapter. Readers who must develop waste-management programs for outpatient facilities should read several excellent reviews of this topic.[102,112,113] We will review a few

TABLE 32-9
QUESTIONS AND ANSWERS ABOUT VANCOMYCIN-RESISTANT ENTEROCOCCUS (VRE)

Q. Is a 10-minute handwash required after caring for a VRE patient?

A. A 10-minute handwash is not required. What is required is thorough handwashing with either a 4% chlorhexidine (Hibiclens, Stuart Pharmaceuticals, Wilmington, Del) or 60% isopropyl alcohol hand wash preparation. If forearms become contaminated wash them as well.

Q. How many people may care for a VRE patient?

A. If the care given to the patient requires physical contact, then one-to-one nursing is the standard. If the care given requires manipulation of intravenous lines, passing of medication, or other nonphysical contact, any qualified healthcare worker (HCW) may provide the care. If physical contact with the patient or the patient's immediate environment (eg, overbed table, linens, bedrails etc.) is needed, the primary nurse should provide the care.

Q. What type of isolation is required?

A. Contact isolation is required. All persons entering the room must use a gown and gloves. All persons exiting the room must wash their hands as described above. The door may be open or shut.

Q. How long do patients have to stay in isolation?

A. Once patients have been identified, they must remain in special organism isolation for the duration of their hospital stay or until three consecutive negative stool or perirectal cultures, which were obtained at least 1 week apart, were negative. Patients whose cultures remain positive at discharge may be cultured during clinic visits to determine whether they are no longer carrying the organism.

Q. What if a patient who was colonized or infected with VRE and then had three negative cultures is readmitted subsequently?

A. This patient would require a private room and either Hibiclens or a 60% alcohol handwashing preparation. A stool culture should be obtained. If the culture results are negative, routine care can be used; if the culture is positive, special organism isolation precautions must be used for the duration of the hospital stay.

Q. What is the protocol for a patient who has to go out of the room?

A. The HCW must gown and glove in the patient's room. The patient is moved to a cart or wheelchair. A clean sheet is placed on the patient. The HCW should remove gloves and gown and wash hands. The HCW should put on a clean gown and gloves outside the room and transport the patient.

Q. Can patients ambulate in the hall?

A. It is preferable that patients not ambulate in the hallways of units where immunocompromised patients are housed. For patients who must ambulate, the patient first should wash hands with 4% chlorhexidine and then put on a clean gown and gloves. The primary nurse for the patient should accompany the patient to ensure that the handrails, doorknobs, elevator buttons, etc, are not touched. The patient should wash his or her hands after removing the gloves.

Q. Do patients with VRE require isolation trays for meals?

A. No, patients do not require isolation trays.

Q. Are head covers or booties required?

A. Head covers are not required. Booties or shoe covers typically are not required, unless the patient has profuse diarrhea or is incontinent of stool.

Q. How should patient equipment be handled?

A. Equipment such as stethoscopes, wheelchairs, etc, should remain in the patient room. Any equipment (eg, glucometer, Doppler, x-ray machine) that must be used on other patients should be wiped down with a hospital-approved disinfectant (Virex, SC Johnson & Son Inc, Racine, WI) and allowed a 10-minute contact time before the item can be used for other patients.

Q. How often should the room be cleaned?

A. The rooms should be cleaned twice per day, usually once on the day shift and once on the evening shift. After the patient has been discharged, housekeeping will utilize a clean-reclean method.

Q. What about discharge planning?

A. A nurse epidemiologist or designee is available on beeper to answer any questions and to assist with discharge planning for a patient with VRE.

TABLE 32-10

CLINIC VISITS FOR PATIENTS INFECTED OR COLONIED WITH VANCOMYCIN-RESISTANT *ENTEROCOCCUS*

- The patient should go directly to the examination room after being encountered
- The patient should not sit in the waiting room
- The room should have a linoleum floor and not carpeting
- Use only plastic, vinyl, or leather-covered furniture that can be wiped down with a germicidal cleaner
- Gown and gloves should be used by anyone having contact with the patient
- Staff should be cohorted as much as possible
- The healthcare worker (HCW) assigned to primary care should wear scrub clothes in addition to the gown and gloves
- Handwashing is of the utmost importance
- A 4% chlorhexidine gluconate (CHG) solution, such as Hibiclens (Stuart Pharmaceuticals, Wilmington, DE), or a solution with 60% alcohol must be used for handwashing
- Once the patient is gone, the room must be decontaminated with an approved cleaner such as Virex (SC Johnson & Son Inc, Racine, WI), Envy (SC Johnson & Son Inc), or End Bac II (SC Johnson & Son Inc)
- A 10-minute contact time should be allowed before wiping down the surfaces
- 60% alcohol also is effective in decontamination of equipment
- Surfaces such as the examination table, chairs, floors, commode, sink, etc, should be wiped down
- If the primary HCW *must* assist with other patients, have the primary HCW change scrub clothes and then scrub his or her arms and hands with the CHG or alcohol solution before contact with other patients
- Because immunosuppressed patients are at highest risk for acquiring this organism, extreme care must be taken so that transmission does not occur
- Sharing of equipment (including electronic thermometers, blood pressure cuffs, stethoscopes, intravenous line poles, bedside commodes and wheelchairs) is not permitted
- Personal equipment (eg, stethoscopes, scissors) should not be used
- Disposable blood pressure cuffs are available in stores

---

of the basic principles, most of which were discussed by Morrison in his review of the topic.[112]

The control plan must meet city, county, state, and federal regulations. Healthcare organizations must comply with all regulatory requirements; penalties can be imposed for noncompliance.

Infection control personnel should help other staff to do the following:

- Define which items are noninfectious waste and which are infectious.
- Develop protocols and procedures for separating infectious waste from noninfectious waste, labeling the infectious waste properly, and transporting, storing, and disposing of infectious waste safely.
- Develop contingency plans for managing waste spills and inadvertent exposures of visitors or healthcare workers.
- Develop programs to teach staff to handle infectious waste.

Infection control personnel also could help staff identify ways to minimize infectious waste. Examples include the following:

- Stop discarding noninfectious waste, such as wrappers and newspapers, in infectious waste containers.
- Substitute products that do not require special modes of disposal (eg, needleless intravenous systems) for those that must be discarded in the infectious waste (eg, needles).
- Substitute reusable items for the single-use items.

Infection Control in Special Settings

Dialysis Centers

Background

Dialysis centers can be associated with hospitals (on-site or at a distance), or they can be freestanding. In the former case, the infection control staff should ensure that the policies and procedures in the unit are consistent with those in the hospital. Infection control staff would be wise to educate the staff in the dialysis unit about basic infection control guidelines, including standard precautions. The freestanding dialysis units resemble other freestanding medical facilities in that they usually are for-profit organizations, and they rarely have trained infection control staff.

Bloodborne Pathogens

The primary infection control issue in dialysis centers is transmission of bloodborne pathogens, such as HBV, HCV, and HIV. To date, transmission of HBV has been the most common problem. Use of good infection control precautions and the hepatitis B vaccine have decreased the risk of transmission substantially in this setting. Staff members always should use standard precautions when they handle blood and other specimens, such as peritoneal fluid, which can contain high levels of HBsAg and HBV.[114]

In this section, we will review some basic infection control precautions for dialysis units by summarizing the main points from an excellent chapter by Favero et al.[114] Infection control personnel who need detailed information should read that chapter and several other articles.[114-117]

Infection control precautions designed to prevent transmission of hepatitis B in dialysis centers include the following[114]:

- Patients and staff members should be screened for HBsAg and anti-HBsAg when they enter the unit.
- Dialysis centers should survey susceptible

patients and healthcare workers routinely for HBsAg and anti-HBsAg to determine whether transmission of HBV has occurred in the unit.

- Patients who are HBsAg carriers should undergo dialysis in a separate room designated only for use by such patients. If this is impossible, patients who are HBsAg carriers should be dialyzed on dedicated machines in an area that is separated from the area in which HBV-seronegative patients are dialyzed.
- Medications in multidose vials should not be shared among patients.
- Staff members should not care for patients who carry HBsAg and for seronegative patients during the same shift.
- Ideally, the same hemodialysis equipment should not be used for both HBsAg-seropositive and HBsAg-seronegative patients. However, when this is not possible, the machines should be disinfected using conventional protocols, and the external surfaces should be cleaned or disinfected using soap and water or a detergent germicide.
- HBsAg-positive patients should not participate in dialyzer reuse programs.
- Centers that do peritoneal dialysis should separate HBsAg-positive patients from those who are HBsAg-negative and should observe precautions similar to those used for hemodialysis patients, because peritoneal fluid can transmit HBV to susceptible persons.

Hepatitis D virus (HDV) has been transmitted in dialysis centers. Therefore, patients who are infected with HDV should be dialyzed on dedicated machines in an area that is separated from all other dialysis patients, especially those who are HBsAg-positive.[114] If there is evidence that HDV has been transmitted within the unit, patients should be screened for delta antigen and antibody to delta antigen.

Hepatitis C virus has caused outbreaks in dialysis centers.[118] However, Favero et al do not recommend using specific precautions for patients who have antibody to HCV or for those who are infected with HIV.[114] These authors also do not recommend routine screening for HCV. Rather, they recommend the following:

- Staff should use precautions that limit exposure to blood and body fluids.[118]
- Staff always should clean and disinfect all instruments and environmental surfaces that are touched routinely.[118]
- Articles should not be shared among patients.[118]
- The center should measure liver enzymes for all patients to determine whether any patients have evidence of non-A, and non-B hepatitis, including HCV.[114]
- If liver enzymes from several patients increase during a short time period, staff should identify the etiology of each patient's hepatitis, so that the staff can determine whether an outbreak exists.[114]
- Hemodialysis centers could conduct serological surveys of their patient and staff populations to determine the baseline prevalence of hepatitis C in their center and to determine whether the prevalence has changed over time.[114]

If transmission of bloodborne pathogens occurs in a dialysis unit, staff must determine how the organism was transmitted and what infection control procedures have been violated. To facilitate such investigations, Favero et al have recommended that dialysis centers maintain detailed records on the following[114]:

- The lot number of all blood and blood products used.
- All mishaps such as needlesticks, blood leaks or spills, and dialysis machine malfunctions.
- The location, name, or number of the dialysis machine used for each dialysis session.
- The names of staff members who connect and disconnect the patient to and from a machine.
- Results of serologic tests for hepatitis.
- All accidental needle punctures and similar accidents sustained by staff members and patients.[114]

Staphylococcus aureus

Patients on dialysis have high rates of S aureus nasal carriage. Reports in the literature indicate that 32% to 81% of hemodialysis patients[119] and 23% to 67% of patients on continuous ambulatory peritoneal dialysis (CAPD) carry this organism.[120] S aureus causes 70% to 92% of vascular-access-site infections in patients on hemodialysis[119] and 25% to 85% of exit-site infections in patients treated with CAPD.[119] S aureus also is the leading cause of tunnel infections in patients on CAPD. Moreover, the risk of S aureus infection is significantly higher for dialysis patients who carry this organism in their nares than for patients who do not carry it.[119,120]

Most dialysis patients are infected by the unique S aureus strains that they carry in their nares.[121,122] Thus, the most effective preventive strategies involve decolonization of the nares. Several investigators have documented that prophylactic use of rifampin[119] or mupirocin[123] can prevent S aureus infections in patients on hemodialysis, and use of mupirocin can prevent exit-site infections in patients on CAPD.[124]

Approximately 10% to 20% of S aureus infections in patients on CAPD occur in noncarriers or are caused by strains other than those carried by the patients. To date, the source of these infections has not been identified. One case report suggested that family members who care for the patient might be a source of the infecting organism.[125] In addition, there is molecular epidemiological evidence that patients on CAPD can share the same strain of S aureus.[126] Thus, healthcare workers in dialysis units, family members, and home healthcare staff must practice basic infection control precautions to prevent spread of *S aureus* to dialysis patients.

Outbreaks in Dialysis Centers

Numerous outbreaks have occurred in dialysis centers (see Tables 32-1, 32-2, and 32-7). Most of the outbreaks that we reviewed were caused by major deficiencies in basic infection practices. The primary errors were inadequate or improper disinfection processes, poor compliance with precautions to prevent spread of bloodborne pathogens, and allowing HBsAg-positive and HBsAg-negative patients to share multidose vials of medications.

Infection Control in Physical Therapy

Physical therapy facilities can be located in hospitals, in clinics, or can be freestanding. Many of these facilities provide services to outpatients. Physical therapy facilities have not been documented to be the source of outbreaks except in the case of infections associated with hydrotherapy. However, the absence of data is no cause to be sanguine, because all the elements necessary for transmission of pathogens exist in physical therapy centers. In addition, few investigators have looked rigorously for evidence of transmission in this setting.

The Association for Professionals in Infection Control and Epidemiology has published the only recommendations for infection control in physical therapy.[127] However, these recommendations provide limited guidance, because little information is available regarding appropriate infection control precautions for this setting.[128] The following text outlines a few basic infection control principles for physical therapy centers that are summarized from an excellent review written by Linnemann.[128] Readers who are interested in a more in-depth discussion should read that review.

Infection control professionals who advise physical therapy units should ensure that the staff implement the following recommendations[128]:

- All mats, table tops, and equipment handles should be covered with impervious materials, so that these items can be cleaned frequently.
- Cleaning supplies should be stored where they are readily accessible, so that staff can clean the equipment whenever necessary, not just at the scheduled times.
- Handwashing sinks should be located such that therapists can wash their hands easily after each patient or between patients if they are helping more than one patient at a time.
- Physical therapists should be educated regarding standard precautions and the mechanisms by which organisms are transmitted.
- Physical therapists should understand that they could transmit infectious agents as they move from patient to patient and should know what precautions are necessary to prevent spread of pathogens.
- Therapists should wear gloves and gowns when they could contaminate their hands or clothing.
- Patients who have active infections caused by transmissible organisms or who are infected or colonized with resistant organisms should not use the facility. If such patients are allowed to use the facility, the staff must use appropriate precautions to prevent spread of these organisms.
- Physical therapists should have annual skin tests for tuberculosis and should be up to date on all of their immunizations.

Outbreaks in the Outpatient Setting

The overall incidence of infection in the outpatient setting may be quite low. However, numerous serious outbreaks have occurred in facilities that provide care for patients who are not hospitalized. We anticipate that outbreaks will occur more frequently in this setting as the proportion of outpatient care increases and as the competition for business becomes more fierce.

Goodman and Solomon reviewed published articles and identified 53 reports of transmission that occurred in the outpatient setting between 1961 and 1990.[129] The outbreaks occurred in general medical offices, clinics, and emergency departments (n = 23); ophthalmologists' offices and clinics (n = 11); dental offices (n = 13); and alternative-care settings (n = 6). These investigators concluded that the outbreaks frequently were associated with "lack of adherence to established infection control procedures."[129] Goodman and Solomon determined that the following several factors accounted for most of the outbreaks:

- Inadequate disinfection and sterilization.
- Absent or inappropriate use of barrier precautions.
- Absent or inappropriate work restrictions for infected healthcare workers.
- Inadequate handwashing.

These investigators also felt that personnel in the outpatient setting may not be familiar with infection control precautions and recommendations. In addition, several features of the setting, such as the following, may be conducive to poor compliance with good infection control practice:

- Numerous patients are seen in the outpatient setting.
- Healthcare workers have contact with the patients for only brief periods of time.
- Patients may wait and healthcare workers may work in confined spaces.[129]

On the basis of our review of the literature, we agree with the conclusions drawn by Goodman and Solomon, and we would add the following:

- Contaminated multidose vials are an important source of outbreaks in the outpatient setting.
- Ophthalmology clinics are high-risk areas for transmission of adenovirus.
- Dialysis units are high-risk areas for transmission of bloodborne pathogens and for bacterial infections, pyrogenic reactions, or

hypotension caused by inadequately disinfected dialyzers or tainted water.

- Endoscopy suites are areas in which staff frequently violate recommended disinfection protocols.
- Inadequate screening for infectious agents, particularly those that are spread through the air or by droplets, allows agents such as measles virus or *M tuberculosis* to spread in the outpatient setting.

We have included eight tables that provide details on selected outbreaks in the outpatient setting, so that infection control professionals will know the common organisms that have caused outbreaks, the deficiencies in infection control practice that have been associated with many outbreaks, and the settings where outbreaks have occurred most often.

OSHA Inspections in the Outpatient Setting

A full discussion of OSHA inspections in the ambulatory setting is beyond the scope of this chapter. However, infection control personnel must understand that OSHA's regulations also apply to facilities that provide care to outpatients. Persons who must ensure that their outpatient facility complies with OSHA's regulations must understand the Bloodborne Pathogen Standard[4] and the tuberculosis recommendations.[5]

Outpatient facilities associated with hospitals might be at greater risk of an OSHA inspection than are physicians' offices. However, OSHA does inspect offices operated by doctors of medicine and osteopathy.[130,131] Between July 6, 1992, and December 31, 1992, OSHA inspected 56 medical offices and imposed $139,881 in penalties.[131] Most inspections result from complaints filed by employees, but some "are conducted from a planned inspection guide."[131] Common violations in physicians' offices "involve personal protective equipment such as gloves and gowns, employee information and training requirements, records of training sessions, storage of those records, development of an exposure control plan, and procedures for laundering of personal protective equipment."[131] Other violations have involved chemicals that are kept on the premises and exposures to ethylene oxide.[131]

Conclusion

By now, you probably are overwhelmed completely and are wondering where to begin. Obviously, one person or one program cannot assess all of the areas that we have discussed in this chapter. Thus, we would recommend that infection control staff assess their own institutions to determine the following:

- What type of outpatient facilities are present in your medical center (eg, only hospital-based clinics, units that provide services to both inpatients and outpatients, only freestanding clinics, or a mixture of on-site and off-site clinics owned by the medical center)?
- What types of patients are seen in the outpatient facilities (eg, young children, immunocompromised patients, healthy preoperative patients)?
- What types of procedures are performed in the outpatient facilities?
- Which procedures are performed most commonly?
- What types of infectious diseases are diagnosed and treated in the outpatient facilities?
- What resources are available for infection control?
- Do the administration and the clinicians support the infection control program?

Once you have identified the primary characteristics of your facility, you should review the policies and procedures in the major areas and conduct walking rounds to answer the following questions:

- Does the area have policies, procedures, and engineering controls to prevent transmission of bloodborne pathogens?
- Does the area have appropriate screening, triage, isolation protocols, and engineering controls to prevent the spread of airborne agents?
- Does the area have appropriate screening, triage, and isolation for patients who may be infected or colonized with other infectious agents?
- Does the area have appropriate exposure management plans for bloodborne pathogens, measles virus, *M tuberculosis*, VZV, *B pertussis*, lice, and scabies?
- Does the staff understand and practice principles of asepsis, including those required to use multidose vials safely?
- Does the staff understand and practice appropriate cleaning, disinfection, and sterilization?
- Are the policies and procedures in this area consistent in content and intent with those from other areas in the medical center?
- Does the area have educational programs to teach staff precautions for *M tuberculosis*, bloodborne pathogens, and other infectious agents? Do they document these programs adequately?

Once you have answered these questions, you should set priorities. We would suggest that all outpatient facilities should focus first on the following preventive measures:

- Ensure that the staff complies with the tuberculosis recommendations and Bloodborne Pathogen Standards published by the CDC and OSHA, respectively.
- Develop screening protocols for other airborne diseases to prevent unnecessary exposures.
- Ensure that the staff and patients have been vaccinated appropriately.
- Ensure that the staff practices good aseptic

technique when handling multidose vials and that protocols and practices for cleaning, disinfection, and sterilization are appropriate.

Once they have addressed these priorities, infection control personnel then can address other issues, including whether or not to develop surveillance for surgical site infections after ambulatory surgery. For example, infection control personnel might be able to work with home-healthcare agencies to identify infections that are associated with inpatient medical care or with treatments given in hospital-based clinics or ambulatory-surgery centers.

Infection control personnel who begin to address infection control needs in the ambulatory setting have not only a huge task to accomplish but also an enormous opportunity. Infection control personnel who take on this challenge will help to improve the quality of patients' care and the safety of healthcare workers and will help their institutions survive in this extraordinarily competitive environment. In addition, those intrepid persons will help shape the course of healthcare over the next decade.

Acknowledgments

The authors thank Jean Pottinger for providing important references, reviewing several drafts of the manuscript, and giving us excellent suggestions that improved its content and structure. We also thank Patsy McAtee for typing countless references and ensuring that the format was correct.

References

1. Lamkin L. Outpatient oncology settings: a variety of services. *Seminars in Oncology Nursing.* 1994;10:227, 229-235.

2. Perl TM, Stevens D, Roy M-C, Herwaldt LA, Lemke J. Are current surveillance activities keeping pace with changing clinical practices? *Infect Control Hosp Epidemiol.* 1996;17(suppl):P22. Abstract.

3. Meier PA. Infection control issues in same-day surgery. In: Wenzel RP, ed. *Prevention and Control of Nosocomial Infections.* 3rd ed. Philadelphia, Pa: Williams & Wilkins; 1997:262-282.

4. Department of Labor, Occupational Safety and Health Administration. 29 CFR Part 1920.1030, Occupational exposure to bloodborne pathogens, final rule. Federal Register December 6, 1991;56:64,004-64,182.

5. Centers for Disease Control and Prevention. Guidelines for preventing the transmission of *Mycobacterium tuberculosis* in health care facilities, 1994. *MMWR.* 1994;43:1-133.

6. Joint Commission on Accreditation of Healthcare Organizations. Leadership Standard. In: *Comprehensive Accreditation Manual for Hospitals: The Official Handbook.* Oakbrook Terrace, Ill: JCAHO; 1996:LD-1-LD-52.

7. Wade BH. Outpatient/out of hospital care issues. In: Wenzel RP, ed. *Prevention and Control of Nosocomial Infections.* 3rd ed. Philadelphia, Pa: Williams & Wilkins; 1997:243-259.

8. Smith PW, Roccaforte JS. Epidemiology and prevention of infections in home health care. In: Mayhall CG, ed. *Hospital Epidemiology and Infection Control.* Philadelphia, Pa: Williams & Wilkins; 1996:1171-1176.

9. Molinari JA. Dental office. In: Olmsted RN, ed. *APIC Infection Control and Applied Epidemiology: Principles and Practice*, Part I Section C, Practice Settings. St Louis, Mo: Mosby-Year Book, Inc; 1996:88-1-88-20.

10. Kelen GD, Hansen KN, Green GB, Tang N, Ganguli C. Determinants of emergency department procedure- and condition-specific Universal (barrier) Precaution requirements for optimal provider protection. *Ann Emerg Med.* 1995;25:743-750.

11. Kelen GD, Green GB, Purcell RH, et al. Hepatitis B and hepatitis C in emergency department patients. *N Engl J Med.* 1992;326:1399-1404.

12. Kelen GD, Green GB, Hexter DA, et al. Substantial improvement in compliance with universal precautions in an emergency department following institution of policy. *Arch Intern Med.* 1991;151:2051-2056.

13. Thurn J, Willenbring K, Crossley K. Needlestick injuries and needle disposal in Minnesota physicians' offices. *Am J Med.* 1989;86:575-579.

14. Miller KE, Krol RA, Losh DP. Universal precautions in the family physician's office. *J Fam Pract.* 1992;35:163-168.

15. Kent GP, Brondum J, Keenlyside RA, LaFazia LM, Scott HD. A large outbreak of acupuncture-associated hepatitis B. *Am J Epidemiol.* 1988;127:591-598.

16. Stryker WS, Gunn RA, Francis DP. Outbreak of hepatitis B associated with acupuncture. *J Fam Pract.* 1986; 22:155-158.

17. Canter J, Mackey K, Good LS, et al. An outbreak of hepatitis B associated with jet injections in a weight reduction clinic. *Arch Intern Med.* 1990;150:1923-1927.

18. Alter MJ, Ahtone J, Maynard JE. Hepatitis B virus transmission associated with a multiple-dose vial in a hemodialysis unit. *Ann Intern Med.* 1983;99:330-333.

19. Danzig LE, Tormey MP, Sinha SD, et al. Common source transmission of hepatitis B virus infection in a hemodialysis unit. *Infect Control Hosp Epidemiol.* 1995;16(suppl):P19. Abstract.

20. Rosenberg J, Gilliss DL, Moyer L, Vugia D. A double outbreak of hepatitis B in a dialysis center. *Infect Control Hosp Epidemiol.* 1995;16(suppl):P19. Abstract.

21. Hlady WG, Hopkins RS, Ogilby TE, Allen ST. Patient-to-patient transmission of hepatitis B in a dermatology practice. *Am J Public Health.* 1993;83:1689-1693.

22. Drescher J, Wagner D, Haverich A, et al. Nosocomial hepatitis B virus infections in cardiac transplant recipients transmitted during transvenous endomyocardial biopsy. *J Hosp Infect.* 1994;26:81-92.

23. Reingold AL, Kane MA, Murphy BL, Checko P, Francis DP, Maynard JE. Transmission of hepatitis B by an oral surgeon. *J Infect Dis.* 1982;145:262-268.

24. Ciesielski C, Marianos D, Ou CY, et al. Transmission of human immunodeficiency virus in a dental practice. *Ann Intern Med.* 1992;116:798-805.

25. Velandia M, Fridkin SK, Cardenas V, et al. Transmission of HIV in dialysis centre. *Lancet.* 1995;345:1417-1422.

26. Chant K, Lowe D, Rubin G, et al. Patient-to-patient transmission of HIV in private surgical consultating rooms. *Lancet.* 1993;342:1548-1549. Letter.

27. Haley CE, McDonald RC, Rossi L, Jones WD, Haley RW, Luby JP. Tuberculosis epidemic among hospital personnel. *Infect Control Hosp Epidemiol.* 1989;10:204-210.

28. Centers for Disease Control. *Mycobacterium tuberculosis* transmission in a health clinic—Florida, 1988. *MMWR.* 1989;38:256-258, 263-264.

29. Calder RA, Duclos P, Wilder MH, Pryor VL, Scheel WJ. *Mycobacterium tuberculosis* transmission in a health clinic. *Bulletin of the International Union Against Tuberculosis and Lung Disease.* 1991;66:103-106.

30. Fischl MA, Uttamchandani RB, Daikos GL, et al. An outbreak of tuberculosis caused by multiple-drug-resistant tubercle bacilli among patients with HIV infection. *Ann Intern Med.* 1992;117:177-183.

31. Couldwell DL, Dore GJ, Harkness JL, et al. Nosocomial outbreak of tuberculosis in an outpatient HIV treatment room. *AIDS.* 1996;10:521-525.

32. Moore M, the Investigative Team. Evaluation of transmission of tuberculosis in a pediatric setting—Pennsylvania. Presented at the 46th Annual Epidemic Intelligence Service Conference; April 14-18, 1997; Atlanta, Ga; p 53.

33. Agerton TB, Valway S, Gore B, Poszik C, Onorato I. Transmission of multidrug-resistant tuberculosis via bronchoscopy. Presented at the 46th Annual Epidemic Intelligence Service Conference; April 14-18, 1997; Atlanta, Ga; p 54.

34. Griffith DE, Hardeman JL, Zhang Y, Wallace RJ, Mazurek GH. Tuberculosis outbreak among healthcare workers in a community hospital. *Am J Respir Crit Care Med.* 1995;152:808-811.

35. Sokolove PE, Mackey D, Wiles J, Lewis RJ. Exposure of emergency department personnel to tuberculosis: PPD testing during an epidemic in the community. *Ann Emerg Med.* 1994;24:418-421.

36. Sepkowitz KA. AIDS, tuberculosis, and the health care worker. *Clin Infect Dis.* 1995;20:232-242.

37. Moran GJ, McCabe F, Morgan MT, Talan DA. Delayed recognition and infection control for tuberculosis patients in the emergency department. *Ann Emerg Med.* 1995;26:290-295.

38. Moran GJ, Fuchs MA, Jarvis WR, Talan DA. Tuberculosis infection-control practices in United States emergency departments. *Ann Emerg Med.* 1995;26:283-289.

39. Davis RM, Orenstein WA, Frank JA, et al. Transmission of measles in medical settings: 1980 through 1984. *JAMA.* 1986;255:1295-1298.

40. Istre GR, McKee PA, West GR, et al. Measles spread in medical settings: an important focus of disease transmission? *Pediatrics.* 1987;79:356-358.

41. Centers for Disease Control. Measles—Washington, 1990. *MMWR.* 1990;39:473-476.

42. Bloch AB, Orenstein WA, Ewing WM, et al. Measles outbreak in a pediatric practice: airborne transmission in an office setting. *Pediatrics.* 1985;75:676-683.

43. Centers for Disease Control. Measles—Hawaii. *MMWR.* 1984;33:702, 707-711.

44. Miranda AC, Falcao JM, Dias JA. Measles transmission in health facilities during outbreaks. *Int J Epidemiol.* 1994;23:843-848.

45. Centers for Disease Control and Prevention. Measles among children of migrant workers—Florida. *MMWR.* 1983;32:471-472, 477-478.

46. Remington PL, Hall WN, Davis IH, Herald A, Gunn RA. Airborne transmission of measles in a physician's office. *JAMA.* 1985;253:1574-1577.

47. Krause PJ, Gross PA, Barrett TL, et al. Quality standard for assurance of measles immunity among health care workers. *Clin Infect Dis.* 1994;18:431-436.

48. Gladstone JL, Millian SJ. Rubella exposure in an obstet-

ric clinic. *Obstet Gynecol.* 1981;57:182-186.

49. Fliegel PE, Weinstein WM. Rubella outbreak in a prenatal clinic: management and prevention. *Am J Infect Control.* 1982;10:29-33.

50. Centers for Disease Control and Prevention. Exposure of patients to rubella by medical personnel—California. *MMWR.* 1978;27:123.

51. Pellitteri OJ, Fried JJ. Epidemic keratoconjunctivitis report of a small office outbreak. *Am J Ophthalmol.* 1950;33:1596-1599.

52. Thygeson P. Office and dispensary transmissions of epidemic keratoconjunctivitis. *Am J Ophthalmol.* 1957;43:98-101.

53. Dawson C, Darrell R. Infections due to adenovirus type 8 in the United States, I: an outbreak of epidemic keratoconjunctivitis originating in a physician's office. *N Engl J Med.* 1963;68:1031-1034.

54. D'Angelo LJ, Hierholzer JC, Holman RC, Smith JD. Epidemic keratoconjunctivitis caused by adenovirus type 8: epidemiologic and laboratory aspects of a large outbreak. *Am J Epidemiol.* 1981;113:44-49.

55. Keenlyside RA, Hierholzer JC, D'Angelo LJ. Keratoconjunctivitis associated with adenovirus type 37: an extended outbreak in an ophthalmologist's office. *J Infect Dis.* 1983;147:191-198.

56. Buehler JW, Finton RJ, Goodman RA, et al. Epidemic keratoconjunctivitis: report of an outbreak in an ophthalmology practice and recommendations for prevention. *Infect Control.* 1984;5:390-394.

57. Craven ER, Butler SL, McCulley JP, Luby JP. Applanation tonometer tip sterilization for adenovirus type 8. *Ophthalmology.* 1987;94:1538-1540.

58. Koo D, Bouvier B, Wesley M, Courtright P, Reingold A. Epidemic keratoconjunctivitis in a university medical center ophthalmology clinic: need for re-evaluation of the design and disinfection of instruments. *Infect Control Hosp Epidemiol.* 1989;10:547-552.

59. Centers for Disease Control and Prevention. Epidemic keratoconjunctivitis in an ophthalmology clinic—California. *MMWR.* 1990;39:598-601.

60. Warren D, Nelson KE, Farrar JA, et al. A large outbreak of epidemic keratoconjunctivitis: problems in controlling nosocomial spread. *J Infect Dis.* 1989;160:938-943.

61. Colon LE. Keratoconjunctivitis due to adenovirus type 8: report on a large outbreak. *Annals of Ophthalmology.* 1991;23:63-65.

62. Jernigan JA, Lowry BS, Hayden FG, et al. Adenovirus type 8 epidemic keratoconjunctivitis in an eye clinic: risk factors and control. *J Infect Dis.* 1993;167:1307-1313.

63. Smith D, Gottsch J, Froggatt J, Dwyer D, Karanfil L, Groves C. Performance improvement process to control epidemic keratoconjunctivitis transmission. *Infect Control Hosp Epidemiol.* 1996;17(suppl):P36. Abstract.

64. American Academy of Ophthalmology. *Updated recommendations for Ophthalmic Practice in Relation to the Human Immunodeficiency Virus and Other Infectious Agents.* San Francisco, Calif: AAO; 1992.

65. Dailey JR, Parnes RE, Aminlari A. Glutaraldehyde keratopathy. *Am J Ophthal.* 1993;115:256-258.

66. Christie CDC, Marx ML, Marchant CD, Reising SF. The 1993 epidemic of pertussis in Cincinnati. Resurgence of disease in a highly immunized population of children. *N Engl J Med.* 1994;331:16-21.

67. Hardy IRB, Strebel PM, Wharton M, Orenstein WA. The 1993 pertussis epidemic in Cincinnati. *N Engl J Med.* 1994;331:1455-1455.

68. American Society for Gastrointestinal Endoscopy. Infection control during gastrointestinal endoscopy: guidelines for clinical application. *Gastrointest Endosc.* 1988;34(suppl):37S-40S.

69. Members of the American Society for Gastrointestinal Endoscopy Ad Hoc Committee on Disinfection. Position statement. Reprocessing of flexible gastrointestinal endoscopes. *Gastrointest Endosc.* 1996;43:540-546.

70. Rutala WA. APIC guideline for selection and use of disinfectants. *Am J Infect Control.* 1996;24:313-342.

71. Spach DH, Silverstein FE, Stamm WE. Transmission of infection by gastrointestinal endoscopy and bronchoscopy. *Ann Intern Med.* 1993;118:117-128.

72. Ayliffe GA. Nosocomial infections associated with endoscopy. In: Mayhall CG, ed. *Hospital Epidemiology and Infection Control.* Philadelphia, Pa: Williams & Wilkins; 1996:680-693.

73. Weber DJ, Rutala WA. Nosocomial infections associated with respiratory therapy. In: Mayhall CG, ed. *Hospital Epidemiology and Infection Control.* Philadelphia, Pa: Williams & Wilkins; 1996:748-758.

74. Muscarella LF. Advantages and limitations of automatic flexible endoscope reprocessors. *Am J Infect Control.* 1996;24:304-309.

75. Reynolds CD, Rhinehart E, Dreyer P, Goldmann DA. Variability in reprocessing policies and procedures for flexible fiberoptic endoscopes in Massachusetts hospitals. *Am J Infect Control.* 1992;20:283-290.

76. Foss D, Monagan D. A national survey of physicians' and nurses' attitudes toward endoscope cleaning and the potential for cross-infection. *Gastroenterology Nursing.* 1992;15:59-65.

77. Beecham JH III, Cohen ML, Parkin WE. *Salmonella typhimurium*: transmission by fiberoptic upper gastrointestinal endoscopy. *JAMA.* 1979;241:1013-1015.

78. Dwyer DM, Klein EG, Istre GR, Robinson MG, Neumann DA, McCoy GA. *Salmonella newport* infections transmitted by fiberoptic colonoscopy. *Gastrointest Endosc.* 1987;33:84-87.

79. Struelens MJ, Rost F, Deplano A, et al. *Pseudomonas aeruginosa* and *Enterobacteriaceae* bacteremia after biliary endoscopy: an outbreak investigation using DNA macrorestriction analysis. *Am J Med.* 1993;95:489-498.

80. Classen DC, Jacobson JA, Burke JP, Jacobson JT, Evans RS. Serious pseudomonas infections associated with endoscopic retrograde cholangiopancreatography. *Am J Med.* 1988;84:590-596.

81. Low DE, Micflikier AB, Kennedy JK, Stiver HG. Infectious complications of endoscopic retrograde cholangiopancreatography: a prospective assessment. *Arch Intern Med.* 1980;140:1076-1077.

82. Earnshaw JJ, Clark AW, Thom BT. Outbreak of *Pseudomonas aeruginosa* following endoscopic retrograde cholangiopancreatography. *J Hosp Infect.* 1985;6:95-97.

83. Langenberg W, Rauws EAJ, Oudbier JH, Tytgat GNJ. Patient-to-patient transmission of *Campylobacter pylori* infection by fiberoptic gastroduodenoscopy and biopsy. *J Infect Dis.* 1990;161:507-511.

84. Akamatsu T, Tabata K, Hironga M, Kawakami H, Uyeda M. Transmission of *Helicobacter pylori* infection via flexible fiberoptic endoscopy. *Am J Infect Control.* 1996;24:396-401.

85. Birnie GG, Quigley EM, Clements GB, Follet EAC, Watkinson G. Endoscopic transmission of hepatitis B virus. *Gut.* 1983;24:171-174.

86. Singh S, Singh N, Kochhar R, Mehta SK, Talwar P. Contamination of an endoscope due to *Trichosporon beigelli*. *J Hosp Infect.* 1989;14:49-53.

87. Wheeler PW, Lancaster D, Kaiser AB. Bronchopulmonary cross-colonization and infection related to mycobacterial contamination of suction valves of bronchoscopes. *J Infect Dis.* 1989;159:954-985.

88. Wang H-C, Liaw Y-S, Yang P-C, Kuo S-H, Luh K-T. A pseudoepidemic of *Mycobacterium chelonae* infection caused by contamination of a fibreoptic bronchoscope suction channel. *Eur Respir J.* 1995;8:1259-1262.

89. Nye K, Shadha DK, Hodgkin P, Bradley C, Hancox J, Wise R. *Mycobacterium chelonei* isolation from bronchoalveolar lavage fluid and its practical implications. *J Hosp Infect.* 1990;16:257-261.

90. Pappas SA, Schaaff DM, DiCostanzo MB, King FW Jr, Sharp JT. Contamination of flexible fiberoptic bronchoscopes. *Am Rev Respir Dis.* 1983;127:391-392. Letter.

91. Steere AC, Corrales J, von Graevenitz A. A cluster of *Mycobacterium gordonae* isolates from bronchoscopy specimens. *Am Rev Respir Dis.* 1979;120:214-416.

92. Kolmos HJ, Lerche A, Kristoffersen K, Rosdahl VT. Pseudo-outbreak of *Pseudomonas aeruginosa* in HIV-infected patients undergoing fiberoptic bronchoscopy. *Scand J Infect Dis.* 1994;26:653-657.

93. Umphrey J, Raad I, Tarrand J, Hill LA. Bronchoscopes as a contamination source of Pseudomonas putida. *Infect Control Hosp Epidemiol.* 1996;17(suppl):P42. Abstract.

94. Hoffmann KK, Weber DJ, Rutala WA. Pseudo-outbreak of Rhodotorula rubra in patients undergoing fiberoptic bronchoscopy. *Am J Infect Control.* 1989;17:99. Abstract.

95. Reeves DS, Brown NM. Mycobacterial contamination of fibreoptic bronchoscopes. *J Hosp Infect.* 1995;30(suppl): 531-536.

96. Van Gossum A, Loriers M, Serruys E, Cremer M. Methods of disinfecting endoscopic material: results of an international survey. *Endoscopy.* 1989;21:247-250.

97. Kaczmarek RG, Moore RM, McCrohan J, et al. Multistate investigation of the actual disinfection/sterilization of endoscopes in health care facilities. *Am J Med.* 1992;92:257-261.

98. Axon ATR, Cockel R, Banks J, Deverill CEA, Newmann C. Disinfection in upper-digestive-tract endoscopy in Britain. *Lancet.* 1981;1:1093-1094.

99. Rutala WA, Clontz EP, Weber DJ, Hoffmann KK. Disinfection practices for endoscopes and other semicritical items. *Infect Control Hosp Epidemiol.* 1991;12:282-288.

100. Gorse GJ, Messner RL. Infection control practices in gastrointestinal endoscopy in the United States: a national survey. *Infect Control Hosp Epidemiol.* 1991;12:289-296.

101. Favero MS. Strategies for disinfection and sterilization of endoscopes: the gap between basic principles and actual practice. *Infect Control Hosp Epidemiol.* 1991;12:279-281.

102. Rutala WA. Disinfection, sterilization, and waste disposal. In: Wenzel RP, ed. *Prevention and Control of Nosocomial Infections.* 3rd ed. Philadelphia, Pa: Williams & Wilkins; 1997:539-593.

103. Alfa MJ, DeGagne P, Olson N, Puchalski T. Comparison of ion plasma, vaporized hydrogen peroxide, and 100% ethylene oxide sterilizers to the 12/88 ethylene oxide gas sterilizer. *Infect Control Hosp Epidemiol.* 1996;17:92-100.

104. Rutala WA, Weber DJ. Low-temperature sterilization technologies: do we need to redefine "sterilization"? *Infect Control Hosp Epidemiol.* 1996;17:87-91.

105. Food and Drug Administration. Compliance policy guide 7124.16. 9/24/87. Available from FDA Kansas City Regional Office.

106. Greene VW. Reuse of disposable devices. In: Mayhall CG, ed. *Hospital Epidemiology and Infection Control.* Philadelphia, Pa: Williams & Wilkins; 1996:946-954.

107. Association for the Advancement of Medical Instrumentation. AAMI—Good Hospital Practice: Flash Sterilization—Steam Sterilization of Patient Care Items for Immediate Use (ST37). Arlington, Va: AAMI Steam Sterilization Hospital Practices Working Group, AAMI Sterilization Standards Committee; 1996.

108. Association for the Advancement of Medical Instrumentation. AAMI—Good Hospital Practice: Guidelines for the Selection and Use of Reusable Rigid Sterilization Container Systems (ST33). Arlington, Va: AAMI Steam Sterilization Hospital Practices Working Group of the Thermal Sterilization Subcommittee, AAMI Sterilization Standards Committee; 1996.

109. Longfield R, Longfield J, Smith LP, Hyams KC, Strohmer ME. Multidose medication vial sterility: an in-use study and a review of the literature. *Infect Control.* 1984;5:165-169.

110. Melnyk PS, Shevchuk YM, Conly JM, Richardson CJ. Contamination study of multiple-dose vials. *Ann Pharmacother.* 1993;27:274-277.

111. Hospital Infection Control Practices Advisory Committee, Centers for Disease Control and Prevention. Recommendations for preventing the spread of vancomycin resistance. *Infect Control Hosp Epidemiol.* 1995;16:105-113.

112. Morrison AJ Jr. Infection control in the outpatient setting. In: Wenzel RP, ed. *Prevention and Control of Nosocomial Infections.* 2nd ed. Philadelphia, Pa: Williams & Wilkins; 1993:89-92.

113. Reinhardt PA, Gordon JG, Alvarado CJ. Medical waste management. In: Mayhall CG, ed. *Hospital Epidemiology and Infection Control.* Philadelphia, Pa: Williams & Wilkins; 1996:1099-1108.

114. Favero MS, Alter MJ, Bland LE. Nosocomial infections associated with hemodialysis. In: Mayhall CG, ed. *Hospital Epidemiology and Infection Control.* Philadelphia, Pa: Williams & Wilkins; 1996:693-714.

115. Alter MJ, Favero MS, Moyer LA, Bland LA. National surveillance of dialysis-associated diseases in the United States, 1989. *Transactions American Society for Artificial Internal Organs.* 1991;37:97-109.

116. Band JD. Nosocomial infections associated with peritoneal dialysis. In: Mayhall CG, ed. *Hospital Epidemiology and Infection Control.* Philadelphia, Pa: Williams & Wilkins; 1996:714-725.

117. Garcia-Houchins S. Dialysis. In: Olmsted RN, ed. APIC *Infection Control and Applied Epidemiology: Principles and Practice,* Part I Section C, Practice Settings. St Louis, Mo: Mosby-Year Book, Inc; 1996:89-1-89-15.

118. Niu MT, Alter JM, Kristensen C, Margolis HS. Outbreak of hemodialysis-associated non-A, non-B hepatitis and correlation with antibody to hepatitis C virus. *Am J Kidney Dis.* 1992;19:345-352.

119. Yu VL, Goetz A, Wagener M, Smith PB, et al. *Staphylococcus aureus* nasal carriage and infection in patients on hemodialysis: efficacy of antibiotic prophylaxis. *N Engl J Med.* 1986;315:91-96.

120. Luzar MA, Coles GA, Faller B, et al. *Staphylococcus aureus* nasal carriage and infection in patients on continuous ambulatory peritoneal dialysis. *N Engl J Med.* 1990;322:505-509.

121. Ena J, Boelaert JR, Boyken L, Van Landuyt HW, Godard CA, Herwaldt LA. Epidemiology of *Staphylococcus aureus* infections in patients on hemodialysis. *Infect Control Hosp Epidemiol.* 1994;15;78-81.

122. Pignatari A, Pfaller M, Hollis R, Sesso R, Leme I, Herwaldt L. *Staphylococcus aureus* colonization and infection in patients on continuous ambulatory peritoneal dialysis. *J Clin Microbiol.* 1990;28:1898-1902.

123. Boelaert JR, Van Landuyt HW, Godard CA, et al. Nasal mupirocin ointment decreases the incidence of *Staphylococcus aureus* bacteraemias in haemodialysis patients. *Nephrol Dial Transplant.* 1993;8:235-239.

124. The Mupirocin Study Group. Nasal mupirocin prevents *Staphylococcus aureus* exit-site infection during peritoneal dialysis. *J Am Soc Nephrol.* 1996;7:2403-2408.

125. Dryden MS, McCann M, Phillips I. Housewife peritonitis: conjugal transfer of a pathogen. *J Hosp Infect.* 1991;17:69-70. Letter.

126. Herwaldt LA, Boyken LD, Coffman S. Epidemiology of S aureus nasal carriage in patients on continuous ambulatory peritoneal dialysis who were in a multicenter trial of mupirocin. Presented at the 36th Interscience Conference on Antimicrobial Agents and Chemotherapy; September 15-18, 1996; New Orleans, La; p 233. Abstract.

127. Temple RS. Physical medicine and rehabilitation/occupational therapy/speech. In: Olmsted RN, ed. APIC *Infection Control and Applied Epidemiology: Principles and Practice*, Part I Section D, Support Services and Facilities Management. St Louis, Mo: Mosby-Year Book, Inc; 1996:114-1-114-5.

128. Linnemann CC. Nosocomial infections associated with physical therapy, including hydrotherapy. In: Mayhall CG, ed. *Hospital Epidemiology and Infection Control*. Philadelphia, Pa: Williams & Wilkins: 1996:725-730.

129. Goodman RA, Solomon SL. Transmission of infectious diseases in outpatient health care settings. *JAMA*. 1991;265:2377-2381.

130. Zuber TJ, Geddie JE. Occupational safety and health administration regulations for the physician's office. *J Fam Pract*. 1993;36:540-550.

131. Favero MS, Sadovsky R. Office infection control, OSHA, and you. *Patient Care*. 1993;27:117-121.

132. Inman PM, Beck A, Brown AE, Stanford JL. Outbreak of injection abscesses due to *Mycobacterium abscessus*. *Arch Dermatol*. 1969;100:141-147.

133. Borghans JGA, Stanford JL. Mycobacterium chelonei in abscesses after injection of diphtheria-pertussis-tetanus-polio vaccine. *Am Rev Respir Dis*. 1973;107:1-8.

134. Jackson PG, Keen H, Noble CJ, Simmons NA. Injection abscesses in a diabetic due to Mycobacterium chelonei var abscessus. *British Medical Journal*. 1980;281:1105-1106.

135. Newman PE, Goodman RA, Waring GO III, et al. A cluster of cases of *Mycobacterium chelonei* keratitis associated with outpatient office procedures. *Am J Ophthalmol*. 1984;97:344-348.

136. Lowry PW, Jarvis WR, Oberle AD, et al. *Mycobacterium chelonae* causing otitis media in an ear-nose-and-throat practice. *New Engl J Med*. 1988;319:978-982.

137. Wenger JD, Spika JS, Smithwick RW, et al. Outbreak of *Mycobacterium chelonae* infection associated with use of jet injectors. *JAMA*. 1990;264:373-376.

138. Weems JJ Jr, Usry G, Schwab U. Infection due to rapidly-growing mycobacteria associated with ultrasound directed prostrate biopsy. *Infect Control Hosp Epidemiol*. 1996;17(suppl):P50. Abstract.

139. Centers for Disease Control and Prevention. Infection with *Mycobacterium abscessus* associated with intramuscular injection of adrenal cortex extract—Colorado and Wyoming, 1995-1996. *MMWR*. 1996; 45:713-715.

140. Kothari T, Reyes MP, Brooks N, Brown WJ, Lerner AM. *Pseudomonas cepacia* septic arthritis due to intra-articular injections of methylprednisolone. *Can Med Assoc J*. 1977;116:1230, 1232. Letter.

141. Huang A, Stamler D, Edelstein P, Skalina D, Brennan PJ. Isolation of Pseudomonas pickettii in a sinus clinic. Program of the Third Annual Meeting of the Society for Hospital Epidemiology of America; April 18-20, 1993; Chicago, IL; p A29. Abstract.

142. Pegues DA, Carson LA, Anderson Rl, et al. Outbreak of *Pseudomonas cepacia* bacteremia in oncology patients. *Clin Infect Dis*. 1993;16:407-411.

143. Climo M, Pastor A, Wong E. Outbreak of P aeruginosa infections related to contaminated urodynamic testing equipment. *Infect Control Hosp Epidemiol*. 1996; 17(suppl):P48. Abstract.

144. Arsan AK, Adisen A, Duman S, Aslan B, Kocak I. Acute endophthalmitis outbreak after cataract surgery. *J Cataract Refract Surg*. 1996;22:1116-1120.

145. Ginsburg CM, Henle G, Henle W. An outbreak of infectious mononucleosis among the personnel of an outpatient clinic. *Am J Epidemiol*. 1976;104:571-575.

146. Istre GR, Kreiss K, Hopkins RS, et al. An outbreak of amebiasis spread by colonic irrigation at a chiropractic clinic. *N Engl J Med*. 1982;307:339-342.

147. Greaves WL, Hinman AR, Facklam RR, Allman KC, Barrett CL, Stetler HC. Streptococcal abscesses following diphtheria-tetanus toxoid-pertussis vaccination. *Pediatr Infect Dis J*. 1982;1:388-390.

148. Kantor RJ, Carson LA, Graham DR, Petersen NJ, Favero MS. Outbreak of pyrogenic reactions at a dialysis center: association with infusion of heparinized saline solution. *Am J Med*. 1983;74:449-456.

149. Stetler HC, Garbe PL, Dwyer DM, et al. Outbreaks of group A streptococcal abscesses following diphtheria-tetanus toxoid-pertussis vaccination. *Pediatrics*. 1985;75:299-303.

150. Rutala WA, Weber DJ, Thomann CA. Outbreak of wound infections following outpatient podiatric surgery due to contaminated bone drills. *Foot Ankle Int*. 1987;7:350-354.

151. Nakashima AK, McCarthy MA, Martone MJ, Anderson RL. Epidemic septic arthritis caused by *Serratia marcescens* and associated with a benzalkonium chloride antiseptic. *J Clin Microbiol*. 1987;25:1014-1018.

152. O'Mahony MC, Stanwell-Smith RE, Tillett HE, et al. The Stafford outbreak of legionnaires' disease. *Epidemiol Infect*. 1990;104:361-380.

153. Gordon SM, Drachman J, Bland LA, Reid MH, Favero M, Jarvis WR. Epidemic hypotension in a dialysis center caused by sodium azide. *Kidney Int*. 1990;37:110-115.

154. Longfield RN, Wortham WG, Fletcher LL, Nauscheutz WF. Clustered bacteremias in a hemodialysis unit: cross-contamination of blood tubing from ultrafiltrate waste. *Infect Control Hosp Epidemiol*. 1992;13:160-164.

155. Flaherty JP, Garcia-Houchins S, Chudy R, Arnow PM. An outbreak of gram-negative bacteremia traced to contaminated O-rings and reprocessed dialyzers. *Ann Intern Med*. 1993;119:1072-1078.

156. Beck-Sague CM, Jarvis WR, Bland LA, Arduino MJ, Aguero SM, Verosic G. Outbreak of gram-negative bacteremia and pyrogenic reactions in a hemodialysis center. *Am J Nephrol.* 1990;10:397-403.

157. Fridkins SK, Kremer FB, Bland LA, Padhye A, McNeil MM, Jarvis W. *Acremonium kiliense* endophthalmitis that occurred after cataract extraction in an ambulatory surgical center and was traced to an environmental source. *Clin Infect Dis.* 1996;22:222-227.

158. Hopkins DP, Cicirello H, Dievendorf G, Kondracki S, Morse D. An outbreak of culture-negative peritonitis in dialysis patients—New York. Presented at the 46th Annual Epidemic Intelligence Service Conference; April 14-18, 1997; Atlanta, Ga.

Other Resources

American Society of Gastrointestinal Endoscopy (ASGE) and the Society of Gastroenterology Nurses and Associates. *Reprocessing of Flexible Gastrointestinal Endoscopes.* A white paper publication, December 1995. This document may be accessed through the ASGE home page http://www.asge.org. Select position papers, then select this title. Original copies may be obtained by writing to ASGE or by calling 508-526-8330.

American Academy of Ophthalmology's Updated Recommendations for Ophthalmic Practice in Relation to the Human Immunodeficiency Virus and Other Infectious Agents may be obtained from that society at 655 Beach St, San Francisco, Calif 94109; telephone, 415- 561-8500; fax, 415-561-8533; web site, http://www.eyenet.org.

Centers for Disease Control. (CDC). Guidelines for preventing the transmission of tuberculosis in health-care settings, with special focus on HIV-related issues. *MMWR.* 1990;39.

Core Curriculum On Tuberculosis. *What the Clinician Should Know.* 3rd ed. CDC, National Center for Prevention Services, Division of Tuberculosis Elimination, US Department of Health and Human Services, Atlanta Ga; 1994.

Department of Labor, OSHA. Occupational exposure to tuberculosis. *Federal Register.* 1997;62(201).

Diosegy AJ, MC Lord. What physicians need to know about OSHA: how to avoid tough new penalties. *North Carolina Medical Journal.* 1993;54:251-254.

ECRI Special Report. *Reuse of Single-Use Medical Devices.* 1997, ECRI 5200 Butler Pike, Plymouth Meeting, Pa 19462; telephone 610-825-6000; fax, 610-834-1275; e-mail ecri@hslc.org.

Heroux DL. Ambulatory care. In: Olmsted RN, ed. *APIC Infection Control and Applied Epidemiology: Principles and Practice*, Part I Section C, Practice Settings. St Louis, Mo: Mosby-Year Book, Inc; 1996:83-1-83-15.

Heroux D, Garris J, Nahan J, Vivolo P. Ambulatory Care Infection Control Manual. © 1993, Group Health Cooperative, Group Health Cooperative of Puget Sound, 1809 Seventh Ave, Suite 1003, Seattle, Wash 98101. Publishing coordination and production by Laing Communications Inc., Redmond, Washington.

The Reuse of Single-Use Medical Devices. 1996, Canadian Healthcare Association, CHA Press, 17 York St, Suite 100, Ottawa, Ontario K1N 9J6, Canada.

CHAPTER 33

OSHA Inspections

August J. Valenti, MD, Michael D. Decker, MD, MPH

Abstract

The Occupational Safety and Health Act of 1970 requires that every worker be provided with a safe and healthful workplace and authorizes the Occupational Safety and Health Administration (OSHA) to conduct workplace inspections. OSHA conducts workplace inspections in hospitals and checks for compliance with the Bloodborne Pathogens Standard, the Enforcement Policy and Procedures for Occupational Exposure to Tuberculosis, and the Hazardous Chemicals Standards, among others. The hospital epidemiologist bears considerable responsibility for developing and implementing plans to protect employees from occupational exposures to infectious hazards such as bloodborne pathogens and tuberculosis. To prepare for an inspection, the hospital epidemiologist must understand the basis on which OSHA operates and must proceed in a thoughtful, coordinated manner.

Introduction

The Occupational Safety and Health Administration (OSHA) published its *Occupational Exposure to Bloodborne Pathogens Final Rule* in the December 6, 1991, *Federal Register*.[1] By now, healthcare institutions should have instituted all parts of the standard. Moreover, on October 8, 1993, OSHA stated its intention to enforce policies and procedures for occupational exposure to tuberculosis (TB) based on the Centers for Disease Control and Prevention's (CDC) 1994 revised guidelines for preventing transmission of TB in healthcare settings.[2,3] The hospital epidemiologist must understand the functions of OSHA, OSHA's inspection process, and OSHA's requirements for compliance with its standards.

You should study carefully the material cited above. SHEA has published articles that focus on the key elements of these documents.[4,5] Pamphlets on occupational exposure to bloodborne pathogens (OSHA 3127), OSHA's inspection process (OSHA 2098), and OSHA's consultation services (OSHA 3047) are available from the OSHA Publications Office, 200 Constitution Ave NW, Room N3101, Washington, DC 20210; telephone (202) 219-4667. The American Hospital Association also has published a special briefing on the Bloodborne Pathogens Standard.[6]

TABLE 33-1

US States With OSHA-Approved Occupational
Safety and Health Programs

- Alaska
- Arizona
- California
- Connecticut
- Hawaii
- Indiana
- Iowa
- Kentucky
- Maryland
- Michigan
- Minnesota
- Nevada
- New Mexico
- New York
- North Carolina
- Oregon
- Puerto Rico
- South Carolina
- Tennessee
- Utah
- Vermont
- Virgin Islands
- Virginia
- Washington
- Wyoming

Understanding OSHA

OSHA is authorized to conduct workplace inspections to determine whether employers are complying with the agency's safety and health standards. The General Duty Clause of the Occupational Safety and Health Act of 1970 requires that employers provide every worker with a safe and healthful workplace. In the case of bloodborne pathogens, OSHA has adopted a specific standard on which it bases its protection enforcement policy. When a specific standard does not yet exist, such as for protection against occupational exposure to TB, OSHA's efforts rely on the General Duty Clause. OSHA can issue citations under that clause if its inspectors can demonstrate that the employer failed to keep the workplace free of a recognized hazard that was causing, or was likely to cause, death or serious physical harm, and that a feasible and useful method of abatement existed. In addition, OSHA expects TB control programs to be in compliance with its standards for respiratory protection (29 CFR 1910.134), record-keeping (29 CFR 1910.20, which requires access to employee exposure and medical records, and 29 CFR 1904, which requires a log and summary of occupational injuries and illnesses [called the OSHA 200 log]), and hazard notification (29 CFR 1910.145; which requires that warnings be posted outside TB isolation rooms).

Regional Offices

OSHA has 10 regional offices. Some US territories, commonwealths, and states administer their own OSHA-approved occupational safety and health programs (Table 33-1). In Connecticut and New York, state programs cover public employees, and OSHA covers private employees.

The Bloodborne Pathogens Standard and the Language of OSHA

A program meeting the Bloodborne Pathogens Standard must include the following:

- A written exposure control plan that is accessible to all workers and includes a list of all job categories having occupational exposure to blood or other potentially infectious materials (OPIM), outlines a schedule for implementing all provisions of the standard, and states a procedure for reporting and investigating exposure incidents.
- Protocols that mandate that healthcare workers practice universal precautions (now included in standard precautions), describe how to implement work practice and engineering controls, and describe housekeeping

schedules for cleaning and decontamination of equipment and disposal of regulated wastes.

- A program to provide personal protective equipment.
- A hepatitis B vaccination program.
- A postexposure evaluation and follow-up program.
- A comprehensive hazard communication program that includes specific labels for regulated waste and for containers used to store or transport blood or OPIM, material safety data sheets, and programs to train employees.
- A recordkeeping system that is well maintained, is accessible to OSHA and employees, and includes records of training programs and employees' medical records.

If your institution has HIV or HBV research laboratories or production facilities, OSHA specifies additional requirements.[7]

OSHA and TB Control

Under the General Duty Clause and standards such as the Respiratory Protection Standard, OSHA may cite hospitals for failing to protect employees from TB even though a specific TB protection standard has not yet been adopted (a specific standard currently is under development). The General Duty Clause requires that hospitals implement any (if necessary, every) method of abatement (intervention) that is feasible and effective. OSHA relies on CDC's recommendations to guide its judgment as to which interventions are considered feasible and effective.[8] OSHA has listed the following as examples of useful abatement methods:

- A written TB control plan that documents all aspects of the program and identifies persons responsible for the program.
- A protocol for the early identification of individuals with active TB.

- A system of medical surveillance (free of charge for employees).
- Baseline screening for all employees, and repeat screening workers who have high risk of exposure every 6 months.
- A program (free of charge) for evaluating and managing employees with TB exposures, positive skin tests, skin-test conversions, and clinical TB.
- Properly exhausted or HEPA-filtered, negative-pressure rooms for isolating known or suspected cases of TB and for performing high-hazard procedures such as sputum induction or bronchoscopy.
- TB training programs for employees.
- Site-specific protocols that specify the purpose and proper use of controls such as respirators.

Respiratory protection programs must be in place at worksites in which employees could be exposed to individuals with confirmed or suspected cases of infectious TB or in which employees are involved in high-hazard procedures that increase the likelihood of exposure. National Institute for Occupational Safety and Health-approved HEPA particulate respirators had been the minimum acceptable respiratory protective devices, until regulations permitting new classes of respirators were issued in June 1995. Hospitals must instruct employees how to use, clean, maintain, and dispose of these devices properly. The program must fit-test each employee periodically to ensure that the respirator forms a proper seal around the nose and mouth. In addition, the program must train employees to check the fit of the respirator each time they use it. Healthcare workers who are unable to achieve an adequate seal with a negative-pressure respirator (bearded workers, for example) may require a positive-pressure respirator such as a powered air-purifying respirator (or they may be required to shave). Clearly marked signs indicating the presence of a TB hazard must be posted outside TB isolation rooms.

OSHA Inspections

OSHA lists its inspection priorities as imminent danger situations, catastrophes and fatal accidents, employee complaints, programmed inspections, and follow-up inspections. Thus far, employee complaints have triggered nearly all hospital inspections. If an employee believes he or she is in imminent danger from a hazard or thinks there is a violation of an OSHA standard that may result in physical harm to workers, the employee may ask for an inspection. OSHA will withhold the employee's name from the employer if the employee so requests. OSHA will inform the employee of any actions taken and also will hold an informal review with an employee of any decision not to inspect.

An inspection consists of three parts: an opening conference, a tour of the facility, and a closing conference. At the opening conference, the compliance safety and health officer (CSHO) first will explain the reasons for the inspection, the scope of the inspection, and the applicable OSHA standards. Although a complaint regarding the Bloodborne Pathogens Standard may have triggered the visit, OSHA almost certainly will conduct a complete survey, including hazardous chemicals, radiation safety, hazard communication, and so on. In some cases, the inspection may be terminated at this point, if the CSHO finds that an exemption is appropriate, as in cases where an OSHA-funded consultation program is in progress (see below). If an employee's complaint triggered the inspection, the CSHO will give a copy of the complaint to the employer. The CSHO will ask the employer to designate an employer representative. An employee representative (selected by the union, employee members of the safety committee, or the employees) is entitled to attend the opening conference and to accompany the CSHO during the inspection. The hospital epidemiologist and infection control professional should accompany the CSHO during the tour to answer technical or clinical questions that may arise (and should, in their interactions with the CSHO, be aware that it is likely they will be viewed by the CSHO as a representative of management, not as independent professionals). Infection control personnel may help to avert a citation simply by clarifying the hospital's protocols.

During the inspection, the CSHO will review policies, procedures, and training records; survey engineering controls; and observe employee practices. The CSHO will interview employees privately about their safety and work practices. The CSHO will review records of work-related injuries, illnesses, and fatalities, and will check the OSHA 200 log, in which should be recorded all workplace injuries, including needlestick injuries, TB (Mantoux) skin-test conversions, cases of TB in employees, etc. During the tour, the CSHO will point out to the employer any unsafe working conditions and may take photographs or measurements to document the problem. The CSHO may specify corrective actions and may allow the hospital to correct the problems at this point. However, OSHA still may cite and fine the hospital for these deficiencies.

At the closing conference, the CSHO will meet with the representatives of the employer and employees to discuss the problems and needs. The CSHO will provide an OSHA document that explains the employer's rights and responsibilities following the inspection. The CSHO will discuss all apparent violations, but will not indicate the proposed penalties at this time (the OSHA area director actually issues citations and proposes penalties). A hospital spokesperson should explain to the CSHO how the employer has attempted to comply with the standards and should provide any information that can help OSHA to determine how much time may be needed to abate an apparent violation.

After the Inspection

The area director will send citations and notices of proposed penalties to the hospital by certified mail. The hospital must post these citations on or near the areas where the alleged violations occurred. Penalties vary according to the seriousness of the violation. The area director may propose substantial fines for willful violations of a standard ($5,000 to $70,000 for each violation). Moreover, repeated violations and failure to comply may lead to very large fines. Both the hospital and the employees have the right to appeal. Employees may request an informal review if OSHA decides not to issue a citation and may contest the time allowed for the hospital to eliminate the hazardous conditions.

If your hospital decides to contest a citation, an abatement period, or a proposed penalty, it must submit a written "Notice of Contest" to the area director within 15 working days from the time of the citation. The area director will forward the objection to the Occupational Safety and Health Review Commission (OSHRC), which operates independently of OSHA and which will assign the case to an administrative law judge. If the hospital fails to file a "Notice of Contest" within 15 days, the citation and proposed penalty will become a final order of the OSHRC that cannot be appealed.

Do not be afraid to contest citations. After one inspection, we were able to reduce our fines substantially by contesting those areas that we felt were cited unfairly. The safety officer, an administrator, the hospital epidemiologist, and an infection control professional met informally with the area director, who is authorized to revise citations and penalties. Because we had demonstrated good faith and because there was room for honest disagreement, we were able to get our penalties reduced.

Tips for Preparing for OSHA

The hospital epidemiologist and the administration must understand that the *employer* is responsible for compliance; employees have no responsibility whatsoever. It is the employer who controls the workplace, and the employer must use that control to ensure that employees comply. Therefore, the

hospital administration must understand, promulgate, and enforce the regulations. The infection control department, the safety committee, and the employee health unit will bear much of the responsibility for developing and implementing the exposure control plan and the TB protection program.

Each institution will have its own best approach to managing these responsibilities. At Maine Medical Center, we have established an Infection Control Working Group (separate from the Infection Control Committee) comprised of key people in management, nursing, infection control, and quality assurance. Representatives (usually department heads) from clinical and nonclinical departments, such as engineering, laundry, and housekeeping, are invited as needed. This working group meets bimonthly and is responsible for developing, reviewing, and revising the exposure control plan. A TB oversight committee answers to the working group. We choose to involve the administrators at this level because they learn about important issues, they can smooth interdepartmental communications, and they can speed the implementation of new policies and procedures. During an actual inspection, members of the working group communicate with hospital representatives accompanying the compliance officer and provide additional information when needed. After the inspection, members of the working group implement proposed corrective measures and help to prepare responses to any citations.

The hospital epidemiologist must understand the key elements of the standards. The epidemiologist may want to conduct periodic surveys (mock OSHA inspections) of hospital departments to ensure compliance, check documentation, and identify problem areas. A checklist will help the epidemiologist to evaluate each of the areas subject to inspection (see the *SHEA Newsletter*, Spring 1992, Appendix I, page 15, for key requirements and a table that will help infection control personnel to design a checklist). The infection control department should maintain records of these inspections.

The management of employee exposures to blood, OPIM, and TB will vary according to each institution's plan, but infection control, employee health, and occupational medicine should work together to establish a postexposure prophylaxis protocol. Infection control personnel should develop policies for handling prehospital exposures of nonemployed emergency medical personnel, visitors, students, and nonemployee physicians and their personnel. These policies should be reviewed by the administration and the legal department.

In larger institutions, the infection control department will not be able to assume the entire burden of initial employee training and the required annual updates. One widely used approach is termed "train the trainer." OSHA coordinators are designated in each department and are responsible for implementing regulations and teaching personnel about the standards that apply to their departments. If individuals at the departmental level are interested, their staff are more likely to understand the regulations and to comply.

Videotapes made by the infection control department or commercially available videos, such as those prepared by the American Medical Association, may be helpful. If you decide to use videotapes as part of the training process, you must include site-specific information, and a knowledgeable individual must be present to answer questions. OSHA specifically warns that commercially produced bloodborne pathogen training packages may not meet the training requirements adequately. Training sessions must be conducted during working hours, on the employer's time, and must cover topics specific to the employer's workplace, including details of the protection plan, names of persons whom the employee must contact after an exposure, and method of medical follow-up.

OSHA has a free consultation service whereby a representative may be invited to evaluate your hospital. We have used it and have found it helpful. The format is the same as for an OSHA inspection. They will inspect your facility for hazards, evaluate your safety and health program, conduct a conference to report their findings to management, provide a written report of recommendations and agreements, assist in implementing recommendations, including training, and conduct a follow-up inspection to determine whether the hospital corrected the problems appropriately. If you receive a comprehensive consultation visit, correct all specified hazards, and institute the core elements of an effective safety and health program, your hospital may be exempt from general schedule enforcement inspections for 1 year. However, if an employee files a complaint or if a fatality or catastrophe occurs within the year, OSHA may inspect your hospital. The exemption provision applies only to states under the federal OSHA program, but some states that have their own enforcement plans have adopted similar provisions. You cannot be fined under this program, and consultants do not report violations to the OSHA enforcement staff. However, OSHA requires that the hospital correct all identified hazards. Consultation visits do not guarantee that your hospital will pass a federal or state OSHA inspection. This process (discussed in OSHA pamphlet 3047) provides an opportunity to have OSHA answer your questions and to clarify their regulations.

We strongly recommend a pro-active approach. Hospital epidemiologists should seek to develop a cordial working relationship with their regional or state OSHA. By understanding the occupational health paradigm,[9] finding common ground, and promoting dialogue, hospitals can decrease the unpleasantness inevitably associated with these bureaucratic incursions.

References

1. US Department of Labor, Occupational Health and Safety Administration. Occupational exposure to bloodborne

pathogens: final rule. *Federal Register.* December 6, 1991;56:64004-64182.

2. Clark RA. Enforcement Policy and Procedures for Occupational Exposure to Tuberculosis. Washington, DC: Occupational Safety and Health Administration; October 8, 1993. US Department of Labor. Memorandum to Regional Administrators.

3. Centers for Disease Control and Prevention. Guidelines for preventing the transmission of *Mycobacterium tuberculosis* in health-care facilities, 1994. *MMWR.* 1994;43(RR-13).

4. Decker MD. The OSHA bloodborne hazard standard. *Infect Control Hosp Epidemiol.* 1992;13:407-417.

5. Decker MD. OSHA enforcement policy for occupational exposure to TB. *Infect Control Hosp Epidemiol.* 1993;14: 689-693.

6. American Hospital Association. *OSHA's Final Bloodborne Pathogens Standard: A Special Briefing.* February 1992. Item 155904.

7. US Department of Health and Human Services. *Biosafety in Microbiological and Biomedical Laboratories.* May, 1988; publication no. NIH 88-8395.

8. Centers for Disease Control. Guidelines for preventing the transmission of TB in health-care settings, with special focus on HIV-related issues. *MMWR.* 1990;(RR-17) 39.

9. Geberding JL. Occupational infectious diseases or infectious occupational diseases? Bridging the views on TB control. *Infect Control Hosp Epidemiol.* 1993;14:686-688.

CHAPTER 34

Preparing for and Surviving a JCAHO Inspection

Mary D. Nettleman, MD, MS

Abstract

The Joint Commission on Accreditation of Healthcare Organizations (JCAHO) has been a major force in shaping the national approach to quality in the healthcare setting. In 1986, the JCAHO announced that it would establish an "Agenda for Change" designed to improve the measurement of quality. The result is that hospitals now are being held to a new set of standards, creating opportunity, uncertainty, and anxiety. This chapter is designed as a primer to help epidemiologists and infection control professionals prepare for JCAHO visits.

Getting Started

The best advice is to start early and work continuously to prepare for a JCAHO visit. Most standards require that compliance be documented for at least 1 year prior to the survey. Several resources are available to assist the epidemiologist (Table 34-1).

The *Comprehensive Accreditation Manual for Hospitals*, published annually by JCAHO, is an ideal place to begin preparing for a survey.[1] The accreditation manual contains standards that hospitals are expected to meet, as well as scoring guidelines and rules for accreditation. All sections that apply to the epidemiologist should be read. In some institutions, the epidemiologist's responsibilities are confined to infection control. In other institutions, the responsibilities have been broadened to include most of the functions described in the accreditation manual. It is helpful to go over each standard individually and consider how compliance will be documented.

One caution is that standards for infection control are not limited to the section labeled "Surveillance, Prevention, and Control of Infection." It is expected that infection control activities also will conform to standards outlined in the section "Improving Organizational Performance." Standards in the "Management of Information" section also may apply to the dissemination and presentation of surveillance data.

JCAHO sponsors many educational events and conferences. These conferences are helpful, and the speakers often have insight into changes planned for the future. For the novice, these events are a valuable introduction to the standards and to the survey process.

TABLE 34-1

TIPS FOR PREPARING FOR A JCAHO SURVEY

- Read the *Comprehensive Accreditation Manual for Hospitals*
- Read the *JCAHO* report from the last visit to your facility
- Telephone or write JCAHO if there are questions
- Attend educational events
- Perform "mock" site visits
- Contact facilities that have recently been accredited

It is usual for the JCAHO surveyors to focus on areas that have caused problems in other facilities. At conferences, one can discuss the standards with experts and with healthcare workers who have been surveyed recently. The results of these discussions can help the epidemiologist anticipate common problems and identify standards that are being emphasized.

It is especially useful to contact facilities that have been reviewed by the same survey team (physician, nurse, and administrator) that will review your hospital. A "multi-hospital system option" is available for chains of at least two hospitals. Under this option, a single survey team may review all hospitals in a chain. This option allows the chain to orient the team to the structure and practices of the system, potentially making the survey process more effective and efficient. An added bonus is the ability to communicate key findings and areas of concern from one hospital to hospitals that have not yet been surveyed.

Finally, the epidemiologist should read the evaluation and recommendations from the last JCAHO visit. Surveyors will not hesitate to concentrate on areas that caused problems in the past.

Specific Standards and Indicators

Details of how to establish a quality improvement program are beyond the scope of this chapter. It is best to review each standard individually to assess compliance. There should be evidence that the leadership is willing to spend time and money on quality improvement, as well as to provide direction and support for the program. Committee minutes are one of the major resources used by the JCAHO to document compliance with standards. The epidemiologist should make certain that the minutes reflect discussion, conclusions, actions, and results of actions. There should be evidence that projects have improved the quality of care and patient outcome. Under no circumstances should minutes be altered after they have been approved by the committee. Falsification of data is considered grounds to deny accreditation.

The infection control program must be managed by an individual who is qualified by virtue of education, training, certification, licensure, or experience. For infection control professionals, certification by the Certification Board for Infection Control would fulfill this requirement. For hospital epidemiologists, training in infectious diseases and active membership in the Society for Healthcare Epidemiology of America (SHEA) would fulfill this requirement. Many other qualifications also would fulfill the requirement.

Common Pitfalls in Infection Control

After working hard to comply with the intent of every standard, it can be very disappointing to be caught on a technicality. For example, surveyors will look for detailed documentation proving that the elements of the infection control program are described and evaluated annually. This is accomplished most efficiently through the infection control committee minutes. The minutes should include a discussion of:

- The definitions of nosocomial infections (or a statement saying that they were reviewed and where the definitions are kept).
- The rationale for selecting a specific surveillance system and the time frame over which that system will be used.
- The patient population characteristics.
- The data collection methodology.

- How the system is reviewed for accuracy.
- Who is responsible for data collection, analysis, and follow-up.
- The method of reporting and follow-up.
- Requirements for reporting to public health authorities.
- Documentation of significant infections among employees.

It must be documented that the elements of the program are reviewed annually in conjunction with the results of data analysis and infection control activities. Goals for the future should be described.

Infection control committees will be expected to show that their actions have resulted in improved delivery of care and improved patient outcome. Attendance by committee members, including administrative members, should be good.

Inservices regarding standard precautions and fire and safety training currently are mandatory, and attendance records are required to document compliance. When asked by surveyors, all healthcare workers should be able to describe standard precautions, should confirm attendance at annual inservices, and should confirm that they have been vaccinated against hepatitis B and are immune to rubeola (or at least have been offered the vaccines).

If other regulators mandate training for infection control, the JCAHO may ask to see appropriate documentation. Thus, employees who use respirators may be asked about training and fit testing. The draft guidelines for prevention of nosocomial pneumonia from the Centers for Disease Control and Prevention recommend that healthcare workers be educated "regarding nosocomial bacterial pneumonia and infection control procedures to prevent their occurrence."[2] Educational activities dealing with specific epidemics or problems should be documented.

Mock Site Visits

In between triennial surveys, many hospitals have found it useful to stage mock site visits. A multidisciplinary team usually is chosen to review each clinical area and to score compliance with JCAHO standards. Some hospitals hire outside agencies to perform the mock site visit. The purpose of the review is to identify problem areas and to give healthcare workers an opportunity to improve their presentation skills.

In the 1997 manual, the JCAHO emphasizes performance and outcome. In other words, it is not enough to have well-written policies. Hospitals must show that their performances are in accordance with their policies. Surveyors may find a nurse or physician or house staff member and ask them how to clean up a blood spill or dispose of infectious waste. Surveyors might ask healthcare workers when they last attended inservice training for standard precautions (required annually) or were tested for tuberculosis. They might ask a physician what he or she would do if the needle disposal box were too full to use. Surveyors may also talk with patients to ensure that educational goals have been met. To allow healthcare workers to gain experience and to identify problem areas, hospitals may want to stage mock interviews before the actual survey occurs.

Tips for Surviving the Survey

All surveyors bring with them their own experiences and personalities. Surveyors often spend long amounts of time away from home and frequently endure stressful, even hostile, situations. Courtesy and hospitality will create a good working environment. Most surveyors appreciate time at the end of the day to summarize their work and begin written reports. Schedules are usually tight, so meetings and tours should begin on time. Staff should be prompt. Committee minutes and policies should be organized and accessed easily. Presentations should be concise and given by knowledgeable individuals. Whenever possible, data should be shown in graphic form.

In general, there are too many standards and not enough time. Survey teams often will focus on areas that have caused problems in other hospitals or areas in which they have a particular interest. As discussed above, contacting hospitals that recently have been surveyed by the same team may make it possible to identify surveyors' areas of interest and help to gauge the surveyors' personalities. Some surveyors are especially irritated if meetings are late. Some may prefer that the schedule be arranged in a certain way. Others may have personal preferences for their environment (room temperature, amount of walking, etc.) or pet peeves that can be avoided.

Surveyors don't know ahead of time what types of projects a specific hospital has initiated. Don't allow the surveyor to overlook your best projects. Bring your best projects to the attention of the surveyor. Modesty has no place during a survey. Tell the surveyor that your hospital is especially proud of these projects, and tell him or her why.

The Survey Schedule

Healthcare organizations are surveyed every 3 years. The usual survey team consists of a physician, a nurse, and an administrator, who review all areas of the hospital. In 1994, the JCAHO began unannounced, 1-day surveys on a 5% random sample of hospitals. The unannounced surveys take place about 18 months after the triennial survey and concentrate on areas found to cause the most problems in the previous survey. The JCAHO will also conduct an unscheduled or unannounced survey when it becomes aware of potentially serious patient care or safety issues. The JCAHO usually give the organizations 24 to 48 hours advance notice of an unscheduled survey.

Publicity

Increasingly, the results of the JCAHO surveys will become available to the public. Detailed descriptions of compliance with standards may be available to the media. Unfortunately, negative findings may receive more attention in the press than positive findings, and noncompliance with a small number of minor standards may overshadow an exemplary record of quality care.

The Future: The Indicator Measurement System

The JCAHO has developed the Indicator Measurement System, which is anticipated to augment on-site accreditation surveys in the future. Hospitals will collect data continuously for a specified set of indicators and transmit the data electronically to JCAHO. JCAHO will aggregate and analyze the data and will give comparative performance data to hospitals.

A major source of concern is whether the Indicator Measurement System will have a positive impact on the quality of patient care. For example, inhospital mortality rates will be monitored for patients who present with an acute myocardial infarction. Because all hospitals will be compared with each other, some will be "high" outliers. Because crude mortality rates are influenced by so many factors, it will be difficult for outlier hospitals to determine if a problem exists. In the future, results of the Indicator Measurement System may be made public. After years of study showing that publication of hospital-specific crude or adjusted mortality rates had no impact on patient outcome, the Health Care Financing Agency has moved from mortality as a measurement of quality.[3] Clearly, the JCAHO must be careful not to repeat past mistakes.

Some monitors are straightforward. For example, charts of patients who have primary breast cancers resected will have to be monitored by the hospital to ensure that a pathologist's report is present. Unfortunately, hospitals that show they are highly compliant with this standard still will be required to collect data for continuous monitoring. In implementing this system, the JCAHO must ensure that the administrative burden of monitoring does not eliminate the resources available to address new and important problems.

Infection control monitors that have been approved are:

- Surgical site infection rates.
- Pneumonia in ventilated patients.
- Primary bloodstream infection rates.

There are no indicators that would measure the sensitivity or specificity of the infection control surveillance system. This may have the unintended, paradoxical effect of making hospitals with poor surveillance systems (eg, that identify only a small proportion of infections) look better than hospitals with good surveillance systems.

JCAHO requires that hospitals participate in at least one "reference database" to compare the results of quality monitoring with data from similar facilities in a type of benchmarking process. Hospitals may participate voluntarily in the Indicator Measurement System from the JCAHO to fulfill this requirement.

Conclusion

Foresight and planning can reduce stress associated with a JCAHO survey. Important resources for the epidemiologist include the *Comprehensive Accreditation Manual for Hospitals*, recommendations from previous JCAHO surveys, and educational meetings. Communication with colleagues who have been reviewed recently is an invaluable means of preparing for future surveys. Finally, although JCAHO accreditation is important, it is equally important to realize that the primary purpose of quality improvement programs is to improve the structure, process, and outcome of care.

References

1. Joint Commission on Accreditation of Healthcare Organizations. *Comprehensive Accreditation Manual for Hospitals. The Official Handbook*. Chicago, Ill: JCAHO; 1996.
2. Centers for Disease Control and Prevention. Draft guideline for prevention of nosocomial pneumonia: notice of comment period. *Federal Register*. 1994;59:4980-5022.
3. Jencks SF, Wilensky GR. The health care quality improvement initiative: a new approach to quality assurance in Medicare. *JAMA*. 1992;268:900-903.

CHAPTER 35

Product Evaluation

William M. Valenti, MD, Loreen A. Herwaldt, MD

Abstract

As healthcare budgets shrink, infection control personnel must become more involved in the process by which their institutions choose products and equipment. This chapter suggests an approach that individuals or programs can use to assess products in a consistent and thorough manner.

Introduction

The current healthcare environment is dominated by managed care and capitated reimbursement, which have reduced the financial resources available to healthcare facilities substantially. More than ever, clinicians and administrators must spend healthcare dollars wisely, without sacrificing the quality of care or safety. In addition, nosocomial infections increase the cost of healthcare substantially, and the cost of these infections is not reimbursed under capitated programs. Thus, hospitals now have tremendous incentive to lower nosocomial infection rates. In theory, one way to reduce the incidence of nosocomial infections is to use devices that have a lower risk of infection than other products. Over the past few years, manufac-

turers have released a staggering number of products purported to decrease infections. These products usually cost more than the standard products. Administrators and staff in healthcare facilities must evaluate such devices and other products that may affect infection rates to determine whether they are efficacious and thus worth the added cost.

Transmission of Nosocomial Pathogens

Experts in infection control agree that most pathogens acquired in healthcare facilities are transmitted by people and medical devices. The so-called inanimate environment, (eg, walls, floors, countertops, food, and water) play a minor role in transmission of pathogens. In general, infection control professionals agree that the environment should be cleaned and maintained routinely as part of the healthcare facility's overall strategy to control infection. However, infection control activities designed to decrease infections should focus on the role of people, invasive procedures, and medical devices such as catheters, endoscopes, and surgical-room equipment. Thus, when evaluating a product, healthcare workers should consider the

TABLE 35-1
MODES OF INFECTION TRANSMISSION

Mode	Example
Airborne	Varicella-zoster virus, *Mycobacterium tuberculosis*
Contact	
Direct (person-to-person)	
Fecal-oral	Hepatitis A virus
Contact with other infectious material	Respiratory syncytial virus
Indirect	
Contaminated equipment	Endoscopes contaminated with hepatitis B virus
Droplets (close contact)	Influenza virus, group A streptococcus
Common Vehicle	
Bloodborne	Human immunodeficiency virus, hepatitis B virus
Foodborne	*Campylobacter jejuni*, *Shigella* sp

various modes by which pathogens are transmitted (Table 35-1) to determine whether the device might facilitate or decrease transmission of important nosocomial pathogens.

The infection control literature describes numerous outbreaks and pseudo-outbreaks attributed to problems with disinfection and sterilization of equipment and invasive devices. Table 35-2 describes five outbreaks that demonstrate several ways in which medical devices can become contaminated. Some outbreaks have occurred because the equipment was designed poorly or because the instructions for cleaning and disinfection were inadequate.

Healthcare workers who determine whether to purchase invasive medical devices and equipment should do the following:

- Look for design flaws that could make the device hard to clean and disinfect.
- Determine whether the instructions for cleaning and disinfection meet current standards.
- Determine whether the healthcare facility actually can clean and disinfect the device adequately (ie, the facility has the equipment needed to reprocess the device; the staff have been, or will be, trained to reprocess the device; and the staff have adequate time to reprocess the device properly).
- Review the literature to see whether similar devices have caused outbreaks at other institutions and what factors (eg, design flaw, improper use, improper disinfection) caused the outbreaks.

Other equipment-related outbreaks have occurred because staff did not know how to clean and disinfect the equipment, took short cuts to save time or money, or did not maintain the device properly. In this era of cost containment, staff may be tempted to save time and money by changing disinfection and sterilization protocols and procedures. Not all of the outbreaks described in Table 35-2 were caused by cost-saving efforts. However, the outbreaks illustrate the types of infection control errors that can result from efforts to decrease costs. These outbreaks also emphasize that the basic, time-honored principles of infection control, such as proper reprocessing of reusable patient-care devices, regular maintenance of equipment, and effective staff education, are as important (or perhaps more important) than purchasing expensive, high-tech devices touted to lower infection rates.

A Standardized Method for Analyzing Products

The Centers for Disease Control and Prevention (CDC) recently published a new guideline for isolation precautions in hospitals.[1] This document provides a framework that the product assessment team (described below) can apply when evaluating products and equipment (Table 35-3). The isolation guideline ranks procedures according to whether or not scientific data support their use. Each new product or device does not need to be assessed with this rigor. However, the similar hierarchical ranking may help the team evaluate

TABLE 35-2
EXAMPLES OF OUTBREAKS CAUSED BY CONTAMINATED EQUIPMENT

Author	Problem	Equipment	Error	Resolution
Lemaitre et al[10]	Patients colonized or infected with *Sphingomonas paucimobilis*	Reusable nickel-plated temperature probes in ventilator circuits	The manufacturer's recommendation to wipe the probe with alcohol before reuse was inadequate	The probes were replaced with a more expensive probe that could be cleaned manually and gas sterilized
Takigawa et al[11]	Pseudoepidemic of *Mycobacterium chelonae*	Automatic bronchoscope washer and bronchoscope	The automatic bronchoscope washer was defective	The procedure was modified to include disinfection with 70% alcohol
			The bronchoscopes were not prepared adequately before they were placed in the automatic washer	The concentration of glutaraldehyde was increased
Bennett et al[12]	Pseudoepidemic of *Mycobacterium xenopi*	Bronchoscopes, endoscopes, brushes	The tap water was contaminated	A submicron filter was installed on the water supply
Dolce et al[13]	Outbreak of proctocolitis caused by glutaraldehyde	Endoscopes	The staff did not follow the manufacturer's instructions regarding how long the endoscopes should be rinsed to remove the glutaraldehyde	Staff in the endoscopy suite were trained to clean and disinfect endoscopes according to the manufacturer's instructions
Rudnick et al[14]	Gram-negative bacteremia in open-heart surgery patients	Pressure-monitoring equipment	Pressure-monitoring equipment that was left uncovered overnight in the operating room became contaminated when housekeepers sprayed disinfectant on the floor	Pressure-monitoring equipment was assembled just before the procedure, and housekeepers stopped spraying disinfectant solutions while cleaning

whether specific products and equipment could benefit the institution in general and the overall infection control effort in particular. This approach allows the healthcare facility to determine whether published data apply to their situation, and it allows personnel to use their common sense and experience when definitive scientific data are not available (categories 2 and 3). In addition to ranking products on the basis of published data, members of the product assessment team must assess a product's priority for implementation in that institution.

Healthcare providers may have difficulty evaluating whether products and equipment will be cost-effective in their institution. The task is especially difficult if the manufacturers do not provide peer-reviewed publications to support their claims, but only provide advertisements and promotional materials. We recommend that the healthcare facility form a multidisciplinary team that will do the following:

- Define priorities based on the facility's rates of infections, rates of sharps injuries, or other pertinent data.

TABLE 35-3
CATEGORIES FOR VALUE ANALYSIS

Category 1

This product is strongly recommended for all hospitals and strongly supported by well-designed experimental or epidemiologic studies

Category 2

This product is strongly recommended for all hospitals and viewed as effective by experts in the field, based on a strong rationale and suggestive evidence, even though definitive studies have not been done

Category 3

This product is suggested for implementation in many hospitals and supported by suggestive clinical or epidemiologic studies, a strong theoretical rationale, or definitive studies This product is applicable to some, but not all, hospitals

Category 4

The role of this product has not been defined, because the evidence is insufficient or consensus has not been reached

Category 5

This product is unnecessary; recommendations that healthcare facilities use this product conflict with current data and the opinions of most experts in infection control

Adapted from Garner J et al.[1]

- Develop criteria regarding product design and performance.
- Assess published data regarding the product or similar products.
- Gather information regarding the experience of similar institutions.
- Plan a trial period for the product in the appropriate clinical settings to determine whether the product functions well.
- Assess the results of the trial period.
- Analyze the cost benefit or cost-effectiveness in their institution.

The multidisciplinary team should include members from the purchasing and stores department, central sterile supply, the infection control program, and at least one representative of the staff who will use the product. In some situations, repre-sentatives from the hospital administration and from the finance department also should participate. Infection control personnel can help the team by assessing the product's effect on important parameters such as the rates of infections and sharps injuries. The person who represents the primary users should assess whether the product is likely to meet their needs and to be accepted.

After the multidisciplinary team has identified products or equipment that meet the predefined criteria, the members should decide whether these items must be tested before the institution purchases them. Chiarello states that healthcare workers are likely to reject new devices, despite infection control or safety advantages, if the staff do not like to use them.[2] The team should assess the results of the trial period, including cost, staff satisfaction, adverse reactions, rates of infection, rates of injuries, the frequency of malfunction, the ease of cleaning and disinfection, and other appropriate information, before deciding whether or not to recommend the product.

In this era of managed care, the cost and the cost-effectiveness of a product have become increasingly important. The assessment of the cost-effectiveness is easy if the same product is cheaper when obtained from a different supplier or if an equivalent product, which is made by another company, is cheaper. In these situations, the multidisciplinary team could discuss the substitution, inform the primary users of the minor change, and work with the purchasing and stores department to ensure a seamless transition.

The multidisciplinary team may need to analyze more thoroughly some products or equipment, particularly those that are more expensive than the products currently used in the institution. Cost-effectiveness analysis (CEA) is a method that many healthcare facilities have used for this purpose.[3] CEA allows the team to determine a ratio of the incremental costs for devices to the expected change in outcomes. This method forces the members to consider the cost of the product, the change in outcome that the product should produce, and the scientific principles of disease transmission before the team determines whether a product should be purchased. Furthermore, CEA can help the multidisciplinary team convince the administration that a more expensive product should be purchased, because the expected outcome would be improved significantly or because the complication rate would be decreased significantly and, thus the overall cost to the institution would be decreased.

Laufer and Chiarello used CEA to evaluate three devices designed to prevent needlesticks.[3] They used the following formula to estimate the cost of preventing a needlestick injury with each of the devices.

$$\frac{\text{Incremental costs of devices}}{(\text{Injuries without devices}) - (\text{Injuries with devices})}$$

The cost to prevent a needlestick injury varied substantially with the device evaluated. The authors estimated the cost of preventing one needlestick injury would be $984 if protective injection equipment was used, $1,574 if an intravenous system with recessed needles was used, or $1,877 if a needleless intravenous system was used. To date, no one has determined whether such devices, which cost more money than most systems currently in use, will be cost-effective if used long-term.

Examples

In the following paragraphs, we will discuss several products that are purported to reduce the risk of infection in healthcare facilities. We will assign these interventions to the categories adapted from the CDC's isolation guidelines. In addition, Table 35-4 gives examples of products that the manufacturers claim will reduce infection rates and the classification that we assigned to the devices. However, a caveat is necessary. The literature in this field changes rapidly. Therefore, infection control personnel who must purchase products should not rely on our assessment, but should review the literature before they make their decision.

TABLE 35-4

ASSESSMENT OF DEVICES PURPORTED TO DECREASE THE RISK OF INFECTION

Device	Supporting Evidence	Category
Needleless devices	Some preliminary evidence is available	2
Antibiotic-coated intravenous catheters	Some preliminary evidence is available	3
Silver-coated intravenous catheters	Not available	3
Antibiotic-coated urinary catheters	Not available	3
Copper-based paint or other antibacterial paint	Not available	5

Protecting Healthcare Workers from Bloodborne Pathogens

Hepatitis B vaccine reduces the risk of hepatitis B infection in healthcare workers exposed to patients' blood and body fluids. Therefore, hepatitis B vaccine is a Category 1 intervention (see Table 35-3).

In the era of human immunodeficiency virus (HIV) infections, equipment that reduces the risk of accidental needlesticks may be worth the extra expense, because these injuries are a primary mode by which this virus is transmitted to healthcare workers. Many companies market devices designed to prevent needlesticks. The manufacturers usually claim that their products reduce the risk of sharps injuries and therefore reduce the risk of infection with HIV and other bloodborne pathogens. Devices that prevent needlestick injuries would be useful for all healthcare facilities in which needles are used. Several studies indicate that needlestick prevention systems might decrease needlestick accidents.[4] However, these studies also have found that healthcare workers may not use these devices or may use them incorrectly, thereby increasing the risk of injury.[4] Further studies must be done to document the efficacy of these devices.

Therefore, use of these devices would be a Category 2 intervention (see Table 35-3).

Because data from controlled clinical trials are limited, a hospital's multidisciplinary team must assess other data to determine whether the needlestick prevention devices should be introduced into their healthcare facility. First, the multidisciplinary team should review the literature on needlestick injuries and on transmission of bloodborne pathogens, so that the team can base their program on current data. To date, the literature indicates that the risk of transmission of HIV via needlestick is relatively low—approximately one half of 1% or less.[5] Although the risk of transmission is low, HIV infection is chronic, and, up to now, fatal. Thus, all healthcare facilities should strive to maximize the healthcare workers' safety by minimizing the risk of exposure to infectious material. Second, the multidisciplinary team should know the epidemiology of needlestick injuries in their hospital, so that the team can develop a program that will be efficacious. Thus, the team must know how, where, and when needlestick injuries occur, and what devices and procedures are associated most frequently with these accidents. Third, they should evaluate any available data on several different devices that might lower the rate of the most common injuries or the rates of injuries having the highest risk of transmitting bloodborne pathogens in their hospital. Fourth, the team should know the incidence of infection with bloodborne pathogens in their patient population and should identify the areas in the facility that treat these patients most frequently. The team should use these data to determine which, if any, needlestick-prevention devices to introduce into their hospital.

Protecting Patients, Healthcare Workers, and Visitors From Pathogens in the Environment

Manufacturers often claim that their products will reduce the risk of infection from organisms found in the environment. Occasionally, some of these claims find their way into credible publications, only to confuse individuals who are assessing the value of these products for their hospitals. A recent manuscript on the bactericidal effects of copper-based paints illustrates this point.[6] The author showed that copper-based paints kill bacteria and then concluded that "such paints could be used to render surfaces self-disinfecting in strategic locations where environmental causation of nosocomial infections is suspected."[6] This conclusion conflicts with current infection control thought on the role of the environment in infection transmission. In an accompanying editorial, Rutala and Weber wisely point out that walls always harbor bacteria, but they never have been linked by scientific data to nosocomial infection.[7] At best, self-disinfecting paint would be a Category 4 intervention. We think that self-disinfecting paint is more likely to be a Category 5 intervention: use of this product is unnecessary and is in conflict with current infection control thought.

Companies that produce disinfectants may try to capitalize on healthcare workers' fears of HIV infection by claiming that their products kill HIV on contact. However, most agents that are used to clean floors, countertops, and other surfaces readily kill HIV. In addition, HIV is inactivated rapidly by several products that are inexpensive and readily available, including 10% chlorine bleach, 50% ethanol, 35% isopropyl alcohol, hydrogen peroxide, and soap and water.[8] Thus, an expensive new product is not needed to clean areas contaminated by blood, because existing products are cheaper and do the job adequately. Thus, a new product designed specifically for this purpose would be in Category 5. Rather than buying an expensive new product, personnel from the infection control program and from the housekeeping department should teach healthcare workers how to manage blood spills, and should develop policies and procedures that clearly specify when and how to clean the environment and how to manage blood spills and other emergencies.

Preventing Transmission of *Mycobacterium tuberculosis*

In some instances, the multidisciplinary team must consider the big picture when evaluating the infection-associated risks and benefits of particular products. For example, when developing their tuberculosis control program, healthcare facilities must consider the nature of the individual facility, the frequency with which tuberculosis patients are seen in the facility, and skin-test conversion rates of employees. Institutions also must comply with the guidelines from regulatory or advisory agencies, such as the Occupational Safety and Health Administration and the CDC.

Data in the literature indicate that ultraviolet (UV) lights kill *M tuberculosis*. However, most experts do not think that UV light alone is adequate, and the CDC's guidelines state that UV lights cannot substitute for proper air handling units, but could be used as an adjunctive measure.[9] Thus, UV light would be a Category 4 strategy, because a consensus has not been reached.

Conclusion

In many cases, the purchaser cannot choose a product solely on the manufacturer's claims or on the cost. We recommend that healthcare facilities develop a multidisciplinary team to evaluate products carefully. The team would review the literature, the experience of other hospitals, and the manufacturer's materials to determine whether the product could do the required functions, has an equal or lower risk of infection compared with the current product, and would be cost-effective. Products that meet these criteria should be tested by the staff who will use them to ensure that the products will be accepted and used properly after they are introduced into general use.

Infection control personnel will find the process of evaluating products to be quite complex and time-consuming. However, we feel that this task will assume greater importance as managed care increases its presence in healthcare delivery. Infection control personnel must ensure that the risk of infections does not increase as healthcare facilities drastically reduce the cost of care. Many infection control programs already are being asked whether their hospitals can cut costs by substituting one product for another or one procedure for another. Other, less fortunate, infection control programs have discovered that changes had been made only when an investigation of increased infection rates identified the substitution of a cheaper product. Infection control personnel who help their institutions to assess products carefully will enable these healthcare facilities to survive the current financial crisis without sacrificing the quality of care or employee safety.

Note

Sections of this chapter are reprinted and revised in part with permission from *Infection Control and Sterilization Technology,* June 1996, Vol 2, No. 6, Mayworm Associates, 507 N Milwaukee Ave, Libertyville, IL 60048.

References

1. Garner J, the Hospital Infection Control Practices Advisory Committee. Guideline for isolation precautions in hospitals, part II: recommendations for isolation precautions in hospitals. *Infect Control Hosp Epidemiol.* 1996;17:60-80.
2. Chiarello LA. Selection of needle stick prevention devices: a conceptual framework for approaching product evaluation. *Am J Infect Control.* 1995;23:386-395.
3. Laufer FN, Chiarello LA. Application of cost-effectiveness methodology to the consideration of needle stick prevention technology. *Am J Infect Control.* 1994;22:75-82.
4. L'Ecuyer PB, Schwab EO, Iademarco E, Barr N, Aton EA, Fraser VJ. Randomized prospective study of the impact of three needleless intravenous systems on needlestick injury rates. *Infect Control Hosp Epidemiol.* 1996;17:803-808.
5. Centers for Disease Control and Prevention. Case-control study of HIV seroconversion in healthcare workers after percutaneous exposure to HIV infected blood. *MMWR.*

1995;44:929-932.

6. Cooney TE. Bactericidal activity of copper and noncopper paints. *Infect Control Hosp Epidemiol.* 1995;16:444-446.

7. Rutala WA, Weber DJ. Environmental interventions to control nosocomial infections. *Infect Control Hosp Epidemiol.* 1995;16:442-443.

8. Centers for Disease Control and Prevention. Recommendations for preventing transmission of HTLV III/LAV in the workplace. *MMWR.* 1985;34:682-686.

9. Valenti WM. Tuberculosis in the HIV era: everything old is new again. *Am J Infect Control.* 1992;20:35-36.

10. Lemaitre D, Elaichouni A, Hundhausen M, et al. Tracheal colonization with *Sphingomonas paucimobilis* in mechanically ventilated neonates due to contaminated ventilator temperature probes. *J Hosp Infect.* 1996;32:199-206.

11. Takigawa K, Fujita J, Negayama K, et al. Eradication of contaminating *Mycobacterium chelonae* from bronchofiberscopes and an automated bronchoscope disinfection machine. *Respir Med.* 1995;89:423-427.

12. Bennett SN, Peterson DE, Johnson DR, et al. Bronchoscopy-associated *Mycobacterium xenopi* pseudoinfections. *Am J Respir Crit Care Med.* 1994;150: 245-250.

13. Dolce P, Gourdeau M, April N, Bernard PM. Outbreak of glutaraldehyde-induced protocolitis. *Am J Infect Control.* 1995;23:34-39.

14. Rudnick JR, Beck-Sague CM, Anderson R, et al. Gram-negative bacteremia in open-heart–surgery patients traced to probable tap-water contamination of pressure-monitoring equipment. *Infect Control Hosp Epidemiol.* 1996;17:281-285.

Recommended Reading

Centers for Disease Control and Prevention. Evaluation of safety devices for preventing percutaneous injuries among health-care workers during phlebotomy procedures—Minneapolis-St. Paul, New York City, and San Francisco, 1993-1995. *MMMR.* 1997;46(2):21-29.

Index